Biomedical Aspects of Histamine

Mohammed Shahid · Nancy Khardori ·
Rahat Ali Khan · Trivendra Tripathi
Editors

Biomedical Aspects of Histamine

Current Perspectives

Springer

Editors
Associate Professor Mohammed Shahid
Department of Microbiology
Jawaharlal Nehru Medical College & Hospital
Aligarh Muslim University
202002 Aligarh
India
shahidsahar@yahoo.co.in

Prof. Nancy Khardori
Division of Infectious Diseases
Department of Internal Medicine
School of Medicine
Southern Illinois University
N. Rutledge 751
62702 Springfield
IL, USA
nkhardori@siumed.edu

Prof. Rahat Ali Khan
Department of Pharmacology
Jawaharlal Nehru Medical College & Hospital
Aligarh Muslim University
202002 Aligarh
India
drrakhan@yahoo.co.in

Dr. Trivendra Tripathi
Department of Biochemistry
Jawaharlal Nehru Medical College & Hospital
Aligarh Muslim University
202002 Aligarh
India
tripathiamu@gmail.com

ISBN 978-90-481-9348-6 e-ISBN 978-90-481-9349-3
DOI 10.1007/978-90-481-9349-3
Springer Dordrecht Heidelberg London New York

Library of Congress Control Number: 2010935671

Printed on acid-free paper

Springer is part of Springer Science+Business Media (www.springer.com)

Foreword

Histamine enjoys a wide spectrum of actions spanning across many organ systems. It is a biogenic amine formed by decarboxylation of the amine acid histidine. Its actions are mediated through a specific receptor of which four isoforms have been characterized so far. All these are seven transmembrane G-protein coupled receptors. Medical students often get introduced to actions of histamine following study of '*wheal and flare*' phenomenon associated with histamine release in the skin, and to a lesser extent following study of gastric acid output. The receptor involved in the former is H1 isoform whereas H2 isoform is involved in the latter. The finding that histamine is a major mediator of allergic response resulted in the discovery of first antagonist by Bovet and Staub in 1937. Soon the drugs inhibiting actions began to appear in 1940s. Initially these were classified as 'antihistamines' but now they are classified according to their receptor isoform specificity.

In the last decade two additional receptor isoforms have been characterized and each subtype finds a wide tissue distribution. H1 isoform was at first thought to be strictly confined to the vascular endothelium and smooth muscle cells. Now we know it to exist in neural tissue also. In the tubero-mamillary nucleus of the hypothalamus, it acts as an autoreceptor inhibiting further release of histamine. Here it is possibly involved in control of circadian rhythm and wakefulness. Similarly existence of H2 receptor in cardiac muscle, mast cells in addition to gastric mucosa points to possible role of histamine in cardiac function. Relative new entrants are the H3 and H4 receptors. The former are found distributed in the central nervous system and to a lesser extent in the peripheral nervous tissue, gastric mucosa, and bronchial smooth muscle while H4 isoform is distributed across bone marrow, basophils, thymus, spleen, small intestine and colon.

Histamine exists in two pools (*slow turning over pool* located primarily in the mast cells and basophils; and *rapidly turning over pool* located in gastric enterochromaffin like cells [ECL] and the histaminergic neurons in CNS). Unlike the mast cells and basophils, ECL and histaminergic neurons do not store histamine. Instead a physiologic stimulus is required to turn on the synthesis. Thus ingestion of food is needed for activation of histidine decarboxylase in the gut. These observations should allow for more nuanced approach in dealing with histamine blockade/modulation.

The latest kid on the block H4 is already raising hopes for developing a drug that would have impact in mitigating adverse side effects of chemotherapy in patients being treated with anti-neoplastic drugs. For instance H4 isoform being expressed in bone marrow may have an important role in erythropoiesis. H4 activation prevents the induction of cell cycle genes through a cAMP/PKA dependent pathway not associated with apoptosis. The arrest of G1/GS transition (induced by growth factor) protects progenitor cells from the toxicity of cell cycle dependent chemotherapy drug like Ara-C [Petit-Berton AF et al. *Plos One* 2009; 4(8):e6504].

Histamine and histaminergic neurons/storage cells being widely distributed, it is not surprising that the biologic effects are wide spread and diverse. Elucidation of receptor isoforms and the functions they sub serve has opened up new vistas particularly in understanding signal transduction and the biologic consequences thereof. Understanding this new and evolving biology opens up doors for pharmacologic manipulations that could be harnessed to benefit patients.

In this compendium the editors have commissioned twenty chapters addressing classical and emerging pharmacology. Emerging role in sleep disorders, sexual/reproductive function, pain and itching are some areas that are bound to evoke curiosity in readers-even those not vested in histamine biology. This compendium will be an important resource for those dealing with consequences of histamine storage/release disorders.

Springfield, Illinois, USA

Romesh Khardori

Preface

Histamine, discovered in 1910 by Sir Henry H. Dale, has become one of the most important multifunctional biogenic amines in the field of biomedicine. Histamine has been known to play the broadest spectrum of activities in various physiological and pathological conditions.

While searching the literature, compiled in the form of a book, on above-mentioned important aspects related to histamine, histamine receptors (H1–H4) and role of their agonists/antagonists, we still found scarcity of knowledge, especially unveiling the recent developments in the current field. The published books on H3- and H4-receptors are limited, while H3- and H4-receptors are noble histamine receptors in histaminergic pharmacology and it is assumed that within the next few years the H3- and H4-receptors antagonists will be freely available in the market as antagonists for H1- and H2-receptors.

Therefore, we realized that there is an urgent need to compile the newly discovered data on H1–H4 receptors related to biomedical facets in the form of a significant book, covering all aspects of histamine and histamine receptors.

We have discussed these issues, and decided to edit a book in the larger interest of students and researchers so as to fill the gap in book publications. Here we have worked to bring together experts in the field to contribute a series of chapters spanning a cross-section of the field. It is our hope and intent that the outcome of these efforts in the form of *Biomedical Aspects of Histamine: Current Perspectives* will serve as a valued resource to the entire scientific/academic community. We hope that this text not only encapsulates the recent literature in the field, but will also illuminate related issues for the benefits of teaching, research and drug discovery.

This book consists of 20 chapters in 12 themes which address various aspects of histamine in biomedical science. Part I "Histamine Biology and Physiology" provides an overview of histamine synthesis, regulation, metabolism and its clinical aspects in biological system in Chapter 1, and Chapter 2 discusses regulation of mammalian histamine synthesis- histidine decarboxylase. Part II "Enzymology in Histamine Biology" discusses enzymology in histamine biogenesis in Chapter 3. Part III "Pharmacology of Histamine Noble Receptors and Their Ligands in

Drug Development" deals with biological and pharmacological aspects of histamine receptors and their ligands (Agonists/antagonists) in Chapter 4. Part IV "Histamine Role in Immune Modulation and Regulation" discusses the role of histamine in immunoregulation in context of T-regulatory and invariant NKT cells in Chapter 5, and immune regulation by various facets of histamine in immunomodulation and allergic disorders in Chapter 6. Part V "Histamine in Regulation of Cell Proliferation and Differentiation" discusses effects of histamine on lymphocytes in Chapter 7, and histamine aspects in acid peptic diseases and cell proliferation in Chapter 8. Part VI "Histamine Role in Pathogenesis and Diagnosis of Allergic, Inflammatory, Autoimmune and Cancer Diseases" deals the role of histamine in pathogenesis of autoimmune, allergic, inflammatory and malignant diseases in Chapter 9, and biological characteristics of histamine receptors in airways disease management in Chapter 10. Part VII "Histamine Role in Inflammation and Allergy" discusses mast cells as a source and target for histamine in Chapter 11, and histamine H1 receptor gene expression mechanism as a novel therapeutic target of allergy in Chapter 12. Part VIII "Histamine in the Nervous System" deals the neuronal histamine and its receptors as new therapeutic targets for food intake and obesity in Chapter 13, and implications of histaminergic system in brain histamine dysfunction in Chapter 14. Part IX "Histamine H3 Receptor: A Target for Momentous Brain Research" discusses pre-synaptic control by histamine H3 Receptors of neurotransmitter release in Chapter 15. Part X "Histamine H4 Receptor: A Noble Target for Inflammatory and Immune Research" deals expression of histamine H4 receptor in human synovial cells and dermal tissues in Chapter 16. Part XI "Role of Histamine in Reproductive Function" discusses novel role for histamine through classical H1 and H2 receptors: regulation of leydig cell steroidogenesis and its implications for male reproductive function in Chapter 17, and possible effects of histamine in physiology of female reproductive function in Chapter 18. Part XII "Other Biomedical Aspects of Histamine Agonists, Antagonists, and Inverse Agonists" deals histamine role in malaria in Chapter 19, and histamine-cytokine and histamine-antibody network in immune regulation in Chapter 20.

We have made our sincere efforts to provide good scientific content in this book. It is our hope that this book will be useful to graduates and post-graduates medical students, teachers, researchers and clinicians. However, there may also be some shortcomings. We invite you to communicate your experiences with the book to us.

We thank all the contributors/experts for timely submission of their excellent contributions and for their overall cooperation. We also thank many leading scientists in this field who may not have contributed directly, but encouraged or guided us towards successful completion of this project.

The technical and scientific advice received from the Springer book editorial team, especially from Meran Owen, Peter Butler and Tanja van Gaans (Springer Science + Business Media B. V., Dordrecht, The Netherlands) and Ms. Anandhi Bashyam, Project Manager, Integra Software Services Pvt. Ltd., Pondicherry, India, is thankfully acknowledged. Finally we acknowledge the Almighty God, who provided all the positive thoughts and channels needed for completion of this book project.

Aligarh, India — Mohammed Shahid
Springfield, Illinois — Nancy Khardori
Aligarh, India — Rahat Ali Khan
Aligarh, India — Trivendra Tripathi
September 2010

Contents

List of Figures

List of Tables

Contributors

Jameel Ahmad Department of Pharmacology, Jawaharlal Nehru Medical College and Hospital, Aligarh Muslim University, Aligarh 202002, UP, India, ahmad.drjameel@gmail.com

Aijaz Ahmed Khan Department of Anatomy, Jawaharlal Nehru Medical College and Hospital, Aligarh Muslim University, Aligarh 202002, UP, India, aijazahmedkhan7@live.com

Rahat Ali Khan Department of Pharmacology, Jawaharlal Nehru Medical College and Hospital, Aligarh Muslim University, Aligarh 202002, UP, India, drrakhan@yahoo.co.in

Hamdan Ibrahim Al-Mohammed Section of Microbiology, Department of Biomedical Sciences, College of Medicine, King Faisal University, Al Hassa 31982, Kingdom of Saudi Arabia, al-mohammed@hotmail.co.uk

Abdulrahman A. Alsultan Section of Microbiology, Department of Biomedical Sciences, College of Medicine, King Faisal University, Al Hassa 31982, Kingdom of Saudi Arabia, aalsultan10@hotmail.com

Ali Ibrahim Al-Sultan Section of Endocrinology, Department of Internal Medicine, College of Medicine, King Faisal University, Al Hassa 31982, Kingdom of Saudi Arabia, dean-medicinehassa@kfu.edu.sa

Miguel Ángel Medina Departamento de Biología Molecular y Bioquímica, Universidad de Málaga Facultad de Ciencias, Campus de Teatinos, Malaga 29071, Spain; "CIBER de Enfermedades Raras" (CIBERER), Valencia, Spain, medina@uma.es

José-Antonio Arias-Montaño Departamento de Fisiología, Biofísica y Neurociencias, Cinvestav-IPN, México, D.F. 07000, México, jaarias@fisio.cinvestav.mx

Sandeep Bhattacharya Department of Physiology, C.S.M. Medical University, Erstwhile King George's Medical University, Lucknow, UP, India, dr.sabhattacharya@gmail.com

Ewa Brzezińska-Błaszczyk Department of Experimental Immunology, Medical University of Łódź, Pomorska 251, 92-213 Łódź, Poland, ewab@csk.umed.lodz.pl

Varun Dwivedi Food Animal Health Research Program (FAHRP), Ohio Agricultural Research and Development Center (OARDC), The Ohio State University, 1680, Madison Avenue, Wooster, OH 44691, USA, dwivedi.6@osu.edu

Abdul Faiz Faizy Department of Biochemistry, Jawaharlal Nehru Medical College and Hospital, Aligarh Muslim University, Aligarh 202002, UP, India, abul.faiz@gmail.com

Hiroyuki Fukui Department of Molecular Pharmacology, Institute of Health Biosciences, The University of Tokushima Graduate School, 1-78-1 Shomachi, Tokushima 770-8505, Japan, hfukui@ph.tokushima-u.ac.jp

Renukaradhya J. Gourapura Food Animal Health Research Program (FAHRP), Ohio Agricultural Research and Development Center (OARDC), The Ohio State University, 1680, Madison Avenue, Wooster, OH 44691, USA, gourapura.1@osu.edu

Anwar Huq Maryland Pathogen Research Institute, Bioscience Research Building, University of Maryland, MD 20742, USA, huq@umd.edu

Atsushi Ichikawa Institute for Biosciences, Mukogawa Women's University, Kyuban-cho 11-68, Nishinomiya, Hyogo 663-8179, Japan, aichikaw@mukogawa-u.ac.jp

Priyanka Jain Department of Pulmonary Medicine, C.S.M. Medical University, Erstwhile King George's Medical University, Lucknow, UP, India, jainpriyanka10@gmail.com

Haris M. Khan Department of Microbiology, Jawaharlal Nehru Medical College and Hospital, Aligarh Muslim University, Aligarh 202002, UP, India, harismk2003@hotmail.com

Manzoor M. Khan Department of Pharmaceutical Sciences, Creighton University Medical Center, Omaha, NE 68178, USA, mmkhan@creighton.edu

Nancy Khardori Division of Infectious Diseases, Department of Internal Medicine, School of Medicine, Southern Illinois University, Springfield, IL, USA, nkhardori@siumed.edu

Anil Kumar Department of Pharmacology, Jawaharlal Nehru Medical College and Hospital, Aligarh Muslim University, Aligarh 202002, UP, India, drakumar10@gmail.com

Takayuki Masaki Department of Internal Medicine, Oita University, 1-1 Idaigaoka, Yufu-Hasama, Oita, 879-5593 Japan, masaki@med.oita-u.ac.jp

Yoshiko Matsuda Department of Geriatric Pharmacology and Therapeutics, Graduate School of Pharmaceutical Sciences, Chiba University, 1-8-1 Inohana, Chuo-ku, Chiba 260-8675, Japan, y-ikawa@umin.ac.jp

Monika Misra Department of Pharmacology, Jawaharlal Nehru Medical College and Hospital, Aligarh Muslim University, Aligarh 202002, UP, India, drmonikamisra@gmail.com

Hiroyuki Mizuguchi Department of Molecular Pharmacology, Institute of Health Biosciences, The University of Tokushima Graduate School, 1-78-1 Shomachi, Tokushima 770-8505, Japan, guchi003@ph.tokushima-u.ac.jp

Shagufta Moin Department of Biochemistry, Jawaharlal Nehru Medical College and Hospital, Aligarh Muslim University, Aligarh 202002, UP, India, shagufta.moin@yahoo.com

Carolina Mondillo Laboratory of Molecular Endocrinology and Signal Transduction, Institute of Biology and Experimental Medicine (IByME – CONICET), Vuelta de Obligado 2490, C1428ADN, Buenos Aires, Argentina, mondillo@dna.uba.ar

Aurelio A. Moya-García Departamento de Biología Molecular y Bioquímica, Universidad de Málaga Facultad de Ciencias, Campus de Teatinos, Malaga 29071, Spain; "CIBER de Enfermedades Raras" (CIBERER), Valencia, Spain, amoyag@uma.es

Takao Namiki Department of Japanese-Oriental "KAMPO" Medicine, Graduate School of Medicine, Chiba University, 1-8-1 Inohana, Chuo-ku, Chiba 260-8670, Japan, tnamiki@faculty.chiba-u.jp

Nasreen Noor Department of Obstetrics and Gynaecology, Jawaharlal Nehru Medical College and Hospital, Aligarh Muslim University, Aligarh 202002, UP, India, nasreen_71@rediffmail.com

Angélica Osorio-Espinoza Departamento de Fisiología, Biofísica y Neurociencias, Cinvestav-IPN, México, D.F. 07000, México, aosorio@fisio.cinvestav.mx

Richa Pandey Department of Immunology, National JALMA Institute for Leprosy and Other Mycobacterial Diseases (ICMR), Tajganj Agra 282001, UP, India, richapandeyindia@gmail.com

Omar Pedro Pignataro Laboratory of Molecular Endocrinology and Signal Transduction, Institute of Biology and Experimental Medicine (IByME – CONICET), Vuelta de Obligado 2490, C1428ADN, Buenos Aires, Argentina; Department of Biological Chemistry, School of Sciences, University of Buenos Aires (UBA), Argentina, pignatar@dna.uba.ar

Almudena Pino-Ángeles Departamento de Biología Molecular y Bioquímica, Universidad de Málaga Facultad de Ciencias, Campus de Teatinos, Malaga 29071, Spain; “CIBER de Enfermedades Raras” (CIBERER), Valencia, Spain, apino@uma.es

Judith Ramos-Jiménez Colegio de Ciencia y Tecnología, Universidad de la Ciudad de México, Av. La Corona No. 320, Col. Loma La Palma, México, D.F. 07160, México, jurji_2000@yahoo.com

Adil Raza Department of Microbiology, Jawaharlal Nehru Medical College and Hospital, Aligarh Muslim University, Aligarh 202002, UP, India, dradil786_786@yahoo.co.in

Waseem Rizvi Department of Pharmacology, Jawaharlal Nehru Medical College and Hospital, Aligarh Muslim University, Aligarh 202002, UP, India, waseemrizvi76@hot.com

Francisca Sánchez-Jiménez Department of Molecular Biology and Biochemistry, Universidad de Málaga Facultad de Ciencias, Campus de Teatinos, Malaga 29071, Spain; “CIBER de Enfermedades Raras” (CIBERER), Valencia, Spain, kika@uma.es

Mohammed Shahid Department of Microbiology, Jawaharlal Nehru Medical College and Hospital, Aligarh Muslim University, Aligarh, UP, 202002, India; Section of Microbiology, Department of Biomedical Sciences, College of Medicine, King Faisal University, Al Hassa, 31982, Kingdom of Saudi Arabia, shahidsahar@yahoo.co.in

Fatima Shujatullah Department of Microbiology, Jawaharlal Nehru Medical College and Hospital, Aligarh Muslim University, Aligarh 202002, UP, India, sfatima777@gmail.com

Rajni Kant Shukla Department of Pulmonary Medicine, C.S.M. Medical University, Erstwhile King George’s Medical University, Lucknow, UP, India, rickylkw2006@gmail.com

Mashiatullah Siddiqui Department of Biochemistry, Jawaharlal Nehru Medical College and Hospital, Aligarh Muslim University, Aligarh 202002, UP, India, mashiat2005@rediffmail.com

Anuradha Singh Department of Microbiology, Jawaharlal Nehru Medical College and Hospital, Aligarh Muslim University, Aligarh 202002, UP, India, anubiotech@indiatimes.com

Farrukh Sobia Department of Microbiology, Jawaharlal Nehru Medical College and Hospital, Aligarh Muslim University, Aligarh 202002, UP, India, sobia.asghar@yahoo.com

Masahiko Suzuki Department of Orthopaedic Surgery, Graduate School of Medicine, Chiba University, 1-8-1 Inohana, Chuo-ku, Chiba 260-8670, Japan, masahiko@faculty.chiba-u.jp

Satoshi Tanaka Department of Immunochemistry, Division of Pharmaceutical Sciences, Okayama University Graduate School of Medicine, Dentistry and Pharmaceutical Sciences, Tsushima-naka, Okayama 700-8530, Japan, tanaka@pharm.okayama-u.ac.jp

Trivendra Tripathi Department of Biochemistry, Jawaharlal Nehru Medical College and Hospital, Aligarh Muslim University, Aligarh 202002, UP, India, tripathiamu@gmail.com

Koichi Ueno Department of Geriatric Pharmacology and Therapeutics, Graduate School of Pharmaceutical Sciences, Chiba University, 1-8-1 Inohana, Chuo-ku, Chiba 260-8675, Japan, kueno@p.chiba-u.ac.jp

Katsunori Yamaura Department of Geriatric Pharmacology and Therapeutics, Graduate School of Pharmaceutical Sciences, Chiba University, 1-8-1 Inohana, Chuo-ku, Chiba 260-8675, Japan, yamaura@p.chiba-u.ac.jp

About the Editors

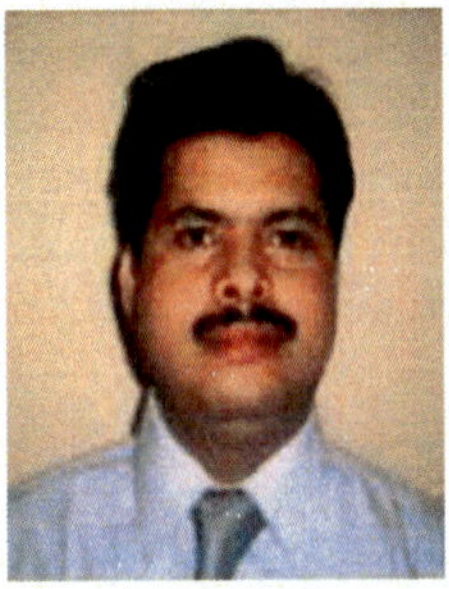

Dr. Mohammed Shahid, M.B.B.S., M.D., Ph.D., MNZIMLS (New Zealand), is Associate Professor in the Department of Microbiology of J.N. Medical College & Hospital, Aligarh Muslim University, India. He has recently been awarded the Young Scientist Award by the Department of Science & Technology, Ministry of Science & Technology, Govt. of India. He was also been awarded a Commonwealth Academic Fellowship by the British Council and the Association of Commonwealth University, U.K., during 2005–2006 to work with Prof. Peter Hawkey's group on the antibiotics resistance problem. His field of interest and research is confined to mechanism and resistance to beta-lactam antibiotics, with special interest in CTX-M and AmpC β-lactamases, plasmid-mediated drug resistance, and indigenous drugs. He also has research experience on human fungal pathogens such as *Aspergillus and Candida* species. His work on Aspergillosis in patients suffering from bronchogenic carcinoma has received high acclaim and recognition in international scientific community. Moreover, his group is working in the field of histamine-research and produced some pioneer researches related to H1–H4 receptors and their agonists/antagonists. Dr. Shahid has published more than 75 research papers in reputed journals, and has three books to his credit. He is presently the member of many scientific bodies, both international and national. He has also been the member of the reviewer panel and editorial board of various international journals/publication houses, including "The Lancet" published by "Elsevier" and also those of Bentham Science Publications, USA, and Global Science Books, UK. He has worked as an Associate Professor in College of Medicine, King Faisal University, Al-Hassa, Kingdom of Saudi Arabia.

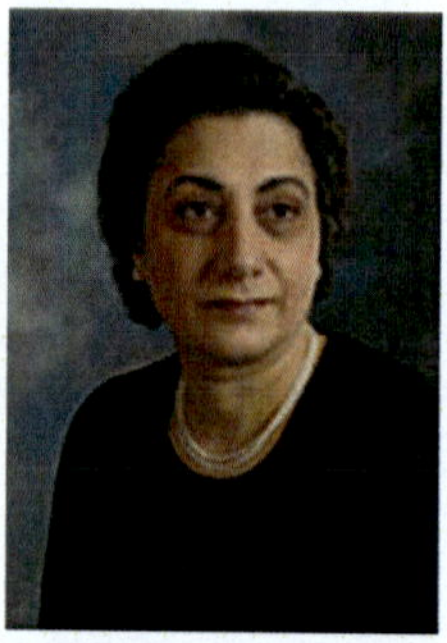

Dr. Nancy Khardori, M.B.B.S., M.D., Ph.D., FACP, FIDSA, is Professor of Medicine and Microbiology/ Immunology, Division of Infectious Diseases, School of Medicine, Department of Internal Medicine, Southern Illinois University, Springfield. She is Chief, Division of Infectious Diseases, and Director, Infectious Diseases Fellowship, and also Adjunct Faculty, Section of Infectious Diseases, Department of Medical Specialties, The University of Texas MD Anderson Cancer Center. Her major area of research is microbial adherence, biofilms and device related infections. In addition, her laboratory works on new antibacterial and antifungal agents and their activity in treating biofilm/device associated infections. She has a clinical interest in Diagnosis and management of infectious diseases, Hepatic diseases, and Microbial adherence infections. Dr. Khardori has several research papers and books to her credit. She is presently the member of many scientific bodies, both international and national. She has also been the member of the reviewer panel and editorial board of various international journals/publication houses.

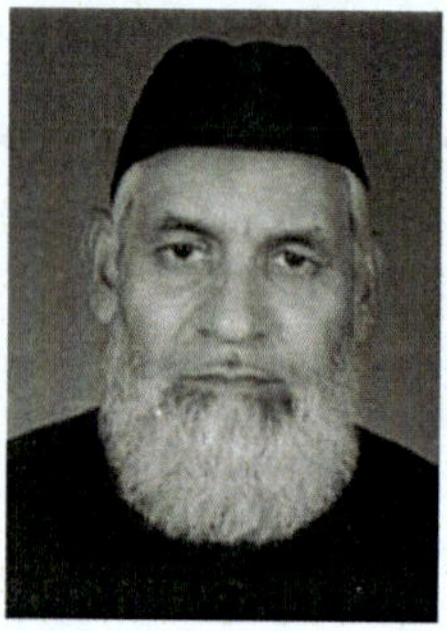

Dr. Rahat Ali Khan, M.B.B.S., M.D., is presently serving as Professor and Chairman, Department of Pharmacology, J. N. Medical College, Aligarh Muslim University, Aligarh, India. He is involved in teaching and research for more than three decades. Thrust areas of his research are Neuropharmacology, Clinical Pharmacology, Immunopharmacology, Trace element studies, Autacoids-Histamine and Indigenous drugs. About 20 theses of M.D. / M.S. / Ph.D. have been guided; 40 research papers, mostly in international journals have been published; More than 80 research papers have been presented in various national and international conferences. He has many book chapters to his credit. He has also been the member of the reviewer panel and editorial board of various International journals, member of various academic bodies and member/convener of Institutional ethical committee, Animal Ethical committee, Bioethical committee of J. N. Medical College, AMU, Aligarh, Director associate in interdisciplinary brain research center JNMC, AMU, Aligarh, member of University court. He has been member of various scientific bodies including addicted treatment welfare society, Pakistan.

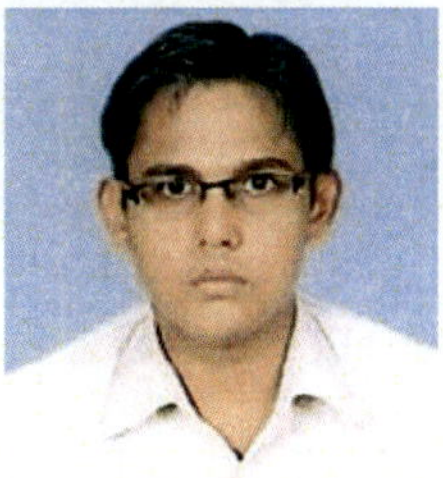

Dr. Trivendra Tripathi, M.Sc., Ph.D., has recently been awarded Doctor of Philosophy in Biochemistry on thesis entitled "To Study the Role of Histamine in Immunomodulation" under supervision of Dr. Mashiat Ullah Siddiqui, Associate Professor, Former Chairman, Department of Biochemistry and Professor Rahat Ali Khan, Chairman, Department of Pharmacology, and Dr. Mohd. Shahid, Associate Professor, Department of Microbiology of J. N. Medical College & Hospital, Aligarh Muslim University, India. He completed his post-graduate in Department of Biotechnology, Janta College, Bakewar, Etawah of Chhatrapati Shahu Ji Maharaj University, Kanpur, India. His M.Sc. thesis was on "Biochemical and Immunological Studies on Reactive Oxygen Species Modified Immunoglobulin-G" under Prof. Rashid Ali, Ex-Chairman, Department of Biochemistry, JNMCH, AMU, Aligarh, India. He completed his graduate study in Chemistry from Department of Chemistry, Aligarh Muslim University, Aligarh, India. Dr. Tripathi's work concerned with in vivo experimentations of Histamine, Histamine-receptors (H1R, H2R, H3R and H4R)-agonists/antagonists in immune modulation and regulation, and their biochemical and histopathological effects in Rabbit model. He has authored several research publications, book chapters and review articles. He has presented his research findings in many national and international conferences and symposia. He is presently the member of many scientific bodies, both international and national. He has also been the member of the reviewer panel of an international journal *Journal of Pediatric Biochemistry* which is published by the Society of Pediatric Science, Yuzuncu Yil University, Turkiye.

Part I
Histamine Biology and Physiology

Chapter 1
An Overview of Histamine Synthesis, Regulation and Metabolism, and its Clinical Aspects in Biological System

Mohammed Shahid, Trivendra Tripathi, Nancy Khardori, and Rahat Ali Khan

Abstract Histamine is an autacoid widespread in plant and animal kingdoms. In the early 1900s, it was identified as a mediator of biological functions by Sir Henry Dale and co-workers and drugs targeting histamine receptors have been in clinical use for more than 60 years. The synthesis of histamine was discovered by Windausa and Vogta in 1907. Its synthesis, regulation and metabolism causes numerous biological effects. This chapter will provide an overview of histamine synthesis, regulation and metabolism, and the biological effects thereof.

Keywords Histamine synthesis · Histamine metabolism · Histamine regulation

Abbreviations

HDC	histidine decarboxylase
ECL	enterochromaffin-like cells
DCs	dendritic cells
IL	interleukin
GM-CSF	granulocyte monocyte-colony stimulating factor
TNF	tumour necrosis factor
LPS	lipopolysaccharide
BMMCs	bone marrow derived mast cells
IgE	immunoglobulin-E
PKC	protein kinase C
cDNAs	complementary deoxyribonucleic acids
PMA	phorbol 12-myristate 13-acetate
MAP	mitogen-activated protein
ERK	extracellular signal-regulated protein kinase
mRNA	messenger ribonucleic acids
ECL	enterochromaffin-like cells

M. Shahid (✉)
Department of Microbiology, Jawaharlal Nehru Medical College and Hospital, Aligarh Muslim University, Aligarh, UP, 202002, India
e-mail: shahidsahar@yahoo.co.in

M. Shahid et al. (eds.), *Biomedical Aspects of Histamine*,
DOI 10.1007/978-90-481-9349-3_1,

HMT	histamine N^{τ}-methyltransferase
DAO	diamine oxidase
H1R	histamine H1-receptor
H2R	histamine H2-receptor
H3R	histamine H3-receptor
H4R	histamine H4-receptor

Contents

1.1 Introduction

Histamine molecule exhibits two basic structural moieties, i.e. primary aliphatic amine (pK_{a1} 9.4) and imidazole (pK_{a2} 5.8). These make the monocation with different tautomers; the preferred form at physiologic pH value (96%) with a minor dicationic fraction (3%) and a very small amount of the neutral form (Cooper et al. 1990). The nomenclature for histamine positions may be highly significant for histamine biology including synthesis, regulation, metabolism, and also histamine derivatives; see Fig. 1.1.

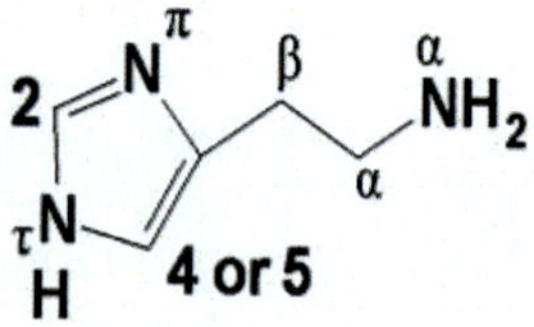

Fig. 1.1 Specific nomenclature for histamine positions

1.2 Synthesis of Histamine

Histamine was first identified as an autacoid having potent vasoactive properties. It is a low molecular weight amine synthesized from L-histidine exclusively by L-histidine decarboxylase (HDC) (E.C. 4.1.1.22 or E.C. 4.1.1.26), which is dependent on the cofactor pyridoxal-5′-phosphate to a putative binding site (TFNPSKW) on the protein. Histamine cannot be generated by another enzymatic pathway (Dy and Schneider 2004, Parsons and Ganellin 2006). Histidine decarboxylase (HDC) is an enzyme that is expressed in various cells through out the body, including central nervous system (neurons), gastric-mucosa (parietal cells), mast cells (~3 pg/cell histamine), and basophils (~1 pg/cell histamine). Histamine has an important role in human physiology, and exerts its diverse biologic effects by 4 types of receptors (Akdis and Blaser 2003, Lovenberg et al. 1999, MacGlashan 2003, Oda et al. 2000, Schneider et al. 2002). Histamine is synthesized by enterochromaffin-like cells (ECL) in the stomach and plays an important role in gastric acid secretion. Only basophils and mast cells can store the amine in specific granules. In the hematopoietic system, histamine is closely associated with anionic proteoglycans heparin (in mast cells) and chondroitin-4-sulfate (in basophils). In this specific form, histamine can be released in large amounts during degranulation in response to various immunological (immunoglobulin E, or cytokines) or non-immunological (compound 48/80, calcium ionophore, mastoparin, substance P, opioids, or hypo-osmolar solutions) stimuli (Dy and Schneider 2004). Histamine synthesis in Golgi apparatus can be inhibited by α-fluoromethylhistidin (Hill et al. 1997).

Recently, many myeloid and lymphoid cell types that do not store histamine have been shown to have HDC activity and are capable of synthesis of large amounts of histamine (Szeberényi et al. 2001). This so called "neo synthesized histamine," has been shown in various cells, including hematopoietic progenitors, macrophages, neutrophils, platelets, dendritic cells (DCs) and T cells (Dy and Schneider 2004, Ghosh et al. 2002, Shiraishi et al. 2000, Tanaka et al. 2004, Yokoyama et al. 2004). Histamine synthesis in non-mast cells was first confirmed using W/W^V mice, which genetically lack mature mast cells, upon stimulation with a phorbol ester (Taguchi et al. 1982). HDC activity is demonstrated in vitro through cytokines, such as interleukin (IL)-1, IL-3, IL-12, IL-18, GM-CSF, macrophage-colony stimulating factor, TNF-α, and calcium ionophore (Schneider et al. 1987, Yoshimoto et al. 1999). In vivo HDC activity has been shown to be modulated by LPS stimulation, inflammation, infection and graft rejection (Dy et al. 1981).

The generation of HDC-knockout mice provides a tool to study the role of endogenous histamine in a broad range of normal and disease processes. Such mice demonstrate diminished numbers of mast cells and significantly decreased granule content, which suggests that histamine might affect the production of mast cell granule proteins (Ohtsu et al. 2001). In a recent study, interleukin-3 (IL-3)-dependent bone marrow derived mast cells (BMMCs) have been found to be activated by certain immunoglobulin-E (IgE) clones in absence of specific antigen, leading to their survival, cytokine secretion, histamine production, adhesion, and migration (Kawakami and Kitaura 2005). In addition to this study, Tanaka et al. (2002) has shown a drastic and transient induction of HDC (~ 200-fold in activity) in BMMCs stimulated by IgE alone, which was much higher than that after antigen stimulation. This induction resulted in the increase in stored histamine. Another study suggested that the anti-apoptic effects of monomeric IgE on BMMCs were mediated by IL-3 in an autocrine fashion (Kohno et al. 2005). Although Schneider et al. (1987) found the potential role of IL-3 to induce HDC in bone marrow cells, it is clearly indicated that monomeric IgE-induced histamine synthesis may not be mediated through

IL-3 (Kohno et al. 2005). Since stimulation of histamine synthesis occurs upon IgE-mediated antigen induction, and this remains controversial if these two modes of FcεRI activation share a common signal transduction pathway. However, many recent studies have demonstrated the qualitative differences between both modes: such as monomeric IgE-induced Ca^{2+} influx is mediated by a distinct channel from that activated upon antigen stimulation (Tanaka et al. 2005), and protein kinase C β-II (PKCβII) plays a significant role in monomeric IgE-induced histamine synthesis in mast cells, but not upon antigen stimulation (Liu et al. 2005). Since, only small levels of increase in histamine synthesis were found by monomeric IgE both in purified rat peritoneal mast cells and in vitro maturated BMMCs, inducing effects of monomeric IgE on mast cells may be limited to immature mast cells (Tanaka et al. 2005). However, Tanaka and Ichikawa (2006) has suggested that monomeric IgE-induced histamine synthesis exacerbates the symptoms of chronic allergy, while drastic increases in the levels of serum IgE are often observed in such diseases.

1.3 Regulation of Histamine

Histamine is synthesized only by HDC enzyme. Therefore, histamine regulation is dependent on the gene of HDC enzyme, which is expressed in the cells throughout the body. The complementary deoxyribonucleic acids (cDNAs) of HDC enzyme have been isolated from mouse mastocytoma, fetal rat liver, erythroleukemia cells and human basophil leukemia cells. Based on structural studies, mouse and human genes are composed of 12 exons spanning approximately 24 kb. The 2.4 kb single transcript is produced by mouse gene, whereas two splice variants of 3.4 and 2.4 kb exist in humans, and latter encode the functional HDC (Yatsunami et al. 1994). HDC gene is found on chromosome 2 in mice and chromosome 15 in humans and its expression is controlled by lineage-specific transcription factors. These factors interact with a promoter region consisting of a GC box, four GATA consensus sequences, a c-Myb-binding motif and four CACC boxes (Nakagawa et al. 1997). It has been demonstrated in several studies that the HDC transcription is regulated by various factors in gastric cancer cells such as gastrin, oxidative stress and PMA, through a Ras-independent, Raf-dependent mechanism, MAP kinase/ERK and a protein kinase C (PKC) pathway functioning on three overlapping cis acting elements (GAS-RE 1, GAS-RE 2 and GAS-RE3) known as gastrin response elements (Höcker et al. 1998, Raychowdhury et al. 2002). The negative control on HDC expression in gastric epithelial cell line is exerted by expression of the transcription factors GATA-4 and GATA-6 (Watson et al. 2002). This is well known that the expression of HDC in basophils and mast cells is a consequence of the state of CpG methylation in the promoter region (Kuramasu et al. 1998). Many studies on the mast cell line HMC1 and the pluripotent hematopoietic cell line UT7D1 have demonstrated that HDC-gene expression is subject to post-transcriptional control. Therefore, the chromosomal configuration and methylation of the HDC-promoter is likely to account for its cell-specific expression (Maeda et al. 1998, Oh et al. 2001). It has also been reported that PMA stimulates a strong increase in HDC activity which is affected by actinomycin D and that is not paralleled by enhanced HDC mRNA expression. Similar effect was noted in cell lines (HEL and CMK) with megakaryocyte/basophil differentiation potential (Dy et al. 1999). In addition to this effect, a mechanism that accounts for the strong enhancement of HDC activity in ECL cells in response to gastrin is explained by a translation control of HDC expression (Zhao et al. 2003).

Two essential mechanisms of translational control have been explained in hematopoietic cells:

(i) a rapamycin dependent pathway that is linked to phosphoinositide 3-kinase (PI3K), FRAP/mTOR and phosphorylation/dephosphorylation of repressor of translation 4E-binding protein (4E-Bps),
(ii) ERK- and p38-dependent pathway that controls the 4E-BP expression by the induction of Egr-1 (Rolli-Derkinderen et al. 2003).

The multiple carboxy-truncated isoforms are formed due to post-translational processing of HDC gene; the gene is initially translated 73–74 kDa protein in mammals, and originally it was assumed that enzymes purified from native sources corresponded to a dimer of two processed isoforms of 53 and 55 kDa. According to Fleming and Wang (2003), the biosynthesis of histamine involves primarily the 55 kDa isoform and it is being acknowledged that many other isoforms generated from 74 kDa primary translation product can also be active. It is also being documented that enhancing the histidine decarboxylase activity might cause reduction in messenger RNA (mRNA) degradation by amino acid carboxyl-terminal PEST (proline-glutamic acid-serine-threonine) domains (Fleming and Wang 2000). Here is a need to completely understand the negative feed back regulation of HDC activity that differs from one cell type to another. It has been shown in AGS-B cells that over expression of the HDC protein inhibit histidine decarboxylase promoter activity by downregulation of ERK signals (Colucci et al. 2001).

However, in gastrin-stimulated ECL cells, this type of feedback mechanism was not observed. It was also demonstrated that in the hematopoietic cells, as well as in the stomach, negative feedback signals could be produced through high cytosolic histamine concentration (Rolli-Derkinderen et al. 2003). Histamine reuptake mechanism comparable to that of the other aminergic neurotransmitters has not been observed (Masahito et al. 2006).

1.4 Metabolism of Histamine

It is noteworthy that only a small amount of released histamine (2–3%) is excreted unchanged. The remaining histamine (more than 97%) is metabolized by two enzymatic pathways: histamine N^{τ}-methyltransferase (HMT) (EC2.1.1.8) and diamine oxidase (DAO) (EC1.4.3.6) before excretion (Hill et al. 1997, Maintz and Novak 2007, Fig. 1.2). DAO is the main enzyme for the metabolism of ingested histamine.

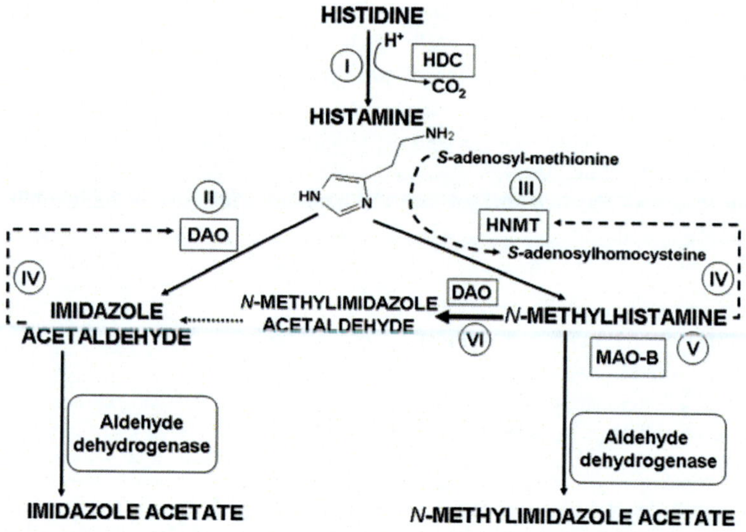

Fig. 1.2 Summary of the histamine metabolism. (I) Histamine is synthesized by decarboxylation of histidine catalyzed by *L*-histidine decarboxylase (HDC). (II) Histamine can be metabolized by extracellular oxidative deamination of the primary amino group by diamine oxidase (DAO) or (III) intracellular methylation of the imidazole ring by histamine-*N*-methyltransferase (HNMT). (IV) Thus, insufficient enzyme activity caused by enzyme deficiency or inhibition may lead to accumulation of histamine. Both enzymes can be inhibited by their respective reaction products in a negative feedbackloop. (V) *N*-Methylhistamine is oxidatively deaminated to *N*-methyl-imidazole acetaldehyde by monoamine oxidase B (MAO B) or (VI) by DAO. Because the methylation pathway takes place in the cytosolic compartment of cells, MAO B (V) has been suggested to catalyze this reaction in vivo (Maintz and Novak 2007, Tsujikawa et al. 1999)

It has been documented that DAO, when functioning as a secretory protein, may be responsible for scavenging extra-cellular histamine after mediator release. Conversely, HMT, the other important enzyme inactivating histamine, is a cytosolic protein that can convert histamine only in the intracellular space of cells (Maintz and Novak 2007). HMT metabolizes the majority of histamine (50–80%) to *N*-methyl histamine, which is further metabolized to the primary urinary metabolite *M*-methylimidazole acetic acid by monoamine oxidase. DAO metabolizes the histamine (15–30%) to imidazole acetic acid (Akdis and Blaser 2003). The study of the former pathway was greatly facilitated by the availability of a potent and highly specific inhibitor of DAO, aminoguanidine. HMT appears to be the most important enzyme responsible for the degradation of histamine in the airways, because blockers of HMT (such as SKF 91488) increase the bronchoconstricting action of histamine in vitro and in vivo, whereas DAO inhibition remained unaffected (Sekizawa et al. 1993). However, recently, it has been documented that impaired histamine degradation based on reduced DAO activity and the resulting histamine excess may cause several symptoms mimicking an allergic reaction. The ingestion of histamine-rich food or of alcohol or drugs that release histamine or block DAO may provoke diarrhea, headache, rhinoconjunctival symptoms, asthma, hypotension, arrhythmia, urticaria, pruritus, flushing, and other conditions in patients with histamine intolerance. Symptoms can be reduced by a histamine-free diet or be eliminated by antihistamines (Maintz and Novak 2007).

HMT is expressed in airway epithelial cells and may therefore be responsible for the local metabolism of histamine released from airway mast cells. Mechanical removal of airway epithelium enhances the bronchoconstriction response to histamine in vitro (Barnes et al. 1985, Flavahan et al. 1985, Knight et al. 1990); this might be the result, in part, of loss of the metabolizing enzyme. Furthermore, experimental viral infections resulted in reduced epithelial HMT activity in association with increased responsiveness to inhaled histamine (Nakazawa et al. 1994). The half-life of pharmacologically active doses of histamine is less than 10 s in the rat and 20–30 s in the dog. In earlier studies, histamine levels were measured by bioassay, but subsequently fluorometric and radio-enzymatic techniques were developed (Parsons and Ganellin 2006).

1.5 Biological Effects of Histamine

Histamine is a known mediator of several biological reactions through differential expression of four types of histamine receptors (H1R, H2R, H3R and H4R). These affect secretion by effector cells (mast cells and basophils) through various immunological [such as triggering of degranulation of mast cells by crosslinking of the FcϵRI receptor by specific allergens] or non-immunological stimuli [such as neuropeptides, complement factors (i.e., C3a and C5a), cytokines, hyperosmolarity, lipoproteins, adenosine, superoxidases, hypoxia, chemical and physical factors (extreme temperatures and traumas), or alcohol and certain food and drugs, may activate mast cells] (Maintz and Novak 2007, Shahid et al. 2009). Histamine causes smooth muscle cell contraction, vasodilatation, increased vascular permeability and mucus secretion, tachycardia, alterations of blood pressure, and arrhythmias. It stimulates gastric acid secretion and nociceptive nerve fibers. It also plays a potent role in hematopoiesis, neurotransmission, immunomodulation, day-night rhythm, wound healing, and the regulation of cell proliferation and angiogenesis in tumor models and intestinal ischemia (Maintz and Novak 2007, see Fig. 1.3). Basal plasma histamine concentrations of 0.3 to 1.0 ng/mL are considered normal (Dyer et al. 1982). Histapenia (deficiency of histamine) and histadelia (abundance of histamine) can cause both neurological and physical disorders. Histapenia may be caused by excess copper levels, as this decreases blood histamine levels. Exceeding the individual histamine tolerance causes concentration-dependent histamine mediated symptoms (Dyer et al. 1982, Maintz and Novak 2007). Scromboid poisoning studies have shown that healthy persons may develop severe headache or flushing due to ingestion of massive amounts of histamine (Morrow et al. 1991). It has been documented that inhibition of DAO followed by oral histamine administration may induce severe and even life-threatening reactions, such as hypotension, bronchospasm or shock

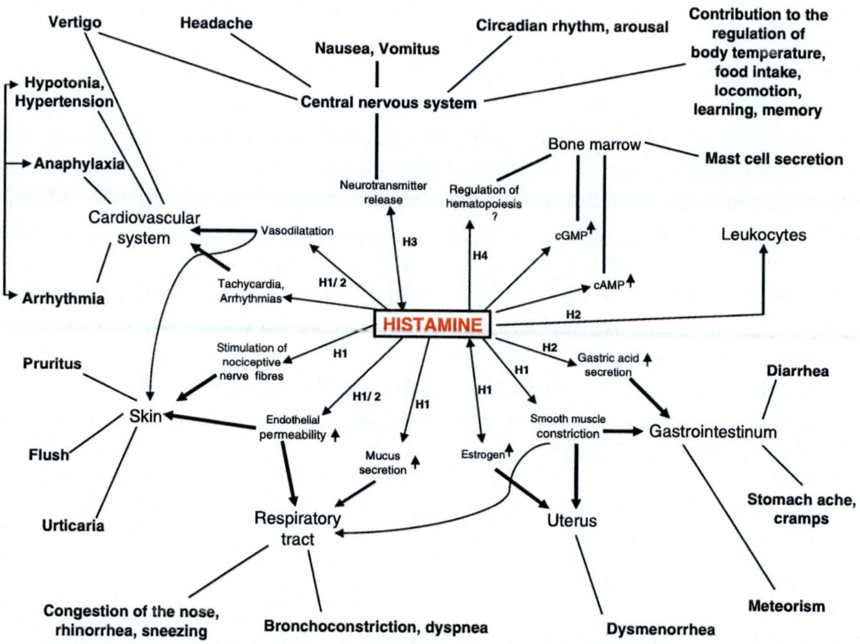

Fig. 1.3 Histamine-mediated symptoms. Modified from Maintz et al. (2006)

(Maintz and Novak 2007). Patients with hyperhistaminemia showed recurrent anaphylactic reactions (Hershko et al. 2001). The ingestion of the small amounts of histamine causes reduced DAO activity in histamine-sensitive patients that are well tolerated by healthy persons. Classical symptoms of histamine intolerance comprise gastrointestinal disorders, sneezing, rhinorrhea and congestion of the nose, headache, dysmenorrhea, hypotonia, arrhythmias, urticaria, pruritus, flushing, and asthma (Maintz and Novak 2007, see Fig. 1.3).

1.6 Conclusion

The pleiotropic effects of histamine in biological system depend on its synthesis, regulation and metabolism. Under physiological conditions, H1 and H2 isoforms of histamine are involved in vaso regulation, smooth muscle cell contraction, circadian rhythm and wakefulness, gastric acid output and possibly in cardiac function. No symptoms or constellation of symptoms have clearly been lived to lower than basal levels of histamine, therefore the role of histamine agonists in pharmacotherapy has not been explored. On the other hand, there is a clear role for histamine antagonists in allergic disease and peptic ulcer disease. The detection of H3 and H4 receptors in nervous system, bronchial smooth muscle and bone marrow has raised hopes for further pharmacotherapy related to histamine.

Acknowledgement Trivendra Tripathi acknowledges University Grants Commission, New Delhi, India for providing UGC Fellowship [UGC letter DON F. 19-33/2006 (CU)].

References

Akdis CA, Blaser K (2003) Histamine in the immune regulation of allergic inflammation. J Allergy Clin Immunol 112:15–22

Barnes PJ, Cuss FM, Palmer JB (1985) The effect of airway epithelium on smooth muscle contractility in bovine trachea. Br J Pharmacol 86:685–691

Colucci R, Fleming JV, Xavier R et al (2001) L-Histidine decarboxylase decreases its own transcription through down regulation of ERK activity. Am J Physiol 281:G1081–G1091

Cooper DG, Young RC, Durant GJ et al (1990) Histamine receptors. In: Hansch C, Emmett JC (eds) Comprehensive medicinal chemistry. Pergamon, Oxford, pp 323–421

Dy M, Lebel B, Kamoun P et al (1981) Histamine production during the anti-allograft response: demonstration of a new lymphokine enhancing histamine synthesis. J Exp Med 153:293–309

Dy M, Pacilio M, Arnould A et al (1999) Modulation of histidine decarboxylase activity and cytokine synthesis in human leukemic cell lines: relationship with basophilic and/ or megakaryocytiv differentiation. Exp Hematol 27:1295–1305

Dy M, Schneider E (2004) Histamine-cytokine connection in immunity and hematopoiesis. Cytokine Growth Factor Rev 15:393–410

Dyer J, Warren K, Merlin S et al (1982) Measurement of plasma histamine: description of an improved method and normal values. J Allergy Clin Immunol 70:82–87

Flavahan NA, Aarhus LL, Rimele TJ et al (1985) Respiratory epithelium inhibits bronchial smooth muscle tone. J Appl Physiol 58:834–838

Fleming JV, Wang TC (2000) Amino acid carboxy-terminal PEST domains mediate gastrin stabilization of rat L-histidine decarboxylase isoforms. Mol Cell Biol 20:4932–4947

Fleming JV, Wang TC (2003) The production of 53–55 kDa isoforms is not required for rat L-histidine decarboxylase activity. J Biol Chem 278:686–694

Ghosh AK, Hirasawa N, Ohtsu H et al (2002) Defective angiogenesis in the inflammatory granulation tissue in histidine decarboxylase-deficient mice but not in mast cell-deficient mice. J Exp Med 195:973–982

Hershko AY, Dranitzki Z, Ulmanski R et al (2001) Constitutive hyperhistaminaemia: a possible mechanism for recurrent anaphylaxis. Scand J Clin Lab Invest 61:449–452

Hill SJ, Ganellin CR, Timmerman H et al (1997) International Union of pharmacology. XIII. Classification of histamine receptors. Pharmacol Rev 49:253–278

Höcker M, Rosenberg I, Xavier R et al (1998) Oxidative stress activates the human histidine decarboxylase promoter in AGS gastric cancer cells. J Biol Chem 273:23046–23054

Kawakami T, Kitaura J (2005) Mast cell survival and activation by IgE in the absence of antigen: a consideration of the biological mechanisms and relevance. J Immunol 175:4167–4173

Knight DA, Adcock JA, Phillips MJ et al (1990) The effect of epithelium removal on human bronchial smooth muscle responsiveness to acetylcholine and histamine. Pulm Pharmacol 3:198–202

Kohno M, Yamasaki S, Tybulewicz VL et al (2005) Rapid and large amount of autocrine IL-3 production is responsible for mast cell survival by IgE in the absence of antigen. Blood 105:2059–2065

Kuramasu A, Saito H, Suzuki S et al (1998) Mast cell-/basophil-specefic transcriptional regulation of human L-histidine decarboxylase gene by CpG methylation in the promoter region. J Biol Chem 273:31607–31614

Liu Y, Furuta K, Teshima R et al (2005) Critical role of PKC βII in activation of mast cells by monomeric IgE. J Biol Chem 280:38976–38981

Lovenberg TW, Roland BL, Wilson SJ et al (1999) Cloning and functional expression of the human histamine H3 receptor. Mol Pharmacol 55:1101–1107

MacGlashan D Jr (2003) Histamine: a mediator of inflammation. J Allergy Clin Immunol 112:S53–S59

Maeda K, Taniguchi H, Ohno I et al (1998) Induction of L-histidine decarboxylase in a human mast cell line, HMC-1. Exp Hematol 26:325–331

Maintz L, Novak N (2007) Histamine and histamine intolerance. Am J Clin Nutr 85:1185–1193

Maintz L, Benfadal S, Allam JP et al (2006) Evidence for a reduced histamine degradation capacity in a subgroup of patients with atopic eczema. J Allergy Clin Immunol 117:1106–1112

Masahito O, Kohei Y, Yoh-Ichi S et al (2006) Recent advances in molecular pharmacology of the histamine system: organic cation transporter as a histamine tranporter and histamine metabolism. J Pharmacol Sci 101:24–30

Morrow JD, Margolies GR, Rowland J et al (1991) Evidence that histamine is the causative toxin of scombroid-fish poisoning. N Engl J Med 324:716–720

Nakagawa S, Okaya Y, Yatsunami K et al (1997) Identification of multiple regulatory elements of human L-Histidine decarboxylase gene. J Biochem 121:935–940

Nakazawa H, Sekizawa K, Morkkawa M et al (1994) Viral respiratory infection causes airway hyperresponsiveness and decreases histamine *N*-methyltransferase activity in guinea pigs. Am J Respir Crit Care Med 149:1180–1185

Oda T, Morikawa N, Saito Y et al (2000) Molecular cloning and characterization of a novel type of histamine receptor preferentially expressed in leukocytes. J Biol Chem 275:36781–36786

Oh CK, Filler SE, Cho SH (2001) Eukaryotic translation initiation factor 6 enhances histamine and IL-2 production in mast cells. J Immunol 166:3606–3611

Ohtsu H, Tanaka S, Terui T et al (2001) Mice lacking histidine decarboxylase exhibit abnormal mast cells. FEBS Lett 502:53–56

Parsons ME, Ganellin CR (2006) Histamine and its receptors. Br J Pharmacol 147:S127–S135

Raychowdhury R, Fleming JV, Mclaughlin JT et al (2002) Identification and characterization of a third gastrin response element (GAS-RE3) in the human histidine decarboxylase gene promoter. Biochem Biophys Res Commun 297:1089–1095

Rolli-Derkinderen M, Machavoine F, Baraban JM et al (2003) ERK and p38 inhibit the expression of 4E-BP1 repressor of translation through induction of Egr-1. J Biol Chem 278:18859–18867

Schneider E, Pollard H, Lepault F et al (1987) Histamine-producing cell-stimulating activity. Interleukin 3 and granulocyte-macrophage colony-stimulating factor induce de novo synthesis of histidine decarboxylase in hemopoietic progenitor cells. J Immunol 139:3710–3717

Schneider E, Rolli-Derkinderen M, Arock M et al (2002) Trends in histamine research: new functions during immune responses and hematopoiesis. Trends Immunol 23:255–263

Sekizawa K, Nakazawa H, Ohrui T et al (1993) Histamine *N*-methyltransferase modulates histamine and antigen-induced bronchoconstriction in guinea pigs *in vivo*. Am Rev Respir Dis 147:92–96

Shahid M, Tripathi T, Sobia F et al (2009) Histamine, histamine receptors and their role in immunomodulation: an updated systematic review. The Open Immunol J 2:9–41

Shiraishi M, Hirasawa N, Oikawa S et al (2000) Analysis of histamine-producing cells at the late phase of allergic inflammation in rats. Immunology 99:600–606

Szeberényi JB, Pállinger E, Zsinkó M et al (2001) Inhibition of effect of endogenously synthesized histamine disturbs *in vitro* human dendritic cell differentiation. Immunol Lett 76:175–182

Taguchi Y, Tsuyama K, Watanabe T et al (1982) Increase in histidine decarboxylase activity in skin of genetically mast-cell deficient W/W^{v} mice after application of Phorbol myristate 13-acetate: evidence for the presence of histamine producing cells without basophilic granules. Proc Natl Acad Sci USA 79:6837–6841

Tanaka S, Deai K, Konomi A et al (2004) Expression of L-histidine decarboxylase in granules of elicited mouse polymorphonuclear leukocytes. Eur J Immunol 34:1472–1482

Tanaka S, Ichikawa A (2006) Recent advances in molecular pharmacology of the histamine systems: immune regulatory roles of histamine produced by leukocytes. J Pharmacol Sci 101:19–23

Tanaka S, Mikura S, Hashimoto E et al (2005) $Ca2^{+}$ influx- mediared histamine synthesis and IL-6 release in mast cells activated by monomeric IgE. Eur J Immunol 35:460–468

Tanaka S, Takasu Y, Mikura S et al (2002) Antigen independent induction of histamine synthesis by immunoglobulin E in mouse bone marrow derived mast cells. J Exp Med 196:229–235

Tsujikawa T, Uda K, Ihara T et al (1999) Changes in serum diamine oxidase activity during chemotherapy in patients with hematological malignancies. Cancer Lett 147:195–198

Watson F, Kiernan RS, Dimaline R (2002) GATA proteins are potential negative regulators of HDC gene expression in the gastric epithelium. Biochem Biophys Acta 1576:198–202

Yatsunami K, Ohtsu H, Tsuchikawa M et al (1994) Structure of the L hidtidine decarboxylase gene. J Biol Chem 269:1554–1559

Yokoyama M, Yokoyama A, Mori S et al (2004) Inducible histamine protects mice from P. acnes-primed and LPS-induced hepatitis through H2-receptor stimulation. Gastroenterology 127:892–902

Yoshimoto T, Tsutsui H, Tominaga K et al (1999) IL-18, although antiallergic when administered with IL-12, stimulates IL-4 and histamine release by basophils. Proc Natl Acad Sci USA 96:13962–13966

Zhao CM, Chen D, Yamada H et al (2003) Rat stomach ECL cells: mode of activation of histidine decarboxylase. Regul Pept 114:21–27

Chapter 2
Regulation of Mammalian Histamine Synthesis: Histidine Decarboxylase

Satoshi Tanaka and Atsushi Ichikawa

Abstract Histamine plays a wide variety of physiological and pathological responses, such as immediate allergy, inflammation, gastric acid secretion, neurotransmission, and immune modulation. Histamine synthesis is mediated by the enzyme, L-histidine decarboxylase (HDC), which catalyzes decarboxylation of L-histidine. In contrast to extensive investigation and development of specific antagonists for histamine receptors, regulation of histamine synthesis remains to be clarified. We review here a series of studies about regulation of histamine synthesis, with a particular attention to the rate-limiting enzyme, HDC. We describe and discuss about the findings on various aspects of HDC, such as transcriptional regulation, post-translational regulation, and novel functions identified with the gene targeted mouse strain for HDC. It should be surely required for better understanding of the physiological roles of histamine to clarify the regulation of histamine synthesis, since accumulating evidence has indicated the critical roles of newly-formed histamine in health and disease.

Keywords Histamine synthesis · Histamine regulation · HDC

Abbreviations

HDC	histidine decarboxylase
ECL	enterochromaffin-like
PACAP	pituitary adenylyl cyclase-activating protein
CML	chronic myeloid leukemia
GM-CSF	granulocyte-macrophage colony stimulating factor
VMAT2	vesicular monoamine transporter 2
PEST	proline (P), glutamic acid (E), serine (S) and threonine (T)

S. Tanaka (✉)
Department of Immunochemistry, Division of Pharmaceutical Sciences, Okayama University Graduate School of Medicine, Dentistry and Pharmaceutical Sciences, Tsushima-naka, Okayama 700-8530, Japan
e-mail: tanaka@pharm.okayama-u.ac.jp

M. Shahid et al. (eds.), *Biomedical Aspects of Histamine*,
DOI 10.1007/978-90-481-9349-3_2, © Springer Science+Business Media B.V. 2010

Contents

2.1 Introduction

Histamine is involved in a wide variety of physiological and pathological responses, such as immediate allergy, inflammation, gastric acid secretion, neurotransmission, and immune modulation (Haas et al. 2008, Jutel et al. 2005, Leurs et al. 2005, Schubert 2007, Thurmond et al. 2008). In accord with prominent success of various histamine receptor antagonists as therapeutic drugs for immediate allergy and peptic ulcer diseases, significant progress has been made in understanding the functions of histamine H1 and H2 receptors. Identification of novel histamine receptors, H3 and H4, has enhanced our understanding of various roles of histamine (Lovenberg et al. 1999, Oda et al. 2000). In contrast to the long history of histamine receptor study, biosynthesis of histamine remained to be clarified.

Histidine decarboxylase (L-histidine decarboxylase, HDC, EC 4.1.1.22) is the rate limiting enzyme for mammalian histamine synthesis. Histamine synthesis had long been evaluated through measurement of enzymatic activity of HDC in various tissues and cells, whereas many groups tried to purify this enzyme (Watanabe and Wada 1983). In 1990, HDC cDNA was cloned for the first time in rats, and consequently researches with genetic approaches started (Joseph et al. 1990). Identification of the HDC gene enabled us to investigate the transcriptional regulation of histamine synthesis. Cloning of HDC cDNA revealed that HDC is translated as the 74-kDa precursor protein and might be post-translationally cleaved to the 53–55-kDa species. This post-translational processing of HDC was found to be accompanied by increase in the enzymatic activity in several histamine-forming cells. In 2001, the gene targeted mouse strain for HDC was established (Ohtsu et al. 2001), and a series of novel functions of histamine has been identified using this strain.

In general, histamine synthesis is transient, and therefore induction and/or enzymatic activation of HDC plays key roles in a diverse array of histamine-mediated responses. Accumulating experimental evidence about HDC has consolidated and enriched our comprehension of the physiological roles of histamine. Novel functions of histamine have often been identified using HDC as a probe.

This review covers the areas of studies related to regulation of HDC. We regret that we could not cite many excellent papers in this field owing to limits of the space.

2.2 Purification and cDNA Cloning of HDC

HDC mediates decarboxylation of L-histidine to histamine, which requires pyridoxal 5′-phosphate as the cofactor (Schayer 1978, Shore et al. 1959). HDC has been regarded as the only enzyme that forms histamine, which has been recently confirmed by the gene targeted mouse strain (Ohtsu et al. 2001). Since fluorometric detection of histamine is sensitive and convenient, it has been used extensively in measurement of histamine content (Palacios et al. 1978). Early studies demonstrated that active histamine synthesis was observed in fetal liver, pregnant mouse kidney, mastocytoma, and stomach, although it was difficult to purify the enzyme due to its instability. A suicide inhibitor of HDC, α-fluoromethylhistidine, made a significant contribution to characterization of tissue histamine synthesis (Maeyama et al. 1982). Several groups tried to purify HDC from various sources, such as fetal liver, and kidney (Martin and Bishop 1986, Taguchi et al. 1984, Tran and Snyder 1981). In 1984, Watanabe et al. demonstrated for the first time the presence of hisatminergic neuron using the specific antibody raised against partially purified rat HDC protein (Watanabe et al. 1984). The presence of histaminergic neuron was also confirmed by Panula et al. using the specific antibody raised against histamine (Panula et al. 1984). A majority of these trials to purify HDC protein revealed that HDC consisted of two identical subunit, of which molecular mass was ∼55-kDa. Ohmori et al. succeeded in identification of partial amino acid sequence of HDC purified from mouse mastocytoma cell line, P-815 (Ohmori et al. 1990). On the other hand, cDNA of rat HDC was genetically identified for the first time through analysis of androgen binding protein (ABP) (Joseph et al. 1990, Sullivan et al. 1991). Although it remains unknown whether the fusion transcript of ABP and HDC is physiologically relevant, full length cDNA of rat HDC was identified using this fusion transcript as a probe. After that time, mouse and human HDC cDNAs were cloned in succession (Yamamoto et al. 1990, Zahnow et al. 1991). Cloning of HDC revealed that HDC might be initially translated as the precursor form, of which molecular mass is 74-kDa, and raised the possibility that HDC might undergo post-translational processing. Amino terminal approximately 55-kDa region of HDC is highly homologous between species and shares homology with the other amino acid decarboxylase, such as DOPA decarboxylase (DDC, also known as aromatic L-amino acid decarboxylase).

2.3 Transcriptional Regulation of HDC

Constitutive expression of HDC has been observed in the limited kinds of cells, such as histamine-containing neuron, mast cells, and basophils. Although histamine is one of the essential mediators in gastric acid secretion, prolonged fasting has been reported to virtually abolish the expression of HDC in the enterochromaffin-like (ECL) cells. Since histamine synthesis is often regulated through transcriptional regulation of the HDC gene, it should be required for better understanding of physiological roles of histamine to clarify the transcriptional regulation of the HDC gene.

2.3.1 Stomach

In 1972, Black et al. reported that histamine stimulated gastric acid secretion via the histamine H2 receptor, and then they successfully developed selective H2 antagonists (Black et al. 1972). H2 receptor antagonists had been the principal therapeutic agent for peptic ulcer and gastroesophageal reflux disease, both of which resulted from gastric acid hypersecretion until proton pump inhibitors were developed. HDC was found to be expressed in the ECL cells, and newly-formed histamine induces gastric acid secretion from parietal cells by acting on the H2 receptors. Although both gastrin and pituitary adenylyl cyclase-activating protein (PACAP) are the major stimulus of histamine release from ECL cells (Prinz et al. 2003), transcriptional regulation of HDC upon gastrin stimulation has been intensively studied.

Following cDNA cloning, gastrin-mediated induction of HDC was demonstrated in rat fundus (Dimaline and Sandvik 1991). Kölby et al. demonstrated that hypergastrinemia and ECL tumor formation drastically induced mRNA expression of HDC (Kölby et al. 1996). Transcriptional regulation of human and rat HDC gene was investigated in detail by Wang's group. Three GC-rich gastrin responsive elements were located downstream of the transcription initiation site of human HDC gene, and one of the nuclear factors bound to these elements was identified as Kruppel-like factor 4, which was involved in repression of HDC gene expression (Ai et al. 2004, Höcker et al. 1997, Raychowdhury et al. 1999, Zhang et al. 1996). A transcription factor, YY1, was found to repress HDC promoter activity in co-operation with SREBP-1a, and gastrin down-regulated mRNA expression of SREBP-1a, indicating that gastrin-mediated induction of HDC might be attributed at least in part to down-regulation of SREBP-1a (Ai et al. 2006). In process of these researches, they revealed that oxidative stress, such as hydrogen peroxide, could induce transcriptional activation of HDC gene through the gastrin responsive element (Höcker et al. 1998). They also demonstrated the differences of promoter activity of human HDC gene in PC12 cells, which stably expressed the human gastrin/CCK-2 receptor, upon stimulation of gastrin and PACAP (McLaughlin et al. 2004). Gastrin-mediated transcriptional activation was also reported in rat HDC gene (Höcker et al. 1996).

2.3.2 Mastocytoma

Transcriptional activation of mouse HDC gene was investigated in a mouse mastocytoma cell line, P-815, since purification and cDNA cloning were performed using this cell line. Although histamine synthesis was found to be suppressed by glucocorticoid in several reports (Zahnow et al. 1998), dexamethasone drastically induced HDC in combination with phorbol ester in P-815 cells (Kawai et al. 1992, Ohgoh et al. 1993). Transcriptional activation of mouse HDC gene was also observed in the cells stimulated with the combination of Ca^{2+} ionophore and cyclic AMP elevating agents (Miyazaki et al. 1992). Expression of HDC in P-815 cells was induced when the cells were transplanted into the peritoneal cavity of the syngenic BDF1 mice. Although it remains to be clarified which humoral factors are involved in such induction, Ohtsu et al. (1996) suggested that down-regulation of NF-E2 should lead to transcriptional activation of mouse HDC gene.

2.3.3 Tissue/Cell Specific Expression

Since expression of HDC is not ubiquitous but limited in specific cell types, gene expression of HDC should be spatiotemporally regulated. Yatsunami et al. determined the structure of human HDC gene (Yatsunami et al. 1994). Investigation of the 5′-lanking region of human HDC gene suggested that the c-Myb binding motif is involved in the specific expression of HDC in human basophilic leukemia, KU-812-F (Nakagawa et al. 1997). Kuramasu et al. found that mast cell- or basophil-specific expression of human HDC is regulated by CpG methylation in the promoter region (Kuramasu et al. 1998). DNA methylation-mediated regulation was also found in the cell type-specific expression of mouse HDC (Suzuki-Ishigaki et al. 2000). Recently, Aichberger et al. demonstrated that the chronic myeloid leukemia (CML)-specific oncoprotein BCR/ABL was involved in induction of histamine synthesis and that H1 receptor antagonists with binding potential to cyp450 can suppress proliferation of human chronic myeloid leukemia cell lines, such as K562 and KU-812 (Aichberger et al. 2006).

One of the tissues that exhibit highest HDC activity is fetal liver. HDC is drastically induced in the fetal liver immediately before parturition, indicating that histamine plays a critical role in fetal hematopoiesis (Héron et al. 2001, Karlstedt et al. 2001). However, it remains largely unknown how expression of HDC is transcriptionally regulated in hematopoietic lineage cells except mast cells and basophils.

2.4 Post-Translational Regulation of HDC

HDC might be initially translated as the precursor, of which molecular mass is 74-kDa, whereas the molecular mass of the enzyme purified from various sources was ∼55-kDa (Fig. 2.1). Several groups including us focused on the significance of the post-translational processing of HDC in regulation of histamine synthesis. In contrast to cytosolic distribution of DDC, the presence of insoluble and membrane-bound enzymatic activity of HDC had been recognized in various tissues (Baudry et al. 1973, Toledo et al. 1991). The recombinant HDC proteins were characterized in various expression systems, soon after its cDNA cloning. The

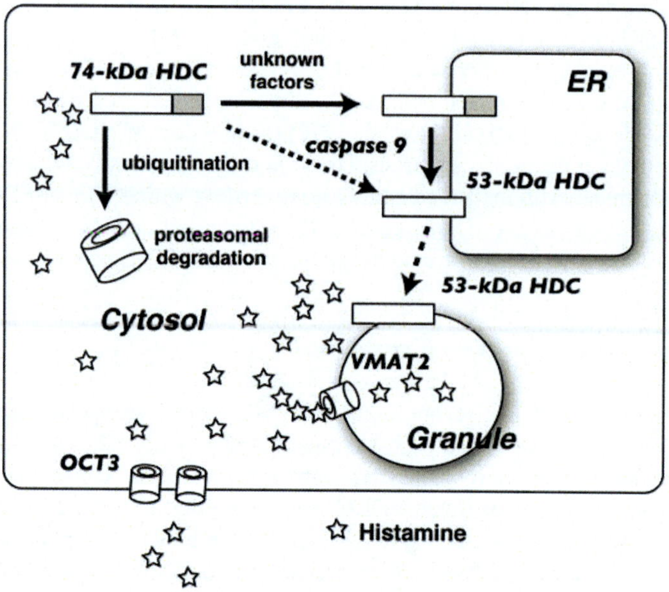

Fig. 2.1 Post-translational regulation of HDC. HDC is initially translated as the precursor 74-kDa form, which is enzymatically active. The 74-kDa HDC then undergoes proteolytic cleavage to yield the 53-kDa mature form. The post-translational processing was found to be mediated by caspase-9 and was accompanied by enzymatical activation in a mouse mastocytoma cell line. On the other hand, the residual 74-kDa HDC might be degraded through the ubiquitin-proteasome system. The carboxyl-terminal region has a potential to target HDC to the ER, although it remains unknown how the ER targeting occurs. In mast cells and neutrophils, the 53-kDa HDC was found to be localized in the granules, which may contribute to efficient uptake and storage of histamine via vesicular monoamine transporter-2 (VMAT-2). Accumulated cytosolic histamine is exported via organic cation transporter-3 (OCT3)

recombinant 74-kDa HDC was largely distributed in the insoluble fraction of the insect cell expression system, whereas the recombinant carboxyl-terminal deleted 54-kDa HDC in the soluble fraction (Yamamoto et al. 1993, Yatsunami et al. 1995). The 74-kDa HDC was enzymatically active in spite of its insoluble nature. Although no significant differences in specific activities were detected in between human 74-kDa and 54-kDa forms, proteolytic cleavage of mouse 74-kDa HDC resulted in formation of the 53-kDa soluble enzyme and increased enzyme activity (Tanaka et al. 1995). Dartsch et al. (1998) reported that the recombinant 74-kDa rat HDC exhibited lower enzyme activity whereas the carboxyl-terminal truncated 54-kDa was an active enzyme in COS-7 cells. However, Fleming and Wang demonstrated that proteolytic cleavage of rat HDC did not affect the enzyme activity and suggested that amino acid residues, $S^{502}K^{503}D^{504}$, which is not conserved in mouse and human, is the processing site in mammalian expression system with COS cells (Fleming and Wang 2003). They also reported that the carboxyl-terminal region of rat HDC contains a region, which hinders substrate binding (Fleming et al. 2004).

We have recently identified the processing sites and the responsible protease for the post-translational processing of mouse HDC in a mouse mastocytoma, P-815 cells (Furuta et al. 2007). Alanine scanning mutation analysis revealed that tandem di-aspartic acid residues ($D^{517}D^{518}$, and $D^{550}D^{551}$), which are completely conserved among mouse, rat, and human, are the potential candidates for the processing sites. We demonstrated that caspase-9 played a critical role in the post-translational processing and enzymatical activation of HDC. Combination of butyrate and a Zn^{2+} chelator, TPEN, augmented the enzyme activity of caspase-3 and -9 and lead to increased histamine synthesis, but no obvious apoptic cell death was observed in the cells.

The relationship between the molecular species and the intracellular localization of HDC is complicated. A series of studies in various expression systems have indicated that the 74-kDa HDC is localized at least in part in the insoluble fraction (Yamamoto et al. 1993, Yatsunami et al. 1995). However, the 74-kDa HDC was found to be localized mainly in the cytosol in a rat basophilic/mast cell line, RBL-2H3, where as the mature 53-kDa HDC in the granule compartments (Tanaka et al. 1998). In COS-7 cells, the carboxyl-terminal region mediated accumulation of mouse HDC protein in the ER, and in vitro translation system with reticulocyte lysate, the nascent 74-kDa mouse HDC was post-translationally targeted to the microsomal membranes whereas the carboxyl-terminal 54-kDa HDC was not (Suzuki et al. 1998). In casein-elicited activated mouse neutrophils, a rapid post-translational processing of HDC was observed and the 53-kDa HDC was localized in the granules (Tanaka et al. 2004). It is plausible that insoluble 74-kDa HDC found in the expression systems results from over expression and the absence of the endogenous partner proteins required for further post-translational processing. Viguera et al. predicted based on the sequence comparison that instability of HDC protein might be mediated by two PEST sequences (Viguera et al. 1994), which are enriched in proline (P), glutamic acid (E), serine (S) and threonine (T) and target proteins for rapid destruction (Rechsteiner and Rogers 1996). Indeed, the 74-kDa mouse HDC was found to be modified by ubiquitin and to undergo proteasomal degradation (Tanaka et al. 1997). In rat HDC protein, two PEST sequences were also involved in rapid degradation, and gastrin contributed to stabilization of multiple forms of HDC proteins (Fleming and Wang 2000).

2.5 Histamine Forming Cells

Specific antibodies raised against the recombinant HDC protein have made a significant contribution to identification of histamine-forming cells. Accumulating evidence suggests that a diverse array of cells can produce histamine in addition to mast cells, basophils, ECL cells, and neuron (Table 2.1).

Drastic increase in histamine synthesis in fetal liver just before parturition indicates that histamine may be involved in regulation of fetal hematopoiesis. Watanabe et al. demonstrated that such increase in histamine synthesis was abolished in *W/W*

Table 2.1 Histamine synthesis in various kinds of cells

Cell type	Function	Reference(s)
Mast cell	Immediate allergy, Inflammation	Metcalfe et al. (1997)
Basophil	Immediate allergy, Inflammation	Sullivan and Locksley (2009)
Macrophage	Immune suppression	Kawaguchi-Nagata et al. (1985), Takamatsu et al. (1996), Yokoyama et al. (2004)
Microglia	Neurotransmission?	Katoh et al. (2001)
Neutrophil	Inflammation	Shiraishi et al. (2000), Tanaka et al. (2004), Xu et al. (2006)
Neuron	Neurotransmission	Haas et al. (2008), Panula et al. (1984), Watanabe et al. (1984)
ECL cell	Gastric acid secretion	Prinz et al. (2003), Rubin and Schwartz (1979)
Male germ cells	Fertilization?	Safina et al. (2002)
Mammary epithelial cell	?	Wagner et al. (2003)
Epithelial cells (uterus)	Implantation	Paria et al. (1998)
Unidentified (kidney, during pregnancy)	Vasodilation?	Morgan et al. (2006)

mice, which suggested that c-kit-dependent cell lineage expressed HDC in fetal liver (Watanabe et al. 1981). Histamine synthesis in non-mast cells was also exhibited in the skin upon phorbol ester stimulation (Taguchi et al. 1982). Dy et al. (1981) demonstrated that histamine synthesis was induced upon allograft rejection. They have focused on histamine synthesis during hematopoiesis, in particular interleukin-3-dependent hematopoietic progenitor cells (Dy et al. 1993, 1996, Schneider et al. 1993). One of the potential candidates for non-mast cell histamine-forming cells is macrophages (Kawaguchi-Nagata et al. 1985). Takamatsu et al. (1996) first demonstrated that bone marrow-derived macrophages can produce histamine in response to endotoxin. Histamine synthesis was found to be induced by phorbol ester and thapsigargin in a mouse macrophage cell line, RAW264.7, in which the 74-kDa HDC was dominantly expressed (Hirasawa et al. 2001, Shiraishi et al. 2000). Accumulating evidence suggests that nascent histamine produced by macrophages plays critical roles in suppression of immune responses mainly by acting on the H2 receptor (Yokoyama et al. 2004). The H2 receptor-mediated suppression might be important feedback system of immune responses (Elenkov et al. 1998, van der Pouw Kraan et al. 1998, Vannier et al. 1991). Hirasawa et al. (1987) reported that histamine synthesis occurred in the late phase of anaphylactic inflammation in addition to rapid degranulation of mast cells in the immediate phase. Histamine synthesis in the late phase of allergic inflammation was accompanied by elicited neutrophil accumulation (Shiraishi et al. 2000). Based on these remarks, we demonstrated that activated neutrophils express HDC in the casein-induced peritonitis model and that granulocyte-macrophage colony stimulating factor (GM-CSF) has a potential to induce HDC in immature neutrophils (Tanaka et al. 2004). Xu et al. (2006) demonstrated that mycoplasma pneumonia directly stimulated histamine synthesis in naïve neutrophils, which provoked lung and airway inflammation. We observed that activated neutrophils infiltrated into tumor tissues produced histamine, which might down-regulate local cytokine production, such as TNF-α and IFN-γ, by acting on the H2 receptor in the tumor tissues (Takahashi et al. 2001, 2002). Ghosh et al. (2002) demonstrated that histamine promoted angiogenesis in inflammatory granulation tissues, which was mediated by the H2 receptor. Angiogenesis induced by histamine was also observed in the W/W^V mice, suggesting that the source of histamine might be macrophages or neutrophils.

2.6 Gene Targeting of HDC

Ohtsu et al. reported establishment of the gene targeted mouse strain for HDC for the first time (Ohtsu et al. 2001), and thereafter, a wide variety of histamine-mediated responses has been identified, a part of which could not be attributed to the specific histamine receptor functions. The gene targeted mice for HDC and histamine receptors will certainly provide us with a deeper insight into the physiological roles of histamine. We discuss here a part of recent findings obtained with the HDC deficient ($HDC^{-/-}$) mice. Ohtsu and Watanabe also summarized the studies using the $HDC^{-/-}$ mice (Ohtsu and Watanabe 2003).

Histamine plays a central role in immediate allergic responses and many H1 receptor antagonists have been developed for therapeutic drugs for type I allergy (Du Buske 1996, Thurmond et al. 2008). The $HDC^{-/-}$ mice were resistant to IgE-mediated passive cutaneous and systemic anaphylaxis (Makabe-Kobayashi et al. 2002, Ohtsu et al. 2002). However, the impaired allergic responses in the $HDC^{-/-}$ mice could not be attributed solely to lack of histamine as a critical proinflammatory mediator, since mast cells in the skin and peritoneal cavity in the $HDC^{-/-}$ mice exhibited severe morphological abnormality in the granules (Ohtsu et al. 2001). The scarce electron density of the mature mast cells in the $HDC^{-/-}$ mice indicated that histamine is involved in granule maturation of mast cells. We previously reported that a part of IgE clones have a potential to induce histamine synthesis in immature mast cells in the absence of the antigens (Tanaka et al. 2002b). It is plausible that autocrine loop of histamine promotes granule maturation and exacerbates allergic inflammation in chronic allergy with elevated serum IgE concentrations. Since histamine is also produced by intestinal bacteria, it is difficult to completely exclude the trace amount of histamine in the $HDC^{-/-}$ mouse tissues. Indeed, dietary supplemented histamine was accumulated in the granules of mast cells and macrophages and it might affect the phenotype of the $HDC^{-/-}$ mice (Ohtsu et al. 2002, Tanaka et al. 2003). Schneider et al. (2005) demonstrated that transport of histamine across the plasma membrane was mediated by organic cation transporter 3 (OCT3), whereas granule storage of histamine was found to be mediated solely by vesicular monoamine transporter 2 (VMAT2) (Travis et al. 2000). These systems may be involved in cellular uptake of dietary supplemented histamine.

A series of studies with the H1- and H2-deficient mice highlighted the critical role of histamine in immune modulation. Jutel et al. demonstrated that histamine augmented Th1 responses through the H1 receptor and suppressed both Th1 and Th2 responses by acting on the H2 receptors (Jutel et al. 2001). Modulatory roles of histamine in helper T cells and dendritic cells through the H1 and H2 receptors should be taken into consideration of the immunological phenotype of the $HDC^{-/-}$ mice (Jutel et al. 2002). In experimental autoimmune encephalomyelitis, an animal model for multiple sclerosis, lack of HDC resulted in disease exacerbation (Musio et al. 2006). Although it remains to be determined which kinds of histamine receptors are involved, it is likely that impaired production of IFN-γ and TNF-α was mediated by the H2 receptor. Beghdadi et al. recently demonstrated that the $HDC^{-/-}$ mice were highly resistant to severe malaria through the preserved blood-brain barrier integrity, the absence of infected erythrocyte aggregation, and a lack of sequestration of $CD4^+$ and $CD8^+$ T cells (Beghdadi et al. 2008). They also revealed that the H1 and H2 receptors were involved in the pathogenesis using the gene targeted mice and the specific antagonists. Co-operative action of the H1 and H2 receptors has often been found in histamine-mediated immune modulation. The $HDC^{-/-}$ mice exhibited accelerated bacterial clearance in peritoneal cavity, and this histamine-mediated suppression of bacterial clearance was inhibited by the H1 and H2 antagonists (Hori et al. 2002). In an ovalbumin-induced allergic asthma model, airway eosinophilia was significantly suppressed in the $HDC^{-/-}$ mice whereas airway hyperresponsiveness was not affected (Koarai et al. 2003). These findings might be related to histamine-mediated leukocyte chemotaxis, which is mediated by the H1 and H4 receptors (Thurmond et al. 2008, Zampeli and Tiligada 2009).

Parietal cells undergo gastric acid secretion upon activation of the H2 receptor. In the H2 receptor deficient ($H2R^{-/-}$) mice, gastric acid secretion induced by histamine or gastrin was completely abolished but that by carbachol remained intact (Kobayashi et al. 2000). The $H2R^{-/-}$ mice exhibited a marked hypertrophy in gastric mucosa and elevated serum gastrin levels. We found that the $HDC^{-/-}$ mice also exhibited moderate hypergastrinemia and that they were sensitive to carbachol but not to gastrin in acid secretion (Furutan et al. 2003, Tanaka et al. 2002a). The $HDC^{-/-}$ mice were hypersensitive to exogenous histamine in acid secretion, which were reminiscent of rebound acid hypersecretion after the abrupt withdrawal of prolonged H2 receptor blockade. Gastric hyperplasia was also observed in the $HDC^{-/-}$ mice, which was not so severe as in the $H2R^{-/-}$ mice (Nakamura et al. 2004).

In addition to these phenotypes in immune and gastrointestinal systems, many studies have indicated the pathological and physiological roles of histamine. The $HDC^{-/-}$ mice should provide us with a deeper insight in functions of histamine.

2.7 Conclusion

In contrast to extensive research for the specific receptors of histamine, regulation of histamine synthesis remained to be clarified in detail. Cloning of HDC enabled us to raise specific antibodies against the recombinant HDC protein and to characterize a variety of histamine-forming cells. Identification of histamine-forming cells has lead to better understanding of the function of histamine. Furthermore, various unexpected functions of histamine have been found using the HDC deficient mouse strain, a part of which could not be attributed simply to a single receptor-mediated response. Comparison between and combinatorial use of the HDC deficient and the histamine receptor deficient mice should make a significant contribution to the field of histamine research.

References

Ai W, Liu Y, Langlois M et al (2004) Kruppel-like factor 4 (KLF4) represses histidine decarboxylase gene expression through an upstream Sp1 site and downstream gastrin responsive elements. J Biol Chem 279:8684–8693

Ai W, Liu Y, Wang TC (2006) Yin yang 1 (YY1) represses histidine decarboxylase gene expression with SREBP-1a in part through an upstream Sp1 site. Am J Physiol Gastrointest Liver Physiol 290:G1096–G1104

Aichberger KJ, Mayerhofer M, Vales A et al (2006) The CML-related oncoprotein BCR/ABL induces expression of histidine decarboxylase (HDC) and the synthesis of histamine in leukemic cells. Blood 108:3538–3547

Baudry M, Martres MP, Schwartz JC (1973) The subcelluar localization of histidine decarboxylase in various regions of rat brain. J Neurochem 21:1301–1309

Beghdadi W, Porcherie A, Schneider BS et al (2008) Inhibition of histamine-mediated signaling confers significant protection against severe malaria in mouse models of disease. J Exp Med 205:395–408

Black JW, Duncan WA, Durant CJ et al (1972) Definition and anatgonism of histamine H_2-receptors. Nature 236:385–90

Dartsch C, Chen D, Persson L (1998) Multiple forms of rat stomach histidine decarboxylase may reflect posttranslational activation of the enzyme. Regul Pept 77:33–41

Dimaline R, Sandvik AK (1991) Histidine decarboxylase gene expression in rat fundus is regulated by gastrin. FEBS Lett 281:20–22

Du Buske LM (1996) Clinical comparison of histamine H_1-receptor antagonist drugs. J Allergy Clin Immunol 98:S307–S318

Dy M, Arnould A, Lemoine FM et al (1996) Hematopoietic progenitors and interleukin-3-denpendent cell line synthesize histamine in response to calcium ionophore. Blood 87:3161–3169

Dy M, Lebel B, Kamoun P et al (1981) Histamine production during the anti-allograft response. J Exp Med 153:293–309

Dy M, Machavoine F, Lebel B et al (1993) Interleukin 3 promotes histamine synthesis in hematopoietic progenitors by increasing histidine decarboxylase mRNA expression. Biochem Biophys Res Commun 192:167–173

Elenkov IJ, Webster E, Papanicolaou DA et al (1998) Histamine potently suppresses human IL-12 and stimulates IL-10 production via H_2 receptors. J Immunol 161:2586–2593

Fleming JV, Fajardo I, Langlois MR et al (2004) The C-terminus of rat L-histidine decarboxylase specifically inhibits enzymic activity and disrupts pyridoxal phosphate-dependent interactions with L-histidine substrate analogues. Biochem J 381:769–778

Fleming JV, Wang TC (2000) Amino- and carboxy-terminal PEST domains mediate gastrin stabilization of rat L-histidine decarboxylase isoforms. Mol Cell Biol 20:4932–4947

Fleming JV, Wang TC (2003) The production of 53–55-kDa isoforms is not required for rat L-histidine decarboxylase activity. J Biol Chem 278:686–694

Furuta K, Nakayama K, Sugimoto Y et al (2007) Activation of histidine decarboxylase through post-translational cleavage by caspase-9 in a mouse mastocytoma P-815. J Biol Chem 282:13438–13446

Furutan K, Aihara T, Nakamura E et al (2003) Crucial role of histamine for regulation of gastric acid secretion ascertained by histidine decarboxylase-knockout mice. J Pharmacol Exp Ther 307:331–338

Ghosh AK, Hirasawa N, Ohtsu H et al (2002) Defective angiogenesis in the inflammatory granulation tissue in histidine decarboxylase-deficient mice but not in mast cell-deficient mice. J Exp Med 195:973–982

Haas HL, Sergeeva OA, Selbach O (2008) Histamine in the nervous system. Physiol Rev 88:1183–1241

Héron A, Rouleau A, Cochois V et al (2001) Expression analysis of the histamine H_3 receptor in developing rat tissues. Mech Dev 105:167–173

Hirasawa N, Murakami A, Ohuchi K (2001) Expression of 74-kDa histidine decarboxylase protein in a macrophage-like cell line RAW264.7 and inhibition by dexamethasone. Eur J Pharmacol 418:23–28

Hirasawa N, Ohuchi K, Watanabe M et al (1987) Role of endogenous histamine in psotanaphylactic phase of allergic inflammation in rats. J Pharmacol Exp Ther 241:967–973

Höcker M, Rosenberg I, Xavier R et al (1998) Oxidative stress activates the human histidine decarboxylase promoter in AGS gastric cancer cells. J Biol Chem 273:23046–23054

Höcker M, Zhang Z, Fenstermacher DA et al (1996) Rat histidine decarboxylase promoter is regulated by gastrin through a protein kinase C pathway. Am J Physiol Gastrointest Liver Phyiol 270:G619–G633

Höcker M, Zhang Z, Merchant JL et al (1997) Gastrin regulates the human histidine decarboxylase promoter through an AP-1-dependent mechanism. Am J Physiol Gastrointest Liver Physiol 272:G822–G830

Hori Y, Nihei Y, Kurokawa Y et al (2002) Accelerated clearance of Escherichia coli in experimental peritonitis of histamine-deficient mice. J Immunol 169:1978–1983

Joseph DR, Sullivan PM, Wang YM et al (1990) Characterization and expression of the complementary DNA encoding rat histidine decarboxylase. Proc Natl Acad Sci USA 87:733–737

Jutel M, Blaser K, Akdis CA (2005) Histamine in allergic inflammation and immune modulation. Int Arch Allergy Immunol 137:82–92

Jutel M, Watanabe T, Akdis M et al (2002) Immune regulation by histamine. Curr Opin Immunol 14:735–740

Jutel M, Watanabe T, Klunker S et al (2001) Histamine regulates T-cell and antibody responses by differential expression of H_1 and H_2 receptors. Nature 413:420–425

Karlstedt K, Nissinen M, Michelsen KA et al (2001) Multiple sites of L-histidine decarboxylase expression in mouse suggest novel developmental functions for histamine. Dev Dyn 221:81–91

Katoh Y, Niimi M, Yamamoto Y et al (2001) Histamine production by cultured microglial cells of the mouse. Neurosci Lett 305:181–184

Kawaguchi-Nagata K, Okamura H, Tamura T et al (1985) Induction of histidine decarboxylase activity in the spleen of mice treated with staphylococcal enterotoxin A and demonstration of its non-mast cell origin. Biochem Biophys Res Commun 129:187–192

Kawai H, Ohgoh M, Emoto S et al (1992) Synergistic effects of 12-O-tetradecanoylphorbol-13-acetate and dexamethasone on de novo synthesis of histidine decarboxylase in mouse mastocytoma P-815 cells. Biochim Biophys Acta 1133:172–178

Koarai A, Ichinose M, Ishigaki-Suzuki S et al (2003) Disruption of L-histidine decarboxylase reduces airway eosinophilia but not hyperresponsiveness. Am J Respir Crit Care Med 167:758–763

Kobayashi T, Tonai S, Ishihara Y et al (2000) Abnormal functional and morphological regulation of the gastric mucosa in histamine H_2 receptor-deficient mice. J Clin Invest 105:1741–1749

Kölby L, Wängberg B, Ahlman H et al (1996) Histidine decarboxylase expression and histamine metabolism in gastric oxyntic mucosa during hypergastrinemia and carcinoid tumor formation. Endocrinology 137:4435–4442

Kuramasu A, Saito H, Suzuki S et al (1998) Mast cell-/basophil-specific regulation of human L-histidine decarboxylase gene by CpG methylation in the promoter region. J Biol Chem 273:31607–31614

Leurs R, Bakker RA, Timmerman H et al (2005) The histamine H_3 receptor: from gene cloning to H_3 receptor drugs. Nat Rev Drug Discov 4:107–120
Lovenberg TW, Roland BL, Wilson SJ et al (1999) Cloning and functional expression of the human histamine H_3 receptor. Mol Pharamcol 55:1101–1107
Maeyama K, Watanabe T, Taguchi Y et al (1982) Effect of α-fluoromethylhistidine, a suicide inhibitor of histidine decarboxylase, on histamine levels in mouse tissues. Biochem Pharmacol 14:2367–2370
Makabe-Kobayashi Y, Hori Y, Adachi T et al (2002) The control effect of histamine on body temperature and respiratory function in IgE-dependent systemic anaphylaxis. J Allergy Clin Immunol 110:298–303
Martin SAM, Bishop JO (1986) Purification and characterization of histidine decarboxylase from mouse kidney. Biochem J 234:349–354
McLaughlin JT, Ai W, Sinclair NF et al (2004) PACAP and gastrin regulate the histidine decarboxylase promoter via distinct mechanisms. Am J Physiol Gastrointest Liver Physiol 286:G51–G59
Metcalfe DD, Baram D, Mekori YA (1997) Mast cells. Physiol Rev 77:1033–1079
Miyazaki T, Ohgoh M, Ohmori E et al (1992) Synergistic effects of cyclic AMP and Ca^{2+} ionophore A23187 on de novo synthesis of histidine decarboxylase in mastocytoma P-815 cells. Biochim Biphys Acta 1133:179–186
Morgan TK, Montgomery K, Mason V et al (2006) Upregulation of histidine decarboxylase expression in superficial cortical nephrons during pregnancy in mice and women. Kidney Int 70:306–314
Musio S, Gallo B, Scabeni S et al (2006) A key regulatory role for histamine in experimental autoimmune encephalomyelitis: disease exacerbation in histidine decarboxylase-deficient mice. J Immunol 176:17–26
Nakagawa S, Okaya Y, Yatsunami K et al (1997) Identification of multiple regulatory elements of human L-histidine decarboxylase gene. J Biochem 121:935–940
Nakamura E, Kataoka T, Furutani K et al (2004) Lack of histamine alters gastric mucosal morphology: comparison of histidine decarboxylase-deficient and mast cell-deficient mice. Am J Physiol Gastrointest Liver Physiol 287:G1053–G1061
Oda T, Morikawa N, Saito Y et al (2000) Molecular cloning and characterization of a novel type of histamine receptor preferentially expressed in leukocytes. J Biol Chem 275:36781–36786
Ohgoh M, Yamamoto J, Kawata M et al (1993) Enhanced expression of the mouse L-histidine decarboxylase gene with a combination of dexamethasone and 12-O-tetradecanoylphorbol-13-acetate. Biochem Biophys Res Commun 196:1113–1119
Ohmori E, Fukui T, Imanishi N et al (1990) Purification and chracterization of L-histidine decarboxylase from mouse mastocytoma P-815 cells. J Biochem (Tokyo) 107:834–839
Ohtsu H, Kuramasu A, Suzuki S et al (1996) Histidine decarboxylase expression in mouse mast cell line P-815 is induced by mouse peritoneal cavity incubation. J Biol Chem 271: 28439–28444
Ohtsu H, Kuramasu A, Tanaka S et al (2002) Plasma extravasation induced by dietary supplemented histamine in histamine-free mice. Eur J Immunol 32:1698–1708
Ohtsu H, Tanaka S, Terui T et al (2001) Mice lacking histidine decarboxylase exhibit abnormal mast cells. FEBS Lett 502:53–56
Ohtsu H, Watanabe T (2003) New functions of histamine found in histidine decarboxylase gene knockout mice. Biochem Biphys Res Commun 305:443–447
Palacios JM, Mengod G, Grau M et al (1978) Pyridoxal 5′-phosphate as a cofactor for rat brain histidine decarboxylase. J Neurochem 30:213–216
Panula P, Yang HY, Costa E (1984) Histamine-containing neurons in the rat hypothalamus. Proc Natl Acad Sci USA 81:2572–2576
Paria BC, Das N, Das SK et al (1998) Histidine decarboxylase gene in the mouse uterus is regulated by progesterone and correlates with uterine differentiation for blastocyst implantation. Endocrinology 139:3958–3966

Prinz C, Zanner R, Gratzl M (2003) Physiology of gastric enterochromaffin-like cells. Annu Rev Physiol 65:371–382

Raychowdhury R, Zhang Z, Höcker M et al (1999) Activation of human histidine decarboxylase gene promoter activity by gastrin is mediated by two distinct nuclear factors. J Biol Chem 274:20961–20969

Rechsteiner M, Rogers SW (1996) PEST sequences and regulation by proteolysis. Trends Biochem Sci 21:267–271

Rubin W, Schwartz B (1979) Electron microscopic radioautographic identification of the ECL cell as the histamine-synthesizing endocrine cell in the rat stomach. Gastroenterology 77:458–467

Safina F, Tanaka S, Inagaki M et al (2002) Expression of L-histidine decarboxylase in mouse male germ cells. J Biol Chem 277:14211–14215

Schayer RW (1978) Biogenesis of histamine. In Rocha e Silva M (ed) Handbook of experimental pharmacology, vol 18/2 Springer, Berlin Heidelberg New York

Schneider E, Machavoine F, Pléau JM et al (2005) Organic cation transporter 3 modulates murine basophil functions by controlling intracellular histamine levels. J Exp Med 202:387–393

Schneider E, Poemacher RE, Nabarra B et al (1993) Mast cells and their committed precursors are not required for interleukin-3-induced histamine synthesis in murine bone marrow: characteristics of histamine-producing cells. Blood 81:1161–1169

Schubert ML (2007) Gastric secretion. Curr Opin Gastroenterol 23:595–601

Shiraishi M, Hirasawa N, Kobayashi Y et al (2000) Participation of mitogen-activated protein kinase in thapsigargin- and TPA-induced histamine production in murine macrophage RAW264.7 cells. Br J Pharmacol 129:515–524

Shiraishi M, Hirasawa N, Oikawa S et al (2000) Analysis of histamine-producing cells at the late phase of allergic inflammation in rats. Immunology 99:600–606

Shore PA, Burkhalter A, Cohn VH Jr (1959) A method for the fluorometric assay of histamine in tissues. J Pharmacol Exp Ther 127:182–186

Sullivan BM, Locksley RM (2009) Basophils: A nonredundant contributor to host immunity. Immunity 30:12–20

Sullivan PM, Petrusz P, Szpirer C et al (1991) Alternative processing of androgen-binding protein RNA transcripts in fetal rat liver. J Biol Chem 266:143–154

Suzuki S, Tanaka S, Nemoto K et al (1998) Membrane targeting and binding of the 74-kDa form of mouse L-histidine decarboxylase via its carboxyl-terminal sequence. FEBS Lett 437:44–48

Suzuki-Ishigaki S, Numayama-Tsuruta K, Kuramasu A et al (2000) The mouse L-histidine decarboxylase gene: structure and transcriptional regulation by CpG methylation in the promoter region. Nucleic Acids Res 28:2627–2633

Taguchi Y, Tsuyama K, Watanabe T et al (1982) Increase in histidine decarboxylase activity in skin of genetically mast-cell-deficient W/Wv mice after application of phorbol 12-myristate 13-acetate: evidence for the presence of histamine-producing cells without basophilic granules. Proc Natl Acad Sci USA 79:6837–6841

Taguchi Y, Watanabe T, Kubota H et al (1984) Purification of histidine decarboxylase from the liver of fetal rats and its immunochemical and immunohistochemical characterization. J Biol Chem 259:5214–5221

Takahashi K, Tanaka S, Furuta K et al (2002) Histamine H_2 receptor-mediated modulation of local cytokine expression in a mouse experimental tumor model. Biochem Biophys Res Commun 297:1205–1210

Takahashi K, Tanaka S, Ichikawa A (2001) Effect of cimetidine on intratumoral cytokine expression in an experimental tumor. Biochem Biophys Res Commun 281:1113–1119

Takamatsu S, Nakashima I, Nakano K (1996) Modulation of endotoxin-induced histamine synthesis by cytokine in mouse bone marrow-derived macrophages. I Immunol 156:778–785

Tanaka S, Deai K, Inagaki M et al (2003) Uptake of histamine by mouse peritoneal macrophages and a macrophage cell line, RAW264.7. Am J Physiol Cell Physiol 285:C592-C598

Tanaka S, Deai K, Konomi A et al (2004) Expression of L-histidine decarboxylase in granules of elicited mouse polymorphonuclear leukocytes. Eur J Immunol 34:1472–1482

Tanaka S, Fukui T, Yamamoto J et al (1995) Processing and activation of recombinant mouse mastocytoma histidine decarboxylase in the particulate fraction of Sf9 cells by porcine pancreatic elastase. Biochimica Biophys Acta 1253:9–12

Tanaka S, Hamada K, Yamada N et al (2002a) Gastric acid secretion in L-histidine decarboxylase-deficient mice. Gastroenterology 122:145–155

Tanaka S, Nemoto K, Yamamura E et al (1997) Degradation of the 74 kDa form of L-histidine decarboxylase via the ubiquitin-proteasome pathway in a rat basophilic/mast cell line (RBL-2H3). FEBS Lett 417:203–207

Tanaka S, Nemoto K, Yamamura E et al (1998) Intracellular localization of the 74- and 53-kDa forms of L-histidine decarboxylase in a rat basophilic/mast cell line, RBL-2H3. J Biol Chem 273:8177–8182

Tanaka S, Takasu Y, Mikura S et al (2002b) Antigen-independent induction of histamine synthesis by immunoglobulin E in mouse bone marrow-derived mast cells. J Exp Med 196:229–235

Thurmond RL, Gelfand EW, Dunford PJ (2008) The role of histamine H_1 and H_4 receptors in allergic inflammation: the search for new antihistamine. Nat Rev Drug Discov 7:41–53

Toledo A, Rodriguez R, Sabriá J et al (1991) Calcium effects on the solubilization of membrane-bound histidine decarboxylase in the rat brain. J Neurochem 56:380–384

Tran VT, Snyder S (1981) Histidine decarboxylase. Purification from fetal rat liver, immunologic properties, and histochemical localization in brain and stomach. J Biol Chem 256: 680–686

Travis ER, Wang YM, Michael Dj et al (2000) Differential quantal release of histamine and 5-hydroxytryptamine from mast cells of vesicular monoamine transporter 2 knockout mice. Proc Natl Acad Sci USA 97:162–167

van der Pouw Kraan TC, Snijders A, Boeije LC et al (1998) Histamine inhibits the production of interleukin-12 through interaction with H_2 receptors. J Clin Invest 102:1866–1873

Vannier E, Miller LC, Dinarello CA (1991) Histamine suppresses gene expression and synthesis of tumor necrosis factor alpha via histamine H_2 receptors. J Exp Med 174:281–284

Viguera E, Trelles O, Urdiales JL et al (1994) Mammalian L-amino acid decarboxylase producing 1,4-diamines: analogies among differences. Trends Biochem Sci 19:318–319

Wagner W, Ichikawa A, Tanaka S et al (2003) Mouse mammry epithelial histamine system. J Physiol Pharmacol 54:211–223

Watanabe T, Kitamura Y, Maeyama K et al (1981) Absence of increase of histidine decarboxylase activity in mast cell-deficient *W/W* mouse embryos before parturition. Proc Natl Acad Sci USA 78:4209–4212

Watanabe T, Taguchi Y, Shiosaka S et al (1984) Distribution of the histaminergic neuron system in the central nervous system of rats; a fluorescent immunohistochemical analysis with histidine decarboxylase as a marker. Brain Res 295:13–25

Watanabe T, Wada H (1983) Histidine decarboxylase and histamine *N*-methyl transferase. In: Parvez S, Nagatsu T, Nagatsu I, Parvez H (eds) Methods in biogenic amine research. Elsevier Science, Ltd. (Amsterdam, Netherlands) pp 689–720

Xu X, Zhang D, Zhang H et al (2006) Neutrophil histamine contributes to inflammation in mycoplasma pneumonia. J Exp Med 203:2907–2917

Yamamoto J, Fukui T, Suzuki K et al (1993) Expression and characterization of recombinant mouse mastocytoma histidine decarboxylase. Biochim Biphys Acta 1216:431–440

Yamamoto J, Yatsunami K, Ohmori E et al (1990) cDNA-derived amino acid sequence of L-histidine decarboxylase from mouse mastocytoma P-815 cells. FEBS Lett 276:214–218

Yatsunami K, Ohtsu H, Tsuchikawa M et al (1994) Structure of the L-histidine decarboxylase gene. J Biol Chem 269:1554–1559

Yatsunami K, Tsuchikawa M, Kamada M et al (1995) Comparative studies of human recombinant 74- and 54-kDa L-histidine decarboxylase. J Biol Chem 270:30813–30817

Yokoyama M, Yokoyama A, Mori S et al (2004) Inducible histamine protects mice from P. acnes-primed and LPS-induced hepatitis through H_2-receptor stimulation. Gastroenterology 127:892–902

Zahnow C, Panula P, Yamatodani A et al (1998) Glucocorticoid hormones downregulate histidine decarboxylase mRNA and enzyme activity in rat lung. Am J Physiol Lung Cell Mol Physiol 275:L407–L413

Zahnow CA, Yi HF, McBride OW et al (1991) Cloning of the cDNA encoding human histidine decarboxylase from an erythroleukemia cell line and mapping of the gene locus to chromosome 15. DNA Seq 1:395–400

Zampeli E, Tiligada E (2009) The role of histamine H4 receptor in immune and inflammatory disorders. Bt J Pharmacol 157:24–33

Zhang Z, Höcker M, Koh TJ et al (1996) The human histidine decarboxylase promoter is regulated by gastrin and phorbor 12-myristate 13-acetate through a downstream *cis*-acting element. J Biol Chem 271:14188–14197

Part II
Enzymology in Histamine Biology

Chapter 3
Enzymology in Histamine Biogenesis

Almudena Pino-Ángeles, Aurelio A. Moya-García, Miguel Ángel Medina, and Francisca Sánchez-Jiménez

Abstract Histamine is a multifunctional biogenic amine with relevant roles in intercellular communication, inflammatory processes and many emergent pathologies. Histamine biosynthesis depends on the single decarboxylation of the amino acid histidine. In Gram-negative bacteria and animals, this reaction is carried out by a PLP-dependent histidine decarboxylase activity (HDC, EC 4.1.1.22), an enzyme that has been rather difficult to experimentally characterize. Interest in the mammalian HDC has increased due to recent findings on physiological consequences observed in HDC knockout animals. During the last few years, important advances have been made in the study of the structure/function relationship that explains its catalytic behaviour, mainly through a combination of both biophysical and biocomputational approaches. This chapter provides a comprehensive review of the current knowledge on this topic and how this knowledge could be extracted, which could give insights to characterize other unstable and minor proteins with physiopathological relevance. A model for the structure of the enzyme allowed us to understand its topology and to locate the catalytic environment, which was validated by direct-mutagenesis. Hybrid quantum mechanics and molecular mechanics simulations made it possible to understand the decarboxylation reaction at atomic level, as well as the conformational changes of the enzyme caused by the substrate binding. At this point, the search for and design of new and more selective modulators of the activity are possible. We also point out some important outstanding problems: (i) the exact role of the carboxy-terminal portion of the primary translation product; (ii) the putative binding proteins that can explain several intracellular features deduced for this enzyme; and (iii) the need for a deeper comparison to the unsolved PLP-dependent bacterial counterpart and other homologous enzymes.

F. Sánchez-Jiménez (✉)
Department of Molecular Biology and Biochemistry, Universidad de Málaga Facultad de Ciencias, Campus de Teatinos, Malaga 29071, Spain; "CIBER de Enfermedades Raras" (CIBERER), Valencia, Spain
e-mail: kika@uma.es

The authors Almudena Pino-Ángeles and Aurelio A. Moya-García have contributed equally to this work.

M. Shahid et al. (eds.), *Biomedical Aspects of Histamine*,
DOI 10.1007/978-90-481-9349-3_3, © Springer Science+Business Media B.V. 2010

Keywords Histidine · Histamine · Pyruvoyl-dependent reaction · Pyridoxal-dependent reaction · Vitamin B6 · Decarboxylation · Biogenic amines · Food spoiling · Inflammation · Allergy · Neurotransmission · Gastric secretion

Abbreviations

PLP	pyridoxal-5-phosphate
Pyr-	pyruvoyl moiety
DC	amino acid decarboxylase
HDC	histidine decarboxylase
DDC	L-aromatic amino acid/dopa decarboxylase
GDC	glutamate decarboxylase
HME	histidine methylesther
FMH	flurometyhl histidine

Contents

3.1 Introduction

Histamine is the product of the α-decarboxylation of the proteinogenic amino acid histidine. In several animals, including rat and growing humans, the endogenous synthesis of histidine, which is metabolically linked to de novo nucleic acid synthesis, is not enough to accomplish the endogenous synthesis of proteins and other histidine-derived secondary metabolites, so that food intake is the most important source for the endogenous pool of the amino acid (Bender 1985). After protein digestion, histamine can be considered the product of a single step pathway catalysed by the enzyme histidine decarboxylase (HDC, EC 4.1.1.22). In any case, diet can also be an important source of histamine, since microorganisms growing on the raw material of fermented foods, as well as the intestinal flora, can also produce the amine which is assimilated in the gastrointestinal track. Due to these facts, there is a growing demand for consumers and control authorities to reduce the allowable limits of histamine in food and beverages.

Histamine can elicit pleiotropic responses in the human body through different receptors, as it is a mediator of the immune response, gastric secretion and neurotransmission (see other chapters of this book). Its uptake, synthesis, degradation, reception and storage must be strictly controlled since it is, both an essential compound for several physiological functions, and a toxic compound when it is present either in excess or in the wrong metabolic context, as revealed by experiments with knock-out and histamine-treated animals. Histamine has been related to allergies and many other inflammatory responses, peptic ulcers, food intolerance, bone loss, several neurological and fertility disorders and even tumour growth modulation (Csaba et al. 2007a, b, Dere et al. 2004, Jorgensen et al. 2006, Klausz et al. 2004, Liu et al. 2007, Mondillo et al. 2007, Ohtsu 2008, Ohtsu and Watanabe 2003, Pos et al. 2008, Rahman et al. 2007). Consequently, from a biomedical point of view, the characteristics of both bacterial and animal enzymes are interesting and must be taken into account to develop strategies to interfere with histamine metabolism and its undesirable consequences (Medina et al. 2003).

In this chapter, we review the current knowledge about the structural features and function of histidine decarboxylase, new perspectives to control its activity, as well as the approaches used to generate this body of knowledge which combined multiple characteristics that are specially resistant to molecular and mechanistic characterizations, thus complicating the use of this enzyme as a potential target for antihistaminic treatments.

3.2 A Brief Presentation of the Involved Elements and Organisms

Histamine biosynthesis takes places by α-decarboxylation of the L-amino acid histidine:

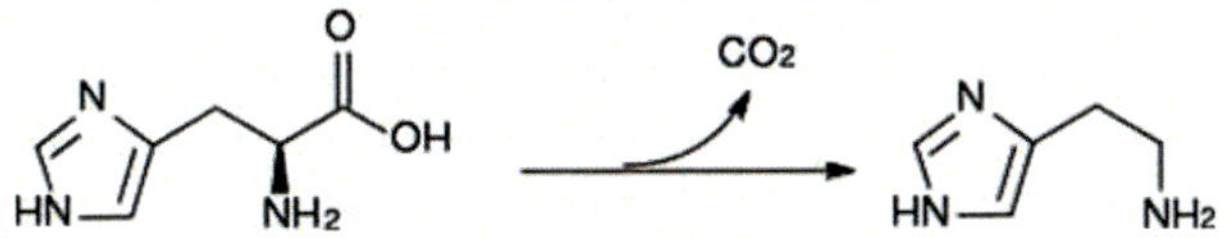

In general, biocatalysis of this reaction proceeds by a covalent mechanism. It involves that a carbonyl group ($R_1R_2C{=}O$) that belong to the reaction cofactor is finally able to form a Schiff base ($R_1R_2C{=}N{-}R_3$) with the α-amino group of the substrate histidine ($H_2N{-}R_3$).

Histamine can be produced by both Gram-negative and Gram-positive bacteria, and in a reduced set of animal cell types. In all cases, the enzyme keeps the same nomenclature and EC number (EC 4.1.1.22). However, the structure and the properties of HDCs present in different organisms differ enormously and are sometimes completely different. In fact, the HDC of Gram positive bacteria has a different evolutionary origin. In Gram-negative bacteria and animals the enzyme requires pyridoxal-5-phosphate (PLP) as a cofactor (see its formula below, Fig. 3.1).

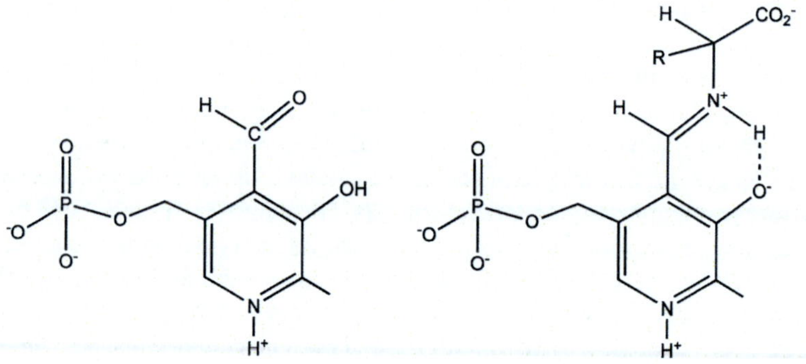

Fig. 3.1 Structures of pyridoxal-5′-phosphate in both its aldehide (*left*) and aldimine (*right*) forms

PLP also seems to be required for the activation of the HDC of Gram-positive bacteria, studied on *Lactobacillus casei* 30a, but after purification, the enzyme does not contain covalently bound PLP. Alternatively, a pyruvoyl (Pyr) residue is located in the catalytic site of *L. casei* 30a (Gallagher et al. 1989).

Most of the molecular and enzymatic features of the Gram-positive bacteria HDC prototype were characterized 20 years ago. This information, together with the microbiological and biotechnological interest shown on this enzyme, has been reviewed recently by different groups. On the contrary, many questions still remain to be solved about the molecular properties and pharmacological usefulness of the PLP-dependent enzymes. A lot of new information, especially concerning the mammalian enzyme, has been collected during the last 20 years especially on the mammalian enzyme.

We dedicate a section to highlight the most relevant features of the Pyr-dependent HDC and the following sections will summarize the advances, as well as the pending questions, on the PLP-dependent HDCs.

This strategy will allow us to show the weak points still required to achieve a full characterization of these enzymes, and how this is being achieved through experimental and in silico approaches.

3.3 Major Structural and Catalytic Properties of Gram-Positive Bacteria HDC

The active enzyme described for *L. casei* 30a comprises twelve polypeptides. Six of these polypeptides (β chains) correspond to the first 81 residues of the inactive primary translation product, whereas the other six subunits (α chains) correspond to the respective carboxy-termini. The self-cleavage of the primary translation product between residues Ser81 and Ser82 followed by the deamination of the newly formed amino-terminal residue gives rise to the pyruvoyl residue necessary for catalysis (the C=O donor). Thus, both types of mature monomers are generated: α (1–81) and β (from Pyruvoyl-moiety82 to the carboxy-terminus) (Gallagher et al. 1993). For clarity, the quaternary structure of the D53,54N mutant of the enzyme is shown in Fig. 3.2, panel A (PDB code: 1IBW). It corresponds to a cup-shaped trimer of αβ subunits (Worley et al. 2002). In the panel B of the same figure, a representation of the active site of this enzyme is detailed, and some of the residues relevant for the catalytic activity are depicted (Gallagher et al. 1989, 1993), as well as both the pyruvoyl residue and the substrate analogue histidine methyl esther (HME). The most relevant molecular and kinetic characteristics of the enzyme are listed in Table 3.1. Its mechanism of action was proposed 20 years ago by van Poelje and Snell (van Poelje and Snell 1990). The enzyme exhibits a hyperbolic behaviour at acidic pH (around 4.8); however, it exhibits a marked sigmoidal behaviour at alkaline pH, which leads to a highly reduced histamine biosynthesis at physiological L-histidine concentrations (Pishko and Robertus 1993). The secondary structure of its active site is extremely sensible to pH alterations, as studied by Schelp et al. (2001). This regulatory mechanism seems to be related to the fact that histamine

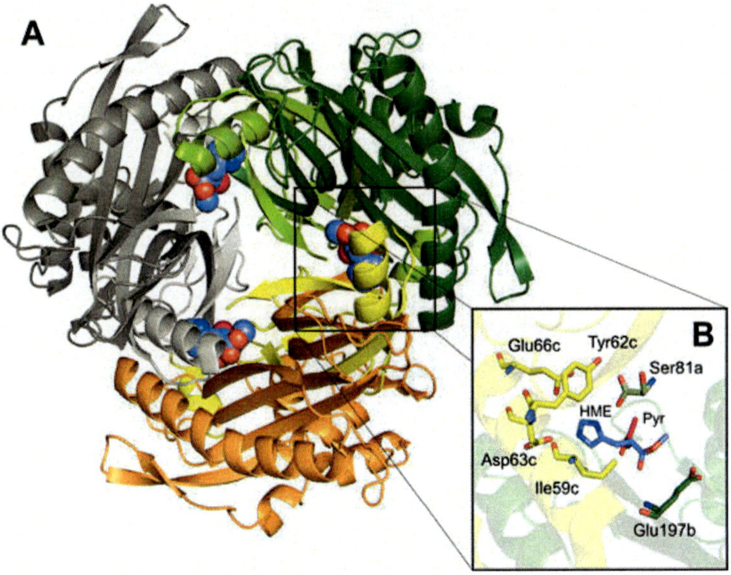

Fig. 3.2 Structure of the Pyr-dependent HDC from *Lactobacillus casei* 30a. (D53,54N mutant, PDB code: 1IBW). (**a**) A view of the quaternary structure of a trimer of αβ subunits. The substrate analog HME and the cofactor are depicted as spheres. The three αβ subunits are depicted in *orange*, *green* and *gray*, and a different gradient of each colour has been used to differ between α and β subunits. (**b**) Detailed view of one of the active sites, in which the most important residues interacting with the external aldimine mentioned in the text are depicted as sticks. The residues are depicted following the colour schema used in the quaternary structure: Ser81a and Glu197b correspond to α and β chain of the green subunit, whereas Ile59, Tyr62, Asp63 and Glu66 belong to the α chain of *yellow*/*orange* subunit. Colors available in the online version of the book

Table 3.1 Relevant molecular and kinetic characteristics of representative histidine decarboxylase enzymes

Enzyme information	*Lactobacillus casei*	*Morganella morganii*	Rat	Human
Precursor MW (kDa)[1]	34	43	74	74[3,m]
Mr of mature enzyme subunit(s) (kDa)	9 (α) + 28 (β)[a]	43[d]	53[(f)]	54[3,m]
Quaternary structure	(αβ)6	α4	α2	α2
Cofactor	Serderived Pyruvoyl-moiety	PLP	PLP	PLP
pI	4.2[b]	3.9[e]	5.1[d]	–
$K_m/S_{0,5}$ (L-histidine) (mM)	0.4–22[4,b,c]	1.1–1.3[b,e]	0.078–0.520[g,h,i,j]	0.27[n]
k_{cat}[2](s^{-1})	296[b]	209–430[5,b,c]	0.077[l]	–

[a]Gallagher et al. (1993); [b]Tanase et al. (1985); [c]Pishko and Robertus (1993); [d]Snell and Guirard (1986); [e]Guirard and Snell (1987); [f]Rodríguez-Caso et al. (2003a); [g]Savany and Cronenberger (1982); [h]Toledo et al. (1988); [i]Chudomelka et al. (1990); [j]Tran and Snyder (1981); [l]Olmo et al. (2002); [m]Yatsunami et al. (1995); [n]Mamune-Sato et al. (1990)
[1]Deduced molecular weight (MW) retrieved from Uniprot (www.uniprot.org)
[2]Calculated from data contained in the mentioned references
[3]Yatsunami et al. (1995) observed similar activities from both the primary translation product and the 53 kDa
[4]Pishko and Robertus (1993) observed an allosteric behaviour for this enzyme; affinity changes by 1–2 orders of magnitude depending on the pH
[5]The higher value was obtained in the presence of bovine serum as a stabilizer of HDC enzyme

is necessary to counteract the acids produced by the bacteria during fermentation and, consequently, it is proposed to be important for keeping an optimum bacterial growth rate (Fernández and Zúñiga 2006).

Homologous enzymes have also been reported in other Gram-positive bacteria. Apart from other *Lactobacillus sp.*, pyruvoyl-dependent HDCs have been detected in *Clostridium perfringens, Micrococcus sp., Oenocococcus oeni, Staphylococcus capitis*, and *Tetragenococcus muriaticus*. A very complete review of the structure, function, expression, metabolic context, regulation and roles of these enzymes in Gram-positive bacteria, has recently been published by Landete et al. (2008).

3.4 General Concepts on PLP-Dependent Histidine Decarboxylases

The catalytic mechanisms of PLP-dependent enzymes, including PLP-dependent α-amino acid decarboxylases, have been extensively studied since the 1950s by Metzler's and Christen's groups, among others (Hayashi 1995, John 1995, Kallen et al. 1985, Metzler et al. 1954).

As mentioned before for all HDCs, PLP-catalysis follows a covalent mechanism involving the formation of a Schiff base between the corbonyl group of pyridoxal and an amino group. In this case, this amino group belongs alternatively to either the enzyme or the substrate. Two different chemical forms can be therefore distinguished for the cofactor (see Fig. 3.1): the pyridoxal form (as its free form, panel A) and the aldimine form (panel B), when linked to the amino group of the enzyme (internal aldimine) or to the amino group of the amino acid substrate (external aldimine).

The first step in the catalytic mechanism of PLP-dependent enzymes is the interconversion between both aldimine species. PLP is bound to an amino group of a cationic residue (usually the ε amino group of a lysine residue) forming a Schiff base known as the internal aldimine. As the substrate (histidine in our case) enters in the catalytic site, its α-amino group acts as a nucleophilic group towards the Schiff base leading to the external aldimine. This transaldimination reaction can occur through two different mechanisms, the currently accepted one involves the formation of a diamine intermediate (Salvá et al. 2002). Once the external aldimine has been formed, it generates a carbanionic intermediate, named the quinoinoid intermediate due to its quinone-like structure (Fig. 3.3). It was proposed that the extended π system of the pyridine ring acts as an electron sink for carbanion stabilization (Eliot and Kirsch 2004, Hayashi 1995, John 1995). However, other authors also claim for an important role for the imine group (Bach et al. 1999, Toney 2001). Our recent study on the reaction mechanisms of HDC suggests that while the PLP acts as an electron sink, which is the role usually assumed for this cofactor, this effect is substantially larger in aqueous solution than in the enzyme (Moya-García et al. 2008). Other chemical characteristics must also contribute to the stabilization of the quinoinoid intermediate, such as the presence of the hydroxyl moiety bound to the ring (French et al. 1965) and the presence of a protonated nitrogen as part of the aromatic heterocycle (Toney 2005). The pyridoxal hydroxyl moiety allows the existence of tautomeric forms (enolimine and ketoenamine forms) that will be discussed later.

The quinoinoid intermediate can proceed via different types of reactions depending on the bond around the Cα atom that is affected, thus determining the function of the different PLP-dependent enzymes: racemases, amino transferases, α and

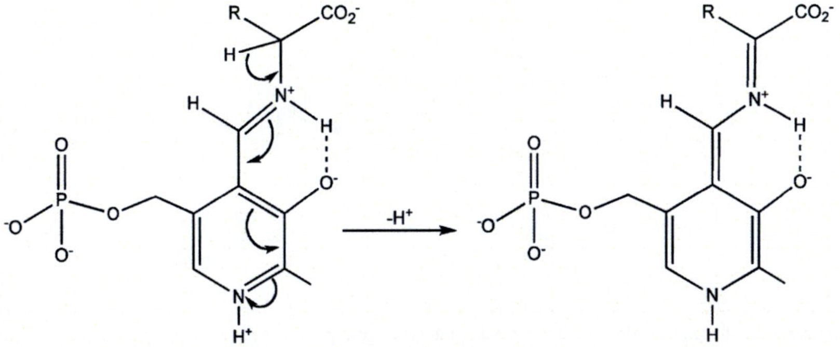

Fig. 3.3 Deprotonation reaction leading to the formation of the quinonoid intermediate during PLP-dependent catalysis

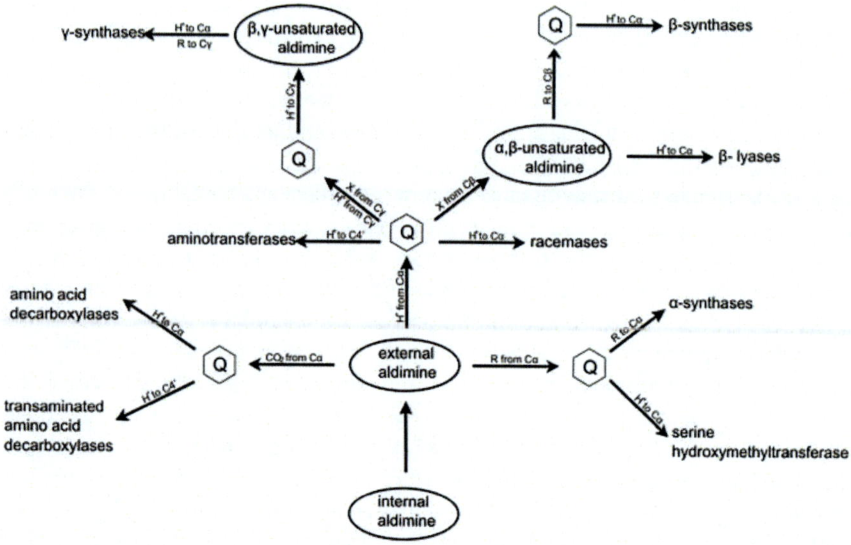

Fig. 3.4 Diversity of the reactions catalysed by PLP-dependent enzymes. Q represents the quinonoid intermediate. C4′ is the carbonyl carbon of PLP. Adapted from Schneider et al. (2000)

β-decarboxylases, synthases, transferases, and lyases (Fig. 3.4, Toney 2005), leading to the so-called Dunathan hypothesis. The Dunathan hypothesis proposes that the Cα bond with the greatest probability of being broken is the one perpendicular (with the highest HOMO-LUMO overlapping) to the plane formed by the π system comprising both the imine group and the pyridine ring. Figure 3.5 illustrates this hypothesis showing the position of the H^+ and carboxyl groups that are removed during the deprotonation and decarboxylation steps. Nevertheless, it has

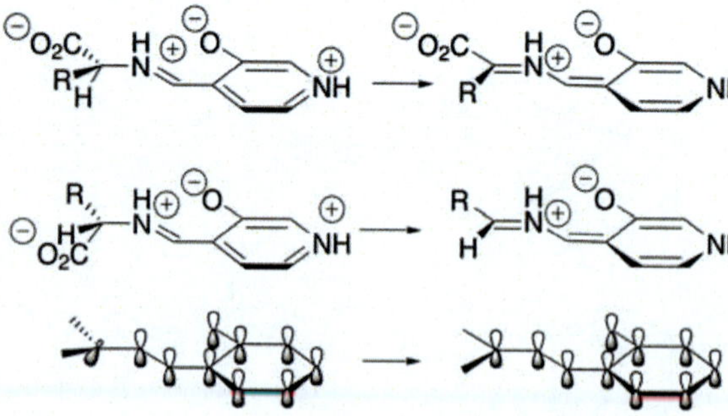

Fig. 3.5 Dunathan's stereoelectronic hypothesis. The substrate binds PLP, so the bond made around the Cα that is going to be broken is aligned with the orbital π of the cofactor (*lower schema*) Through managing the orientation of the substrate, the enzyme can distinguish between deprotonation (*upper schema*) and decarboxylation (*central schema*). Adapted from Eliot and Kirsch (2004)

been confirmed that the enzyme conformation also plays an essential role in defining the final reaction since it drives both the cofactor and the substrate binding site conformations.

Under this assumption, knowledge of the structures of the PLP-dependent HDC becomes essential to fully explain its enzymatic behaviour. Pioneering structural studies on PLP-dependent histidine decarboxylases (Christen and Mehta 2001, Metzler et al. 1954) demonstrated that both the Gram-negative bacteria enzyme and the mammalian enzymes are evolutionary related to other PLP-dependent enzymes. Mehta and Christen (2000) carried out an exhaustive study on the evolution of these enzymes based on more than 30 structures and 700 sequences. The number of different structures currently approaches 250 (Di Giovine 2004). Four independent folding families of paralogous enzymes are currently distinguished:

- Family α: the most numerous (>50) and diverse family from a functional point of view. The enzymes comprising this family diverged from the first ancestral PLP-dependent protein. Aspartate amino transferase is the prototype of this group. PLP-dependent histidine decarboxylases are included in this family.
- Family β: this is a reduced and homogenous family where all the members have a lyase activity. The prototype is tryptophane β synthase.
- D-alanine amino transferase family: this family is interesting for explaining the evolution of the specificity by enantiomers.
- Alanine racemase family: composed of the prototype and other decarboxylases such as the eukaryotic ornithine decarboxylase. Formerly considered as group IV (Grishin et al. 1995).

From this current knowledge we can conclude that the formation of an active PLP-protein complex has occurred several times in nature leading to different lineages of PLP-dependent enzymes. Thus, the functional specialization should have been obtained by the divergent evolution of the protoenzymes.

The presence of multiple evolutionary origins for the PLP-dependent enzymes goes against the mechanistic uniformity detected among them, suggesting that the mechanism is mainly conditioned by the chemical properties of the cofactor, while the type of reaction and substrate specificity must be mainly due to the protein environment.

Nevertheless, some common features among the different families lead us to think about the occurrence of convergent evolution, including the structural similarities in the PLP-binding domain and the existence of PEST regions in the members of independent lineages (Eliot and Kirsch 2004, Schneider et al. 2000, Viguera et al. 1994).

3.5 Phylogenetic Analysis of PLP-Dependent Decarboxylases

At this point, it seems interesting to focus our attention on the positions of both bacterial and mammalian PLP-dependent HDC relative to other PLP-dependent α-amino acid decarboxylases. Taking into account the current difficulties for structural characterization of several PLP-dependent decarboxylases by means of experimental approaches, in silico technologies can provide an alternative approach to obtain a reliable structure (Baker and Sali 2001).

As mentioned above, most α-amino acid decarboxylases (DCs) belong to the folding family α (with an exception mentioned below). However, according to the degree of homology of their sequences, four different groups of PLP-dependent decarboxylases can be distinguished (Mehta and Christen 2000, Sandmeier et al. 1994):

- Group I (DCI): includes only glycine decarboxylase (EC 1.4.4.2)
- Group II (DCII): it includes most of the α-amino acid decarboxylases. In addition to the PLP-dependent histidine decarboxylases, it also includes aromatic α-amino acid/dopa decarboxylase (DDC, EC 4.1.1.28), glutamate decarboxylase (GAD, EC 4.1.1.15) and tyrosine decarboxylase (EC 4.1.1.25).
- Group III (DCIII): includes the prokaryotic cationic amino acid decarboxylases (ornithine, lysine and arginine decarboxylases).
- Group IV (DCIV) includes the eukaryotic cationic amino acid decarboxylases and it belongs to the folding family of alanine racemase, as indicated before.

The pioneering homology analysis on DCIIs, based on 54 available sequences, was carried out by Sandmeier et al. (2004) 15 years ago. Figure 3.6 shows the results of a more recent phylogenetic analysis carried out in our laboratory, using 92 complete sequences (Moya-García 2007). In general, results are coherent with the conclusions achieved by Sandmeier et al. (1994), with some novelties escaping the scope of the present chapter.

Curiously, the mammalian histidine decarboxylase seems to be more closely related to the mammalian aromatic L-amino acid decarboxylase – that is also able to accept histidine as a substrate but with a more reduced efficiency (Lovenberg et al. 1962) – than to the orthologous enzyme of Gram-negative bacteria (Table 3.1). Figure 3.7 shows the alignments of the primary sequences of the *Morganella morganii* HDC, rat HDC and rat DDC. This information will be useful later for describing further structure-function relationship studies.

3.6 Major Structural and Catalytic Properties of the HDC of Gram-Negative Bacteria

PLP-dependent HDC activities have been detected, cloned and characterized in several Gram-negative bacteria: *Enterobacter aerogenes, Erwinia sp., Listonella angillarum, Morganella morganii, Photobacterium phosphoreum, Proteus vulgaris, Pseudomonas fluorescens, and Raoultella ornytolytica and planticola.*

In Table 3.1 the most relevant molecular and kinetic properties of the *M. morganii* HDC are shown. Unfortunately, there is no structural information for any PLP-dependent HDC, in spite of several attempts made by different groups

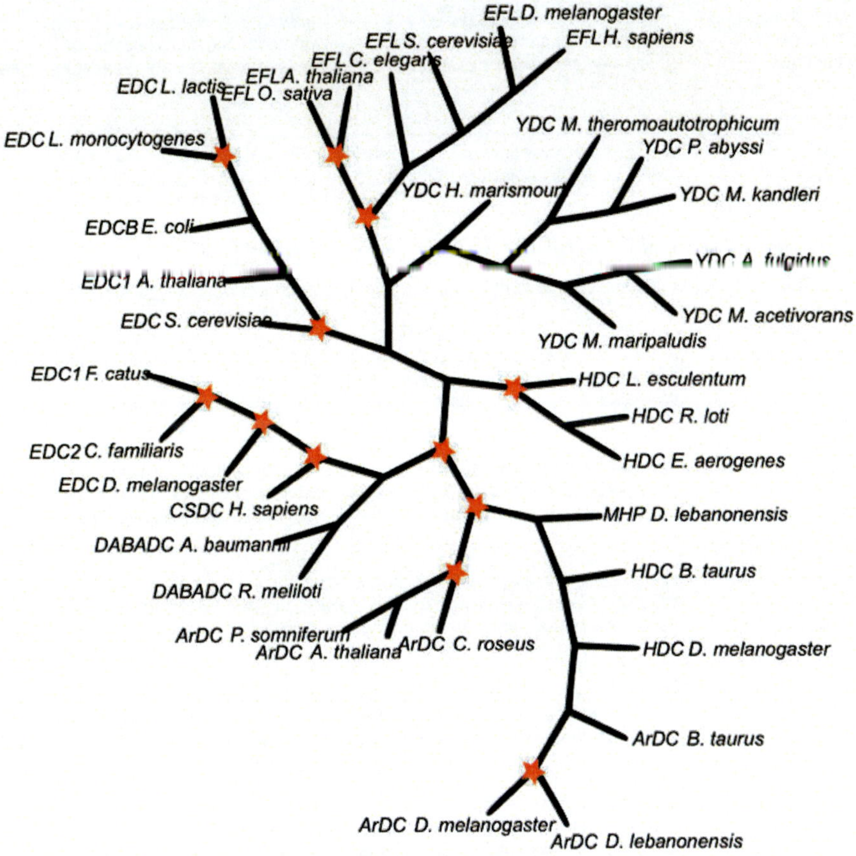

Fig. 3.6 Phylogenetic tree of the PLP-dependent decarboxylases, calculated by the Neighbor-joining method. The stars indicate bootstrap values greater than 95%. Abbreviations used in this figure: ArDC, aromatic L-amino acid decarboxylase; CSDC, cysteine sulfinic acid decarboxylase; DABADC, L-2,4-diaminobutyrate decarboxylase; EDC, glutamate decarboxylase, EFL, sphingosine-1-phophate lyase; HDC, histidine decarboxylase; MHP, α-methyldopa hypersensitive protein; YDC, tyrosine decarboxylase

to reach this goal. Nevertheless, there have been several attempts to model a prototype structure of a bacterial PLP-dependent HDC and to simulate the reaction mechanism (Moya-García et al. 2006, Tahanejad and Naderi-Manesh 2000, Tahanejad et al. 2000), although none of them provide a clear picture of the quaternary structure of the enzyme. The experimental data suggest that these enzymes can conform either homodimers or homotetramers (Snell and Guirard 1986, Tanase et al. 1985). These enzymes present the typical PLP-binding domain composed of several (6–7) β-sheets containing a lysine residue (Lys232 in *M. morganii*, P05034) required to covalently bind the cofactor PLP. However, the conformation of the substrate-binding site still remains unknown (Moya-García et al. 2006).

```
HDC M.morganii  MTLSI---N----DQNKLDAFWAY-----------CVKNQYFNIGYPESAD-------FD   35
HDC Rat         MMEPSEYHEYQARGKEMVDYICQYLSTVRERQVTPNVKPGYLRAQIPSSAPEEPDSWDSI   60
DDC Rat         MDSR----EFRRRGKEMVDYIADYLDGIEGRPVYPDVEPGYLRALIPTTAPQEPETYEDI   56

HDC M.morganii  YTN------------------------------LERFLRFSINNCG-DWGEYCNYLLNSF   64
HDC Rat         FGDIEQIIMPGVVHWQSPHMHAYYPALTSWPSLLGDMLADAINCLGFTWASS----PACT  116
DDC Rat         IRDIEKIIMPGVTHWHSPYFFAYFPTASSYPAMLADMLCGAIGCIGFSWAAS----PACT  112

HDC M.morganii  DFEKEVMEYFADLFKIPFE--------QSWGYVTNGGTEGNMFGCYLGRE----------  106
HDC Rat         ELEMNIMDWLAKMLGLPDFFLHHHPSSQGGGVLQRTVSESTLIALLAARKNKILEMKAHE  176
DDC Rat         ELETVMMDWLGKMLELPEAFLAG-RAGEGGGVIQGSASEATLVALLAARTKMIRQLQAAS  171

HDC M.morganii  -------IFPDGTLYYSKDTHYSVAKIVKLLRIKSQVVESQPNGEIDYDDLMKKIADDKE  159
HDC Rat         PNADESSLNARLVAYASDQAHSSVEKAGLISLVKIKFLPVDDNFSLRGEALQKAIEEDKQ  236
DDC Rat         PELTQAALMEKLVAYTSDQAHSSVERAGLIGGVKIKAIPSDGNYSMRAAALREALERDKA  231

HDC M.morganii  AHPI---IFANIGTTVRGAIDDIAEIQKRLKAAGIKREDYYLHADAALSGMILPFVDDAQ  216
HDC Rat         QGLVPVFVCATLGTTGVCAFDKLSELGPI-----CAREGLWLHVDAAYAGTAFLRPELRG  291
DDC Rat         AGLIPFFVVVTLGTTSCCSFDNLLEVGPI-----CNQEGVWLHIDAAYAGSAFICPEFRY  286

HDC M.morganii  PFTFADGIDSIGVSGHKMIGSPIPCGIVVAKK-ENV-DRISVEIDYIS-AH--DKTITGS  271
HDC Rat         FLKGIEYADSFTFNPSKWMMVHFDCTGFWVKDKYKLQQTFSVNPIYLRH--ANSGVATDF  349
DDC Rat         LLNGVEFADSFNFNPHKWLLVNFDCSAMWVKKRTDLTEAFNMDPVYLRHSHQDSGLITDY  346

HDC M.morganii  RNGHTP-------LMLWEAIRSHSTEEWKRRITRSLDMAQYAVDRMQKA-----------  313
HDC Rat         MHWQIPLSRRFRSIKLWFVIRSFGVKNLQAHVRHGTDMAKYFESLVRSDPVFEIPAERHL  409
DDC Rat         RHWQIPLGRRFRSLKMWFVFRMYGVKGLQAYIRKHVKLSHEFESLVRQDPRFEICTEVIL  406

HDC M.morganii  GINAWRNKNSITVVFPCPSERVWREHCLATSGDVAHLITTAHHLDTVQIDKLI-------  366
HDC Rat         GLVVFRLKGPN-----CLTESVLKE--IAKTGQVFLIPATIQ-------DKLIIRFTVTS  455
DDC Rat         GLVCFRLKGSN-----QLNETLLQR--INSAKKIHLVPCRLR-------DKFVLRFAVCS  452

HDC M.morganii  -----DDVIADFNL--------------------HAA  378
HDC Rat         QFTTKDDILRDWNLIREAANLVLSQHCTSQPSPRAKN  492
DDC Rat         RTVESAHVQLAWEHIRDLASSVLRA--------AEKE  481
```

Fig. 3.7 Multiple alignment of the amino acid full sequences of *Morganella morganii*, rat DDC, and the fragment 1–492 of rat HDC (full rat HDC sequence comprises 656 amino acids) calculated with the T-Coffee server (Notredame et al. 2000). The key residues in rat HDC and its counterparts in the other species are highlighted. Fully conserved H197, D276 and K308 (rat HDC numbering), which are meant to establish key interactions with the PLP, are highlighted in a green box. K202 and N305, which are not conserved in the three enzymes, are included in light blue boxes. Both residues are described as interacting with the phosphate group of PLP according to Moya-García et al. (2008). Finally, the region comprising the flexible loop in rat HDC is included in a light orange box. Y337, a key residue located in the flexible loop fragment and shown to interact with the substrate once it is in the active site, stabilizing the enzyme against proteases degradation is also highlighted in the three sequences, included in a *deep orange box*. Colors available in the online version of the book

The spectroscopical properties of PLP derivatives and how they change depending on their electronic distributions help to provide information on the cofactor position, its environment and the kinetic of the reaction. Thus, the UV absorption properties of these PLP-derivatives, as well as the capacity for fluorescence emission, have been very useful to get important mechanistic information for several PLP-dependent enzymes, including HDC (Boeker and Snell 1972, Chu and Metzler 1994, Hayashi et al. 1986, 1993, 1999, Moore et al. 1996, Olmo et al. 2002). As mentioned before, aldimine can be present in two different tautomeric forms, ketoenamine or enolimine forms, due to the presence of the hydroxyl group bound to the pyridine ring. Ketoenamine absorbs UV light with a maximum around 335 nm and enolimine absorbs around 420 nm. The tautomeric equilibrium can be displaced by the polarity of the environment into the catalytic site. In the bacterial PLP-dependent HDC, the internal aldimine is stabilized mainly as the ketoenamine tautomer (A_{335}/A_{420} ratio around 0.5), which suggest that a hydrophilic environment able to stabilise the tautomer's negative charge (Hayashi et al. 1986, 1990). The internal aldimine of the bacterial enzyme also seems to be very likely to form substituted aldimines with thiols or other nucleophilic reagents suggesting some exposure of the Schiff base outside of the enzyme environment (Tanase et al. 1985).

Some valuable experimentally driven hypotheses on its structure-function relationship are described from the work of Vaaler and Snell (1989) carried out on direct mutants of the enzyme. This work was essential to elucidate that the fragment of residues 229–232 in *M. morganii* must be a part of the catalytic site. This information has been extremely useful to locate key residues and their counterparts in other homologous enzymes (see, for instance, the alignment in Fig. 3.7).

However, the lack of a validated 3D structure is preventing further advances in both the knowledge and the control of this bacterial enzyme that produces major biomedical problems, for instance, the scombroid fish poisoning syndrome caused by several *M. morganii* strains that express HDC, growing on spoiled fish products (Morrow et al. 1991). As in the case of Gram-positive bacteria, the recent review of Landete et al. (2008) provides further information on the genetics, metabolic context and physiopatological role of this enzyme, as well as method to detect its presence in spoiled and/or fermented foods.

3.7 Major Structural and Catalytic Properties of Eukaryotic (Mammalian) HDC

PLP-dependent HDCs have been detected even in protist organisms as *Tetrahymena* (Hegyesi et al. 1998), and they show similar features to those of the animal enzymes. Histidine decarboxylase-like genes have been also detected in fungi and plant genomes and/or cDNA libraries (Erasmus et al. 2003, Picton et al. 1993, Wang et al. 2000). However, functional characterization of the *Arabidopsis* gene revealed that the HDC-like sequence was not able to decarboxylate histidine, but rather serine, producing ethanolamine, which is dedicated to synthesize glycinebetaine and other plant stress-related products (McNeil et al. 2001, Rontein et al. 2001). In any case, scarce or no information exists on the enzymic characteristics of the PLP-dependent histidine decarboxylases of eukaryotic organisms, apart from a few species of mammals, including mice, rats and humans.

In mammals, histidine decarboxylase is expressed in a reduced set of cell types, for example, mast cells and other immune cells, enterochromaffin-like cells and some neurones, and in most cases, these cells are located among other non-histamine producing cell types. Hence, this fact makes it very difficult to purify and characterize the native enzyme. Hundreds of rat fetal livers were necessary to obtain a few hundreds of micrograms of the enzyme (Taguchi et al. 1984). Afterwards, other authors tried the purification from other sources with similar yield problems (Martin and Bishop 1986, Ohmori et al. 1990). In addition, the purified enzyme behaved in an extremely unstable way. Its tendency to be cleaved by proteases unresponsive to usual protease inhibitor cocktails and to make aggregates (with its simultaneous inactivation) has made the characterization of the native enzyme impossible so far.

In 1990, Joseph et al. described the first sequence identified as mammalian histidine decarboxylase, corresponding to the rat enzyme. This allowed the production of purified recombinant versions of the enzyme (Engel et al. 1996, Yamamoto et al. 1990, 1993). However, the primary translation product is longer (74 kDa) than the previously reported monomers from natural sources (53–55 kDa, see Table 3.1). Additionally, most of the published data suggest that the full primary translation product has very low or no HDC activity at all.

Results obtained with both native enzyme and different carboxy terminus-deleted mutants revealed that the fully active mammalian HDC must be a homodimer, whose monomers are carboxy-truncated around the residues 510–520. Nevertheless, other longer versions having 55–70 kDa could also be partially active (Fleming et al. 2004a), as it has also been described in previous studies using ECLC samples (Dartsch et al. 1998, 1999). Neither the structure nor the physiological role of the carboxy-terminal portion (apart from the inhibition of the HDC activity) has been fully clarified, yet. Its sequence and predicted secondary structure do not indicate the existence of any obvious homologous domain with a specific function, although its involvement in the monomer's sorting to the endoplasmic reticulum has been proposed (Furuta et al. 2006, Suzuki et al. 1998). In any case, similar to the behaviour of the full enzyme in vitro and in vivo, the carboxy-terminal region seems to be an extremely unstable polypeptide and the target of many different proteases (Furuta et al. 2007, Olmo et al. 2000, Rodríguez-Agudo et al. 2000, Tanaka et al. 1995).

This is an important feature in mammalian HDC enzymology, since the maximum velocity (V_{max}), defined as a function of the catalytic constant (k_{cat}) and the actual enzyme concentration ([E]), is therefore dependent of both the constant of synthesis (K_s) and the constant of degradation (K_d). Taking into account the extremely low value of mammalian HDC k_{cat} (Table 3.1) and its short half-life value (1–2 h in vivo) (Zhao et al. 2003), it is deduced that histamine synthesis must be an extremely slow process in vivo and must be regulated by many protein-protein interactions controlling the processing, sorting and degradation. However, it is noteworthy that, as far as we know, there are no data concerning protein-protein interaction reported for the mammalian HDC apart from its contact with several proteases. Further important information about the interactions made by this enzyme along with its processing, sorting and life-span remains unknown, yet.

Mammalian HDC polypeptides have been described as substrate for ubiquitin-dependent proteasomal degradation, trypsin-like activities, calpains and caspases, having several motifs and hot-spots for degradation, including PEST regions (Olmo et al. 1999, Viguera et al. 1994), and the cationic residues present in a flexible loop, which are also involved in substrate binding (Fleming et al. 2004b). The susceptibility of this loop to proteolysis was helpful in revealing the participation of its dynamics in the substrate binding event (the Michaelis complex formation), which must be linked to a global conformational change of the protein, which is essential for the catalytic process (Rodríguez-Caso et al. 2003a). The dynamic behaviour of this flexible loop has been recently studied in our group (Pino-Ángeles et al. 2009). Molecular dynamics simulations and essential dynamics analysis have been used in order to unveil whether the flexible loop undergoes a conformational change, as has been suggested previously in the literature (Ishii et al. 1998, Matsuda et al. 2004) as a result of the substrate binding event. Our results are in good agreement with the stated hypothesis derived from experimental data that a movement of the flexible loop towards the active site entrance takes place during the substrate binding process. This movement leads to the protection of the cleavage site located in the loop, hence providing increased enzyme stability against proteases due to substrate binding.

Regarding the rest of the catalysed reaction, the availability of recombinant versions of the enzyme, combined with biophysical and biocomputational approaches, made it possible to unveil the complete reaction mechanism. With the information retrieved by combining UV/visible, fluorescence spectroscopy and circular dichroism techniques, the reaction mechanism can be explained as follows (see Fig. 3.8): The PLP-enzyme internal aldimine is mainly in an enolimine tautomeric form, suggesting an apolar environment around the coenzyme. Michaelis complex formation leads to a polarised, ketoenamine form of the Schiff base. After transaldimination, the coenzyme-substrate Schiff base exists mainly as an unprotonated aldimine, as it has been previously observed for DDC. The cofactor is more resilient to the formation of substituted inactivating derivatives, formed by reacting with thiols or other nucleophilic molecules, than the prokaryotic homologous enzymes and other L-amino acid decarboxylases, suggesting a closer conformation of the catalytic pocket (Olmo et al. 2002).

In agreement with the evolutionary studies of the DCII group, these mechanistic results revealed that the mammalian HDC is more similar to DDC than to its bacterial counterpart, but also less efficient than both homologous DCs. In fact, its k_{cat} is several orders of magnitude lower than both the bacterial PLP-dependent HDC (Table 3.1) and the mammalian DDC (Bertoldi and Borri-Voltattorni 2000). Therefore, structural differences must exist that explain the different substrate specificities among the HDCs and the DDCs and the extremely low catalytic efficiency of the mammalian HDC.

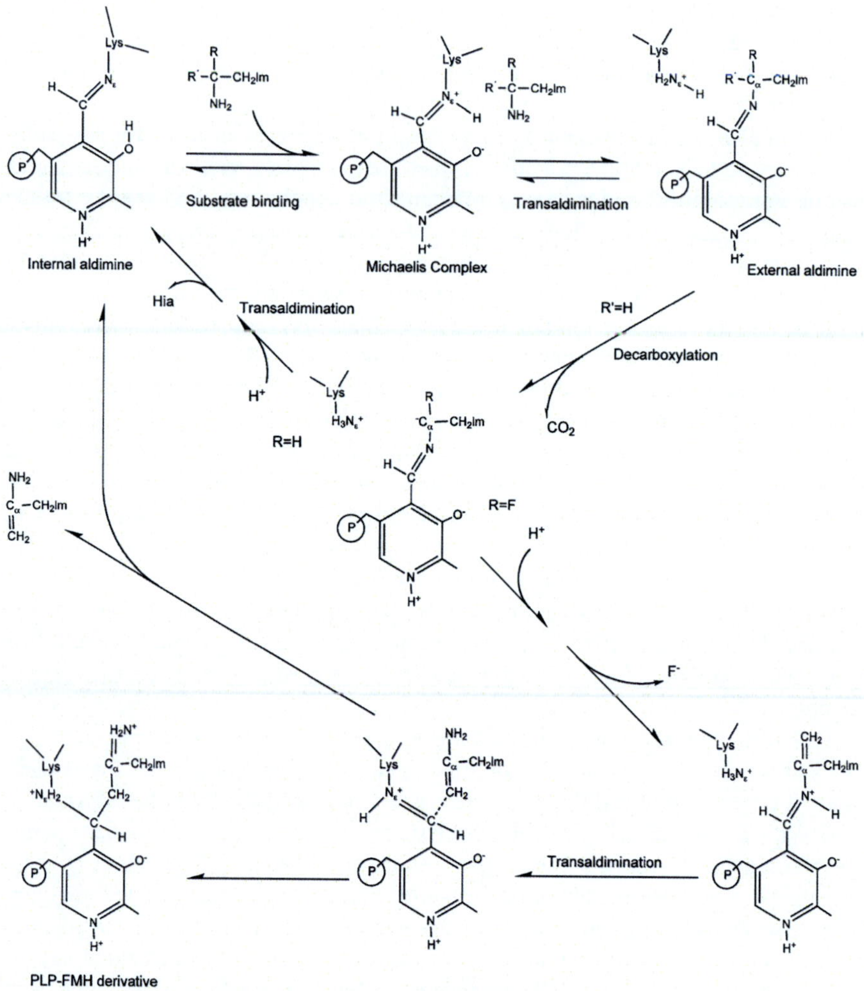

Fig. 3.8 HDC catalytic mechanims with the substrate histidine and the inhibitors α-fluoromethyl histidine and histidine methylester. R can be H (histidine and histidine methylester) or F (α-fluoromethyl histidine). R′ can be H (histidine) or OMe (histidine methylester)

Why then it is so important to know those differences? One of the most important handicaps to control animal histidine decarboxylases in vivo comes from the high degree of identity between the mammalian HDC and DDC and higher than 50% between the common fragments of the active core (residues 1–480). Both are dimeric enzymes with a very similar quaternary structure, a high degree of identity, as can be observed in Figs. 3.6 and 3.7. DDC produces different neurotransmitters, such as dopamine, serotonin and tryptamine, playing very important roles for animal physiology. Any intervention on mammalian HDC should be specific enough to distinguish between both homologous enzymes, as it should also do so with respect to enterobacterial HDC.

As in the case of the bacterial PLP-dependent HDC, all of these mechanistic data were an incomplete puzzle without a 3D structure on which to locate the catalysis-involved elements and the reaction itself. The availability of the first mammalian DDC structure obtained by X-ray diffraction (Burkhard et al. 2001) allowed us to generate the first 3D model of the rat HDC (Rodríguez-Caso et al. 2003a, Fig. 3.9a). The model was validated by more than 20 different direct mutants (Engel et al. 1996, Fleming et al. 2004b), and the first comprehensive review on the structure-function relationships of this enzyme was based on this model (Moya-García et al. 2005). The most relevant features of this emergent information obtained by the integration of biophysical, molecular and computational data were the following:

- The dimerization involves mainly the amino-terminal domain (the one containing a PEST motif for proteasomal degradation) and the PLP-binding domain.
- The catalytic site is located in the dimerisation surface between both dimers, involving the PLP-binding domain of one monomer (A), other residues involved in substrate binding from both monomers and a flexible loop (331–349) of the opposite monomer (B). Figure 3.9b shows a detailed picture of the catalytic site of mammalian HDCs.

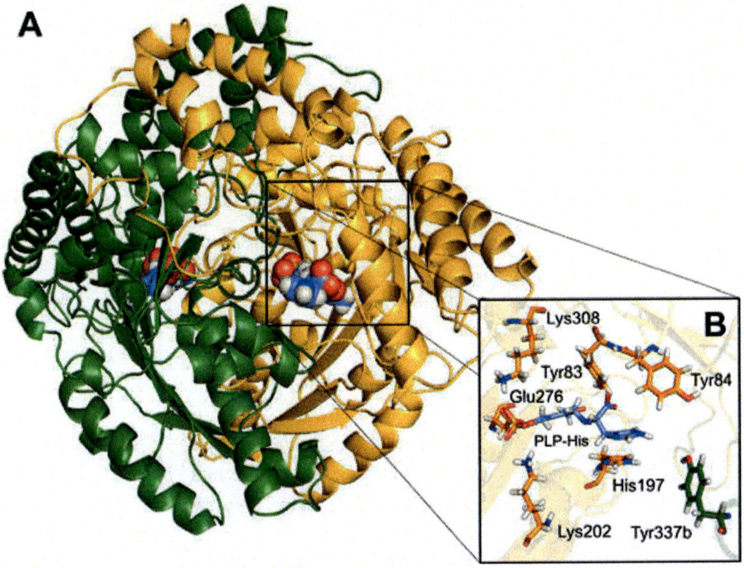

Fig. 3.9 Structure of rat HDC (fragment 5–480). (**a**) Quaternary structure of the rat HDC model in which both monomers are depicted in *green* and *orange* respectively. External aldimine atoms are coloured and shown as spheres. (**b**) Detailed view of one of the active sites in which the most important residues interacting with the cofactor-substrate adduct are depicted as sticks, maintaining the colour schema used for representing the quaternary structure. The residue Y337 is the only one represented that belongs to the green monomer, its label contains the suffix "b". The mammalian HDC structure has been generated by homology modelling, as mentioned in the text, so hydrogen atoms are present in the structure. Colors available in the online version of the book

– There are important differences between HDC and DDC, in particular concerning the active site conformation and some details of the quaternary structure, deserving deeper characterization as potential target for specific inhibition.

More recently, QM/MM simulations have allowed us to model the histidine decarboxylation step, providing accurate information about the position of the external aldimine in the catalytic site, as well as the role of the different residues and functional groups during the reaction (Moya-García et al. 2008).

3.8 PLP-HDC Inhibitors: What We Have, What We Would Like to Have

PLP-dependent HDC inhibition is an important target and has been sought for many years. Figure 3.10 shows the structures of the most potent inhibitors of the HDC activity described thus far for both bacterial and mammalian PLP-dependent HDCs. The mechanisms of action of the substrate analogs histidine methyl ester (HME) and α-fluoromethylhistidine (FMH), were studied mainly by spectroscopic approaches (Hayashi et al. 1986, Kubota et al. 1984, Olmo et al. 2002, Rodríguez-Caso et al. 2003a), and are depicted in Fig. 3.10. HME blocks the reaction before the decarboxylation step, forming an external aldimine cofactor-analogue, while FMH allows the decarboxylation reaction, acting as a suicide analog. Kinetic constants (Ki values

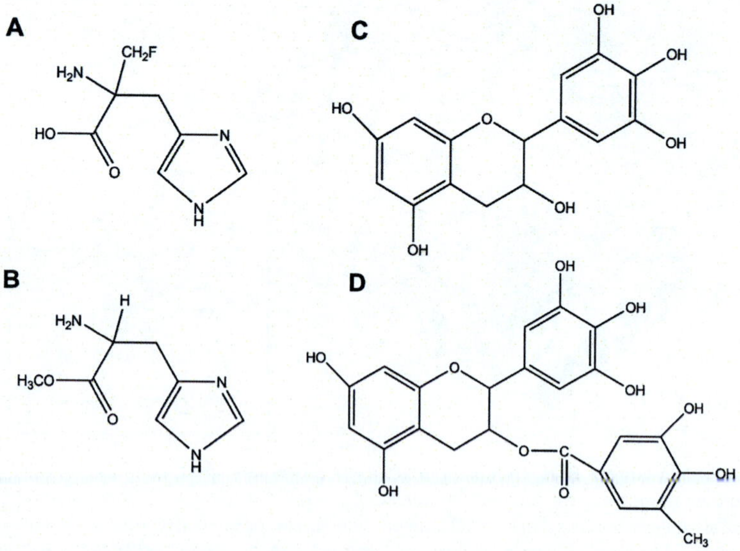

Fig. 3.10 Structures of the most efficient PLP-dependent HDC inhibitors known so far. **(a)** α-fluoromethyl histidine (FMH); **(b)** Histidine methyl ester (HME); **(c)** Epigallocatechin (EGC); **(d)** Epigallocatechin 3-gallate (EGCG)

between 0.1 and 10 μM) obtained with these inhibitors on different PLP-dependent HDC preparations are given in the following references: Chudomelka et al. (1990), Guirard and Snell (1987), Hayashi et al. (1986), Kubota et al. (1984), Yamakami et al. (2000). The epigallocatechines (EGCG/EGC) are also described as HDC direct inhibitors affecting the internal aldimine conformation (Rodríguez-Caso et al. 2003b), but theirs mechanism are still unknown. Nitta et al. (2007) estimated the Ki value of EGCG in 38 ± 8 μM for the human enzyme. None of these inhibitors are specific to the mammalian HDC. FMH and HME also inhibit the bacterial PLP-dependent HDC (Hayashi et al. 1986) and EGCG has also been described as a mammalian DDC inhibitor (Bertoldi et al. 2001, Melgarejo et al. 2009).

More recently, Wu et al. (2008) designed, synthesized and tested analogues of the external aldimine (for instance, pyridoxyl-histidine methyl ester) as inhibitors of the human enzyme. This work can be considered a simple example of a hypothesis-driven way to look for new drugs more efficiently.

In a recently published review, we suggest the usefulness of biocomputational techniques, including molecular modelling and the virtual screening of compound libraries, for identifying new potential inhibitors for the mammalian HDC activity (Moya-García et al. 2009). Virtual screening is currently a computational technique of great interest among the high throughput approaches as a starting point for drug discovery projects. The methodology requires the structure of the protein of interest and a chemical library of compounds, comprising a range from a few tens to millions of small molecules. After a detailed physicochemical characterization of the active site of the protein, in the first stage, every compound in the library is placed into the binding pocket and the energy of binding of the complex is calculated. Afterwards, the best scoring compounds according to these binding energy calculations are then refined by molecular dynamics simulations of the complex. The further refinement of these primary results is possible, enriching the chemical library with compounds structurally similar to the best scoring ones in the previous step. In the last step, a reduced set of potential inhibitors is subjected to experimental validation.

Many reviews on the topic have been also published within the last decade, in which both pros (e.g., its economical efficiency and low consumption of resources), and cons (e.g., the existence of false positives) are highlighted. This approach has been used extensively in recent years, achieving good results in different systems, for instance, in the search of new inhibitors of the HIV protease (Kitchen et al. 2004) and novel ligands for histamine receptor H4 (Kiss et al. 2008).

In our case, the generation, refinement and validation of the mammalian HDC model has set the basis for the identification of new specific inhibitors of its activity through virtual screening.

3.9 The Scope for Future Efforts

As shown in this chapter, the characterization of the enzymatic features of these proteins, specially the PLP-dependent ones, is now possible by using a combination of very different techniques of molecular biology, biophysics and biocomputation, conveying the necessity of multidisciplinar approaches for solving some biological problems completely. We hope that this approach will allow us to locate specific points for the selective intervention of these enzymes. However, the majority of the studies carried out to date have been performed on the isolated enzyme (avoiding other elements of the cell). In order to shed light on all of the questions about the mammalian HDC and the biological meaning of histamine biosynthesis, for instance, whether it is stored in granules or not, its regulatory role in growth, etc (Abrighach et al. 2009, Colucci et al. 2001, Dy and Schneider 2004), the integration of data related to its interaction with other elements in the cell (the membrane, proteases or other polypeptides) is still needed.

Acknowledgements This work was supported by Grant SAF2008-02522 (Ministerio de Ciencia e Innovación), funds to BIO-267 (Plan Andaluz de Investigación), and Grant from Fundación Ramón Areces. CIBERER is an initiative of the Instituto de Salud Carlos III. Thanks to Pedro L. Garrido-López for his help during the preparation of the illustrations.

References

Abrighach H, Fajardo I, Sánchez-Jiménez F et al (2009) Exploring polyamine regulation by nascent histamine in a human transfected cell model. Amino Acids 38:561–573

Bach RD, Canepa C, Glukhovtsev MN (1999) Influence of electrostatic effects on activation barriers in enzymatic reactions: pyridoxal 5′-phosphate-dependent decarboxylation of α-amino acids. J Am Chem Soc 121:6542–6555

Baker D, Sali A (2001) Protein structure prediction and structural genomics. Science 294:93–96

Bender DA (1985) Amino acid metabolism. Wiley, New York

Bertoldi M, Borri-Voltattorni C (2000) Reaction of dopa decarboxylase with L-aromatic amino acids under aerobic and anaerobic conditions. Biochem J 352:533–538

Bertoldi M, Gonsalvi M, Borri-Voltattorni C. (2001) Green tea polyphenols: novel irreversible inhibitors of dopa decarboxylase. Biochem Biophys Res Commun 284:90–93

Boeker EA, Snell EE (1972) Amino acid decarboxylases. The enzymes VI:217–253

Burkhard P, Dominici P, Vorri-Voltattorni C et al (2001) Structural insight into Parkinson's disease treatment from drug-inhibited DOPA decarboxylase. Nat Struct Biol 8:1847–1862

Christen P, Mehta PK (2001) From cofactor to enzymes. The molecular evolution of pyridoxal-5′-phosphate-dependent enzymes. Chem Rec 1:436–447

Chu W, Metzler DE (1994) Enzymatically active truncated cat brain glutamate decarboxylase: expression, purification and absorption spectrum. Arch Biochem Biophys 313:287–295

Chudomelka PJ, Ramaley RF, Murrin LC (1990) Histidine decarboxylase from rat and rabbit brain: partial purification and characterization. Neurochem Res 15:17–24

Colucci R, Fleming JV, Xavier R et al. (2001) L-histidine decarboxylase decreases its own transcription through downregulation of ERK activity. Am J Physiol Gastrointest Liver Physiol 281:1081–1091

Csaba G, Kovács P, Buzás E et al (2007a) Histidine decarboxylase (HDC) knock out mouse immune cells have altered expression of ACTH, triiodothyronine and endorphin. Inflamm Res 56:428–431

Csaba G, Kovács P, Buzás E et al (2007b) Serotonin content is elevated in the immune cells of histidine decarboxylase gene knock out (HDCKO) mice. Focus on mast cells. Inflamm Res 56:89–92

Dartsch C, Chen D, Persson L (1998) Multiple forms of rat stomach histidine decarboxylase may reflect posttranslational activation of the enzyme. Regul Pept 77:33–41

Dartsch C, Chen D, Hakanson R et al (1999) Histidine decarboxylase in rat stomach ECL cells: relationship between enzyme activity and different molecular forms. Regul Pept 81:41–48

Dere E, de Souza-Silva MA, Spieler RE et al (2004) Changes in motoric, exploratory and emotional behaviours and neuronal acetylcholine content in 5-HT turnover in histidine decarboxylase-KO mice. Eur J Neurosci 20:1051–1058

Di Giovine P (2004) PLPMDB: pyridoxal-5′-phosphate dependent enzymes mutants database. Bioinformatics 20:3652–3653

Dy M, Schneider E (2004) Histamine-cytokine connection in immunity and hematopoiesis. Cytokine Growth Factor Rev 5:393–410

Eliot A, Kirsch J (2004) Pyridoxal phosphate enzymes: mechanistic, structural and evolutionary considerations. Annu Rev Biochem 73:383–415

Engel N, Olmo MT, Coleman CS et al (1996) Experimental evidence for structure/function features in common between mammalian histidine decarboxylase and ornithine decarboxylase. Biochem J 320:365–368

Erasmus DJ, van der Merwe GK, van Vuuren HJ (2003) Genome-wide expression analysis: metabolic adaptation of *Saccharomyces cerevisiae* to high sugar stress. FEMS Yeast Res 3:375–399

Fernández M, Zúñiga M (2006) Amino-acid catabolic pathways of lactic acid bacteria. Crit Rev Microbiol 32:155–183

Fleming JV, Fajardo I, Langlois MR et al (2004a) The carboxyl-terminus of rat L-histidine decarboxylase (HDC) specifically inhibits enzymatic activity and disrupts PLP-dependent interactions with L-histidine substrate analogues. Biochem J 381:769–778

Fleming JV, Sánchez-Jiménez F, Moya-García AA et al (2004b) Mapping of catalytically important residues in the rat L-histidine decarboxylase enzyme using bioinformatic and site directed mutagenesis approaches. Biochem J 379:253–261

French TC, Auld DS, Bruice TC (1965) Catalytic reactions involving azomethines. V. Rates and equilibria of imine formation with 3-hydroxypyridine-4-aldehyde and amino acids. Biochemistry 4:77–84

Furuta K, Ichikawa A, Nakayama K et al (2006) Membrane orientation of the precursor 74-kDa of L-histidine decarboxylase. Inflamm Res 55:185–191

Furuta K, Nakayama K, Sugimoto Y et al (2007) Activation of histidine decarboxylase through post-translational cleavage by caspase-9 in a mouse mastocytoma P-815. J Biol Chem 282:13438–13446

Gallagher T, Snell EE, Hackert ML (1989) Pyruvoyl-dependent histidine decarboxylase. Active site structure and mechanistic analysis. J Biol Chem 264:12737–12743

Gallagher T, Rozwarski DA, Ernst SR et al (1993) Refined structure of the pyruvoyl-dependent histidine decarboxylase from *Lactobacillus* 30a. J Mol Biol 230:516–528

Grishin NV, Phillips MA, Goldsmith EJ (1995) Modelling of the spatial structure of eukaryotic ornithine decarboxylases. Protein Sci 4:1291–1304

Guirard BM and Snell EE (1987) Purification and properties of pyridoxal-5′-phosphate-dependent histidine decarboxylases from *Klebsiella planticola* and *Enterobacter aerogenes*. J Bacteriol 169:3963–3968

Hayashi H, Tanase S, Snell EE (1986) Pyridoxal 5′-phosphate-dependent histidine decarboxylase. Inactivation by alpha-fluoromethylhistidine and comparative sequences at the inhibitor- and coenzyme- binding sites. J Biol Chem 261:11003–11009

Hayashi H, Wada H, Yoshimura T et al (1990) Recent topics in pyridoxal 5′-phosphate enzyme studies. Annu Rev Biochem 59:87–110

Hayashi H, Mizuguchi H, Kagamiyama H (1993) Rat liver aromatic L-amino acid decarboxylase: spectroscopic and kinetic analysis of the coenzyme and reaction intermediates. Biochemistry 32:812–818

Hayashi H (1995) Pyridoxal enzymes: mechanistic diversity and uniforminity. J Biochem 118: 463–473

Hayashi H, Tsukiyama F, Ishii S et al (1999) Acid-base chemistry of the reaction of aromatic L-amino acid decarboxylase and dopa analyzed by transient and steady-state kinetics: preferential binding of the subtrate with its amino group unprotonated. Biochemistry 38:15615–15622

Hegyesi H, Kovacs P, Falus A et al (1998) Presence and localization of histidine decarboxylase enzyme (HDC) and histamine in *Tetrahymena*. Cell Biol Int 22:493–497

Ishii S, Hayashi H, Okamoto A et al (1998) Aromatic L-amino acid decarboxylase: conformational change in the flexible region around Arg334 is required during transaldimination process. Protein Sci 7:1802–1810

John RA (1995) Pyridoxal phosphate-dependent enzymes. Biochim Biophys Acta 1248:81–96

Jorgensen EA, Vogelsang TW, Knigge U et al (2006) Increased susceptibility to diet-induced obesity in histamine-deficient mice. Neuroendocrinology 83:289–294

Joseph DR, Sullivan PM, Wang YM et al (1990) Characterization and expression of the complementary DNA encoding rat histidine decarboxylase. Proc Natl Acad Sci 87:733–737

Kallen RG, Korpela T, Martell AE et al (1985) In: Metzler DE and Christen P (eds) Transaminases. Wiley, New York

Kiss R, Kiss B, Könczöi A et al (2008) Discovery of novel human histamine H4 receptor ligands by large-scale structure-based virtual screening. J Med Chem 51:3145–3153

Kitchen DB, Decornez H, Furr JR et al (2004) Docking and scoring in virtual screening for drug discovery: methods and applications. Nat Rev Drug Discov 3:935–949

Klausz G, Buzás E, Scharek P et al (2004) Effects of Helicobacter pylori infection on gastric inflammation and local cytokine production in histamine-deficient (histidine decarboxylase knock-out) mice. Immunol Lett 94:223–228

Kubota H, Hayashi H, Watanabe T et al (1984) Mechanism of inactivation of mammalian L-histidine decarboxylase by (S) α-fluoromethyl histidine. Biochem Pharmacol 33:983–990

Landete JM, De las Rivas B, Marcobal A et al (2008) Updated molecular knowledge about histamine biosynthesis by bacteria. Crit Rev Food Sci Nutr 48:697–714

Lovenberg W, Weissbach H, Udenfriend S (1962) Aromatic L-amino acid decarboxylase. J Biol Chem 237:89–93

Liu L, Zhang S, Zhu Y et al (2007) Improved learning and memory of contextual fear conditioning and hippocampal CA1 long-term potentiation in histidine decarboxylase knock-out mice. Hippocampus 17:634–641

Mamune-Sato R, Tanno Y, Maeyama K et al (1990) Histidine decarboxylase in human basophilic leukemia (KU-812-F) cells. Characterization and induction by phorbol myristate acetate. Biochem Pharmacol 40:1125–1129

Martin SAM, Bishop JO (1986) Purification and characterization of histidine decarboxylase from mouse kidney. Biochem J 234:349–354

Matsuda N, Hayashi H, Miyatake S et al (2004) Instability of the apo form of aromatic L-amino acid decarboxylase in vivo and in vitro: implications for the involvement of the flexible loop that covers the active site. J Biochem 135:33–42

Metzler DE, Ikawa M, Snell EE (1954) A general mechanism for vitamin B6-catalyzed reactions. J Am Chem Soc 76:5648–5652

McNeil SD, Nuccio ML, Ziemak MJ et al (2001) Enhanced synthesis of choline and glycine betaine in transgenic tobacco plants that overexpress phosphoethanolamine N-methyltransferase. Proc Natl Acad Sci 98:10001–10005

Medina MA, Urdiales JL, Rodríguez-Caso C et al (2003) Biogenic amines and polyamines: similar biochemistry for different physiological missions and biomedical applications. Crit Rev Biochem Mol Biol 38:23–59

Mehta PK, Christen P (2000) The molecular evolution of pyridoxal-5′-phosphate-dependent enzymes. Adv Enzymol Relat Areas Mol Biol 74:129–184

Melgarejo E, Medina MA, Sánchez-Jiménez F et al (2009) Epigallocatechin gallate reduces human monocyte mobility and adhesion *in vitro*. Br J Pharmacol 158:1705–1712

Mondillo C, Falus A, Pignataro O et al (2007) Prolongued histamine deficiency in histidine decarboxylase gene knockout mice affects Leydig cell function. J Androl 28:86–91

Moore PS, Dominici P, Borri-Voltattorni C (1996) Cloning and expression of pig kidney dopa decarboxylase: comparison of the naturally occurring and recombinant enzymes. Biochem J 315:249–256

Morrow JD, Margolies GR, Rowland J et al (1991) Evidence that histamine is the causative toxin of scombroid-fish poisoning. N Engl J Med 324:716–720

Moya-García AA, Medina MA, Sánchez-Jiménez F (2005) Mammalian histidine decarboxylase: from structure to function. Bioessays 27:57–63

Moya-García AA, Pino-Ángeles A, Sánchez-Jiménez F (2006) New structural insights to help in the search for selective inhibitors of mammalian pyridoxal-5′-phosphate-dependent histidine decarboxylase. Inflamm Res Suppl 1:S55–S56

Moya-García (2007) Estructura-función de enzimas dependientes de vitamina B_6. Estudio computacional. Universidad de Málaga. PhD Thesis

Moya-García AA, Ruíz-Pernía J, Martí S et al (2008) Analysis of the decarboxylation step in mammalian histidine decarboxylase. A computational study. J Biol Chem 283:12393–12401

Moya-García AA, Pino-Ángeles A, Gil-Redondo R et al (2009) Structural features of mammalian histidine decarboxylase reveal the basis for specific inhibition. Br J Pharmacol 157:4–13

Nitta Y, Kikuzaki H, Ueno H (2007) Food components inhibiting recombinant human histidine decarboxylase activity. J Agric Food Chem 55:299–304

Notredame C, Higgins D, Heringa J (2000) T-Coffee: a novel method for multiple sequence alignments. J Mol Biol 302:205–217

Ohmori E, Fukui T, Imanishi N et al (1990) Purification and characterization of L-histidine decarboxylase from mouse mastocytoma P-815 cells. J Biochem 107:834–839

Ohtsu H, Watanabe T (2003) New functions of histamine found in histidine decarboxylase gene knockout mice. Biochem Biophys Res Commun 305:443–447

Ohtsu H (2008) Progress in allergy signal research on mast cells: the role of histamine in inmunological and cardiovascular disease and transporting system of histamine in the cell. J Pharmacol Sci 106:347–353

Olmo MT, Rodríguez-Agudo D, Medina MA et al (1999) The pest regions containing C-termini of mammalian ornithine decarboxylase and histidine decarboxylase play different roles in protein degradation. Biochem Biophys Res Commun 257:269–272

Olmo MT, Urdiales JL, Pegg E et al (2000) In vitro study of proteolytic degradation of rat histidine decarboxylase. Eur J Biochem 267:1527–1531

Olmo MT, Sánchez-Jiménez F, Medina MA et al (2002) Spectroscopic analysis of recombinant rat histidine decarboxylase. J Biochem 132:433–439

Picton S, Gray JE, Payton S et al (1993) A histidine decarboxylase-like mRNA is involved in tomato fruit ripening. Plant Mol Biol 23:627–631

Pino-Ángeles A, Morreale A, Negri A et al (2009) Substrate uptake and protein stability relationship in mammalian histidine decarboxylase. Proteins 78:154–161

Pishko EJ, Robertus JD (1993) Site-directed alteration of three active-site residues of a pyruvoyl-dependent histidine decarboxylase. Biochemistry 32:4943–4948

van Poelje PD, Snell EE (1990) Pyruvoyl-dependent enzymes. Annu Rev Biochem 59:29–59

Pos Z, Wiener Z, Pocza P et al (2008) Histamine suppresses fibulin-5 and insulin-like growth factor-II receptor expression in melanoma. Cancer Res 68:1997–2005.

Rahman MA, Inoue T, Ishikawa T et al (2007) Involvement of chemical mediators in nasal allergic responses of HDC-KO mice. Eur J Pharmacol 567:245–251

Rodríguez-Agudo D, Sánchez-Jiménez F, Medina MA (2000) Rat histidine decarboxylase is a substrate for m-calpainin vitro. Biochem Biophys Res Commun 271:777–781

Rodríguez-Caso C, Rodríguez-Agudo D, Moya-García AA et al (2003a) Local changes in the catalytic site of mammalian histidine decarboxylase can affect its global conformation and stability. Eur J Biochem 270:4376–4387

Rodríguez-Caso C, Rodríguez-Agudo D, Sánchez-Jiménez F et al (2003b) Green tea epigallocatechin-3-gallate is an inhibitor of mammalian histidine decarboxylase. Cell Mol Life Sci 60:1760–1763

Rontein D, Nishida I, Tashiro G et al (2001) Plant synthesize ethanolamine by direct decarboxylation of serine using pyridoxal phosphate enzyme. J Biol Chem 276:35523–35529

Salvá A, Donoso J, Frau J et al (2002) Theoretical studies on transimination of vitamin B6 analogs. Int J Quant Chem 89:48–56

Sandmeier E, Hale TI, Christen P (1994) Multiple evolutionary origin of pyridoxal-5′-phosphate-dependent aminoacid decarboxylases. Eur J Biochem 221:997–1002

Savany A, Cronenberger L (1982) Isolation and properties of multiple forms of histidine decarboxylase from rat gastric mucosa. Biochem J 205:405–412

Schelp E, Worley S, Monzingo AF et al (2001) pH-induced structural changes regulate histidine decarboxylase activity in *Lactobacillus* 30a. J Mol Biol 306:727–732

Schneider G, Kack H, Lindqvist Y (2000) The manifold of vitamin B6 dependent enzymes. Structure 8:R1–R6

Snell EE, Guirard BM (1986) Pyridoxal-dependent histidine decarboxylase from *Morganella* AM-15. Methods Enzimol 122:139–143

Suzuki S, Tanaka S, Nemoto K et al (1998) Membrane targeting and binding of the 74-kDa form of mouse L-histidine decarboxylase via its carboxyl-terminal sequence. FEBS Lett 437:44–48

Taguchi Y, Watanabe T, Kubota H et al (1984) Purification of histidine decarboxylase from the liver of fetal rats and its immunochemical and immunohistochemical characterization. J Biol Chem 259:5214–5221

Tanaka S, Fukui T, Yamamoto J et al (1995) Processing and activation of recombinant mouse mastocytoma histidine decarboxylase in the particulate fraction of Sf9 cells by porcine pancreatic lactase. Biochim Biophys Acta 1253:9–12

Tanase S, Guirard BM, Snell EE (1985) Purification and properties of pyridoxal 5′-phosphate-dependent histidine decarboxylase from *Morganella morganii* AM-15. J Biol Chem 260:6738–6746

Tahanejad FS, Naderi-Manesh H, Habibinejad B et al (2000) Homology-based molecular modelling of PLP-dependent histidine decarboxylase from *Morganella morganii*. Eur J Med Chem 35:567–576

Tahanejad FS, Naderi-Manesh H (2000) Quantum mechanical study of the intermediate formed following the reaction of the histidine decarboxylase's substrate and inhibitors with coenzyme. Eur J Med Chem 35:283–289

Toledo A, Sabriá J, Rodríeguez R et al (1988) Properties and ontogenic development of membrane-bound histidine decarboxylase from rat brain. J Neurochem 51:1400–1406

Toney MD (2001) Computational studies on nonenzymatic and enzymatic pyridoxal phosphate catalyzed decarboxylation of 2-aminoisobutyrate. Biochemistry 40:1378–1384

Toney MD (2005) Reaction specificity in pyridoxal phosphate enzymes. Arch Biochem Biophys 433:279–287

Tran VT, Snyder SH (1981) Histidine decarboxylase. Purification from fetal rat liver, inmunologic properties and histochemical localization in brain and stomach. J Biol Chem 256:680–686

Vaaler GL, Snell EE (1989) Pyridoxal 5′-phosphate dependent histidine decarboxylase: overproduction, purification, biosynthesis of soluble site-directed mutant proteins, and replacement of conserved residues. Biochemistry 28:7306–7613

Viguera E, Trelles O, Urdiales JL et al (1994) L-amino acid decarboxylases producing 1,4-diamines: analogies among differences. Trends Biochem Sci 19:318–319

Wang R, Guegler K, LaBrie ST et al (2000) Genomic analysis of a nutrient response in *Arabidopsis* reveals diverse expression patterns and novel metabolic and potential regulatory genes induced by nitrate. Plant Cell 12:1491–1509

Worley S, Schelp E, Monzingo AF et al (2002) Structure and cooperativity of a T-state mutant of histidine decarboxylase from *Lactobacillus* 30a. Proteins 46:321–329

Wu F, Yu J, Gehring H (2008) Inhibitory and structural studies of novel coenzyme-substrate analogs of human histidine decarboxylase. FASEB J 22:890–897

Yamakami J, Sakurai E, Kuramasu A et al (2000) L-histidine decarboxylase protein and activity in rat brain microvascular endothelial cells. Inflamm Res 49:231–235

Yamamoto J, Yatsunami K, Ohmori E et al (1990) cDNA-derived amino acid sequence of L-histidine decarboxylase from mouse mastocytoma P-815 cells. FEBS Lett 276:214–218

Yamamoto J, Fukui T, Suzuki K et al (1993) Expression and characterization of recombinant mouse mastocytoma histidine decarboxylase. Biochim Biophys Acta 1216:431–440

Yatsunami K, Tsuchikawa M, Kamada M et al (1995) Comparative studies of human recombinant 74- and 54-kDa L-histidine decarboxylases. J Biol Chem 270:30813–30817

Zhao CM, Chen D, Yamada H et al (2003) Rat stomach ECL cells: mode of activation of histidine decarboxylase. Regul Pept 114:21–27

Part III
Pharmacology of Histamine Noble Receptors and Their Ligands in Drug Development

Chapter 4
Biological and Pharmacological Aspects of Histamine Receptors and Their Ligands

Mohammed Shahid, Trivendra Tripathi, Rahat Ali Khan, Nancy Khardori, Ali Ibrahim Al-Sultan, Hamdan Ibrahim AL-Mohammed, Abdulrahman A. Alsultan, Anwar Huq, Aijaz Ahmed Khan, and Mashiatullah Siddiqui

Abstract Histamine is considered a principle mediator of several physiological and pathological processes. It induces biological activities through differential expression of four types of histamine receptors (H1R, H2R, H3R and H4R). All the histamine receptors are the G protein-coupled receptor (GPCR) family, are expressed on several histamine responsive target tissues and cells, and suggest a potential role of histamine in cell proliferation, differentiation, hematopoiesis, embryonic development, regeneration, wound healing, aminergic neuron-transmission and several brain functions, secretion of pituitary hormones, regulation of gastrointestinal and circulatory functions, cardiovascular system, inflammatory reactions, immunomodulation, functioning of endocrine system and homeostasis. Since H4R has been discovered very recently and there is paucity of comprehensive literature covering new histamine receptors, their agonists/antagonists and role in various diseases. This has prompted a re-evaluation of the actions of histamine, suggesting a new potential for H4R-agonists/antagonists and a possible synergy between histamine receptors-agonists/antagonists in targeting various patho-physiological conditions. This chapter will highlight the biological and pharmacological characterization of histamine, histamine receptors, and their agonists/antagonists in various biomedical aspects.

Keywords Histamine · Histamine receptors · H3-receptor · H4-receptor · Antagonists · Agonists

---

M. Shahid (✉)
Department of Microbiology, Jawaharlal Nehru Medical College and Hospital, Aligarh Muslim University, Aligarh, UP, 202002, India
Section of Microbiology, Department of Biomedical Sciences, College of Medicine, Al Hassa, Kingdom of Saudi Arabia
e-mail: shahidsahar@yahoo.co.in

M. Shahid et al. (eds.), *Biomedical Aspects of Histamine*,
DOI 10.1007/978-90-481-9349-3_4, © Springer Science+Business Media B.V. 2010

Abbreviations

H1R	histamine H1 receptor
H2R	histamine H2 receptor
H3R	histamine H3 receptor
H4R	histamine H4 receptor
GPCR	G protein-coupled receptor
mRNA	messenger RNA
cAMP	cyclic adenosine monophosphate
Bphs	*Bordetella pertussis*-induced histamine sensitization
VAASH	vasoactive amine sensitization elicited by histamine
Hrh1	histamine H1 receptor gene
SDS-PAGE	sodium dodecyl sulfate polyacrylamide gel electrophoresis
CNS	central nervous system
DAC	1, 2-diacylglycerol
NO	nitric oxide
cGMP	cyclic guanosine monophosphate
NFκB	nuclear factor kappa B
CHO	chinese hamster ovary
cDNA	complementary deoxyribonucleic acid
PKC	protein kinase C
TM	transmembrane
cAMP	cyclic adenosine monophosphate
MAPK	mitogen-activated protein kinase
IFN	Interferon
TNF	tumour necrosis factor
IL	interleukin
T-cells	T lymphocytes
MAPK	mitogen-activated protein kinase
CRE	cAMP responsive elements
CYP450	cytochrome P450
DPPE	N, N diethyl-2-(4-(phenylmethyl)phenoxy) ethanamine
HDC	histidine decarboxylase
VMATs	vesicular monoamine transporters
TGF	transforming growth factor
OCT	organic cation transporter
EMT	extraneuronal monoamine transporter

Contents

4.1 Introduction

Histamine (2-{imidazol-4-yl} ethylamine) is one of the monoamines and its name was coined after the Greek word for tissue *histos*. Histamine has a broad spectrum of activity in various physiological and pathological conditions including cell proliferation and differentiation, hematopoiesis, embryonic development, regeneration, wound healing, aminergic neuro transmission and numerous brain functions (sleep/nociception, food intake and aggressive behavior), secretion of pituitary hormones, regulation of gastrointestinal and circulatory functions, cardiovascular system (vasodilatation and blood pressure reduction), as well as inflammatory reactions, modulation of the immune response, endocrine function and homeostasis (Dy and Schneider 2004, Fumagalli et al. 2004, Haas and Panula 2003, Higuchi et al. 1999, Jutel et al. 2002, Schneider et al. 2002, Shahid et al. 2009, Yokoyama 2001). Histamine is probably one of the earliest known "phlogistic" mediators, and even one of the most intensely studied molecules in biological systems (Shahid et al. 2009). It was synthesized in 1907 and characterized in 1910 as a substance ("beta-1"), owing to its significant competence to constrict guinea pig ileum, and its cogent vasodepressor action. However, it took 17 years to demonstrate its presence in normal tissues. The relationship between histamine and anaphylactic reactions was made soon after that in 1929. Histamine was identified as a mediator of anaphylactic reaction in 1932, whereas its connection to mast cells was not made until 1952, and its connection to basophils in 1972 (Shahid et al. 2009). The search for compounds to neutralize the pathological effects of histamine began at the Pasteur Institute in Paris during the 1930s, and these compounds were found to partially block the effects of histamine based on the ethylenediamine structure. The first antihistamine compound was the adrenolytic benzodioxan, piperoxan (933F), reported by Ungar, Parrot and Bovet in 1937 and was shown to block the effect of histamine on the guinea-pig ileum, structurally related to aryl ethers such as the thymol ether (929F) (Bouvet and Staub 1937, Parsons and Ganellin 2006). This antihistamine compound proved to be too toxic for clinical development. However, the replacement of ether oxygen by an amino group led to the discovery of aniline ethylene diamine derivatives. For his research on antihistamines and curare, Bovet was awarded the Nobel Prize in 1957 (Shahid et al. 2009). The significant role of histamine in allergic reactions was further verified by a series of compounds with antihistamine activity which protected guinea pigs from anaphylaxis. However, the clinical use of these compounds in humans was deferred due to their toxicity (Bouvet and Staub 1937).

The first antihistamine, Antergan^{TM} (phenbenzamine, RP 2339) used in humans, was subsequently replaced by Neoantergan^{TM} (mepyramine, pyrilamine, RP 2786), which is still in use to counteract the uncomfortable effects of histamine release in the skin. Many other antihistamines such as diphenhydramine (Benadryl^{TM}), tripelennamine, chlorpheniramine and promethazine are also used in similar manner to counteract the adverse effects of histamine (Parsons and Ganellin 2006). Since 1945, these antihistamines have been widely used in the treatment of various allergic diseases such as hay fever, urticaria, and allergic rhinitis. However, the side effect of sedation is a drawback to their use. On the other hand, another side effect allowed the use of antihistamines such as cyclizine (Marzine^{TM}) and diphenhydramine in the form of its 8-chlorotheophyllinate (Dramamine^{TM}) as antiemetics for travel sickness (Shahid et al. 2009). By 1950 there were 20 compounds available to block the effects of histamine, but advances in histamine receptor (H1R – H4R) knowledge has led to further pharmaceutical developments (Shahid et al. 2009). All these four receptors are members of the 7-transmembrane (heptahelical) spanning family of receptors, are G protein-coupled (GPCR), and are expressed on various histamine responsive target tissues and cells and suggest an important critical role of histamine in many diseases (Dy and Schneider 2004, Jutel et al. 2002, MacGlashan 2003, Parsons Ganellin 2006, Schneider et al. 2002). The antagonists for H1- and H2-receptors are used extensively in clinical medicine. H4R has been discovered very recently and there is paucity of comprehensive literature covering new histamine receptors and their agonists/antagonists. This chapter will highlight the biological and pharmacological characterization of histamine; histamine receptors (H1R – H4R); their agonists/antagonists; and their cellular distribution, functional characterization, structural biology, and signaling mechanisms; non-classical histamine-binding sites such as cytochrome P450; and histamine transporters.

4.2 Histamine Receptors

Histamine is an important biogenic amine and has multiple effects that are mediated through specific surface receptors on specific target cells. Four types of histamine receptors have now been identified. In 1966, histamine receptors were first differentiated into H1 and H2 (Ash and Schild 1966), and it was reported that some responses to histamine were inhibited by low doses of mepyramine (pyrilamine), whereas others were unsympathetic. In 1999, a third histamine receptor subtype was cloned and termed as H3 (Lovenberg et al. 1999). Subsequently in 2000, the fourth histamine receptor subtype was reported which was termed as H4 (Oda et al. 2000) and introduced a significant chapter in the story of histamine effects.

4.2.1 Histamine H1-Receptor

4.2.1.1 Cellular Distribution and Functional Characterization

In different mammalian tissues, the study of the distribution of histamine H1-receptors (H1Rs) has been significantly helped by the development of specific radioligands for this subtype (Shahid et al. 2009). In 1997, [3H]mepyramine a selective radioligand was developed (Table 4.1) (Hill et al. 1977), and since then it has been used to identify H1-receptors in a wide variety of tissues such as gastrointestinal tract, central nervous system, airways and vascular smooth muscle cells, mammalian brain, hepatocytes, nerve cells, endothelial cells, chondrocytes, monocytes, neutrophils, dendritic cells, T and B lymphocytes (Table 4.2), the cardiovascular system and genitourinary system, endothelial cells and adrenal medulla (Shahid et al. 2009). In many pathological processes of allergy, including allergenic rhinitis, atopic dermatitis, conjunctivitis, urticaria, asthma, and anaphylaxis, H1-receptors are involved. The receptors also mediate bronchoconstriction and enhanced vascular permeability in the lung (Haas and Panula 2003, Smit et al. 1999, Togias 2003). It has been noticed that [3H]mepyramine binds to secondary non-H1-receptor sites in various tissues and cells (Arias-Montano and Young 1993, Dickenson and Hill 1994, Leurs et al. 1995a). In addition to [3H]mepyramine, which predominantly binds to a protein homologous with debrisoquine 4-hydroxylase cytochrome P450 in rat liver (Fukui et al. 1990), this nonspecific binding can be blocked by quinine. This investigation led to the demonstration that quinine may be used to block binding to other lower affinity sites (Liu et al. 1992). However, it is clear that not all secondary binding sites for [3H]mepyramine are sensitive to inhibition by quinine. Thus, in DDT1MF-2 cells, a 38–40 kDa protein has been isolated, which binds H1R antagonists with KD values in the micromolar range but which is not sensitive to inhibition by quinine. Nevertheless, DDT1MF-2 cells can be shown to additionally possess [3H]mepyramine binding sites that have the characteristics of H1R (i.e., KD values in the nanomolar range) and to mediate functional responses, which are clearly produced by histamine H1R activation (Hill et al. 1997).

Furthermore, H1R is also responsible for changes in vascular permeability as a result of endothelial cell contraction (Meyrick and Brigham 1983, Svensjo and Grega 1986); in synthesis of prostacyclin (Carter et al. 1988, McIntyre et al. 1985); in platelet-activating factor synthesis (McIntyre et al. 1985); in release of Von Willebrand factor (Hamilton and Sims 1987), and in nitric oxide release (Van de Voorde and Leusen 1993). H1R on human T lymphocytes has been characterized by use of [125I]iodobolpyramine (Shahid et al. 2009, Villemain et al. 1990) (see also Table 4.1). H1R-deficient mice display both strong systemic T-cell and efficient B-cell responses to antigen (Bryce et al. 2006). H1R has also been demonstrated to increase (Ca^{2+})i (Kitamura et al. 1996). The relationship of H1Rs to adrenal medulla which elicits the release of catecholamines has been established many years ago (Noble et al. 1988, Livett and Marley 1986). Thus, histamine can stimulate the release of both adrenaline and noradrenaline (Livett and Marley 1986), and also induce phosphorylation of the catecholamine biosynthesis enzyme tyrosine hydroxylase by a mechanism which mediates release of intracellular calcium from cultured bovine adrenal chromaffin cells (Bunn et al. 1995). Histaminergic effects cause release of leucine- and methionine- enkephalin (Bommer et al. 1987) and a marked increase in mRNA-encoding proenkephalin A after prolonged exposure (Bommer et al. 1987, Wan et al. 1989). Its negative inotropic effects have been observed in human atrial myocardium and also in guinea pig ventricle (Genovese et al. 1988,

Table 4.1 Characterization of histamine receptors agonist, antagonist and radioligand

Receptor subtypes	Agonists with potency	Antagonists with potency	Radioligands with equilibrium constant for dissociation (Kd)
*H1	Histamine(100)[a, b], Dimethylhistaprodifen (240)[a], Methylhistaprodifen (340)[a], Histamine-trifluoromethyl-toluidine (HTMT)[c], 2-(3-trifluoromethylphenyl) histamine (128)[a, b], 2-Thiazolylethylamine (26)[a], 2-Pyridylethylamine (6)[a]	Mepyramine (pA_2 9.4)[a], (+)-Chlorpheniramine (pA_2 9.4)[a], (−)-Chlorpheniramine (pA_2 6.7)[a], *Trans*-triprolidine (pA_2 10.0)[a], Temelastine (pA_2 9.5)[a], Promethazine (pA_2 8.9) [a], Diphenhydramine (pA_2 9.0)[a], Tripelennamine (pA_2 8.5)[a], Chlorpromazine (pA_2 8.9)[a]	$[^{3}H]$-Mepyramine (Kd 0.8 nM: guinea-pig brain, ileum)[a, b], $[^{125}I]$-Iodobolpyramine (Kd 0.01 nM, guinea-pig brain)[a], $[^{125}I]$-Iodoazidophen-pyramine (Kd 0.01 nM, guinea-pig cerebellum)[a, b]
*H2	Histamine(100)[a, b], Arpromidine (10230)[a, b], Impromidine (4810)[a, b], Sopromidine (740)[a, b], Amthamine (150)[a, b], Dimaprit (71)[a, b], 4-Methylhistamine (43)[a, b]	Cimetidine (pA_2 6.1)[a], Ranitidine (pA_2 6.7)[a], Famotidine (pA_2 7.8)[a], Zolantidine (pA_2 7.6)[a], Mifentidine (pA_2 7.6)[a], Titotidine (pA_2 7.8)[a], Iodoaminopotentidine (pA_2 8.6)[a]	$[^{3}H]$-Tiotidine (25 nM)[a, b], $[^{125}I]$-Iodoamino-potentidine (Kd 0.3 nM)[a, b], $[^{125}I]$-Iodoazido-potentidine (Kd 10 nM)[a, b] (all guinea-pig brain membrains)
*H3	Histamine(100)[a, b], Imetit (6200)[a, b], Immepip (2457)[a, b], *R*-α-methylhistamine (1550)[a, b]	*Thioperamide (pA_2 8.4)[a], Iodophenpropit (pA_2 9.6)[a], *Clobenpropit (pA_2 9.9)[a], Ciproxifan (pA_2 9.3)[a], Impentamine (pA_2 8.4)[a], GR174737 (pA_2 8.1)[a, b], Impromidine (pA_2 7.2)[a]	$[^{3}H]$-R-α-methylhistamine (Kd 0.5 nM)[a, b], $[^{3}H]$-N^{α}-methylhistamine (Kd 2.0 nM)[a, b], $[^{125}I]$-Iodophenpropit (Kd 0.3 nm)[a, b], $[^{125}I]$-Iodoproxyfan (Kd 0.065 nM)[a, b], [3H]-GR168320 (Kd 0.1 nM)[a, b] (all rat cerebral cortical membranes in Tris buffer)
*H4	Imetit (pA_2 8.6)[d], Immepip (pA_2 8)[d], **Clobenpropit (pA_2 7.9, partial agonist)[d], 4-Methylhistamine (pA_2 7.3)[d]	JNJ 10191584 (7.6) [d], *Thioperamide (7.6) [d]	None to date

[a]IUPHAR receptor database (2008)
[b]Hill et al. (1997)
[c]Bell et al. (2004)
[d]Alexander et al. (2006)
**These compounds act as agonist/antagonist for different histamine receptors at variable potencies (*Shahid et al. 2009)

Table 4.2 Characteristics of the histamine receptor subtypes

Characteristics	H1-Receptor*	H2-Receptor*	H3-Receptor*	H4-Receptor*
Receptor described, human gene cloned (years)[a, b]	1966, 1993	1972, 1991	1983, 1999	1994, 2000
Receptor proteins in human[a]	487 amino acids, 56 kD	359 amino acids, 40 kD	445 amino acids,70 kD; splice variants	390 amino acids
Chromosomal location in human[a, c]	3p25, 3p14–21	5, 5q35.3	20, 20q13.33	13q11.2
Equilibrium constant for dissociation (Kd)[b]	~10 μmol/L	~30 μmol/L	~10 nmol/L	20–40 nmol/L
Receptor expression[a]	Widespread, including neurons, smooth muscle (e.g., airways, vascular), and other types of cells.*	Widespread, including gastric mucosa parietal cells, smooth-muscle, heart, and other types of cells.*	High expression in histaminergic neurons, low expression elsewhere.	High expression in bone marrow and peripheral hematopoietic cells, low expression elsewhere.
Gene Structure[c]	Intronless	Intronless	Three introns	Two introns
G-protein coupling[a]	Gαq/11	Gαs	Gi/o	Gi/o
Activated intracellular signals (principal signaling effector molecules)[a,b]	Ca^{2+}↑, cGMP, NF-κB, PLC↑, phospholipase A2, and D, cAMP, NOS	cAMP↑, Ca^{2+},protein kinese C, c-fos, phos-pholipase C	Ca^{2+}↑, MAP kinase↑; inhibition of cAMP↓	Ca^{2+}↑, MAP kinase↑; Inhibition of cAMP↓

cAMP cyclic adenosine monophosphate, *cGMP* cyclic guanosine monophosphate, *MAP* mitogen-activated protein, *NF-κB* nuclear factor-κB, *NOS* nitric oxide synthase, *PLC* phospholipase C

*Other types of cells: epithelial, endothelial cells, neutrophils, eosinophils, monocytes, dendritic cells, T-cells, B cells, hepatocytes, and chondrocytes

[a]Simons (2004)

[b]MacGlashan (2003)

[c]Dy and Schneider (2004)

*Shahid et al.(2009).

Guo et al. 1984). Genovese et al. (1988) suggested that the negative inotropic response to histamine in human myocardium is associated with inhibitory effects on heart rate. This can be unmasked when the positive responses of histamine on the heart rate, and force of contraction (due to histamine H2-receptors) are mediated through conjoint administration of adenosine or adenosine A1-receptor agonists. However, histamine produces a positive inotropic effect in guinea pig left atria and rabbit papillary muscle by a specific mechanism which is not related to a rise in adenosine 3c, 5c-cyclic monophosphate (cAMP) levels (Hattori et al. 1988a, b, Shahid et al. 2009). The distribution of H1Rs in mammalian brain shows higher densities in neocortex, hippocampus, nucleus accumbent, thalamus, and posterior hypothalamus (Schwartz et al. 1991), however, cerebellum and basal ganglia have lower densities (Shahid et al. 2009, Yanai et al. 1992). The distribution of H1Rs in rat and guinea pig is very similar (Ruat and Schwartz 1989, Shahid et al. 2009). H1-receptor binding sites and mRNA levels were overlapped in most areas of brain except in hippocampus and cerebellum in which the inconsistency is mostly to reflect the presence of exuberance H1Rs in dendrites of pyramidal and Purkinje cells (Traiffort et al. 1994). The activation of H1R inhibits the firing and hyperpolarization in hippocampal neurons (Haas 1981) and also an apamine sensitive outward current in olfactory bulb interneurons (Jahn et al. 1995), and these effects are mostly generated by intracellular Ca^{2+} release. However, H1R excite various notable factors such as vegetative ganglia (Christian et al. 1989), hypothalamic supraoptic (Hill et al. 1997), brainstem (Khateb et al. 1990), thalamic (McCormick and Williamson 1991), and human cortical neurons (Reiner and Kamondi 1994) through a block of potassium conductance. Histaprodifens are very potent H1R agonists and are more effective than histamine in activating H1R (Elz et al. 2000).

The functional characterization of H1R has benefited from the use of many potent and specific antagonists (see Table 4.1) (Shahid et al. 2009, Sharma and Hamelin 2003). H1-receptor antagonists were developed initially as the anti-allergic drugs with the known side effect of sedation due to the disturbance of circadian rhythms and locomotor activities as well as the impairment of the exploratory behavior by histamine in the brain. Later the so-called "non-sedating" H1 antagonists which cannot cross the blood-brain barrier were designed (Shahid et al. 2009). Some anti-inflammatory effects of H1R antagonists at high doses could be non-specific because of histamine and other inflammatory mediators like leukotriene and platelet activating factors released from basophils in response to certain H1Rs antagonists (Shahid et al. 2009). *Bordetella pertussis*-induced histamine sensitization (Bphs) controls *Bordetella pertussis* toxin (PTX)-induced vasoactive amine sensitization elicited by histamine (VAASH) and has been established an important role of histamine in autoimmunity. The congenic mapping links Bphs to the histamine H1 receptor gene (Hrh1/H1R) and that H1R differs at three amino acid residues in VAASH-susceptible and -resistant mice. $Hrh1^{-/-}$ mice are protected from VAASH, which can be restored by genetic complementation with a susceptible Bphs/Hrh1 allele, and experimental allergic encephalomyelitis and autoimmune orchitis due to immune deviation. Thus, natural alleles of Hrh1 control both the autoimmune T cells and vascular responses regulated by histamine after PTX sensitization. The exact mechanism through which this effect occurs remains unclear and its clinical relevance is still uncertain (Ma et al. 2002). The chemical structure of specific H1R-antagonists and agonists are shown in Figs. 4.1 and 4.2.

4.2.1.2 Structural Biology of Receptor

H1 receptors have been cloned from cows, rats, guinea pigs and also from humans. The H1 receptor contains 486, 488 or 487 amino acids in rat, mouse and humans, respectively. It contains the typical properties of G protein coupled receptor (GPCR), namely, seven transmembrane domains of 20–25 amino acids predicted to form an α-helice which spans the plasma membrane and an extra cellular NH_2 terminal domain with glycosylation site. H1R is encoded by a single exon gene that is located on the distal short arm of chromosome 3p25 in humans see in Fig. 4.1 and

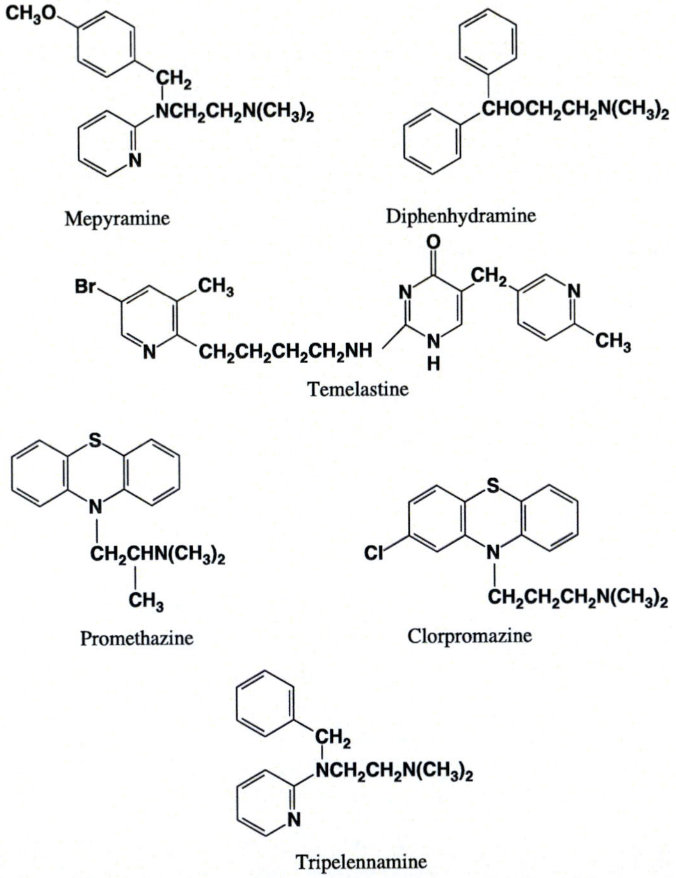

Fig. 4.1 Chemical structures of some histamine H1-receptor antagonists

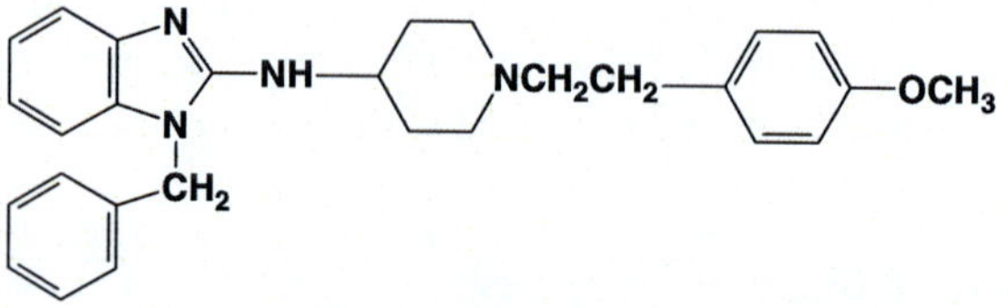

Astemizole

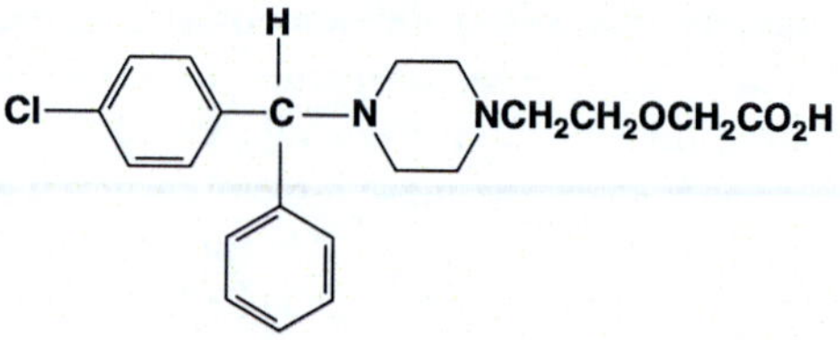

Cetirizine

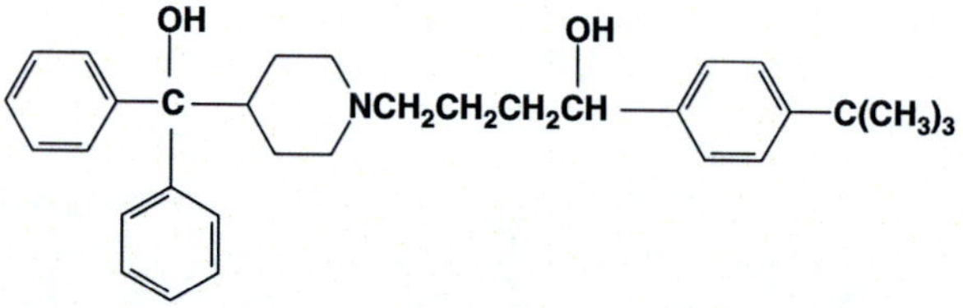

Terfenadine

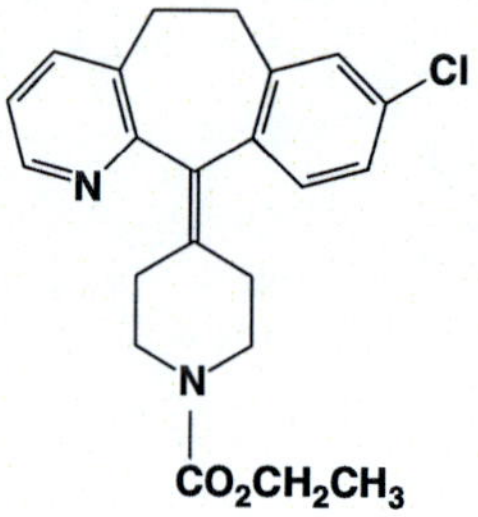

Loratadine

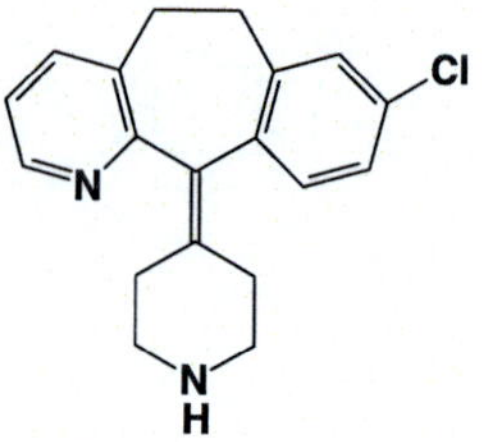

Desloratadine

Fig. 4.1 (continued)

chromosome 6 in mice. Histamine binds to aspartate residues in the transmembrane domain 3 of the H1-receptor, and to asparagine + lysine residues within the transmembrane domain 5 (Shahid et al. 2009). Its structural studies done by photoaffinity binding properties using [125I]iodoazidophenpyramine (Table 4.1) and subsequent sodium dodecyl sulfate polyacrylamide gel electrophoresis (SDS-PAGE) analysis demonstrated that the H1-receptor protein (molecular weight 56 kDa) is found under reducing conditions in the brain of rat, guinea pig, and mouse (Ruat et al. 1990a, Shahid et al. 2009).

Similar studies have also been done by using photoaffinity ligand [3H] azidobenzamide in bovine adrenal medullar membranes and found labeled peptides in the

Fig. 4.1 (continued)

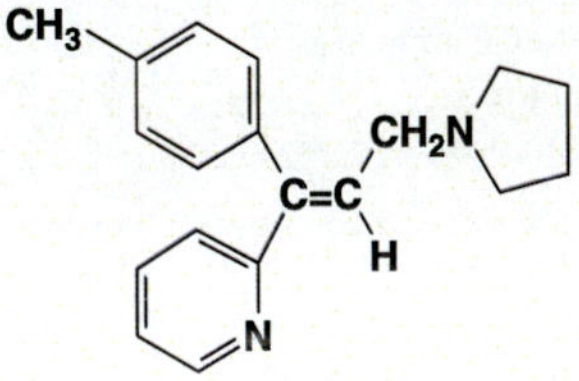

Triprolidine

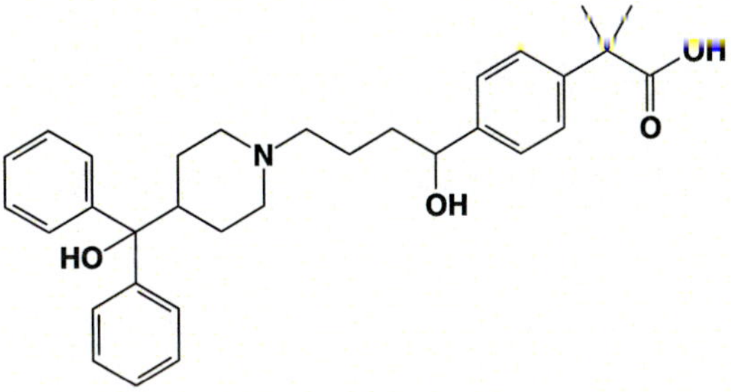

Fexofenadine

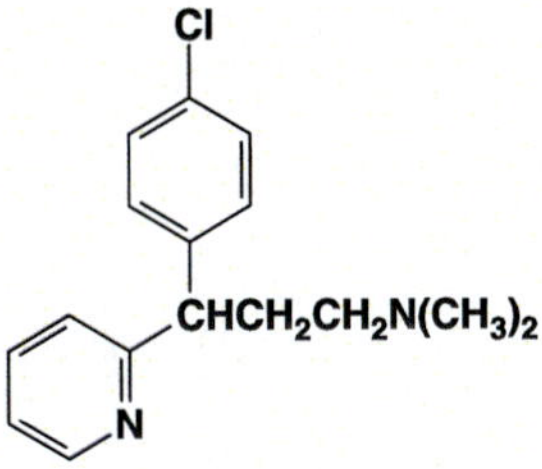

Chlorpheniramine

size range 53–58 kDa (Yamashita et al. 1991). In guinea pig heart, the specifically labeled H1R with [125I]iodoazidophenpyramine was found to contain substantially higher molecular weight, while there was no obvious difference in the characteristics of the H1R in tissues (Table 4.1) (Ruat et al. 1990b). In 1991, H1R was cloned from the bovine adrenal medulla by expression cloning in the *Xenopus* oocyte system. Interestingly, 491 amino acid protein with a calculated molecular weight of 56 kDa was represented by the deduced amino acid sequence (Yamashita et al. 1991); this protein has the seven transmembrane domains expected of a G-protein coupled receptor (GPCR) and contains N-terminal glycosylation sites. The main feature of the proposed H1R structure is the very large 3rd intracellular loop with 212 amino acids and relatively short intracellular C terminal tail with 17 amino acids. The availability of the bovine sequence and lack of introns has enabled the H1-receptor to be cloned from several species including rat (Fujimoto et al. 1993), guinea pig (Horio et al. 1993), mouse (Inove et al. 1996), and human (De Backer et al. 1993, Smit et al. 1996). The human H1-receptor gene has now been localized to chromosome

Fig. 4.2 Chemical structures of some histamine H1-receptor agonist

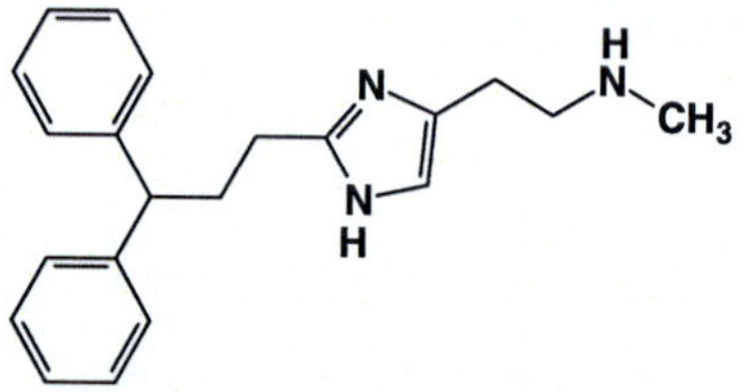

Methylhistaprodifen

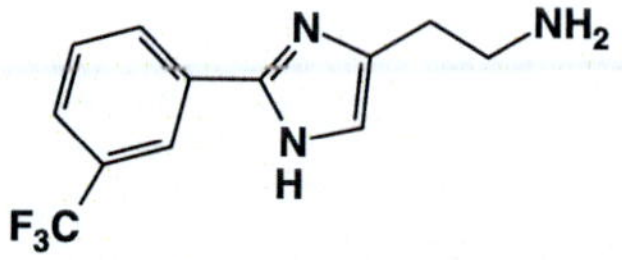

2-[3-(Trifluoromethyl)phenyl]histamine

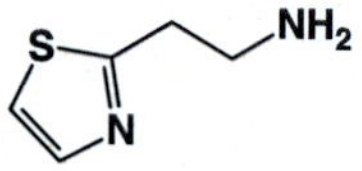

2-(Thiazol-2-yl)ethanamine

3 bands 3p14–p21 (Table 4.2). These clones should be regarded as true species homologues of the H1-receptor, while there are notable variations amongst them in some antagonist potencies (Shahid et al. 2009). Nevertheless, it is clear that the stereoisomers of chlorpheniramine show marked differences between species. For example, the guinea pig H1-receptor has a K_D of 0.9 nM for (1)-chlorpheniramine, whereas for the rat H1-receptor, the value is nearly 8 nM (Shahid et al. 2009). Similar variations for chlorpheniramine and other compounds (mepyramine and triprolidine) have been shown in guinea pig and rat brain, respectively (Shahid et al. 2009). The species differences may explain why compound [125I]iodobolpyramine can label guinea pig CNS H1-receptors, but it is unable to identify H1Rs in the brain of rat (Shahid et al. 2009). In brain membranes of both guinea pig and rat the native H1-receptor protein has been solubilized (Toll and Snyder 1982, Treherne and Young 1988), and the solubilized receptor retains similar differences in H1-antagonist potency for (1)-chlorpheniramine as that detected in membranes (Toll and Snyder 1982). It is important to note that mepyramine seems to be potent antagonist of the recombinant rat H1-receptor (i.e. expressed in C6 cells) than of the native histamine H1-receptor in the brain membrane of rat (Shahid et al. 2009).

In addition, the recombinant studies performed in rat C6 cells (Fujimoto et al. 1993) are complicated by the presence of a low level of endogenous histamine H1-receptors (H1Rs) (Peakman and Hill 1994), but in the functional studies in untransfected C6 cells, a high affinity for mepyramine (K_D 51 nM) has been deduced (Peakman and Hill 1994). The amino acid sequence alignment of the cloned histamine H1- and H2-receptors led to the suggestion that the third and fifth transmembrane domains (TM3 and TM5 respectively) of receptor proteins are responsible for histamine binding (Birdsall 1991, Timmerman 1992). In third transmembrane (TM3) of the human H1-receptor, Aspartate (107) that is conserved in entire aminergic receptors, has appeared to be essential for the histamine binding, and also H1-receptor antagonists to the H1-receptor (Ohta et al. 1994). In H1-receptor, the amino acid residues corresponding to Asparagine (198) and Threonine (194) are in corresponding positions in 5th transmembrane domain (TM5) of the human H1-receptor, while the substitution of an Alanine for Threonine (194) did not influence the binding properties of either agonist or antagonist (Moguilevsky et al. 1995, Ohta et al. 1994). However, the substitution of Alanine (198) for Asparagine (198) decreased agonist affinity, while the affinity of antagonist remained unchanged (Moguilevsky et al. 1995, Ohta et al. 1994). Similar results have been seen in the mutations to the corresponding residues Threonine (203) and Asparagine (207) in the guinea pig-H1R sequence (Leurs et al. 1994a). In addition to these mutations 2-methylhistamine is affected by the Asparagine (207) Alanine mutation, and H1-selective agonists 2-thiazolylethylamine, 2-pyridylethylamine, and 2-(3-bromophenyl) histamine are much less influenced through this mutation (Leurs et al. 1995b). This suggested that Asparagine (207) interacts with the Nt-nitrogen of histamine imidazole ring.

However, it has been shown that Lysine(200) interacts with the Np-nitrogen of histamine ring, and that it is important for the activation of the H1R by histamine and the nonimidazole agonist, 2-pyridylethylamine (Shahid et al. 2009). Furthermore, Leurs et al. (1995b) has demonstrated that the Lysine(200) Alanine mutation did not alter the binding affinity of 2-pyridylethylamine to H1R of guinea pig. Thus, the studies on the organization, genomic structure and promoter function of the human H1R revealed a 5.8 kb intron in the 50 flanking region of this gene, different binding sites for various transcription factors, and the absence of TATA and CAAT sequences at the appropriate locations (De Backer et al. 1998).

4.2.1.3 Signaling Mechanisms

H1-receptor is a Gαq/11-coupled protein with a very large third intracellular loop and a relatively short C-terminal tail see in Fig. 4.3 (Shahid et al. 2009). The main signal induced by ligand binding is the activation of phospholipase C-generating inositol 1, 4, 5-triphosphate and 1, 2-diacylglycerol (DAC) leading to increased cytosolic Ca^{2+} (Shahid et al. 2009). The enhanced intracellular Ca^{2+} levels appear to account for the different pharmacological properties promoted through the receptor including nitric oxide (NO) production, liberation of arachidonic acid from phospholipids, contraction of smooth muscles, dilatation of arterioles and capillaries, vascular permeability in vessels as well as stimulation of afferent neurons, and increased cAMP, and also cGMP levels (Bakker et al. 2002) (see also Table 4.2). This receptor also stimulates nuclear factor kappa B (NFκB) by Gαq/11 and Gβγ upon binding of agonist, while stimulation of NFκB occurs only via Gβγ leading to (pro)inflammatory mediators (Bakker et al. 2001). In a number of tissues and cell

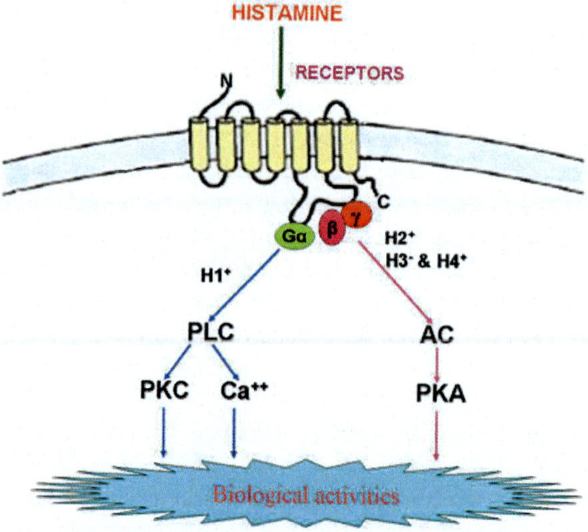

Fig. 4.3 The classical binding sites of histamine and their main signaling pathways such as AC (adenylate cyclase), PKC (protein kinase C), PKA (protein kinase A), PLC (phospholipase C), $H1^+$ or $H2^+$ (stimulation via H1 or H2 receptor), $H3^-$ and $H4^-$ (inhibition via H3 and H4 receptors). (Adapted from Shahid et al. 2009)

types H1R-mediated increases in either inositol phosphate accumulation or intracellular calcium mobilization has been described extensively and further details are provided in several comprehensive reviews (Hill and Donaldson 1992, Leurs et al. 1994b). In Chinese hamster ovary (CHO) cells Ca^{2+} mobilization and [3H]inositol phosphate accumulation has been observed due to stimulation by histamine when CHO cells are transfected with H1R-complementary deoxyribonucleic acid (cDNA) of the human, bovine, and guinea pig origin (Leurs et al. 1994c, Megson et al. 1995).

It is important to note that in some tissues histamine can stimulate inositol phospholipid hydrolysis independently of H1Rs. Thus, in the longitudinal smooth muscle of guinea pig ileum and neonatal rat brain (Claro et al. 1987), a component can be identified in response to histamine that is resistant to inhibition by H1R-antagonists. It is yet to be established whether these effects are due to "tyramine-like" effects of histamine on neurotransmitter release or direct effects of histamine on the associated G-proteins (Bailey et al. 1987, Seifert et al. 1994). In addition to well known effects on the inositol phospholipid signal transduction systems, several other signal transduction pathways can lead to stimulation of H1R and seem to be secondary to changes in intracellular Ca^{2+}concentration or protein kinase C (PKC) activation. Thus, nitric oxide synthase activity (via a Ca^{2+}/calmodulin-dependent pathway), and subsequent stimulation of soluble guanylyl cyclase in a wide variety of various cell types can be activated by histamine (Hattori et al. 1990, Leurs et al. 1991, Schmidt et al. 1990, Yuan et al. 1993). The H1R can stimulate the arachidonic acid release and arachidonic acid metabolite synthesis such as prostacyclin and thromboxane (Muriyama et al. 1990). It has been demonstrated that the histamine-stimulated release of arachidonic acid is partially inhibited (~40%) by pertussis toxin, when CHO-K1 cells transfected with the guinea pig H1R and the same response is also shown in HeLa cell possessing a native H1R to resist pertussis toxin treatment (Shahid et al. 2009). The substantial changes in the intracellular levels of cAMP can be produced by H1-receptor activation, but in most tissues, H1R activation does not stimulate adenylyl cyclase directly, and acts for the amplification of cAMP responses to histamine H2 receptor, adenosine A2 receptor, and also vasoactive intestinal polypeptide receptors (Donaldson et al. 1989, Garbarg and Schwartz 1988, Marley et al. 1991). The role of both intracellular Ca^{2+} ions and protein kinase C has been demonstrated in various cases in this augmentation response (Garbarg and Schwartz 1988). H1R stimulation can also lead to both cAMP responses and to an increase of forskolin-activated cAMP formation when CHO cells are transfected with the bovine or guinea pig H1R (Sanderson et al. 1996, Shahid et al. 2009).

4.2.2 Histamine H2-Receptor

4.2.2.1 Cellular Distribution and Functional Characterization

The H2R is located on chromosome 5 in humans. Similar to what has been demonstrated for H1R, the histamine binds to transmembrane (TM) domains 3 (aspartate) and TM 5 (threonine and aspartate). The short 3rd intra-cellular loop and the long C-terminal tail are also a feature of H2R subtype, and the rat N-terminal extra-cellular tail has N-linked glycosylation sites (Del Valle and Gantz 1997). Similar to H1R, H2R is expressed in different cell types (Table 4.2) (Shahid et al. 2009). It has been documented that H2R is mostly involved in suppressive activities of histamine, while stimulative effects are mediated through H1R. The activation of H2R regulates various functions of histamine including heart contraction, gastric acid secretion, cell proliferation, differentiation and immune response. H2R antagonists, such as zolantidine, are effective in the treatment of stomach and duodenal ulcers and the clinical potency relates to the suppressive effect of these drugs on the secretion of stomach acids (Dy and Schneider 2004, Shahid et al. 2009).

Hill (1990) designed a study to map the distribution of H2Rs by using radiolabeled H2R-antagonists, and achieved more affinity with [3H] titotidine (Table 4.1) for the H2R in guinea pig brain, lung parenchyma, and CHO-K1 cells transfected with the human H2-receptor cDNA (Gajtkowski et al. 1983, Gantz et al. 1991a, Sterk et al. 1986), but it was not successful in the studies of rat brain (Maayani et al. 1982). The most useful H2R-radioligand is [125I]iodoaminopotentidine, which has high affinity (K_D 50.3 nM) for the H2R in brain membranes (Table 4.1) (Hirschfeld et al. 1992, Traiffort et al. 1992a, b) and also in CHO-K1 cells expressing the cloned rat H2R (Traiffort et al. 1992b). This compound has also been used for autoradiographic mapping of H2Rs in the brain of mammal (Traiffort et al. 1992a). [125I]iodoaminopotentidine is also a useful H2R-radioligand (Table 4.1), which was used to map the distribution of H2Rs in human brain with highest densities in the basal ganglia, hippocampus, amygdale, and cerebral cortex, and also lowest densities were identified in cerebellum and hypothalamus (Traiffort et al. 1992a). In guinea pig brain, a similar distribution has been observed (Shahid et al. 2009). Irreversible labeling has also been successfully accomplished by [125I]iodoazidopotentidine (Table 4.1) (Shahid et al. 2009). H2R-stimulated cyclic AMP accumulation or adenylyl cyclase activity in Fig. 4.3 has been shown in various tissues including gastric cells, cardic tissue and brain (Al-Gadi and Hill 1985, 1987) and gastric cells (Johnson 1982). The potent effect of H2Rs have been demonstrated on gastric acid secretion and the inhibition of this secretory process through H2R antagonists had provided evidence for physiological role of histamine in gastric acid secretion (Black and Shankley 1985, Soll and Berglindh 1987). In cardiac tissues of most animal species, high concentrations of histamine were present which can mediate positive chronotropic and inotropic impacts on atrial or ventricular tissues by H2R stimulation (Hescheler et al. 1987, Levi and Alloatti 1988). Also H2R-mediated smooth muscle relaxation has been documented in vascular smooth muscle, uterine muscle and in airways (Foreman et al. 1985, Ottosson et al. 1989).

Hill (1990) had demonstrated that the effects of H2Rs can inhibit a variety of functions within the immune system. H2Rs have been shown to negatively regulate the release of histamine in basophils and mast cells (Plaut and Lichtenstein 1982, Ting et al. 1980). The inhibition of antibody synthesis, T-cell proliferation, cell-mediated cytolysis, and cytokine production were point to the evidence of H2Rs on lymphocytes (Banu Watanabe 1999, Jutel et al. 2001, Melmon and Khan 1987). The chemical structure of specific H2R-antagonist and -agonists are shown in Figs. 4.4 and 4.5.

4.2.2.2 Structural Biology of Receptor

The structural studies of H2R have been conducted using [125I]iodoazidopotentidine and sodium dodecyl sulfate-polyacrylamide gel electrophoresis (SDS-PAGE) and it was suggested that the H2R in guinea pig hippocampus and striatum has a molecular weight of 59 kDa (Shahid et al. 2009). However, comparison with the calculated molecular weights (40.2–40.5 kDa) for the cloned H2Rs indicates that the native H2R in the brain of guinea pig was glycosylated. The cloned H2R proteins possess *N*-glycosylation sites in the N-terminus region (Gantz et al. 1991b, Ruat et al. 1991, Traiffort et al. 1995). Fukushima et al. (1995) has suggested that removal of these glycosylation sites by site-directed mutagenesis showed that *N*-glycosylation of the H2R is not essential for cell surface localization, ligand binding, or coupling via Gs to adenylyl cyclase. Gantz and colleagues for the first time successfully cloned H2R using the polymerase chain reaction to amplify a partial length H2R sequence from canine gastric parietal cDNA using degenerate oligonucleotide primers and this sequence was then used to identify a full length H2R clone following screening of a canine genomic library (Shahid et al. 2009). Following this cloning, many researchers have cloned the rat, human, guinea pig, and mouse H2Rs (Kobayashi et al. 1996, Shahid et al. 2009). These intronless gene (DNA) sequences encode 359 amino acids for

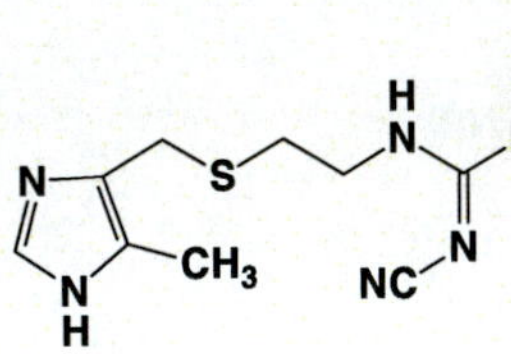

Cimetidine

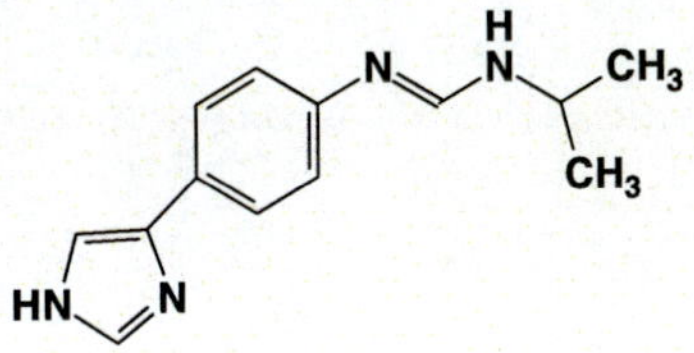

Mifentidine

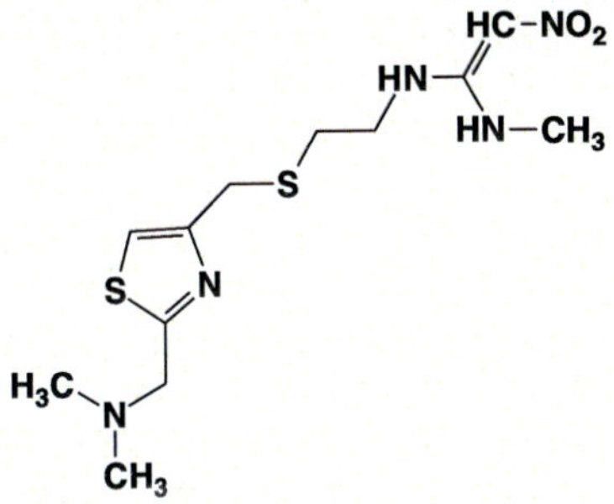

Nizatidine

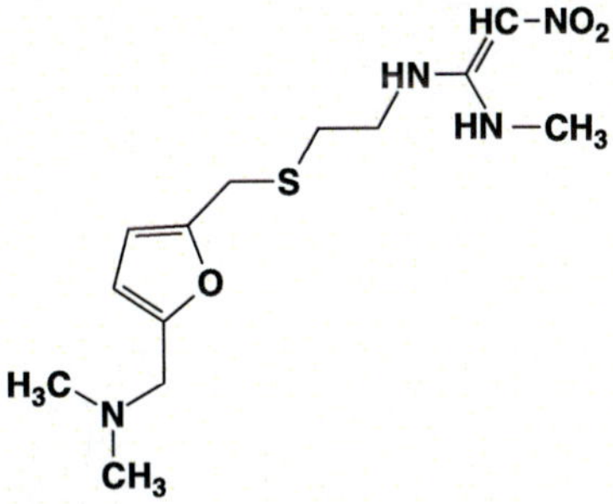

Ranitidine

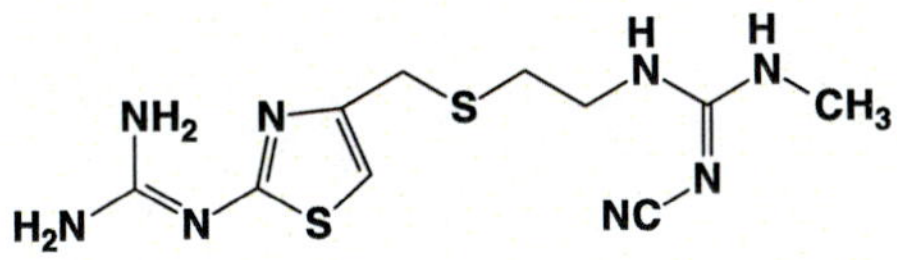

Titotidine

Fig. 4.4 Chemical structures of some histamine H2-receptor antagonists

canine, human, guinea pig or 358 amino acids for rat receptor protein which has the general properties of a G-protein-coupled receptor (GPCR) (Table 4.2). The radioligand binding studies using [125I]iodoaminopotentidine were attempted to show the expression of rat and human H2R proteins in CHO cells and revealed the expected pharmacological specificity as shown in Table 4.1 (Shahid et al. 2009). Chromosomal mapping studies have demonstrated that the H2R gene is localized to human chromosome 5 (Shahid et al. 2009). Birdsall (1991) has compared H2R sequence with other biogenic amine G-protein coupled receptors (GPCRs), and demonstrated that an aspartate in transmembrane (TM) domain 3 and an aspartate and threonine residue in TM 5 were more responsible for histamine binding. Replacement of aspartate (98) by an asparagine residue in the canine H2-receptor results in a receptor that does not bind the antagonist tiotidine and does not stimulate cAMP accumulation in response to histamine (Gantz et al. 1992, Hill et al. 1997). On changing the aspirate (186) residue of TM 5 to an alanine residue,

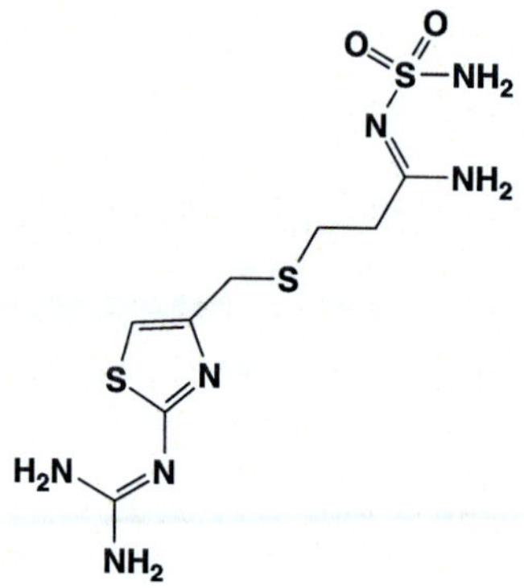

Famotidine

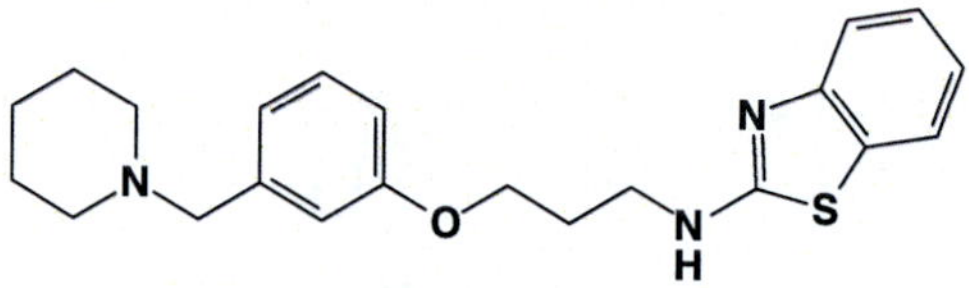

Zolantidine

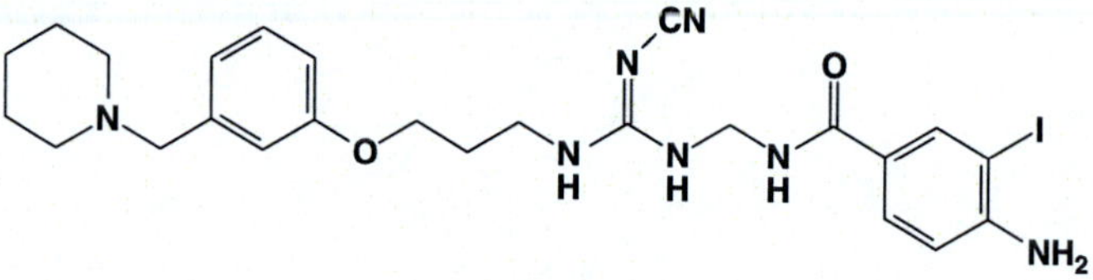

Iodoaminopotentidine

Fig. 4.4 (continued)

there occurs complete loss of the antagonist titotidine binding without affecting the EC 50 for cAMP formation in response to histamine stimulation. Changing the threonine (190) residue to an alanine residue, resulted in a lower K_D for titotidine antagonist and also a reduction in both the histamine EC 50 value and maximal cAMP response (Gantz et al. 1992). Mutation of Asp (186) and Gly (187) residue in the canine histamine H2-receptor to Ala (186) and Ser (187) residue produces a bifunctional receptor, which can be activated through adrenaline, and inhibited via both cimetidine and propranolol (Delvalle et al. 1995). These results indicate that pharmacological specificity of the H2R resides in only limited key amino acid residues.

4.2.2.3 Signaling Mechanisms

H2R is coupled both to adenylate cyclase and phosphoinositide second messenger systems via separate GTP-dependent mechanisms. Receptor binding stimulates

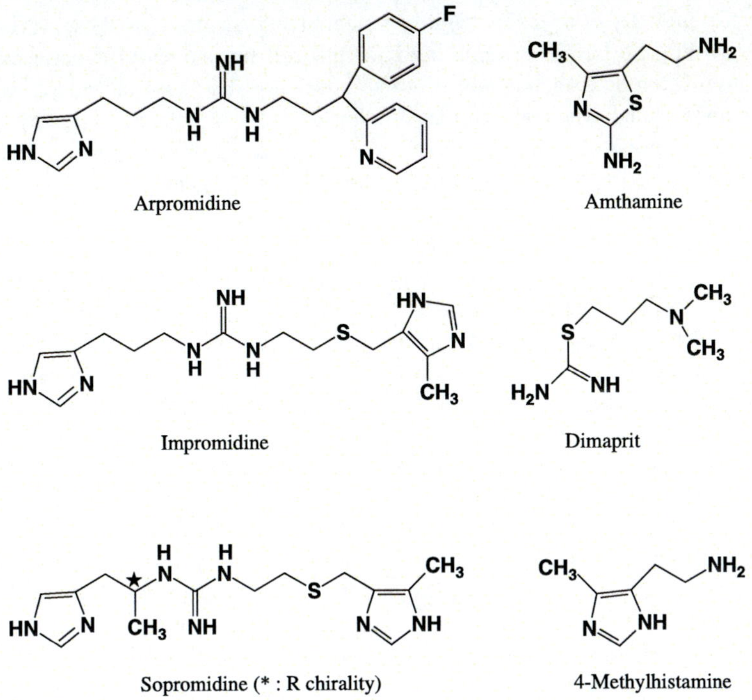

Fig. 4.5 Chemical structures of some histamine H2-receptor agonist

activation of c-Fos, c-Jun, protein kinase C (PKC) and p70 S6 kinase (Shahid et al. 2009) see in Fig. 4.3. Histamine was shown to be a highly potent stimulant of cAMP accumulation in various cells, and H2R-dependent impacts of histamine were predominantly mediated through cAMP, particularly those of central nervous system (CNS) origin (Shahid et al. 2009). Thus, H2R-mediated impacts on cAMP accumulation have been well documented and demonstrated in brain slices, gastric mucosa, fat cells, cardiac myocytes, vascular smooth muscle, basophils and neutrophils (Batzri et al. 1982, Gespach and Abita 1982, Shahid et al. 2009). In addition, H2R-mediated cAMP accumulation had been observed in Chinese hamster ovary (CHO) cells transfected with the rat, canine, or human H2R cDNA (Leurs et al. 1994, Shahid et al. 2009). In both brain and cardiac muscle membranes, the direct stimulation of adenylyl cyclase activity in cell free preparations had been detected (Newton et al. 1982, Olianas et al. 1984).

However, Hill (1990) has suggested used for caution in interpretation of receptor characterization studies using histamine-stimulated adenylyl cyclase activity alone. A most striking feature of studies of H2R-stimulated adenylyl cyclase activity in membrane preparations was the potent antagonism demonstrated with certain neuroleptics and antidepressants (Green 1983). In intact cellular systems, most of the neuroleptics and antidepressants were approximately 2 orders of magnitude weaker as antagonists of histamine-stimulated cAMP accumulation (Kamba and Richelson

1983, Kitbunnadaj 2005). One highly potential explanation for these variations resides within the buffer systems used for the cell-free adenylyl cyclase assays, and some differences in potency of some antidepressants and neuroleptics have been demonstrated when membrane binding of H2Rs has been evaluated using [125I]iodoaminopotentidine (Table 4.1) (Shahid et al. 2009). However, the variations observed in the Ki values deduced from studies of ligand binding in different buffers are not as large as the variations in K_B values obtained from functional studies. For example, in the case of amitriptyline, no difference was observed in binding affinity in Krebs and Tris buffers (Traiffort et al. 1991). In addition to Gs-coupling to adenylyl cyclase, H2Rs are coupled to other signaling systems also. For example, H2R stimulation has been demonstrated to enhance the intracellular free concentration of calcium (Ca^{2+}) ions in gastric parietal cells (Chew and Petropoulos 1991, Delvalle et al. 1992a). In some cell systems, $G\alpha_q$ coupling to PLC and intracellular Ca^{2+} had been demonstrated (Table 4.2). In HL-60 cells, a similar calcium (Ca^{2+}) response to H2R stimulation had been demonstrated (Seifert et al. 1992), and same case was observed in hepatoma-derived cells transfected with the canine H2Rs cDNA (Delvalle et al. 1992b). The influence on $[Ca^{2+}]i$ was accompanied by both an increase in inositol trisphosphate accumulation and a stimulation of cAMP accumulation in these cells (Shahid et al. 2009). Both the H2R-stimulated calcium and inositol trisphosphate responses were inhibited by cholera toxin treatment, whereas cholera toxin produced the expected increase in cAMP levels (Shahid et al. 2009). H2Rs release Ca^{2+} from intracellular calcium stores in single parietal cells (Negulescu and Machen 1988) and no effect of H2R agonists was observed on intracellular calcium levels or inositol phosphate accumulation in CHO cells transfected with the H2R of human. Thus, the effect of H2R stimulation on intracellular Ca^{2+} signaling may be highly cell-specific (Shahid et al. 2009).

The stimulation of H2R produces both inhibition of P2u-receptor-mediated arachidonic acid release and an increase in cAMP accumulation in CHO cells transfected with the rat H2R (Traiffort et al. 1992a). Traiffort et al. (1992b) has demonstrated that the effect on phospholipase A2 activity (i.e., arachidonic acid release) is not mimicked by forskolin, PGE1, or 8-bromo-cAMP, suggesting a mechanism of activation that is independent of cAMP-mediated protein kinase A activity. However, inhibitory effects of H2R stimulation were observed on phospholipase A2 activity in CHO cells transfected with the human H2R. Thus, these cAMP-independent effects might depend on the level of receptor expression or subtle differences between clonal cell lines (Shahid et al. 2009).

4.2.3 Histamine H3-Receptor

4.2.3.1 Cellular Distribution and Functional Characterization

The neurotransmitter function of histamine was established with the discovery of the H3R. This involves brain functions, as well as the peripheral effect of histamine on mast cells via H3Rs, that might be connected to a local neuron-mast cell interaction

(Dimitriadou et al. 1994). Its involvement in cognition, sleep-wake status, energy homeostatic regulation and inflammation led to research as therapeutic approaches mainly for central diseases (Hancock and Brune 2005, Passani et al. 2004). A recent study reported that H3R is presynaptically located as on autoreceptor controlling the synthesis and release of histamine (Leurs et al. 2005). This H3-autoreceptor activation stimulates the negative feedback mechanism that reduces central histaminergic activity (Teuscher et al. 2007). H3R's heterogeneity in binding and its functional studies has been well documented, which suggests more than one H3R subtype. This has been confirmed by demonstration of several H3R variants, generated from the complex H3R gene by alternative splicing. The three functional isoforms have been found in the rat, and they all vary in length of the 3rd intracellular loop, their distinct central nervous system (CNS) localization, and differential coupling to adenylate cyclase and MAPK signaling. Similar results were obtained for humans (Cogé et al. 2001, Drutel et al. 2001, Wellendorph et al. 2002).

Thus, numerous isoforms found in different species and different tissues lead to the assumption that fine-tuning of signaling may be controlled via receptor oligomerization or formation of isoforms (Bongers et al. 2007).

H3R is anatomically localized primarily to the CNS with prominent expression in basal ganglia, cortex hippocampus and striatal area. In the periphery, H3R can be found with low density in gastrointestinal, bronchial and cardiovascular system (Stark 2007). The high apparent affinity of *R*-(α)-methylhistamine for the H3R has enabled the use of this compound as a radiolabeled probe (Table 4.1) (Arrang et al. 1987). In rat cerebral cortical membranes, this compound (*R*-(α)-methylhistamine) has been used to identify a single binding site, which has the important pharmacological characteristics of the H3R (Arrang et al. 1990). In rat brain membranes, [3H]*R*-(α)-methylhistamine binds with high affinity (K_D 50.3 nM), although its binding capacity is low (~30 fmol/mg protein) (Shahid et al. 2009). The autoradiographic studies with [3H]*R*-(α)-methylhistamine have described the presence of specific thioperamide-inhibitable binding in several rat brain regions, especially cerebral cortex, striatum, hippocampus, olfactory nucleus, and the bed nuclei of the stria terminalis, which receive ascending histaminergic projections from the magnocellular nuclei of the posterior hypothalamus (Pollard et al. 1993, Shahid et al. 2009). In human brain and the brain of nonhuman primates, the H3Rs have also been visualized (Martinez-Mir et al. 1990). H3R binding has been characterized using [3H]*R*-(α)-methylhistamine in guinea pig lung (Arrang et al. 1987), guinea pig cerebral cortical membranes (Kilpatrick and Michel 1991), guinea pig intestine and guinea pig pancreas (Korte et al. 1990). *N*α-methylhistamine has been useful as a radiolabeled probe for the H3R (Table 4.1). The relative agonist activity of *N*α-methylhistamine (with respect to histamine) was significantly similar for all three histamine receptor (HRs) subtypes, but the binding affinity of histamine and *N*α-methylhistamine for the H3R was several orders of magnitude higher than for either H1- or H2-receptors (Shahid et al. 2009). Nα-methylhistamine can identify high-affinity H3R sites in both rat and guinea pig brain (Clark and Hill 1995, Korte et al. 1990, West et al. 1990). The binding of H3-receptor-agonists to H3Rs in brain tissues was found to be regulated by guanine nucleotides, implying its relation to heterotrimeric G-proteins (Zweig et al. 1992). Also the binding of H3R agonists appears to be affected by several cations. For example magnesium (Mg^{2+}) and sodium (Na^+) ions inhibit [3H]*R*-(α)-methylhistamine binding in guinea pig and rat brain, and the presence of calcium (Ca^{2+}) ions has been shown to reveal heterogeneity of agonist binding (Shahid et al. 2009). It is important to note that the inhibitory effect of sodium (Na^{2+}) ions on agonist binding means higher B_{max} values that were usually obtained in sodium-free Tris buffers compared with the Na/K phosphate buffers (Clark and Hill 1995). The multiple histamine H3R subtypes exist in rat brain (termed H_{3A} and H_{3B}) on the basis of [^{3}H]N^{α}-methylhistamine binding in rat cerebral cortical membranes in 50 mM Tris buffer (Table 4.1) (West et al. 1990). Based on these conditions, the selective histamine H3-antagonist thioperamide can discriminate two affinity-binding states (West et al. 1990). Heterogeneity of thioperamide binding is sodium (Na^{2+}) ion concentration dependent or depends on guanine nucleotides within the incubation medium. Thus, in the presence of 100 mM sodium chloride, thioperamide binding conforms to a single binding isotherm, and H3R can exist in different conformations which thioperamide, but not agonists or other H3R-antagonists (clobenpropit) can discriminate. This suggests that the equilibrium between these conformations is altered by guanine nucleotides or sodium (Na^{2+}) ions (Shahid et al. 2009). If this speculation is correct, it is likely that the different binding sites represented resting, active, or G-protein-coupled conformations of the H3R. Furthermore, if thioperamide preferentially binds to uncoupled receptors, then this compound should exhibit negative efficacy in functional assays. Radiolabeled H3R antagonist [125I]iodophenpropit, has been used to label histamine H3Rs in rat brain membranes (Table 4.1) (Jansen et al. 1992). The inhibition curves for iodophenpropit and thioperamide were consistent with interaction with a single binding site, but H3R agonists were found to be able to discriminate both high-[4 nM for *R*-(α)-methylhistamine] and low-[0.2 mM for *R*-(α)-methylhistamine] affinity binding sites (Jansen et al. 1992). [^{3}H]GR16820 and [125I]iodoproxyfan have been useful as high-affinity radiolabeled H3R-antagonists (Brown et al. 1994, Ligneau et al. 1994). In rat striatum, in the IUPHAR classification of histamine receptors 267 guanine nucleotides such as guanosine 59*O*-(3-thiotriphosphate) (GTPgS), 40% of the binding sites exhibited a 40-fold lower affinity for H3-agonists, providing further evidence for a potential linkage of H3Rs to G-proteins (Shahid et al. 2009). In rat brain membranes, [^{3}H]thioperamide and [^{3}H]5-methylthioperamide, have both been used to label H3R. However, [^{3}H]thioperamide was shown to bind additionally to low affinity, high-capacity, non H3R sites (Alves-Rodrigues et al. 1996). The localization of H3Rs is based on functional studies, primarily involving inhibition of neurotransmitter release. The H3R was first characterized as an auto receptor regulating histamine synthesis and release from rat cerebral hippocampus, cortex, and striatum. The H3R-mediated inhibition of histamine release has also been demonstrated in human cerebral cortex (Arrang et al. 1988). Differences in the distribution of H3R binding sites and the levels of histidine decarboxylase (an index of histaminergic nerve terminals) suggested at an early stage that H3Rs are not confined to histamine-containing neurons within the mammalian CNS (Van der Werf and Timmerman

1989). It has been demonstrated that H3Rs can regulate neurotransmitter release in mammalian brain as serotonergic, noradrenergic, cholinergic, and dopaminergic (Clapham and Kilpatrick 1992, Schlicker et al. 1989, 1992, 1993). H3R activation inhibits the firing of the histamine-neurons in the posterior hypothalamus by a mechanism different from auto-receptor functions found on other aminergic nuclei, and is presumably a block of Ca^{2+} current (Haas 1992). H3Rs were found to regulate the release of sympathetic neurotransmitters in guinea pig mesenteric artery, human saphenous vein, guinea pig atria, and human heart (Endou et al. 1994, Imamura et al. 1994, 1995, Ishikawa and Sperelakis 1987, Molderings et al. 1992).

An important inhibitory effect of H3R activation on release of neuropeptides (tachykinins or calcitonin gene-related peptide) from sensory C fibers has been reported from airways, meninges, skin, and heart (Ichinose et al. 1990, Imamura et al. 1996, Matsubara et al. 1992, Ohkubo and Shibata 1995). The modulation of acetylcholine, capsaicin, and substance P effects by H3Rs in isolated perfused rabbit lungs has also been reported (Delaunois et al. 1995). There is evidence that H3R activation can inhibit the release of neurotransmitters from nonadrenergic- noncholinergic nerves in guinea pig bronchioles and ileum (Burgaud and Oudart 1994, Taylor and Kilpatrick 1992). In guinea pig ileum, the H3R-antagonists betahistine and phenylbutanoylhistamine were much less potent as inhibitors of H3R-mediated effects on nonadrenergic-noncholinergic transmission than they were as antagonists of histamine release in rat cerebral cortex (Taylor and Kilpatrick 1992).

A similar low potency has been reported for betahistine and phenylbutanoyl (histamine antagonists) for antagonism of H3R-mediated [^{3}H]acetylcholine release from rat entorhinal cortex (Clapham and Kilpatrick 1992), and antagonism of H3R-mediated 5-hydroxytryptamine release from porcine enterochromaffin cells (Schworer et al. 1994). These investigations provide support for the potential existence of distinct H3R subtypes. In addition, it has been shown that phenylbutanoylhistamine can inhibit [^{3}H]acetylcholine release from rat entorhinal cortex slices, and synaptosomes by a nonhistamine receptor mechanism (Arrang et al. 1995). Therefore, the potency of phenylbutanoylhistamine as H3R-antagonist in those preparations can be highly underestimated because of the additional nonspecific activities of the drug (Arrang et al. 1995). The inhibitory effect of H3-receptor stimulation on 5-HT release from porcine enterochromaffin cells in strips of small intestine (Schworer et al. 1994) provides evidence for H3-receptors regulating secretory mechanisms in non-neuronal cells. Hence, it can be concluded that H3R may be present in gastric mast cells or enterochromaffin cells and exerts an inhibitory effect on histamine release and gastric acid secretion. In conscious dogs, H3R activation had been observed to inhibit gastric acid secretion (Soldani et al. 1993). The H3R relaxes rabbit middle cerebral artery by an endothelium-dependent pathway involving both nitric oxide and prostanoid release (Ea Kim and Oudart 1988). H3-receptor stimulation can activate adrenocorticotropic hormone release from the pituitary cell line AtT-20 (Clark et al. 1992). Therefore, H3R provides constitutive properties, which means part of the receptor population spontaneously undergoes allosteric transition leading to a conformation, to which G protein can bind, and also H3R-knock out mice manifest an obese phenotype (characterized by increased body weight, food intake, adiposity, and reduced energy expenditure) (Morisset et al. 2000, Rouleau et al. 2002). Recently, it has been observed that H3R expresses insulin and leptin resistance as well as a diminution of the energy homeostasis-associated genes UCP1 and UCP3 (Takahashi et al. 2002). The chemical structure of specific H3R-antagonists and -agonists are shown in Figs. 4.6 and 4.7.

4.2.3.2 Structural Biology of Receptor

H3R is G protein-coupled receptor (GPCR) and has been cloned (Shahid et al. 2009). Its gene consists of 4 exons spanning 5.5 kb on chromosome 20 (20q13.33) in humans (Table 4.2). Structural studies of H3R are very limited and there are only few reports on its purification studies. By using [^{3}H]histamine as a radioligand, the solubilization of a H3R protein from bovine whole brain has been reported. Size-exclusion chromatography has revealed an apparent molecular mass of 220 kDa. However, because the solubilized receptor retained its guanine nucleotide sensitivity

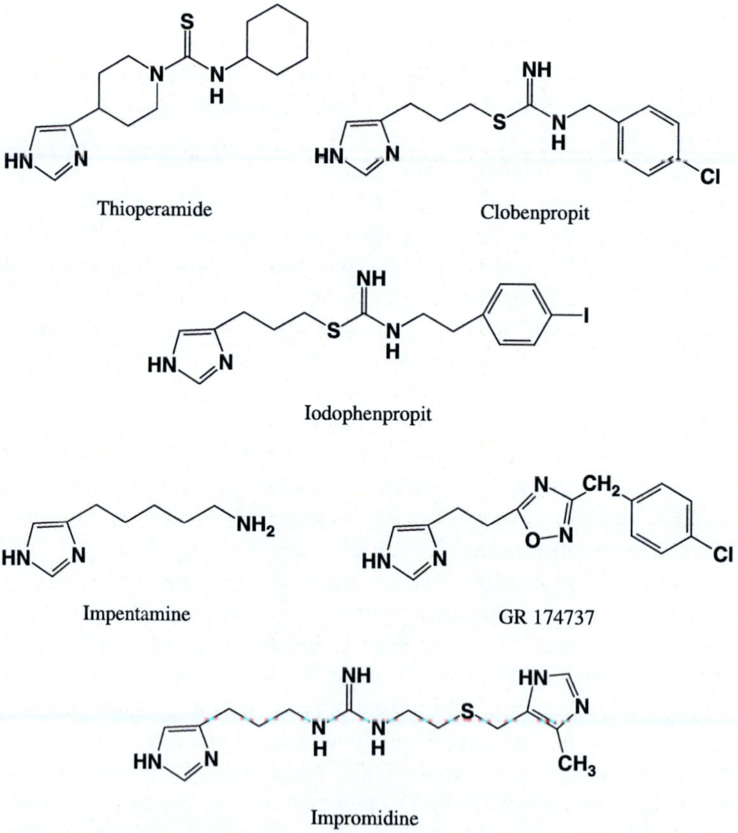

Fig. 4.6 Chemical structures of some histamine H3-receptor antagonists

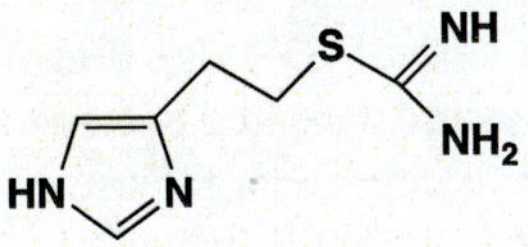

Imetit

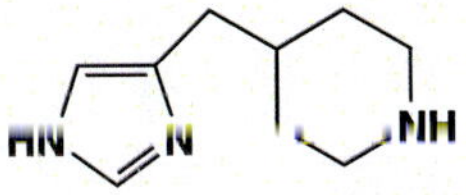

Immepip

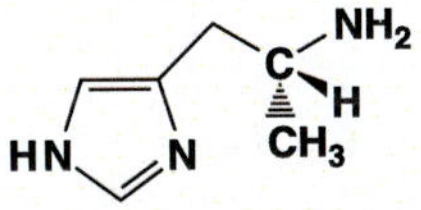

(R)-α-Methylhistamine

Fig. 4.7 Chemical structures of some histamine H3-receptor agonists

and it is likely that the molecular mass of 220 kDa represents a complex of receptor, G-protein, and digitonin (Shahid et al. 2009). Cherifi et al. (1992) have reported the solubilization (with Triton X-100) and purification of the H3-receptor protein from the human gastric tumoral cell line HGT-1. After gel filtration and sepharose-thioperamide affinity chromatography, protein has been purified with a molecular mass of approximately 70 kDa (see Table 4.2).

4.2.3.3 Signaling Mechanisms

The signal mechanisms used by the H3R remain largely subject to speculation, but there is increasing evidence to suggest that this receptor belongs to the G-protein-coupled receptors (Gi/o) (Table 4.2), and its activation leads to inhibition of cAMP formation, accumulation of Ca^{2+} and stimulation of mitogen-activated protein kinase (MAPK) pathway (Shahid et al. 2009), see Fig. 4.3. This evidence has been obtained from ligand-binding studies that involve the modulation by guanine nucleotides of H3R-agonist binding and inhibition of H3R-antagonist binding (Jansen et al. 1994, Shahid et al. 2009). The direct evidence for a functional H3R-G-protein linkage came from studies of [^{35}S]GTPgS binding to rat cerebral cortical membranes (Clark and Hill 1996). In rat cerebral cortical membranes, the presence of H1R- and H2R-antagonists (0.1 mM mepyramine and 10 mM titotidine), and both *R*-(α)-methylhistamine and *N*-(α)-methylhistamine generated a concentration dependent stimulation of [35S]GTPgS binding (EC_{50} = 0.4 and 0.2 nM) (Clark and Hill 1996). Notably, this response was inhibited by pretreatment of membranes with pertussis toxin, implying a direct coupling to a Gi or Go protein (Clark and Hill 1996). The evidence of pertussis toxin-sensitive G-proteins in the response to

H3R stimulation came from studies of H3R signaling in human and guinea pig heart (Shahid et al. 2009). H3R-activation appeared to lead to an inhibition of N-type Ca^{2+} channels responsible for voltage dependent release of noradrenaline in human and guinea pig heart, but several investigations have failed to demonstrate an inhibition of adenylyl cyclase activity in different tissues and cells, which suggest that H3Rs couple to Go proteins (Schlicker et al. 1991, Shahid et al. 2009).

4.2.4 Histamine H4-Receptor

4.2.4.1 Cellular Distribution and Functional Characterization

The discovery of the H4-receptor adds a new chapter to the histamine story. The H4R is preferentially expressed in intestinal tissue, spleen, thymus, medullary cells, bone marrow and peripheral hematopoietic cells, including eosinophils, basophils, mast cells, T lymphocytes, leukocytes and dendritic cells (Shahid et al. 2009). However, moderate positive signals have also been detected in brain, spleen, thymus, small intestine, colon, heart, liver and lung. Although expression studies did not demonstrate H4Rs in the central nervous system (CNS), in situ hybridization studies suggested evidence for their localization human brain in low density (Shahid et al. 2009). The relatively restricted expression of the H4R provides an important role in inflammation, hematopoiesis and immunity by the regulation of H4R expression via stimuli such as IFN, TNF-α and IL-6, IL-10, and IL-13. Basophils and mast cells express H4R-mRNA. The H4R mediates chemotaxis of mast cells and eosinophils as well as controls cytokine release from dendritic cells and T-cells (Shahid et al. 2009).

H4R participates along with the H2R, in the control of IL-16 release from human lymphocytes. The H4R selective antagonist might be useful as anti-inflammatory agents in asthma, arthritis, colitis and pruritis (Shahid et al. 2009). Antagonists, such as JNJ 7777120, have been shown to be effective in various model of inflammation. At this point, very little is known about the biological functions of H4R. There are few reports in the literature, providing evidence for its role in chemotactic activity in mast cells and eosinophils or control of IL-16 production by $CD8^+$ lymphocytes (Shahid et al. 2009). A recent study showed the role of H4R in mast cell, eosinophil, and T cell function, as well as the effects of its antagonist, JNJ 7777120, in a mouse peritonitis model pointing to a more general role for H4R in inflammation. In many diseases such as allergic rhinitis, asthma, and rheumatoid arthritis, conditions where eosinophils and mast cells are involved, H4R antagonists have potential therapeutic utility (Thurmond et al. 2004). The discovery of H4R and its emerging role in inflammation had spurred new interest in the functions of histamine in inflammation, allergy and autoimmune diseases. Early results in animal models suggest that H4R antagonists may have utility in treating various conditions in humans, in particular, in diseases in which histamine is known to be present and H1R antagonists are not clinically effective (Thurmond et al. 2008). Obviously, a better functional characterization of H4R will be possible by new, specific tools,

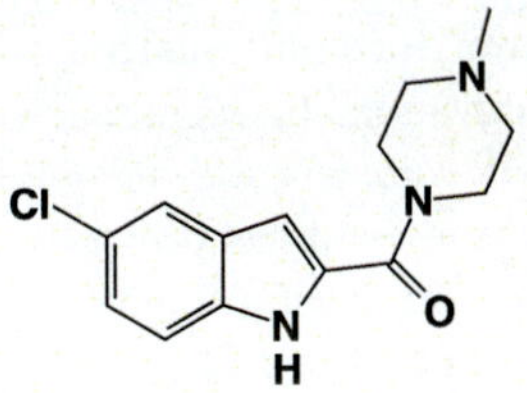

JNJ 7777120

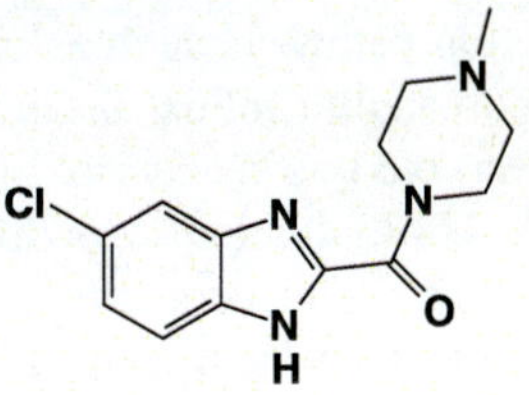

JNJ 10191584

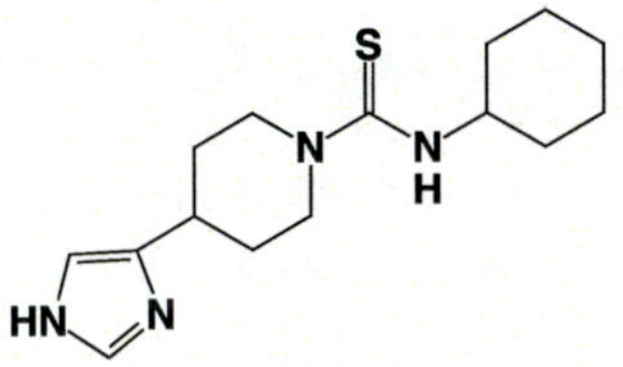

Thioperamide (partial H4R-antagonist)

H4-receptor antagonists

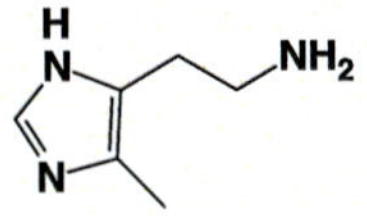

4-Methylhistamine

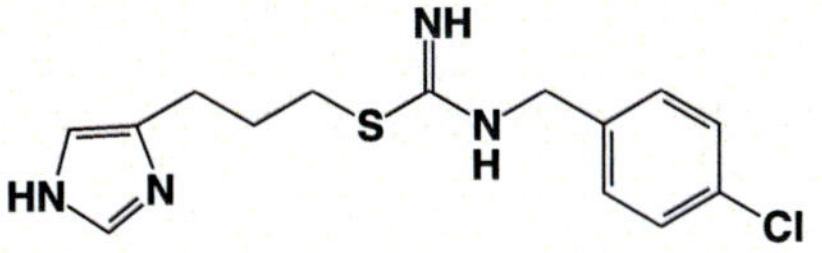

Clobenpropit (partial H4R-agonist)

H4-receptor agonists

Fig. 4.8 Chemical structures of specific H4-receptor-antagonists and -agonists

such as the recently developed potent and selective non-imidazol H4R antagonist (Thurmond et al. 2004). The chemical structure of specific H4R-antagonists and -agonists are shown in Fig. 4.8.

4.2.4.2 Structural Biology of Receptor

The human H4-receptor gene was mapped to chromosome 18q11.2 which encodes a 390 amino acid and related to G-protein coupled receptor (GPCR). It shares 37–43% homology (58% in transmembrane regions) with the H3-receptor and is similar in genomic structure (Shahid et al. 2009). The H4R gene spans more than 21 kbp and contains three exons, separated by two large introns (>7 kb) (Table 4.1) with large interspecies variations from 65 to 72% homology in sequences. Analysis of the 5′ flanking region did not reveal the canonical TATA or CAAT-boxes. The promoter region contains several putative regulatory elements involved in proinflammatory cytokine signaling pathways. H4Rs are coupled to Gi/o, which initiates various transduction pathways such as inhibition of forskolin-induced cAMP formation, enhanced calcium influx and MAPK activation. In accordance with the homology between the two receptors, several H3R-agonists and antagonists were recognized by the H4R, although with different affinities. It has been observed that H3R-agonist *R*-α-methyl histamine acts on H4R with several hundred times less potency. Similar effect has been seen with thioperamide, the classical H3R antagonist which also behaves like a H4R antagonist (Table 4.1), of much lower affinity. Clobenpropit, also a H3R antagonist, exerts agonistic activity on H4R (Shahid et al. 2009).

Histamine binding to H4R is very similar to that reported for the other histamine receptors which show the significance of the Asp94 residue in transmembrane region (TM) 3 and the Glu 182 residue in the TM 5. However, some differences exist and these were exploited to design specific tools. Mouse, rat and guinea pig H4Rs have been cloned and characterized and were found to be only 68, 69, and 65% homologous respectively to their human counterparts. These studies have revealed substantial pharmacological variations between species, with higher affinity of histamine for human and guinea pig receptors than for their rat and mouse equivalents (Liu et al. 2001a, b, Shahid et al. 2009).

4.2.4.3 Signaling Mechanisms

The signal mechanisms used by the H4R are related to the G-protein-coupled receptors (Gi/o), and its activation leads to an inhibition of adenylyl cyclase and downstream of cAMP responsive elements (CRE) as well as activation of mitogen-activated protein kinase (MAPK) and phospholipase C with Ca^{2+} mobilization (Table 4.2); see Fig. 4.3 (Shahid et al. 2009).

4.3 Histamine: Non-Classical Binding Sites

4.3.1 Cytochrome P450

The human cytochrome P450 (CYP450) superfamily comprises 57 genes encoding heme-containing enzymes, which are found in the liver as well as in extrahepatic tissues (adrenals, and peripheral blood leukocytes), where they can be stimulated by various stimuli (Mahnke et al. 1996, Morgan 2001), see Fig. 4.9. They are not only involved in metabolism of large number of foreign substances, but also play an important role in diverse physiological processes [generation, transformation or inactivation of endogenous ligands (steroids and lipids)], which are involved in cell regulation (Nebert and Russell 2002).

Binding of histamine to CYP450 had been shown by Branders, who proposed a second messenger role for intracellular histamine via this binding site. This hypothesis is mainly based on a finding that *N*, *N* diethyl-2-(4-(phenylmethyl)phenoxy)

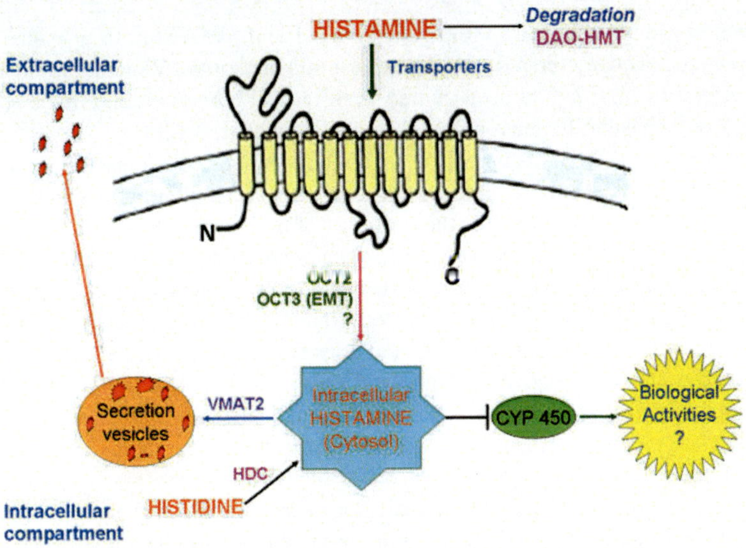

Fig. 4.9 The non-classical histamine binding sites and their main signaling pathways such as DAO: diamine oxidase; HMT: histamine methyl transferase; OCT: organic cation transporter; HDC: histidine decarboxylase; CYP 450: cytochrome P450; VMAT: vesicular monoamine transporter. (Adapted from Shahid et al. 2009)

ethanamine (DPPE), an arylalkylamine analogue of tamoxifen inhibits the binding of histamine to CYP450 (Brandes et al. 2002). DPPE allosterically modifies histamine binding to the heme moiety of CYP450 enzymes and inhibits platelet aggregation, as well as lymphocyte and hematopoietic progenitor proliferation (Labella and Brandes 2000). The effect of DPPE on histamine binding was found to be highly complicated and depends on the nature of the P450 enzymes. Thus, it inhibits the action of histamine on CYP2D6 and CYP1A1, enhances its effect on CYP3A4 and does not affect CYP2B6 (Brandes et al. 2000). The heme moiety of CYP450 binds to several histamine antagonists (Hamelin et al. 1998, Kishimoto et al. 1997), particularly H3R antagonists (thioperamide, clobenpropit and ciproxyfan) (Kishimoto et al. 1997). This property explains some effects of these antagonists, when used at high doses. Notably, histamine interacts with CYP450 and it has been demonstrated that CYP2E1 and CYP3A were upregulated in histidine decarboxylase (HDC)-deficient mice (Tamasi et al. 2003).

4.3.2 Transporters of Histamine

Histamine (2-(1H-imidazol-4-yl) ethanamine) is synthesized in the cytosol and requires a specific transport into secretory vesicles where it is sequestered. Vesicular monoamine transporters (VMATs) are proteins, which accomplish this specific task for several neurotransmitters (Erickson and Varoqui 2000), see Fig. 4.9. The two subtypes of monoamine transporters are VMAT1 and VMAT2 both of which have been cloned and characterized. VMAT2 transports histamine. Vesicular monoamine transporter 2 (VMAT2) had been cloned from rat and human brain, bovine adrenal medulla and a basophilic leukemia cell line (Shahid et al. 2009).

The increased VMAT2 expression in IL-3-dependent cell lines was seen with enhanced histamine synthesis in response to calcium (Ca^{2+})ionophore (Watson et al. 1999). VMAT2 is responsible for the transport of histamine into secretory granules of enterochromaffin-like (ECL) cells. The gene expression of VMAT2 was found to be modulated by cytokines, either positively (TGFα) or negatively (IL-1 and TNF-α) (Kazumori et al. 2004). VMAT2-deleted granules do not release histamine upon activation, even though granule cell fusion does still occur (Travis et al. 2000). The bone marrow-derived mast cells from histidine decarboxylase (HDC)-deleted mice are completely devoid of endogenous histamine but can take up the mediator from histamine-supplemented medium and store it in secretory granules (Shahid et al. 2009). Hence, two transporters are essential to: (i) insure the passage across the plasma membrane, and (ii) cross the vesicular membrane (Shahid et al. 2009). First transporter has not been identified yet, but the second transporter seems to be vesicular monoamine transporter 2 (VMAT2). The non-neuronal monoamine transporters that actively remove monoamines from extracellular space have been described as organic cation transporter 1 (OCT1), OCT2, and extraneuronal monoamine transporter (EMT). EMT was also designated as OCT3. The expression of OCT1 was found to be restricted to liver, kidney and intestine, OCT2 to brain and kidney, while EMT showed a broad tissue distribution. It has been established that OCT1 cannot transport histamine, compared to OCT2 and EMT for which it is a good substrate (Gründemann et al. 1999). Thus, EMT appeared to be a good candidate as histamine transporter in mast cells and basophils, accounting for their capacity to take up the mediator from the environment (Shahid et al. 2009).

4.4 Concluding Remarks

Histamine receptors have been important drug targets for many years. Their physiological and pathological relevance and distribution in various tissues are being documented. The exact role of histamine receptors in immunomodulation is still unclear. The scope of histamine research includes immune responses of both the Th1 and Th2 lymphocytes. The newly discovered H4-receptor plays an important role in inflammation and has opened potential way for the function of histamine in inflammation, allergy and autoimmune diseases. Using known receptor agonists and antagonists, many researchers including some of the authors are involved in understanding and enhancing the therapeutic options involving histamine molecule that has been studied for over 100 years.

Acknowledgments Trivendra Tripathi acknowledges University Grants Commission, New Delhi, India for providing UGC Fellowship [UGC letter DON F. 19-33/2006 (CU)] and M. Shahid is grateful to Department of Science & Technology, Ministry of Science and Technology, Government of India for awarding "Young Scientist Project Award" (FT/SR-L-111/2006).

References

Al-Gadi M, Hill SJ (1985) Characterization of histamine receptors mediating the stimulation of cyclic AMP accumulation in rabbit cerebral cortical slices. Br J Pharmacol 85:877–888

Al-Gadi M, Hill SJ (1987) The role of calcium in the cyclic AMP response to histamine in rabbit cerebral cortical slices. Br J Pharmacol 91:213–222

Alves-Rodrigues A, Leurs R, Tin-Seng WU et al (1996) 3H-Thioperamide as a radioligand for the histamine H3-receptor in rat cerebral cortex. Br J Pharmacol 118:2045–2052

Arias-Montano JA, Young JM (1993) Characteristics of histamine H1-receptors on HeLa cells. Eur J Pharmacol Mol Pharmacol Sect 245:291–296

Arrang JM, Devaux B, Chodkiewicz JP et al (1988) H3-receptors control histamine release in human brain. J Neurochem 51:105–108

Arrang JM, Drutel G, Schwartz JC (1995) Characterization of histamine *H*3-receptors regulating acetylcholine release in rat entorhinal cortex. Br J Pharmacol 114:1518–1522

Arrang JM, Garbarg M, Lancelot JC et al (1987) Highly potent and selective ligands for histamine H3-receptors. Nature (Lond) 327:117–123

Arrang JM, Roy J, Morgat JL et al (1990) Histamine H3-receptor binding sites in rat brain membranes: modulations by guanine nucleotides and divalent cations. Eur J Pharmacol 188:219–227

Ash ASF, Schild HO (1966) Receptors mediating some actions of histamine. Br J Pharmacol 27:427–439

Bailey SJ, Lippe IT, Holzer P (1987) Effect of the tachykinin antagonist [D-Pro4, D-Trp7,9,10] substance P-(4–11) on tachykinin- and histamine-induced inositol phosphate generation in intestinal smooth muscle. Naunyn-Schmiedeberg's Arch Pharmacol 335:296–300

Bakker RA, Schoonus SBJ, Smit MJ et al (2001) Histamine H1-receptor activation of nuclear factor-kB: roles for G gamma- and G alpha/11 subunits in constitutive and agonist mediated signaling. Mol Pharmacol 60:1133–1142

Bakker RA, Timmerman H, Leurs R (2002) Histamine receptors: specific ligands, receptor biochemistry, and signal transduction. Clin Allergy Immunol 17:27–64

Banu Y, Watanabe T (1999) Augmentation of antigen receptor-mediated responses by histamine H1 receptor signaling. J Exp Med 189:673–682

Batzri S, Harmon JW, Thompson WF (1982) Interaction of histamine with gastric mucosal cells: effect of histamine H2-antagonists on binding and biological response. Mol Pharmacol 22: 41–47

Birdsall NJM (1991) Cloning and structure: function of the H2 histamine receptor. Trends Pharmacol Sci 12:9–10

Black JW, Shankley NP (1985) The isolated stomach preparation of the iuphar classification of histamine receptors 271 mouse: a physiological unit for pharmacological analysis. Br J Pharmacol 86:571–579

Bommer M, Liebisch D, Kley N et al (1987) Histamine affects release and biosynthesis of opioid peptides primarily *via* H1-receptors in bovine chromaffin cells. J Neurochem 49:1688–1696

Bongers G, Bakker RA, Leurs R (2007) Molecular aspects of the histamine H3 receptor. Bio Pharmacol 73:1195–1204

Bouvet D, Staub AM (1937) Action protectrice des ethers phenoliques au cours de l'intoxication histaminique. Comp Rend Soc Biol 124:547–549

Brandes LJ, Queen GM, Labella FS (2000) N,N-Diethyl-2-[4-(phenylmethyl) phenoxy] ethanamide (DPPE), a chemopotentiating and cytoprotective agent in clinical trials: interaction with histamine at cytochrome P4503A4 and other isozymes that metabolize antineoplastic drugs. Cancer Chemother Pharmacol 45:298–304

Brandes LJ, Queen GM, Labella FS (2002) Displacement of histamine from liver cells and cell components by ligands for cytochrome P450. J Cell Biochem 85:820–824

Brown JD, O'Shaughnessy CT, Kilpatrick GJ et al (1994) Characterization of the specific binding of the histamine H3-receptor antagonist radioligand 3HGR16820. Br J Pharmacol 114:344

Bryce PJ, Mathias CB, Harrison KL et al (2006) The H1 histamine receptor regulates allergic lung responses. J Clin Invest 116:1624–1632

Bunn SJ, Sim ATR, Herd LM et al (1995) Tyrosine hydroxylase phosphorylation in bovine adrenal chromaffin cells: the role of intracellular Ca21 in the histamine H1-receptorstimulated phosphorylation of Ser (8), Ser (19), Ser (31) and Ser (40). J Neurochem 64: 1370–1378

Burgaud JL, Oudart N (1994) NG-Nitro-L-arginine methyl ester inhibits the effect of an *H*3-histaminergic receptor agonist on Nanc contraction in guinea- pig perfused bronchioles. J Pharm Pharmacol 46:153–155

Carter TD, Hallam TJ, Cusack NJ et al (1988) Regulation of P2ypurinoceptor-mediated prostacyclin release from human endothelial cells by cytoplasmic calcium concentration. Br J Pharmacol 95:1181–1190

Cherifi Y, Pigeon C, Le Romancer M et al (1992) Purification of histamine *H*3 receptor negatively coupled to phosphoinositide turnover in the human gastric cell line HGT1. J Biol Chem 267:25315–25320

Chew CS, Petropoulos AC (1991) Thapsigargin potentiates histamine stimulated HCl secretion in gastric parietal cells but does not mimic cholinergic responses. Cell Regul 2:27–39

Christian EP, Undem BJ, Weinreich D (1989) Endogenous histamine excites neurones in the guinea pig superior cervical ganglion *in vitro*. J Physiol 409:297–312

Clapham J, Kilpatrick GJ (1992) Histamine H3 receptors modulate the release of [3H]-acetylcholine from slices of rat entorhinal cortex: evidence for the possible existence of H3 receptor subtypes. Br J Pharmacol 107:919–923

Clark EA, Hill SJ (1995) Differential effect of sodium ions and guanine nucleotides on the binding of thioperamide and clobenpropit to histamine H3-receptors in rat cerebral cortical membranes. Br J Pharmacol 114:357–362

Clark EA, Hill SJ (1996) Sensitivity of histamine *H*3 receptor agonist stimulated [35S]-GTPgS binding to pertussis toxin. Eur J Pharmacol 296:223–225

Clark MA, Korte A, Myers J et al (1992) High affinity histamine *H*3 receptors regulate ACTH release by AtT-20 cells. Eur J Pharmacol 210:31–35

Claro E, Garcia A, Picacosta F (1987) Histamine-stimulated phosphoinositide hydrolysis in developing rat brain. Mol Pharmacol 32:384–390

Cogé F, Guénin SP, Audinot V et al (2001) Genomic organization and characterization of splice variants of the human histamine H3 receptor. Biochem J 355:279–288

Cogé F, Guénin SP, Rique H et al (2001) Structure and expression of the human histamine H4-receptor gene. Biochem Biophys Res Commun 284:301–309

De Backer MD, Gommeren W, Moereels H et al (1993) Genomic cloning, heterologous expression and pharmacological characterization of a human histamine H1-receptor. Biochem Biophys Res Commun 197:1601–1608

De Backer MD, Loonen I, Verhasselt P et al (1998) Structure of the human histamine H1 receptor gene. Biochem J 335:663–670

Delvalle J, Gantz I (1997) Novel insights into histamine H2 receptor biology. Am J Physiol 273:987–996

Delaunois A, Gustin P, Garbarg M et al (1995) Modulation of acetylcholine, capsaicin and substance P effects by histamine *H*3 receptors in isolated perfused rabbit lungs. Eur J Pharmacol 277:243–250

Delvalle J, Gantz I, Wang LD et al (1995) Construction of a novel bifunctional biogenic amine receptor *via* 2 point mutations of the H2-histamine receptor. Mol Med 1:280–286

Delvalle J, Tsunoda Y, Williams JA et al (1992a) Regulation of [Ca21]i by secretagogue stimulation of canine gastric parietal cells. Am J Physiol 262:G420–G426

Delvalle J, Wang L, Gantz I et al (1992b) Characterization of H2 histamine receptor: linkage to both adenylate cyclase and [Ca2+] signaling systems. Am J Physiol 263:G967–G972

Dickenson JM, Hill SJ (1994) Characteristics of 3H-mepyramine binding in DDT1 MF2 cells: evidence for high binding to a functional histamine H1 receptor. Eur J Pharmacol Mol Pharmacol Sect 268:257–262

Dimitriadou V, Rouleau A, Dam Trung Tuong M et al (1994) Functional relationship between mast cells and C-sensitive nerve fibres evidenced by H3-receptor modulation in rat lung and spleen. Clin Sci 87:151–163
Donaldson J, Brown AM, Hill SJ (1989) Temporal changes in the calcium dependence of the histamine H1-receptor-stimulation of the cyclic AMP accumulation in guinea-pig cerebral cortex. Br J Pharmacol 98:1365–1375
Drutel G, Peitsaro N, Karlstedt K et al (2001) Identification of rat H3 receptor isoforms with different brain expression and signaling properties. Mol Pharmacol 59:1–8
Dy M, Schneider E (2004) Histamine-cytokine connection in immunity and hematopoiesis. Cytokine Growth Factor Rev 15:393–410
Ea Kim L, Oudart N (1988) A highly potent and selective *H*3 agonist relaxes rabbit middle cerebral artery, *in vitro*. Eur J Pharmacol 150:393–396
Elz S, Kramer K, Pertz HH et al (2000) Histaprodifens: synthesis, pharmacological *in vitro* evaluation and molecular modeling of a new class of highly active and selective histamine (H1) receptor agonists. J Med Chem 43:1071–1084
Endou M, Poli E, Levi R (1994) Histamine H3-receptor signalling in the heart: possible involvement of Gi/Go proteins and N-type Ca21 channels. J Pharmacol Exp Ther 269:221–229
Erickson JD, Varoqui H (2000) Molecular analysis of vesicular amine transporter function and targeting to secretory organelles. FASEB J 14:2450–2458
Foreman JC, Norris DB, Rising TJ et al (1985) The binding of 3H-tiotidine to homogenates of guinea-pig lung parenchyma. Br J Pharmacol 86:475–482
Fujimoto K, Horio Y, Sugama K et al (1993) Genomic cloning of the rat histamine H1 receptor. Biochem Biophys Res Commun 190:294–301
Fukui H, Mizuguchi H, Lui YQ et al (1990) Purification of 3Hmepyramine receptor from rat liver and its amino acid sequence homology with debrisoquine-4-hydroxylase cytochrome P-450. Eur J Pharmacol 183:1727–1738
Fukushima Y, Oka Y, Saitoh T et al (1995) Structural and functional analysis of the canine histamine H2-receptor by site-directed mutagenesis: *N*-glycosylation is not vital for its action. Biochem J 310:553–558
Fumagalli F, Baiardini I, Pasquali M et al (2004) Antihistamines: do they work? Further well-controlled trials involving larger samples are needed. Allergy 59:74–77
Gajtkowski GA, Norris DB, Rising TJ et al (1983) Specific binding of [3H]-tiotidine to histamine H2-receptors in guinea pig cerebral cortex. Nature (Lond) 304:65–67
Gantz I, Delvalle J, Wang LD et al (1992) Molecular basis for the interaction of histamine with the histamine-H2 receptor. J Biol Chem 267:20840–20843
Gantz I, Munzert G, Tashiro T et al (1991a) Molecular cloning of the human histamine H2 receptor. Biochem Biophys Res Commun 178:1386–1392
Gantz I, Schäffer M, Del Valle J et al (1991b) Molecular cloning of a gene encoding the histamine H2 receptor. Proc Natl Acad Sci USA 88:429–433
Garbarg M, Schwartz JC (1988) Synergism between histamine H1- and H2-receptors in the cyclic AMP response in guinea-pig brain slices: effect of phorbol esters and calcium. Mol Pharmacol 33:38–43
Genovese A, Gross SS, Sakuma I et al (1988) Adenosine promotes histamine H1-mediated negative chronotropic and inotropic effects on human atrial myocardium. J Pharmacol Exp Ther 247:844–849
Gespach C, Abita JP (1982) Human polymorphonuclear neutrophils. Pharmacological characterisation of histamine receptors mediating the elevation of cyclic AMP. Mol Pharmacol 21:78–85
Green JP (1983) Histamine receptors in brain. Handb Psychopharmacol 17:385–420
Gründemann D, Liebich G, Kiefer N et al (1999) Selective substrates for non-neuronal monoamine transporters. Mol Pharmacol 56:1–10
Guo ZG, Levi R, Graver LM et al (1984) Inotropic effects of histamine in human myocardium: differentiation between positive and negative components. J Cardiovasc Pharmacol 6: 1210–1215

Haas H, Panula P (2003) The role of histamine and the tuberomamillary nucleus in the nervous system. Nat Rev Neurosci 4:121–130

Haas HL (1981) Histamine hyperpolarizes hippocampal neurones *in vitro*. Neurosci Lett 22:75–78

Haas HL (1992) Electrophysiology of histamine receptors. In: Schwartz JC, Haas HL (eds) The histamine receptor: receptor biochemistry and methodology. Wiley-Liss, New York, pp 161–177

Hamelin BA, Gouayad A, Drolet B et al (1998) *In vitro* characterization of cytochrome P450 2D6 inhibition by classic histamine H1 receptor antagonists. Drug Metab Dispos 26: 536–539

Hamilton KK, Sims PJ (1987) Changes in cytosolic Ca21 associated with von Willebrand factor release in human endothelial cells exposed to histamine: study of microcarrier cell monolayers using the fluorescent probe indo-1. J Clin Invest 79:600–608

Hancock AA, Brune ME (2005) Assessment of pharmacology and potential antiobesity properties of H3 receptor antagonists/inverse agonists. Exp Opin Invest Drugs 14:223–241

Hattori Y, Nakaya H, Endou M et al (1990) Inotropic, electrophysiological and biochemical responses in rabbit papillary muscles: evidence for co-existence of H1- and H2-receptors. J Pharmacol Exp Ther 253:250–256

Hattori Y, Nakaya H, Tohse N et al (1988a) Effects of Ca21 channel antagonists and ryanodine on H1-receptor mediated electromechanical response to histamine in guinea-pig left atria. Naunyn Schmiedeberg's Arch Pharmacol 337:323–330

Hattori Y, Sakuma I, Kanno M (1988b) Differential effects of histamine mediated H1- and H2-receptors on contractility, spontaneous rate and cyclic nucleotides in the rabbit heart. Eur J Pharmacol 153:221–229

Hescheler J, Tang M, Jastorff B et al (1987) On the mechanism of histamine induced enhancement of the cardiac Ca21 current. Pflü gers Arch 410:23–29

Higuchi M, Yanai K, Okamura N et al (1999) Histamine H (1) receptors in patients with Alzheimer's disease assessed by positron emission tomography. Neuroscience 1999: 721–729

Hill SJ (1990) Distribution, properties and functional characteristics of three classes of histamine receptor. Pharmacol Rev 42:45–83

Hill SJ, Donaldson J (1992) The H1-receptor and inositol phospholipids hydrolysis. In: Schwartz JC, Haas HL (eds) The histamine receptor. Wiley-Liss, New York, pp 109–128

Hill SJ, Ganellin CR, Timmerman H et al (1997) International Union of pharmacology. XIII. Classification of histamine receptors. Pharmacol Rev 49:253–278

Hill SJ, Young JM, Marrian DM (1977) Specific binding of 3Hmepyramine to histamine H1-receptors in intestinal smooth muscle. Nature (Lond) 270:361–363

Hirschfeld J, Buschauer A, Elz S et al (1992) Iodoaminopotentidine and related compounds: a new class of ligands with high affinity and selectivity for the histamine H2 receptor. J Med Chem 35:2231–2238

Horio Y, Mori Y, Higuchi I et al (1993) Molecular cloning of the guinea-pig histamine H1-receptor gene. J Biochem 114:408–414

Ichinose M, Belvisi MG, Barnes PJ (1990) Histamine *H*3-receptors inhibit neurogenic microvascular leakage in airways. J Appl Physiol 68:21–25

Imamura M, Poli E, Omoniyi AT et al (1994) Unmasking of activated histamine H3-receptors in myocardial ischemia: their role as regulators of exocytotic norepinephrine release. J Pharmacol Exp Ther 271:1259–1266

Imamura M, Seyedi N, Lander HM et al (1995) Functional identification of histamine H3-receptors in the human heart. Circ Res 77:206–210

Imamura M, Smith NCE, Garbarg M et al (1996) Histamine *H*3- receptor-mediated inhibition of calcitonin gene-related peptide release from cardiac C fibers: a regulatory negative feedback loop. Circ Res 78:863–869

Inove I, Taniuchi I, Kitamura D et al (1996) Characteristics of the mouse genomic histamine H1-receptor gene. Genomics 36:178–181

Ishikawa S, Sperelakis N (1987) A novel class (H3) of histamine receptors on perivascular nerve terminals. Nature (Lond) 327:158–160

IUPHAR Receptor database-Histamine receptor, http://www.iuphardb.org/GPCR/chapter Menu forward? chapter ID=1287. Assessed Oct 2009

Jahn K, Haas HL, Hatt H (1995) Histamine activated currents in the olfactory bulb. Naunyn-Schmiedeberg's Arch Pharmacol 352:386–393

Jansen FP, Rademaker B, Bast A (1992) The first radiolabeled histamine H3 receptor antagonist, [125i]iodophenpropit:saturable and reversible binding to rat cortex membranes. Eur J Pharmacol 217:203–205

Jansen FP, Wu TS, Voss HP et al (1994) Characterization of the binding of the first selective radiolabeled histamine H3-receptor antagonist, 125I-iodophenpropit, to rat brain. Br J Pharmacol 113:355–362

Johnson CL (1982) Histamine receptors and cyclic nucleotides. In: Ganellin R, Parsons M (eds) Pharmacology of histamine receptors. Wright and Bristol, England, pp 146–216

Jutel M, Watanabe T, Akdis M et al (2002) Immune regulation by histamine. Curr Opin Immunol 14:735–740

Jutel M, Watanabe T, Klunker S et al (2001) Histamine regulates T-cell and antibody responses by differential expression of H1 and H2 receptors. Nature 413:420–425

Kamba S, Richelson E (1983) Antidepressants are weak competitive antagonists of histamine H2-receptors in dissociated brain tissue. Eur J Pharmacol 94:313–318

Kazumori H, Ishihara S, Rumi MA et al (2004) Transforming growth factor alpha directly augments histidine decarboxylase and vesicular monoamine transporter 2 production in rat enterochromaffin-like cells. Am J Physiol Gastrointest Liver Physiol 286:514

Khateb A, Serafin M, Muehlethaler M (1990) Histamine excites pedunculopontine neurones in guinea pig brainstem slices. Neurosci Lett 112:257–262

Kilpatrick GJ, Michel AD (1991) Characterization of the binding of the histamine H3-receptor agonist [3H] R-α-methyhistamine to homogenates of rat and guinea-pig cortex. Agents Actions 33:69–75

Kishimoto W, Hiroi T, Sakai K et al (1997) Metabolism of epinastine, a histamine H1 receptor antagonist, in human liver microsomes in comparison with that of terfenatine. Res Commun Chem Pathol Pharmacol 98:273–292

Kitamura Y, Arima T, Kitayama Y et al (1996) Regulation of [Ca21]i rise activated by doxepin-sensitive H1-histamine receptors in jurkat cells, cloned human T lymphocytes. Gen Pharmacol 27:289–291

Kitbunnadaj R (2005) Histamine receptors and their ligands. Naresuan Univ J 13:41–53

Kobayashi T, Inove I, Jenkins NA et al (1996) Cloning, RNA expression and chromosomal location of a mouse histamine H2-receptor gene. Genomics 37:390–394

Korte A, Myers J, Shih NY et al (1990) Characterization and tissue distribution of H3-receptors in guinea-pigs by Nα-methylhistamine. Biochem Biophys Res Commun 168:979–986

Labella FS, Brandes LJ (2000) Interaction of histamine and other bioamines with cytochromes P450: implications for cell growth modulation and chemopotentiation by drugs. Semin Cancer Biol 10:47–53

Leurs R, Bakker RA, Timmerman H et al (2005) The histamine H3 receptor: from gene cloning to H3 receptor drug. Nat Rev Drug Disc 4:107–120

Leurs R, Brozius MM, Jansen W et al (1991) Histamine H1-receptor mediated cyclic GMP production in guinea-pig lung tissue is an L-arginine-dependent process. Biochem Pharmacol 42:271–277

Leurs R, Smit MJ, Meeder R et al (1995b) Lysine200 located in the fifth transmembrane domain of the histamine H1-receptor interacts with histamine but not with all H1 agonists. Biochem Biophys Res Commun 214:110–117

Leurs R, Smit MJ, Menge WMBP et al (1994a) Pharmacological characterization of the human histamine H2-receptor stably expressed in Chinese hamster ovary cells. Br J Pharmacol 112:847–854

Leurs R, Smit MJ, Tensen CP et al (1994b) Site directed mutagenesis of the histamine H1-receptor reveals a selective interaction of asparagine207 with subclasses of H1-receptor agonists. Biochem Biophys Res Commun 201:295–301

Leurs R, Smit MJ, Timmerman H (1995a) Molecular pharmacological aspects of histamine receptors. Pharmacol Ther 66:413–463

Leurs R, Traiffort E, Arrang JM et al (1994c) Guinea-pig histamine H1 receptor: II-stable expression in Chinese hamster ovary cells reveals the interaction with three major signal transduction pathways. J Neurochem 62:519–527

Levi RC, Alloatti G (1988) Histamine modulates calcium current in guinea pig ventricular myocytes. J Pharmacol Exp Ther 246:377–383

Ligneau X, Garbarg M, Vizuete ML et al (1994) 125I-Iodoproxyfan, a new antagonist to label and visualize cerebal histamine H3-receptors. J Pharmacol Exp Ther 271:452–459

Liu C, Ma X-J, Jiang X et al (2001a) Cloning and pharmacological characterization of a fourth histamine receptor (H4) expressed in bone marrow. Mol Pharmacol 59:420–426

Liu C, Wilson SJ, Kuel C et al (2001b) Comparison of human, mouse, rat, and guinea pig histamine H4 receptors reveals substantial pharmacological species variation. J Pharmacol Exp Ther 299:121–130

Liu Y, Furuta K, Teshima R et al (1992) Re-examination of 3H mepyramine binding assay for histamine H1-receptor using quinine. Biochem Biophys Res Commun 189:378–384

Livett BG, Marley PD (1986) Effects of opioid peptides and morphine on histamine-induced catecholamine secretion from cultured, bovine adrenal chromaffin cells. Br J Pharmacol 89:327–334

Lovenberg TW, Roland BL, Wilson SJ et al (1999) Cloning and functional expression of the human histamine H3 receptor. Mol Pharmacol 55:1101–1107

Ma RZ, Gao J, Meeker ND et al (2002) Identification of Bphs, an autoimmune disease locus, as histamine receptor H1. Science 297:620–623

Maayani S, Hough LB, Weinstein H et al (1982) Response of the histamine H2-receptor in the brain to antidepressant drugs. In: Costa E, Racagni G (eds) Typical and atypical antidepressants: molecular mechanisms. Raven, New York, pp 133–167

MacGlashan D Jr (2003) Histamine: a mediator of inflammation. J Allergy Clin Immunol 112: S53-S59

Mahnke A, Roos PH, Hanstein WG et al (1996) *In vivo* induction of cytochrome P450 CYP3A expression in rat leukocytes using various inducers. Biochem Pharmacol 51:1579–1582

Marley PD, Thompson KA, Jachno K et al (1991) Histamine induced increases in cyclic AMP levels in bovine adrenal medullary cells. Br J Pharmacol 104:839–846

Martinez-Mir MI, Pollard H, Moreau J et al (1990) Three histamine receptors (H1, H2 and H3) visualized in the brain of human and non-human primates. Brain Res 526:322–327

Matsubara T, Moskowitz MA, Huang Z (1992) UK 14,304, R(-)-α-methylhistamine, and Sms 201–995 block plasma protein leakage within dura mater by prejunctional mechanisms. Eur J Pharmacol 225:145–150

McCormick DA, Williamson A (1991) Modulation of neuronal firing mode in cat and guinea pig LGNd by histamine: possible cellular mechanism of histaminergic control of arousal. J Neurosci 11:3188–3199

McIntyre TM, Zimmerman GA, Satoh K et al (1985) Cultured endothelial cells synthesize both platelet-activating factor and prostacyclin in response to histamine, bradykinin and adenosine triphosphate. J Clin Invest 76:271–280

Megson AC, Dickenson JM, Townsend-Nicholson A et al (1995) Synergy between the inositol phosphate responses to transfected human adenosine A1-receptors and constitutive P2-purinoceptors in CHO-K1 cells. Br J Pharmacol 115:1415–1424

Melmon KL, Khan MM (1987) Histamine and its lymphocyte-selective derivatives as immune modulators. Trends Pharmacol Sci 8:437–441

Meyrick B, Brigham KI (1983) Increased permeability associated with dilation of endothelial cell junctions caused by histamine in intimal explants from bovine pulmonary artery. Exp Lung Res 6:11–25

Moguilevsky N, Varsalona F, Guillaume JP et al (1995) Pharmacological and functional characterization of the wild-type and site-directed mutants of the human H1-histamine receptor stably expressed in CHO cells. J Recept Signal Transduction Res 15:91–102

Molderings GJ, Weibenborn G, Schlicker E et al (1992) Inhibition of noradrenaline release from the sympathetic nerves of the human saphenous vein by presynaptic histamine H3-receptors. Naunyn-Schmiedeberg's Arch Pharmacol 346:46–50

Morgan ET (2001) Regulation of cytochrome P450 by inflammatory mediators: why and how. Drug Metab Dispos 29:207–212

Morisset S, Rouleau A, Ligneau X et al (2000) High constitutive activity of native H3 receptors regulates histamine neurons in brain. Nature 408:860–864

Muriyama T, Kajiyama Y, Nomura Y et al (1990) Histamine-stimulated and GTP-binding protein-mediated phospholipase A2 activation in rabbit platelets. J Biol Chem 265:4290–4295

Nebert DW, Russell DW (2002) Clinical importance of the cytochrome P450. Lancet 360: 1155–1162

Negulescu PA, Machen TE (1988) Intracellular Ca regulation during secretagogue stimulation of the parietal cell. Am J Physiol 254:C130-C140

Newton MV, Hough LB, Azimitia EC (1982) Histamine-sensitive adenylate cyclase in monkey brain. Brain Res 239:639–643

Noble EP, Bömmer M, Liebisch D et al (1988) H1-histaminergic activation of catecholamine release by chromaffin cells. Biochem Pharmacol 37:221–228

Oda T, Morikawa N, Saito Y et al (2000) Molecular cloning and characterization of a novel type of histamine receptor preferentially expressed in leukocytes. J Biol Chem 275: 36781–36786

Ohkubo T, Shibata M (1995) ATP-sensitive K1 channels mediate regulation of substance P release *via* the prejunctional histamine H3-receptor. Eur J Pharmacol 277:45–49

Ohta K, Hayashi H, Mizuguchi H et al (1994) Site-directed mutagenesis of the histamine H1-receptor: roles of aspartic acid107, asparagine198 and threonine194. Biochem Biophys Res Commun 203:1096–1101

Olianas M, Oliver AP, Neff NH (1984) Correlation between histamine induced neuronal excitability and activation of adenylate cyclase in guinea pig hippocampus. Neuropharmacology 23:1071–1074

Ottosson A, Jansen I, Edvinsson L (1989) Pharmacological characterization of histamine receptors in human temporal artery. Br J Clin Pharmacol 27:139–145

Parsons ME, Ganellin CR (2006) Histamine and its receptors. Br J Pharmacol 147:S127-S135

Passani MB, Lin JS, Hancock A et al (2004) The histamine H3 receptor as a novel therapeutic target for cognitive and sleep disorders. Trends Pharmacol Sci 25:618–625

Peakman MC, Hill SJ (1994) Endogenous expression of histamine H1-receptors functionally coupled to phosphoinositide hydrolysis in C6 glioma cells: regulation by cyclic AMP. Br J Pharmacol 113:1554–1560

Plaut M, Lichtenstein LM (1982) Histamine and immune responses. In: Ganellin CR, Parsons ME (eds) The pharmacology of histamine receptors. Wright and Bristol, England, pp 392–435

Pollard H, Moreau J, Arrang JM et al (1993) A detailed autoradiographic mapping of histamine H3-receptors in rat brain. Neuroscience 52:169–189

Reiner PB, Kamondi A (1994) Mechanism of antihistamine induced sedation in the human brain: H1-receptor activation reduces background leakage potassium current. Neuroscience 59: 579–588

Rouleau A, Ligneau X, Tardivel-Lacombe J et al (2002) Histamine H3-receptor-mediated [35S]GTPg[S] binding: evidence for constitutive activity of the recombinant and native rat and human H3 receptors. Br J Pharmacol 135:383–392

Ruat M, Bouthenet ML, Schwartz JC et al (1990a) Histamine H1-receptor in heart: unique electrophoretic mobility and autoradiographic localization. J Neurochem 55:379–385

Ruat M, Schwartz JC (1989) Photoaffinity labeling and electrophoretic identification of the H1-receptor: comparison of several brain regions and animal species. J Neurochem 53: 335–339

Ruat M, Traiffort E, Arrang JM et al (1991) Cloning and tissue expression of a rat histamine H2-receptor gene. Biochem Biophys Res Commun 179:1470–1478
Ruat M, Traiffort E, Bouthenet ML et al (1990b) Reversible and irreversible labeling and autoradiographic localization of thc cerebral histamine H2 receptor using [125i]-iodinated probes. Proc Natl Acad Sci USA 87:1658–1662
Sanderson EM, Iredale PA, Hill SJ (1996) Role of Ca21 ions in the stimulation of cAMP accumulation by histamine in CHO-K1 cells transfected with the bovine H1-receptor. (Abstract) Br J Pharmacol 117:7P
Schlicker E, Behling A, Lummen G et al (1992) Mutual interaction of histamine H3-receptors and a2-adrenoceptors on noradrenergic terminals in mouse and rat brain cortex. Naunyn Schmiedeberg's Arch Pharmacol 345:639–636
Schlicker E, Fink K, Detzner M et al (1993) Histamine inhibits dopamine release in the mouse striatum *via* presynaptic H3-receptors. J Neural Transm 93:1–10
Schlicker E, Fink K, Hinterhaner M et al (1989) Inhibition of noradrenaline release in the rat brain cortex *via* presynaptic H3 receptors. Naunyn-Schmiedeberg's Arch Pharmacol 340: 633–638
Schlicker E, Glaser T, Lümmen G et al (1991) Serotonin and histamine receptor-mediated inhibition of serotonin and noradrenaline release in rat brain cortex under nimodipine treatment. Neurochem Int 19:437–444
Schmidt HHHW, Zernikow B, Baeblich S et al (1990) Basal and stimulated formation and release of L-arginine-derived nitrogen oxides from cultured endothelial cells. J Pharmacol Exp Ther 254:591–597
Schneider E, Rolli-Derkinderen M, Arock M et al (2002) Trends in histamine research: new functions during immune responses and hematopoiesis. Trends Immunol 23:255–263
Schwartz JC, Arrang JM, Garbarg M et al (1991) Histaminergic transmission in the mammalian brain. Physiol Rev 71:1–51
Schworer H, Reimann A, Ramadori G et al (1994) Characterization of histamine *H*3-receptors inhibiting 5-HT release from porcine enterochromaffin cells: further evidence for *H*3-receptor heterogeneity. Naunyn-Schmiedeberg's Arch Pharmacol 350:375–379
Seifert R, Hagelüken A, Hoer A et al (1994) The H1- receptor agonist 2-(3-chlorophenyl) histamine activates Gi proteins in HL-60 cells through a mechanism that is independent of known histamine receptor subtypes. Mol Pharmacol 45:578–586
Seifert R, Hoer A, Schwaner I et al (1992) Histamine increases cytosolic Ca21 in HL-60 promyelocytes predominantly *via* H2 receptors with an unique agonist/antagonist profile and induces functional differentiation. Mol Pharmacol 42:235–241
Shahid M, Tripathi T, Sobia F et al (2009) Histamine, histamine receptors, and their role in immunomodulation: an updated systematic review. The Open Immunol J 2:9–41
Sharma A, Hamelin BA (2003) Classic histamine H1 receptor antagonists: a critical review of their metabolic and pharmacokinetic fate from a bird's eye view. Curr Drug Metab 4:105–129
Simons FER (2004) Advances in H1-Antihistamines. N Engl J Med 351:2203–2217
Smit MJ, Hoffmann M, Timmerman H et al (1999) Molecular properties and signaling pathways of the histamine H1 receptor. Clin Exp Allergy 29:19–28
Smit MJ, Leurs R, Alevijnse AE et al (1996) Inverse agonism of histamine H2-antagonists accounts for up-regulation of spontaneously active histamine receptors. Proc Natl Acad Sci USA 93:6802–6807
Soldani G, Mengozzi G, Intorre L et al (1993) Histamine H3-receptor-mediated inhibition of gastric acid secretion in conscious dogs. Naunyn-Schmiedeberg's Arch Pharmacol 347: 61–65
Soll AH, Berglindh T (1987) Physiology of isolated gastric glands and parietal cells: receptors and effectors regulating function. In: Johnson LR (ed) Physiology of the gastrointestinal tract. Raven, New York, pp 883–909
Stark H (2007) Histamine receptors. Biotrends Rev 1:2–9. http://www.biotrend.com. Accessed Nov 2009

Sterk GJ, Van Der Schaar MWG, Rademaker B et al (1986) Histamine H2-receptor binding on guinea-pig cerebral cortex. Agents Actions 18:231–234

Svensjo E, Grega GJ (1986) Evidence for endothelial cell-mediated regulation of macromolecular permeability by postcapillary venules. Fed Proc 45:89–95

Takahashi K, Suwa H, Ishikawa T et al (2002) Targeted disruption of H3 receptors results in changes in brain histamine tone leading to an obese phenotype. J Clin Invest 110: 1791–1799

Tamasi V, Fulop AK, Egyi K et al (2003) Upregulation of cyp2e1 and cyp3a activities in histamine-deficient histidine decarboxylase gene targeted mice. Cell Biol Int 27:1011–1015

Taylor GJ, Kilpatrick GJ (1992) Characterization of histamine-H3 receptors controlling non-adrenergic non-cholinergic contractions of the guinea pig isolated ileum. Br J Pharmacol 105:667–674

Teuscher C, Subramanian M, Noubade R et al (2007) Central histamine H3 receptor signaling negatively regulates susceptibility to autoimmune inflammatory disease of the CNS. Proc Natl Acad Sci USA 104:10146–10151

Thurmond RL, Desai PJ, Dunford PJ et al (2004) A potent and selective histamine H4 receptor antagonist with anti-inflammatory properties. J Pharmacol Exp Ther 309: 404–413

Thurmond RL, Gelfand EW, Dunford PJ et al (2008) The role of histamine H1 and H4 receptors in allergic inflammation: the search for new antihistamines. Nat Rev Drug Discov 7:41–53

Timmerman H (1992) Cloning of the H1 histamine receptor. Trends Pharmacol Sci 13:6–7

Ting S, Dunsky EH, Zweiman B (1980) Histamine suppression of eosinophilotaxis and histamine release *in vivo*. J Allergy Clin Immunol 65:196–197

Togias A (2003) H1-receptors: localization and role in airway physiology and in immune functions. J Allergy Clin Immunol 112:S60-S68

Toll L, Snyder SH (1982) Solubilization and characterization of histamine H1 receptors in brain. J Biol Chem 257:13593–13601

Traiffort E, Leurs R, Arrang JM et al (1994) Guinea-pig histamine H1-receptor: I-gene cloning, characterization and tissue expression revealed by in situ hybridization. J Neurochem 62: 507–518

Traiffort E, Pollard H, Moreau J et al (1992a) Pharmacological characterization and autoradiographic localization of histamine H2-receptors in human brain identified with 125I-iodoaminopotentidine. J Neurochem 59:290–299

Traiffort E, Ruat M, Arrang JM et al (1992b) Expression of a cloned rat histamine H2 receptor mediating inhibition of arachidonate release and activation of cAMP accumulation. Proc Natl Acad Sci USA 89:2649–2653

Traiffort E, Ruat M, Schwartz JC (1991) Interactions of mianserin, amitriptyline and haloperidol with guinea-pig cerebral histamine H2-receptors studied with 125I-iodoamino-potentidine. Eur J Pharmacol Mol Pharmacol Sect 207:143–148

Traiffort E, Vizuete ML, Tadivellacombe J et al (1995) The guinea-pig histamine H2 receptor-gene cloning, tissue expression and chromosomal localization of its human counterpart. Biochem Biophys Res Commun 211:570–577

Travis ER, Wang YM, Michel DJ et al (2000) Differential quantal release of histamine and 50-hydroxytryptamine from mast cells of vesicular monoamine transporter 2 knockout mice. Proc Natl Acad Sci USA 97:162–167

Treherne JM, Young JM (1988) Temperature dependence of the kinetics of the binding of 3H-(1)-N-methyl-4-methyl diphenhydramine to the histamine H1-receptor: comparison with the kinetics of 3Hmepyramine. Br J Pharmacol 94:811–822

Van de Voorde J, Leusen I (1993) Role of the endothelium in the vasodilator response of rat thoracic aorta to histamine. Eur J Pharmacol 87:113–120

Van der Werf JF, Timmerman H (1989) The histamine H3-receptor: a general presynaptic histaminergic regulatory mechanism? Trends Pharmacol Sci 10:159–162

Villemain FM, Bach JF, Chatenoud LM (1990) Characterization of histamine H1 binding sites on human T lymphocytes by means of [125I] iodobolpyramine. J Immunol 144:1449–1454

Wan DCC, Marley PD, Livett BG (1989) Histamine activates proenkephalin A mRNA but not phenylethanolamine-N methyltransferase mRNA expression in cultured bovine adrenal chromaffin cells. Eur J Pharmacol Mol Pharmacol Sect 172:117–129

Watson F, Deavall DG, MacRo JA et al (1999) Transcriptional activation of vesicular monoamine transporter 2 in the pre-B cell line Ea3.123. Biochem J 337:193–199

Wellendorph P, Goodman MW, Burstein ES et al (2002) Molecular cloning and pharmacology of functionally distinct isoforms of the human histamine H(3) receptor. Neuropharmacology 42:929–940

West RE Jr, Zweig A, Shih NY et al (1990) Identification of two H3-histamine receptor subtypes. Mol Pharmacol 38:610–613

Yamashita M, Fukui H, Sugama K et al (1991) Expression cloning of a cDNA encoding the bovine histamine H1-receptor. Proc Natl Acad Sci USA 88:11515–11519

Yanai K, Ryu JII, Watanabc T ct al (1992) Rcccptor autoradiography with 11C and [3II]-labelled ligands visualized by imaging plates. Neuroreport 3:961–964

Yokoyama H (2001) The role of central histaminergic neurin system as an anticonvulsive mechanism in developing brain. Brain Dev 23:542–547

Yuan Y, Granger HJ, Zawieja DC et al (1993) Histamine increases venular permeability *via* a phospholipase C-NO synthase-guanylate cyclase cascade. Am J Physiol 264:H1734-H1739

Zweig A, Siegel MI, Egan RW et al (1992) Characterization of a digitonin-solubilised bovine brain H3- histamine receptor coupled to a guanine nucleotide-binding protein. J Neurochem 59:1661–1666

Part IV
Histamine Role in Immune Modulation and Regulation

Chapter 5
The Role of Histamine in Immunoregulation in Context of T-Regulatory and Invariant NKT Cells

Varun Dwivedi and Renukaradhya J. Gourapura

Abstract Histamine (HA) is one of the most versatile biogenic amines with multiple physiological functions in the central nervous system (CNS), the respiratory and the intestinal tract due to its ability to induce severe inflammatory reactions. More recently, a number of studies have established that besides its most obvious contribution in allergic reactions, HA also exerts more subtle regulatory functions influencing the orientation of the immune response, thus rekindling interest in this field of investigation. It can influence numerous functions of the cells involved in the regulation of immune responses and hematopoiesis of macrophages, dendritic cells, T lymphocytes, B lymphocytes and endothelial cells. All these cells express histamine receptors and also secrete histamine, which can selectively recruit major effector cells into tissue sites and affect their maturation, activation, polarization, and effector functions leading to chronic inflammation. Histamine regulates antigen-specific T-helper 1 (Th1) and T-helper 2 (Th2) cells, as well as related isotype specific antibody responses. Histamine acts through its receptor called as histamine receptor (H1-H4) subtypes, which positively interferes with the peripheral antigen tolerance induced by T-regulatory cells (Tregs) through several pathways. Natural killer T (NKT) cells are the heterogeneous population of innate immune T cells that have been attracted the attention of many researchers due to their potential to regulate immune responses to a variety of pathogens, tumors, autoimmune diseases etc. A majority of NKT cells in mice are invariant NKT (iNKT) cells and are considered to be immunoregulatory in nature, due to their ability to promptly produce both Th1 and Th2 cytokines rapidly upon activation. In this chapter, we have tried to focus on HA participation in NKT cell activation by functional tuning to ensure optimal cytokine production, which leads to the recruitment and activation of other immune cells involved in inflammatory responses mediated through eosinophils, mast cells, neutrophils, conventional T lymphocytes, dendritic cells etc.

V. Dwivedi (✉)
Food Animal Health Research Program (FAHRP), Ohio Agricultural Research and Development Center (OARDC), The Ohio State University, 1680, Madison Avenue, Wooster, OH 44691, USA
e-mail: dwivedi.6@osu.edu

M. Shahid et al. (eds.), *Biomedical Aspects of Histamine*,
DOI 10.1007/978-90-481-9349-3_5,

Keywords Histamine · Histamine receptors · Immunoregulation · Natural killer T (NKT) cells

Contents

5.1 Introduction

Histamine is a chemical mediator and neurotransmitter belongs to the group of biological amine and plays an important role in physiological functions, and regulation of serious pathological conditions. Histamine is known to participate in all kinds of allergic reaction, inflammation, infection and pain syndrome. Under physiological conditions histamine receptors of all four types are conjugated to guanyl-nucleotide-dependent G-proteins (GPCR) i.e., subtypes H1–H4. A well known co-relation was demonstrated between conformation of histamine molecule and its activity with respect to histamine receptors of different subtypes.

5.2 Histamine Receptors

5.2.1 H1 Histamine Receptors

H1 Histamine receptors are predominantly present on a wide variety of tissues, such as CNS, smooth muscles of gastrointestinal tract, cardiovascular system, and endothelial cells and on lymphocytes. H1 histamine receptors in humans is a glycoprotein that consists of 487 amino acid residues (Arrang et al. 1995). The H1 histamine receptors are conjugated to phospholipase C (PLC); upon activation of PLC (and phospholipase A2 and D) from cell membrane phospholipids, it induces inositol 1, 4, 5 triphosphate (IP3) and 1, 2-diacylglycerol (DAC). Which results in increased release of Ca^{2+} and/or cAMP, cGMP, lead to the formation of nitric oxide, resulting in contraction of smooth muscles, dilation of arterioles and capillaries, increased vascular permeability as well as stimulation of afferent neurons.

5.2.2 H2 Histamine Receptors

H2 histamine receptors are mainly detected on brain cells, gastric parietal cells and cardiac tissues. The human H2 histamine receptor is also a glycoprotein consisting of 359 amino acid residues (Arrang et al. 1995). Accumulation of secondary messenger, cAMP in the cells induces adenylate cyclase which is conjugated to H2 histamine receptors. H2 receptors stimulation mediate positive inotropic and chronotropic effects on atrial and ventricular tissues, but the most prominent effect is the stimulation of gastric acid secretion. In the CNS, H2 histamine receptors inhibit nerve cells function upon hyper-polarization.

5.2.3 H3 Histamine Receptors

The H3 histamine receptors are localized at the pre-synaptic membrane of nerve endings in the CNS and the peripheral nervous system. Histamine has been known as a neurotransmitter only after the discovery of the H3 receptor. As a hetero-receptor, it decreases the synthesis and release of histamine. On the contrary, stimulation of hetero-receptors (Leurs et al. 1995) modulates the release of other neuromediators (acetylcholine, dopamine, nor-adrenaline, and serotonin) (Mochizuki et al. 1994, Schlicker et al. 1989, 1994). A activation of the H3 receptor via G alpha 1 and G alpha 0, results in the inhibition of adenyl cyclase, activation of mitogen activated protein kinase (MAPK), phospholipase A2 (release of arachidonic acid), Akt/GSK-3b kinases, inhibition of Na^+/H^+ anti-porter and K^+ induced Ca^{2+} mobilization.

5.2.4 H4 Histamine Receptors

The histamine H4 receptor has 31–34% overall structural homology to the H3 receptor depending on species. The overall genomic sequence is comparable to that of the H3 receptor with two large introns and three exons, but with large interspecies variations (65–72%). Activation of H4 receptor via G alpha 1 and G alpha 0 leads to inhibition of adenylyl cyclase and downstream cAMP responsive elements (CRE), as well as activation of MAPK and phospholipase C with Ca^{2+} mobilization. H4 receptor distribution has been found in bone marrow and leukocytes, particularly in eosinophils, mast cells, dendritic cells (DC), basophils and T lymphocytes. Moderate level of distribution of this receptor was found in spleen and small intestine, suggesting its regulatory role in inflammatory responses mediated through interferon and cytokines (TNFα, IL-6, IL-10, and IL-13 etc.). The H4 receptor mediates the chemotaxis of mast cells and eosinophils, as well as it controls the cytokine release from DC and T cells (Stark 2007).

5.3 Histamine: Overview on Different Cell Populations

Cells bearing histamine receptors on their surface are capable of secreting histamine, and histamine is critical in the regulation of immune responses. Recent detailed studies confirmed the effect of histamine on function of monocytes, DC, T cells and plasma cells. We are reviewing in this chapter regarding different types of immune cells which gets affected by histamine directly or indirectly, and how it alters various immune responses.

5.3.1 Monocytes and Dendritic Cells

Histamine stimulation of monocytes resulted in much greater increase in cAMP-phosphodiesterase (PDE) activity. Histamine stimulation of PDE activity is mediated predominantly through H1 histamine receptor in monocytes using thiazolylethylamine and chlorpheniramine as H1-agonist and antagonist, respectively, and dimaprit and cimetidine as H2-agonists and antagonists, respectively (Holden et al. 1987). Other studies demonstrated the inhibitory action of histamine on lipopolysaccharide-induced TNF-α production from human blood monocytes (Hotermans et al. 1991).

Histamine is involved not only in the inhibition of apoptosis of monocytes by serum deprivation, CD95/Fas ligation, or dexamethasone treatment in a dose- and time-dependent manner but also, histamine up-regulates the expression of Bcl-2 and Mcl-1 (anti-apoptotic factors), and inhibits the activation of caspase-3 (apoptosis inducer). Histamine induced H2 receptor in turn allows monocytes to prolong their life span and infiltrate to the site of inflammation. This process may contribute to the establishment of chronic allergic disorders, such as atopic dermatitis (AD) (Soga et al. 2007). Upon activation of monocytes by bacterial products, histamine inhibits the production of IL-1α, TNF-α and IL-12, but enhances the secretion of IL-10, mediated through H2R (Elenkov et al. 1998, van der Pouw Kraan et al. 1998, Vannier and Dinarello 1993).

Dendritic cells are the professional antigen (Ag) presenting cells (APC) that play a dominant role in induction and regulation of immune responses. Endogenous histamine is actively synthesized during cytokine-induced DC differentiation and acts in an autocrine and paracrine way (Szeberenyi et al. 2001). Inhibition of histamine synthesis by DC affects its differentiation. In the recent times it is quite evident that histamine affects DC activation and maturation, in preference to Th1/Th2 cell differentiation. Histamine enhances MHC class II and co-stimulatory molecules (CD80 and CD86) expression on DC (Mazzoni et al. 2001). Immature and mature DC express mRNA transcript to H1, H2 and H3 histamine receptors (Caron et al. 2001a, b, Gutzmer et al. 2002, Kapsenberg et al. 1992, Mazzoni et al. 2001). Histamine induces intracellular Ca^{2+} transients, actin polymerization and chemotaxis of immature DC (iDC). Maturation of DC results in loss of these responses; however, in maturing DC, histamine in a dose-dependent manner enhances the intracellular cAMP levels and stimulates IL-10 secretion, while it inhibits the production of IL-12. Specific histamine receptor agonists or antagonists reveal that Ca^{2+} transients, actin polymerization and chemotaxis of iDC is mediated through stimulation of H1R and H3R. Modulation of IL-12 and IL-10 secretion by histamine exclusively involves H2R and H3R (Caron et al. 2001a, b, Gutzmer et al. 2002, Kapsenberg et al. 1992, Mazzoni et al. 2001).

Several reports have shown that histamine directly affects human monocyte-derived DC (Caron et al. 2001a, b, Gutzmer et al. 2002, Idzko et al. 2002, Mazzoni et al. 2001). Histamine induces phenotypic changes, such as CD86 expression in human iDC, and up-regulates the expression of co-stimulatory and accessory molecules, CD40, CD80, CD54 and MHC class II (Caron et al. 2001b). In contrast, Mazzoni et al. (2001) reported that histamine does not significantly affect the phenotype of LPS-driven mature DC. However, histamine alters production of a number of cytokines and chemokines in LPS-matured DC. In particular, histamine increases the IL-10 and IL-8 production and blocks the IL-12 and IL-6 production in LPS-matured human DC (Mazzoni et al. 2001). The downregulation of IL-12 production by histamine in LPS-matured human monocyte-derived DC has also been reported by other investigators (Caron et al. 2001a, b, Gutzmer et al. 2002, Idzko et al. 2002).

5.3.2 Histamine and its Effect on T Lymphocytes

Histamine modulates the activity of immune-competent cells including T lymphocytes by binding to histamine receptors on their cell surface. There is a large variation in response to histamine by human T lymphocyte subsets based on histamine receptors distribution (Khan et al. 1985). Naïve T cell precursors develop into at least two distinct subtypes (Th1 and Th2 cells) on the basis of their different cytokine profiles and functions. Both subsets play distinctive roles in the development, initiation, and regulation of the cell mediated immune responses. The Th1 cells are involved in delayed type hypersensitivity and cytotoxic responses, while Th2 cells regulate allergic diseases and asthma by activating B cells and regulating

IgG and IgE secretion. Th1 cells secrete primarily IL-2, IFN-γ, IL-3, and GM-CSF (granulocyte-monocyte colony stimulating factor), while Th2 cells predominantly secrete IL-3, IL-4, IL-5, IL-10, IL-13 etc. with strong antibody responses and eosinophilia. Histamine down-regulates the proliferation of Th1 lymphocytes. In contrast, histamine up-regulates the proliferation of Th2 lymphocytes (Weltman 2000). Histamine regulates the development of an allergic state by enhancing the secretion of Th2 cytokines such as IL-4, IL-5, IL-10 and IL-13, and by inhibiting the production of Th1 cytokines such as IL-2, IFN-γ and IL-12 (Arad et al. 1996, Carlsson et al. 1985, Dohlsten et al. 1986, Elenkov et al. 1998, Elliott et al. 2001, Krouwels et al. 1998, Osna et al. 2001a, b, Poluektova and Khan 1998, Schmidt et al. 1994, Sirois et al. 2000). Th2 cell-derived cytokines induce an immunoglobulin class switch to IgE (Kapsenberg et al. 1992). The dysregulation of Th1 and Th2 responses results in various immunopathological conditions (Mosmann 1994, O'Garra and Murphy 1993). Atopic diseases are characterized by increase in Th2 cells and IgE antibodies. The diversity of Th1 and Th2 function is not predetermined but depends on signals that drive the cells towards either subset. Histamine has been demonstrated to affect both Th1/Th2 balance and immunoglobulin synthesis (Banu and Watanabe 1999, Elliott et al. 2001, Jutel et al. 2001, Poluektova and Khan 1998). Interestingly, the interaction between histamine and the cytokines is mutual, as some cytokines affect both production and release of histamine as well as histamine receptor expression (Dy et al. 1996). It has been demonstrated that differential patterns of histamine receptor expression on Th1 and Th2 cells determine reciprocal responses following histamine stimulation (Jutel et al. 2001). Th1 cells show predominant but not exclusive expression of H1R, whereas Th2 cells show up-regulation of H2R. However it should be noted that, histamine contributes to the progression of allergic–inflammatory responses by enhancement of secretion of several pro-inflammatory cytokines, such as IL-1α, IL-1β and IL-6, as well as chemokines, RANTES or IL-8, in several cell types and local tissues (Bayram et al. 1999, Jeannin et al. 1994, Meretey et al. 1991, Vannier and Dinarello 1993). On the contrary, production of TNF-α is inhibited by histamine (Vannier et al. 1991).

5.3.3 Antibody Response

Th1 and Th2 cells express different patterns of histamine receptors responsible for generating different T cell responses following histamine stimulation (Jutel et al. 2001). The Th1 cells preferentially express HR1, while Th2 cells express more of HR2. In mice, deletion of HR1 results in suppression of IFN-γ and enhanced secretion of Th2 cytokines (IL-4 and IL-13). HR2-deleted mice show up-regulation of both Th1 and Th2 cytokines. In mice, histamine enhances anti-IgM induced proliferation of B cells, which is abolished in HR1-knockout mice. Also in HR1-knockout mice, antibody production against a T cell-independent antigen-TNP-Ficoll is decreased (Banu and Watanabe 1999), suggesting an important role of HR1 signaling in responses triggered from B cell receptors. Antibody responses to

T cell-dependent antigens like ovalbumin (OVA) show a different pattern (Jutel et al. 2001). HR1-knockout mice produced high OVA-specific IgG1 and IgE in comparison to wild-type mice. In contrast, H2R-knockout mice have decreased serum levels of OVA-specific IgG3 and IgE in comparison to wild-type and H1R knockout mice. Although T cells of H2R knockout mice secreted increased IL-4 and IL-13, OVA-specific IgE was suppressed in the presence of high level of IFN-γ. Thus, H1R and related Th1 responses may play a dominant role the suppression of humoral immune responses (Banu and Watanabe 1999, Jutel et al. 2001).

5.4 T-Regulatory Cells

A key issue in immunology is to understand how the immune system discriminates between self and non-self; inhibits autoimmune responses and elicits only effective immune responses against microbial antigens. Invasion of infectious agents in the host evokes strong humoral and cellular immune responses. Some pathogens are difficult to control and the host response to them often results in tissue damage. This tissue damage might be more intense, were it not for many regulatory mechanisms that restrain the "zeal" of both innate and adaptive effector responses.

The immune system has evolved several mechanisms to establish and sustain unresponsiveness to self antigens (immunological self-tolerance), including physical elimination or functional inactivation of self-reactive lymphocytes (by means of clonal deletion/anergy). There is also a substantial evidence that T cell-mediated active suppression of self-reactive T cells is another essential mechanism of self-tolerance (Coutinho et al. 2001, Maloy and Powrie 2001, Sakaguchi 2004, Shevach 2000). In recent years, however we have witnessed resurgent interest in suppressor or T-regulatory cells (Tregs) in many fields of basic and clinical immunology (Baecher-Allan and Hafler 2004, Sakaguchi 2004). These cells modulate the intensity and quality of immune reactions through attenuation of the cytolytic activities of reactive immune cells. Tregs operate primarily at the site of inflammation where they modulate the immune reaction through three major mechanisms: (a) direct killing of cytotoxic cells through cell-to-cell contact, (b) inhibition of cytokine production by cytotoxic cells, in particular IL-2, (c) direct secretion of immunomodulatory cytokines, in particular TGF-β and IL-10 (Askenasy et al. 2008).

Naturally arising $CD4^+CD25^+Foxp3^+$ Tregs (nTreg) are derived from the thymus and have been extensively studied for their roles in autoimmunity and tolerance. A another population of Tregs generated from the activation and differentiation of mature $CD4^+CD25^-$ T cells in the periphery are called adaptive or inducible Tregs (iTreg) (Sakaguchi 2005).

A cardinal feature of endogenous Tregs is that most if not all are produced by the normal thymus as a functionally distinct and mature T cell subpopulation, and are not induced *de novo* from naive T cells after antigen exposure in the periphery. Most endogenous $CD4^+$ Tregs constitutively express the CD25 molecule [IL-2 receptor α-chain (IL-2Rα)] (Sakaguchi et al. 1995). In addition, they specifically express *Foxp3* which encodes a transcription factor, a key protein in Tregs development and function (Fontenot et al. 2003, Hori et al. 2003, Khattri et al. 2003). With CD25 and Foxp3 as specific cellular markers for detection and manipulation of naturally occurring Tregs, there is now cellular accumulating evidence that the $Foxp3^+CD25^+CD4^+$ Tregs population is actively engaged in the negative control of a variety of physiological and pathological immune responses. Tregs can be exploited not only for the prevention or treatment of autoimmune diseases, but also for the induction of immunological tolerance to non-self antigens (such as transplantation tolerance), negative control of aberrant immune responses (such as allergy and immune-pathology) and for enhancement of host defense mechanisms (such as tumor immunity and microbial immunity) (Sakaguchi 2004).

Natural Tregs however arise during the normal process of maturation in the thymus and survive in the periphery as Tregs. The best characterized "naturally occurring" murine $CD4^+CD25^+Foxp3^+$ T cells that develop in the thymus (Sakaguchi et al. 1995), play a pivotal role in the maintenance of immunological self-tolerance and modulation of immune responses (Fehervari et al. 2006, Malek and Bayer 2004, Nelson 2004). Natural Tregs constitutively express CD25, the T cell inhibitory receptor cytotoxic T lymphocyte-associated antigen 4 (CTLA-4) and the glucocorticoid-inducible tumor necrosis factor receptor (GITR). The unique transcription factor Foxp3 is required for the generation of natural Tregs (Fontenot et al. 2003, Hori et al. 2003, Khattri et al. 2003).

There are several key molecules including CD25 and Foxp3, whose deficiency or functional alteration affects the generation or function of nTregs and thereby causes autoimmune disease. These molecules provide important clues to understand the functions of nTregs in immunological tolerance and immune-regulation. An intriguing feature of natural $CD4^+$ Tregs, whether $CD25^+$ or $CD25^-$, is that they constitutively express CTLA-4, whereas naïve T cells express the molecule only after T cell activation (Read et al. 2000, Salomon et al. 2000, Takahashi et al. 2000b). This raises the issue of what function, if any, the CTLA-4 molecules expressed by natural Tregs have on the control of immune responses. In addition to substantial evidence for CTLA-4-transduced negative signaling in activated effector T cells, several findings also support the possible contribution of CTLA-4 in Tregs-mediated suppression. Blocking of CTLA-4 using monoclonal antibody (mAb) in mice for a short period of time resulted in the autoimmune response, similar to that produced by depletion of $CD25^+CD4^+$ Tregs (Takahashi et al. 2000b). Likewise, treatment with mAb to CTLA-4 abolishes the protective activity of $CD25^+CD4^+$ Tregs in a mouse model of inflammatory bowel disease (Read et al. 2000).

Furthermore, a lethal lympho-proliferative and autoimmune syndrome that spontaneously develops in CTLA-4-deficient mice is not T cell autonomous, but can be inhibited by wild-type T cells (Bachmann et al. 1999). Finally, blockade of CTLA-4 by Fab fragments of CTLA-4 mAb abrogates in vitro $CD25^+CD4^+$ Tregs-mediated suppression in a setting in which Tregs are prepared from wild-type mice and responder T cells are from CTLA-4-deficient mice (Read et al. 2000, Tang et al. 2004). CTLA-4 blockade also abrogates in vitro Tregs-mediated suppression in humans (Manzotti et al. 2002). These results collectively suggest that CTLA-4 on Tregs may transduce co-stimulatory signals via CTLA-4 and TCR interaction, that renders Tregs immunosuppressive. The CTLA-4 blockade prevents Tregs activation and hence attenuates suppression caused in autoimmune diseases.

Among many types of regulatory cells, Foxp3^{+} T cells emerge as key players in maintenance of self-tolerance, and its expression appears to be a more sensitive parameter that dissociates between activated CD4^{+}CD25^{low} T effector cells and CD4^{+}CD25^{high} Tregs. Recent studies demonstrated that some adaptive Tregs loose their CD25 expression in vivo, but retain their FoxP3 expression (Fontenot et al. 2003), suggesting that this transcription factor is a marker with better sensitivity for Tregs identification. However, it is likely that mAb to CD25 and FoxP3 identify different subset of cells, because not all CD25^{high} cells stain positive for FoxP3, and conversely not all the FoxP3^{+} cells are positive for CD25. Although FoxP3 is an inductive transcription factor of CD25 expression, it's up-regulation is secondary to TCR engagement in the presence of TGF-β, and it is not necessarily related to suppressive phenotype of the cells (Tran et al. 2007). In view of the phenotypic infidelity of Tregs, it is questioned whether they share common effector pathways of immune suppression (Miyara and Sakaguchi 2007).

Another possible function of CTLA-4 in Tregs is that it may directly mediate suppression. The CTLA-4 on Tregs triggers induction of indolamine 2, 3-dioxygenase (IDO) by its interaction with CD80 and/or CD86 on DC (Fallarino et al. 2003). This enzyme catalyzes the conversion of tryptophan to kynurenine and other metabolites, which have potent immunosuppressive effects (Munn et al. 2004). The CTLA-4 expressed by Tregs may also ligate CD80 and to a lesser extent CD86 expressed by responder T cells, which directly transduce a negative signal to them (Paust et al. 2004). These possible functions of CTLA-4 in Tregs-mediated suppression, however, need to be further substantiated, as CTLA-4-deficient Foxp3^{+}CD25^{+}CD4^{+} Tregs present in CTLA-4-deficient mice have in vitro suppressive activity equivalent to that of CTLA-4-intact CD25^{+}CD4^{+} Tregs from normal mice (Takahashi et al. 2000b, Tang et al. 2004). Signals through CD28 are critical for thymic generation of CD25^{+}CD4^{+}Tregs and their self-renewal and survival in the periphery. The number of CD25^{+}CD4^{+} T cells is substantially reduced in the thymus and periphery of CD28- or B7-deficient mice (Salomon et al. 2000, Takahashi et al. 2000b, Tang et al. 2003).

5.4.1 Site of Action of Tregs

Regulatory T cells operate primarily at the site of inflammation, in close spatial proximity to and through direct interaction with the effector cells. A requirement of cell-to-cell contact to achieve Tregs-mediated immune-modulation was convincingly demonstrated in in vitro experiments (Piccirillo et al. 2002). Direct interaction with the pathogenic cells places the Tregs at the sites of inflammation, despite weaker chemotactic responses of naïve CD25^{+} Tregs as compared to the chemotaxis of CD25$^{-/low}$ pathogenic T cells (Gavin et al. 2002). This pattern of behavior was nicely demonstrated by the inefficient penetration of Tregs into the pancreas of NOD and SCID mice without co-transfer of diabetogenic T cells (Chen et al. 2005), suggesting that inflammatory signals were required to attract the regulatory cells (Siegmund et al. 2005). Signals of inflammation from the pancreatic lymph nodes and islets, along with physical co-localization with effector T cells is essential to achieve a suppressive activity in a number of diabetes models in vivo (Green et al. 2002, Siegmund et al. 2005). This evolving scenario implies that Tregs are attracted to sites of inflammation after effector T cells homing. Subsequently, the chemotactic receptors of Tregs are down-regulated and adhesive interactions arrest their migration (Lim et al. 2006). From the experimental point of view this is a very important aspect, because analysis is frequently performed on cells harvested from the spleen or mesenteric lymph nodes that contain large number of cells. However, these sites may not adequately reflect the activity of Tregs and may include generalized reactive modulation of immunity, secondary to an ongoing inflammation at a remote site.

5.4.2 Evidence for Human Natural Tregs in Self-Tolerance

The X-linked immunodeficiency syndrome IPEX (immune dys-regulation, polyendocrinopathy, enteropathy, X-linked syndrome) is associated with autoimmune disease in multiple endocrine organs (such as type I diabetes and thyroiditis), inflammatory bowel disease, severe allergy including atopic dermatitis and food allergy, and fatal infection (Gambineri et al. 2003). IPEX in mice is caused by mutations in *Foxp3* gene which encodes the forkhead-winged-helix family transcription factor Foxp3. Mutation in *Foxp3* was first identified as being responsible for an X-linked recessive inflammatory disease in scurfy mutant mice, and subsequently for IPEX in humans (Bennett et al. 2001, Brunkow et al. 2001, Chatila et al. 2000, Wildin et al. 2001).

The Foxp3 is crucial in the development and function of natural $CD25^{+}CD4^{+}$ Tregs (Fontenot et al. 2003, Hori et al. 2003, Khattri et al. 2003). For example, $CD25^{+}CD4^{+}$ peripheral T cells and $CD25^{+}CD4^{+}CD8^{-}$ thymocytes specifically express Foxp3, whereas other thymocytes, T cells, B cells, natural killer cells and natural killer T cells do not (Fontenot et al. 2003, Hori et al. 2003). Notably, in contrast to the stable expression of Foxp3 in nTregs, activated naive T cells or differentiated Th1 or Th2 cells do not express Foxp3, indicating that its expression is highly specific to Tregs (Fontenot et al. 2003, Hori et al. 2003, Khattri et al. 2003). Foxp3-deficient mice fail to develop $CD25^{+}CD4^{+}$ Tregs and succumb to scurfy-like inflammatory disease, which can be prevented by adoptive transfer of normal $CD25^{+}CD4^{+}$ Tregs (Fontenot et al. 2003). Furthermore, retroviral transduction or transgenic expression of *Foxp3* in $CD25^{-}CD4^{+}$ T cells or $CD8^{+}$ T cells phenotypically and functionally converts them to natural Treg-like cells; for example, *Foxp3*-transduced $CD25^{-}CD4^{+}$ T cells are able to suppress proliferation of other T cells in vitro as well as suppress the development of autoimmune diseases and inflammatory bowel disease in vivo (Fontenot et al. 2003, Hori et al. 2003, Khattri et al. 2003). Transduction of *Foxp3* also suppresses IL-2 production but up-regulates the expression of Tregs-associated molecules, such as CD25, CTLA-4 and GITR (Hori et al. 2003). Thus, *Foxp3* seems to be a "master control gene" responsible for the development and function of natural $CD25^{+}CD4^{+}$ Tregs.

The establishment of immunological tolerance requires both induction of clonal deletion/anergy and active immune suppression. Immune suppression has been shown to be mediated by unique subsets of T cells called Tregs (Sakaguchi 2005). In multiple systems of allograft tolerance, the importance of these Tregs population to long-lived allograft survival has been revealed by the fact that depletion of Tregs before, and even after the induction of transplantation results in rapid graft rejection (Quezada et al. 2005, Taylor et al. 2001). However, despite the increasing body of knowledge about Tregs, the mechanisms by which these cells mediate immune suppression and prevent graft rejection are not well resolved.

5.4.3 *Mast Cells and Tregs in Tolerance*

Mast cells are derived from haematopoietic stem cells, which migrate into vascularized tissues and serosal cavities where they complete their maturation (Galli et al. 2005). They are best known as primary responders in allergic reactions such as anaphylaxis and asthma. Previously, extensive serial analysis of gene expression (SAGE) in tolerant tissues revealed that genes predominantly expressed by mast cells were over-expressed in cultures of activated Tregs and in tolerant allografts (Zelenika et al. 2001). These unexpected results ties mast cells, to tolerance promping us to note the potential functional role of mast cells in the establishment of Tregs-mediated allograft tolerance.

It is known that host-derived TGF-β is crucial for peripheral immune-suppression mediated by Tregs. It is tempting to speculate that Tregs-activated mast cells are responsible for TGF-β production, or the liberation and activation of TGF-β via other known or unknown factors that mast cells secrete (Mesples et al. 2005). In addition, tryptophan hydroxylase isoform (TPH1), like IDO, is an enzyme that can metabolize tryptophan and create a tryptophan-deficient environment (Lee et al. 2002). As such, this may be a mechanism used by mast cells to limit T-cell activation. Secondly, recruitment of mast cells into sites of peripheral tolerance may be a common mechanism to control long-lived immune unresponsiveness at that site. In addition to allograft tolerance, a number of tumor models have documented the accumulation of mast cells, as well as Tregs at the tumor sites. Also, it has been shown that mast cells may contribute to tumor growth and metastasis (Theoharides and Conti 2004, Wedemeyer and Galli 2005). Thus, like in the allograft model, the Tregs-mast cell partnership may also have an immunosuppressive role in dampening the immune response to tumors. In addition, both nTregs and iTregs may secrete IL-9, and through IL-9 and other effector molecules they may mediate the activities of mast cells in vivo. Hence, IL-9, mast cells and their other gene products may become attractive therapeutic targets to ameliorate the impact of Tregs in vivo.

Active suppression/regulation by Tregs is essential to establish and sustain self-tolerance. The finding that mast cells are critical in Tregs-dependent allograft tolerance, this further expands the knowledge of the interplay of different cellular components in controlling immune responses. Future studies will continue to unravel this pathway and will allow us to understand other mediators and cells that ultimately control peripheral immune suppression.

5.4.4 Tregs and Histamine Interaction

Although mast cells are traditionally viewed in the context of allergy and asthma, the ability of mast cells to become activated by diverse stimuli and to produce a wide variety of mediators makes them important players also in many other physiological processes (Bischoff 2007). Mast cells are an important component of the innate immune system, acting as sentinel cells that detect infecting microorganisms via pattern recognition molecules such as toll-like receptors (TLR) (Marshall 2004). The wide variety of cytokines, chemokines, and other mediators, including histamine, that are produced and released by mast cells following their activation are believed to promote the recruitment of other immune effector cells and thus modulate their activity. Since mast cells are first-line responders to microbial infections and are present in environments that may also contain endogenous Tregs, it seems likely that mast cells and Tregs might affect each others' function. However, only limited information is available on the interactions that take place between mast cells and Tregs. In a mouse model of sepsis, adoptive transfer of Tregs correlates with an increase in mast cell numbers in the peritoneum (Heuer et al. 2005), whereas mast cell recruitment to skin allografts in response to IL-9 produced by Tregs is essential for the establishment of tolerance to alloantigens (Lu et al. 2006).

In addition, a recent study (Kashyap et al. 2008) showed that Tregs downregulate FcεRI expression by mast cells in vitro through a contact-dependent mechanism and also downregulate IgE-mediated leukotriene C_4 production by mast cells. Although, these studies indicate that Tregs possess the capacity to recruit mast cells and regulate their activation, the effect(s) that mast cells have on Tregs suppressor function has not yet been investigated.

In this study, we review for the first time that histamine released by activated murine bone marrow-derived mast cells (BMMC) inhibited the suppressor function of $CD4^+CD25^+$ Tregs by signaling through H1 receptor. In addition, the histamine-induced decrease in Tregs suppressor function was associated with reduced expression of CD25 and the Tregs-specific transcription factor Foxp3. Activation-induced release of histamine by mast cells may promote the development of protective immune responses to infecting microorganisms by transiently down-regulating endogenous Tregs activity.

Although both $CD4^+CD25^+$ Tregs and $CD4^+CD25^-$ T cells (Tresp) express H1 receptors, histamine acts on the Tregs rather than on responder CD4 T (Tresp) cells, which renders them refractory to Tregs-mediated suppression. The proliferation of Tresp cells that were pretreated with histamine was potently suppressed by untreated Tregs, where as Tregs that were pretreated with histamine did not inhibit the proliferation of untreated Tresp cells.

In recent studies, Forward's group demonstrated that, histamine released by FcR-activated BMMC abrogated the suppressor function of $CD4^+CD25^+$ Tregs. It has been shown in the study that activated BMMC potently inhibit the suppressor function of $CD4^+CD25^+$ Tregs through a mechanism that involved H1 histamine receptor signaling. Furthermore, the H1 receptor agonist, histamine, 2-pyridylethylamine (2-PEA) mimicked histamine-mediated inhibition of Tregs functions. In contrast, H2 receptor antagonism with famotidine did not substantially block the activated BMMC, or histamine-mediated inhibition of Tregs function. The H2 receptor agonist ADHB had little effect on Tregs function. Histamine signaling through the H1 receptor is reported to enhance proliferative responses and IFN-production by $CD4^+$ Th1 cells (Jutel et al. 2001). However, increased $CD4^+$ T cell proliferation and cytokine production may have been caused by histamine H1 receptor-mediated inhibition of endogenous $CD4^+CD25^+$ Tregs contained within the $CD4^+$ responder T cell population. These observations underscore the need to consider the possible effect(s) of endogenous $CD4^+CD25^+$ Tregs when using $CD4^+$ T cells that are heterogeneous in terms of their CD25 expression as a readout system. We suggest that at an early stage of infection-induced inflammation, mast cells are activated and degranulate in response to microbial products. In this regard, streptococcal exotoxin B stimulates human mast cells to release histamine (Watanabe et al. 2002), whereas FimH from *Escherichia coli* is a potent stimulator of mouse mast cell de-granulation (Malaviya et al. 1994). Histamine signaling through the H1 receptor leads to a transient reduction in the suppressor function of endogenous $CD4^+CD25^+$ Tregs, which allows for optimal activation of effector $CD4^+$ and $CD8^+$ T cells. As the infectious agent is cleared, mast cell stimulation by microbial products is reduced and local histamine levels decline. At this point, Tregs suppressor function is restored, and the immune response is down-regulated to minimize bystander damage to healthy tissues. Interestingly, intra-tracheal administration of the H4 receptor agonist 4-methyl histamine is associated with the accumulation of $Foxp3^+$ T cells in the lung in a mouse model of airway hypersensitivity (Morgan et al. 2007), suggesting that histamine may also act via H4 receptors to recruit Tregs to resolve acute inflammation.

5.5 NKT Cells

A subset of T lymphocytes recognize lipid antigens presented by conserved CD1 molecules (Group 1: CD1a, CD1b, CD1c; and Group 2: CD1d). CD1 molecules are non-polymorphic MHC-class-I-like glycoproteins, present endogenous self lipids as well as exogenous microbial and plant pollen derived lipid antigens to the respective CD1-restricted T cells (Agea et al. 2005, Barral and Brenner 2007,

Brutkiewicz 2006, Burdin and Kronenberg 1999, Porcelli and Modlin 1999). CD1a, b and c are expressed on cortical thymocytes and DC in both lymphoid and non-lymphoid organs, and are inducible by exposure to GM-CSF (Porcelli et al. 1992). Also they are abundantly found on langerhans cells (CD1a) and macrophages (Mϕ) in multiple sclerosis patients (CD1b) (Battistini et al. 1996), and B cells (CD1c) (Porcelli 1995). CD1d molecules are expressed on the surface of DC, Mϕ, B cells, subset of activated T cells, γδ T cells, cortical thymocytes, and non-hematopoietic cells (keratinocytes, hepatocytes, intestinal and lung epithelial cells) (Barral and Brenner 2007, Blumberg et al. 1991, Bonish et al. 2000, Eguchi-Ogawa et al. 2007, Exley et al. 2000, Lalazar et al. 2006, Looringh van Beeck et al. 2009, Russano et al. 2007). Pigs are immunologically more similar to humans and they too have both group 1 and group 2 CD1 genes and their mRNA transcripts (Eguchi-Ogawa et al. 2007). CD1-restricted T cells are important players in both innate and adaptive immune responses (Barral and Brenner 2007, Bendelac et al. 2007, Brutkiewicz 2006, Brutkiewicz and Sriram 2002, Godfrey and Kronenberg 2004, Godfrey et al. 2000).

Natural killer T (NKT) cells are CD1d-restricted and are widely studied due to their important role in the host's immunity, and due to availability of appropriate immunological tools to study them. NKT cells are present in all mammals except ruminants (Looringh van Beeck et al. 2009, Van Rhijn et al. 2006). They respond to CD1d bound lipid antigens with a unique α-anomerically linked sugar, one such well studied universal super agonist is α-Galactosylceramide (α-GalCer) (Kawano et al. 1997, Spada et al. 1998). NKT cells are positively selected by CD1d molecules. Majority of NKT cells are called as invariant NKT (iNKT), because they express a highly conserved invariant TCR (Vα14Jα18 in mice and Vα24Jα18 in humans), preferentially paired with Vβ chain of limited diversity. α-GalCer is derived from the marine sponge *Agelas mauritanius*, and it induces rapid cytokine production from iNKT cells both in vivo and in vitro (Metelitsa et al. 2001, Nakagawa et al. 1998, Nieda et al. 2001, Yamaguchi et al. 1996). All the α-GalCer reactive NKT cells are called iNKT or Type I NKT. Other NKT cell subsets are Type II and III NKT cells, both possess diverse TCRα chain, but they also recognize glycolipids (Matangkasombut et al. 2009). We and others have studied distinct roles of Type I and Type II NKT cells in a murine model of T and B cell lymphomas (Godfrey and Kronenberg 2004, Godfrey et al. 2000, Renukaradhya et al. 2006, 2008b, Terabe and Berzofsky 2007). The important role of NKT cells to many viral and bacterial infections have also been reported by us and others (Broxmeyer et al. 2007, Huber et al. 2003, Johnson et al. 2002, Lalazar et al. 2006, Renukaradhya et al. 2005, 2008a).

It has been found that a larger population of NKT cells exists that can be identified by the co-expression of natural killer (NK) surface receptors such as NKP,-P1 (NKI.1 in C57BL/6 mouse strain). In addition to CD4 and CD8 double negative (DN) NKT cells, there are CD4 single-positive (SP) (Arase et al. 1992, Bendelac et al. 1994, Takahama et al. 1991), but not CD8β SP cells are present in mice (Bendelac et al. 1994). NKT cells TCR bias is a concern, as the majority of iNKT cells use a single invariant TCRα chain (Lantz and Bendelac 1994).

NKT cells are found in thymus where they account for 10–20% of adult mature (HSA lo) thymocyte compartment, i.e., upto 0.5% of thymus. In the periphery, particularly in liver they account for 15–50% of the T cells in mice. They are also found to a lesser degree in the spleen (1% of total T-cells) and peripheral lymph nodes (0.3% of T cells) (Bendelac et al. 1994, Ohteki and MacDonald 1994, Yoshimoto and Paul 1994). NKT cells display two sets of unusual biological functions. First, upon primary activation they secrete a large array of both Thl and Th2 cytokines. In this aspect, they resemble activated effector T cells (with which they share a $CD44^{hi}$ $LECAM\text{-}1^{lo}$ $3GII^{lo}$ phenotype) (Bendelac et al. 1992, 1994, Hayakawa et al. 1992, Lantz and Bendelac 1994) rather than conventional naive T cells (Arase et al. 1993, Bendelac and Schwartz 1991, Hayakawa et al. 1992, Yoshimoto and Paul 1994). The cytokine release is particularly impressive, because it occurs rapidly in vivo within hours of TCR engagement (Yoshimoto and Paul 1994). As the early secretion of IL-4 strongly promotes the Th2 class of $CD4^+$ T cell responses (Seder and Paul 1994), the recruitment of NKT cells is likely to have immunoregulatory consequences. In addition to the markers of activated/memory T cells, they also express most known NK receptors, including NKR-P1, Ly-49A and Ly49C, IL-2 receptor α chain and the surface protein recognized by 3A4 mAb (Bendelac et al. 1994, Koyasu 1994, Lantz and Bendelac 1994, Sykes 1990).

Although NKT cells could potentially influence both Thl/Th2 immune responses, they act as natural suppressors of graft-versus-host disease (Palathumpat et al. 1992, Yankelevich et al. 1989), and regulate autoimmune symptoms in lupus (Mozes et al. 1993, Takeda and Dennert 1993) and diabetes (Rapoport et al. 1993). There are as yet no biological phenomena with which they have been directly associated. The key characteristic features of NKT cells include heavily biased TCR gene usage, CD1d restriction and high levels of cytokine production, particularly IL-4 and IFN-γ. In mice, these cells are commonly defined as $NK1.1^+\alpha\beta TCR^+$. As cells bearing these markers are phenotypically and functionally heterogeneous, it is appropriate to compare the different subsets of cells encompassed within this population. Most of the studies covered in this review relate to NKT cells in mice, unless otherwise specified.

5.5.1 NKT Cell Subsets

Although the term NKT was only recently applied, these cells were first described in 1987. Most of the earlier studies in mice were focused on thymic $\alpha\beta TCR^+$ T cells that were CD4 and CD8 double negative (αβDN) with highly biased Vβ8.2 usage. A major subset of these cells was found to express NK1.1, previously associated with NK cells, and to have the potential to secrete high amounts of cytokines. A population of $NK1.1^+$ $CD4^+$ T cells was also identified with similar characteristics (Bendelac 1995, Bendelac et al. 1997, MacDonald 1995). Subsequent reports showed that both populations predominantly express TCR Vα14Jα281 and that their development was dependent on the MHC class I-like, β_2-microglobulin-associated molecule, CD1d. These findings strongly suggested that $NK1.1^+\alpha\beta DN$ and $NK1.1^+CD4^+$ T cells were part of the same lineage (Bendelac 1995, Bendelac et al. 1997, MacDonald 1995). Thus, in recent years NKT cells are usually identified by the co-expression of αβTCR and NK1.1.

Several studies have shown that $CD4^+$, DN and $CD8\alpha^+$ $NK1.1^+$ T cells are present in most tissues and are phenotypically and functionally distinct. Furthermore, peripheral $NK1.1^+$ T-cell subsets differ from their thymic counterparts. Thymus and liver $CD4^+$ and DN NKT cells are generally alike, although those in the liver have greatly reduced expression of the MHC class-I ligands Ly49 A, C/I and G2 (Robson MacDonald et al. 1998). Spleen, lymph nodes and bone-marrow NKT cells are far more heterogeneous. For example, although splenic $CD4^+$ NKT cells are similar to thymic NKT cells, many splenic DN NKT cells are not CD1d-dependent (Benlagha et al. 2000, Eberl et al. 1999b), and they have a more heterogeneous TCR repertoire (Apostolou et al. 2000, Eberl et al. 1999a, Hammond et al. 1999), and produce lower levels of cytokines following short-term in vitro stimulation (Hammond et al. 1999). The likelihood that splenic DN $NK1.1^+$ T cells include two distinct subsets is supported by the bimodal expression of other cell-surface markers and by bimodal reactivity with CD1d-α-GalCer tetramers (Benlagha et al. 2000). Splenic $CD8\alpha^+$ $NK1.1^+$ T cells are CD1d and thymus-independent, express heterogeneous TCR, and do not produce IL-4 rapidly. In addition, some $NK1.1^-CD4^+$ T cells closely resemble cells of the NKT-cell family in their CD1d-reactivity, TCR Vβ8-bias, and high IL-4-production (Benlagha et al. 2000, Chen and Paul 1998, Hameg et al. 1999, Moodycliffe et al. 1999). One explanation for this might be that NK1.1 can be downregulated upon NKT-cell activation (Chen et al. 1997).

5.5.2 Thymus Dependence on NKT Cells

Considering the controversy surrounding the developmental origin of NKT cells, some of the studies showed clear differences between NKT cell subsets; one possibility was that these subsets may have distinct developmental origins. Neonatal thymectomy leads to a specific reduction in NKT cell numbers in peripheral tissues of adult mice (Hammond et al. 1998a). More detailed analysis indicates that both $CD4^+$ and DN NKT cells were significantly reduced, accounting for the drop in total NKT cell numbers, whereas $CD8\alpha^+$ NKT cells in the spleen and liver were not affected in neonatally thymectomized mice. Thus, either $CD8\alpha^+$ NKT cells are a thymus-independent population, or they develop in and leave the thymus prior to day 3 of birth and are maintained in the periphery in a thymus-independent fashion thereafter. The latter possibility seems less likely, as NKT cells are not detected in the neonatal thymus until at least day 7 (Hammond et al. 1998b) and $CD8\alpha^+$ NKT cells are not detected in the thymus of adult mice.

5.5.3 Migration of NKT Cells from Thymus to Periphery

A straightforward approach to determine the thymic origin of NKT cell subsets is to test whether these cells are present amongst recent thymic emigrants (RTE). In one particular study FITC was injected into thymic lobes and $FITC^+$ cells were analyzed in peripheral organs for the presence of NKT cell subsets after 16–36 h. The proportion of $FITC^+$ RTE detected in these experiments was between 0.5 and 1.5%, as expected from the previous studies (Hammond et al. 1999). $NK1.1^+$ cells represented 1.1% of splenic RTE and as in the thymus, both $CD4^+$ and $CD4^-$ subsets were present. In some experiments the $CD4^-$ $NK1.1^+$ RTE cells were further subdivided on the basis of αβTCR expression. Of $CD4^-NK1.1^+$ RTE, 40% were $CD4^-$ $\alpha\beta TCR^+$ (DN NKT cells) and 38% were $CD4^-$ αβ TCR^- (NK) cells. Very few $NK1.1^+$ cells were found among RTE homing to the lymph nodes as expected, since this is not a tissue in which NKT cells normally reside. Moreover, $NK1.1^+$ cells comprised 4.4% of this population and the majority were $\alpha\beta TCR^+$ (75%), including $CD4^+$ and $CD4^-$ cells. This was an important observation as the liver is proposed to be a site of extra-thymic NKT cell development (Makino et al. 1993, Sato et al. 1999). As all livers were perfused via the hepatic portal veins in situ, the level of blood contamination was extremely low and could account for less than 1% of liver RTE which directly demonstrated that at least some liver NKT cells are thymus derived.

5.5.4 NKT Cells in Humans

Humans also have NKT cells with very similar characteristics to mouse NKT cells including DN (Dellabona et al. 1994, Exley et al. 1997) and $CD4^+$ subsets (Davodeau et al. 1997). Both subsets react with mice CD1d and produce high levels of IL-4 and IFN-γ when stimulated (Takahashi et al. 2000a). Significantly, human NKT cells express the homologous TCR gene rearrangement (Vβ11, the homologue of mouse Vβ8.2; and Vα24JαQ, the homologue of mouse Vα14Jα281). Furthermore, human NKT cells can recognize mouse CD1d and vice versa, indicating highly conserved specificity (Burdin et al. 1999).

5.5.5 Factors Influencing NKT-Cell Development

In addition to CD1d, several other factors are known to influence NKT-cell development. Thymic stromal-cell-derived cytokines IL-15 and IL-7 are required for development of normal numbers and IL-4-producing potential, respectively. Of both $CD4^+$ and DN NKT cells (Ohteki et al. 1997, Vicari et al. 1996), an intact thymic structure is also important (Elewaut et al. 2000, Iizuka et al. 1999, Nakagawa et al. 1997). In contrast to conventional T cells, NKT cell development requires an interaction with membrane lymphotoxin expressing cells (Elewaut et al. 2000, Iizuka et al. 1999). Interestingly, lymphotoxin deficiency affected all three populations ($CD4^+$, DN and $CD8^+$) of $NK1.1^+$ T cells, suggesting at least some commonality to the development of these subsets (Elewaut et al. 2000). NKT cell development is also absolutely dependent on pre-Ta signaling (Eberl et al. 1999a) and partly dependent on GM-CSF signaling (Sato et al. 1999). Fyn-deficient mice show a selective defect in the development of CD1d-dependent NKT cells, but not conventional T cells, or $CD8^+NK1.1^+$ T cells (Eberl et al. 1999c, Gadue et al. 1999). Analysis of NKT cells in common cytokine receptor γ-chain-deficient mice revealed at least two stages in NKT cell development (Lantz et al. 1997). Such mice generate thymocytes expressing normal amounts of Vα14Jα281 mRNA and develop IL-4 producing DN cells suggesting the presence of NKT cells, yet these cells fail to express the NK receptors NK1.1 and Ly49, and are not exported to the periphery. Thus, intra-thymic selection and development of IL-4-producing capacity seem to be an earlier processes, whereas acquisition of the NK surface phenotype and emigration to the periphery are later common γ-chain-dependent events.

5.5.6 NKT Cell Ligands

The expression of CD3/αβTCR by NKT cells suggests that they require TCR-specific recognition to get activated. The biased TCR gene usage of mouse and human NKT cells probably reflects the fact that they are restricted to CD1d during their development and possibly their activation (Bendelac et al. 1997, Hong et al. 1999). The TCR-bias and CD1d-dependence of mouse $NK1.1^+$ T cells varies between subsets and different tissues. The target of the non-TCR-biased, CD1-independent $NK1.1^+$ T cells is unknown, but their more diverse TCR expression (Eberl et al. 1999b, Hammond et al. 1999) suggests it is a conventional MHC–peptide complex. Most NKT cells seem to recognize CD1d in conjunction with hydrophobic ligands (probably glycolipids) (Benlagha et al. 2000, Burdin and Kronenberg 1999), although the precise nature of these ligands is not yet clear. One candidate family of natural ligands might be the glycosylphosphatidylinositol (GPI)-anchors (Joyce et al. 1998, Schofield et al. 1999) and phosphoinositol mannosides (Apostolou et al. 1999), although this issue remains contentious (Burdin et al. 1998, Molano et al. 2000). The ability of NKT cells to respond to tumor-derived lipid extracts (including phospholipids) in the context of CD1d suggests that they might see a natural lipid ligand, possibly altered in tumor tissue (Gumperz et al. 2000). There are obviously several possibilities that need not be mutually exclusive. Given that NKT cells appear to show tissue specificity in their recognition of CD1d (Hong et al. 1999), it seems likely that these cells can recognize a diverse array of hydrophobic ligands in conjunction with CD1d, indicating the potential for antigen-specific activation, and perhaps even self-tolerance of these cells.

5.5.6.1 α-Galactosylceramide (α-GalCer)

α-GalCer is derived from a marine sponge, binds CD1d and strongly stimulates both $CD4^+$ and DN NKT cells (Hong et al. 1999, Kawano et al. 1997). Although GalCers are a major constituent of some mammalian tissues, particularly in the central nervous system, the majority appear to be β-linked galactosylceramides (β-GalCers), rather than α-linked GalCers. The nature of the galactosyl linkage might be a critical point, since α-GalCers show stronger immune-stimulatory activities than β-GalCers (Motoki et al. 1995). It is therefore probably significant that the genes encoding a 3–1 galactosyl transferases, which are thought to be responsible for synthesizing such α-linked carbohydrate moieties are defective in humans and some other old-world primates (Galili and Swanson 1991, Larsen et al. 1990), suggesting on face value that α-GalCer cannot be a normal product of human cells. However, as this carbohydrate moiety also defines the human "B" blood group, this is clearly an area requiring more systematic study. If α-GalCer is not a product of human cells, it might either mimic a natural ligand, or displace CD1d-bound glycolipids through high-affinity interactions with CD1d.

5.5.7 *Role of NKT Cells in Immune Responses*

The range of actions attributed to NKT cells is extremely diverse. Many studies have suggested that an important natural function for NKT cells might be to protect self-tissues (particularly vital organs) from damaging inflammatory-type immune responses. There is also clear evidence that they can control immune responses to infection and some tumors.

5.5.7.1 Th1 Inhibition

In some systems, NKT cells suppress Th1-associated cell-mediated immunity (Hammond et al. 1998b, Sonoda et al. 1999, Wang et al. 1997, Zeng et al. 1999) through production of IL-4, IL-10 and/or TGF-β. NKT cells are essential for controlling anterior chamber-associated immune-deviation (ACAID), believed to prevent the eye from damage by inflammatory immune responses. This phenomenon was originally found to be thymus-dependent, and specifically regulated by thymic αβDN cells (Wang et al. 1997), and more recently, it was associated with NKT cells (Sonoda et al. 1999). Interestingly, the latter study also showed restoration of ACAID using adoptive transfer of NKT cells from spleen, in apparent contrast with the thymus-dependent population identified in an earlier study. Bone-marrow DN NKT cells were observed to be important in preventing graft-versus-host disease following allogeneic bone-marrow transplantation in an IL-4-dependent manner (Zeng et al. 1999), which might reflect a natural role for these cells in preventing inflammatory immune responses in the bone marrow.

5.5.7.2 Th2 Induction

The strong capacity to produce IL-4 has led to a speculation that NKT cells might drive the differentiation of Th2 responses (Bendelac 1995, Bendelac et al. 1997, MacDonald 1995). Although demonstrated in few studies, most investigations using NKT-deficient (CD1d$^{-/-}$ or β2 M$^{-/-}$) (Bendelac et al. 1997) mice do not support an essential role for these cells in such responses (Bendelac et al. 1997, Hong et al.

1999). However, this does not exclude them as important players in some Th2-associated responses. For example, Vα14 TCR transgenic mice, which have tenfold increased NKT-cell numbers have elevated serum IgE and IL-4 levels (Bendelac et al. 1996), and NKT-cell activation in vivo promotes Th2-associated immunity (Burdin et al. 1999, Kitamura et al. 2000, Singh et al. 1999).

5.5.8 Relationship Between Histamines and NKT Cells

Histamine involvement in modulation of cytokines secreted by iNKT cells was demonstrated (Lisbonne et al. 2003). As rapid production of cytokines (IL-4 and IFN-γ) in response to TCR cross-linking constitutes a typical feature of iNKT cells. In this study, α-GalCer was injected to wild-type and histamine deficient (HDC) mice to determine its capacity to specifically activate and promptly induce these cytokines. HDC is the enzyme which is required to synthesize HA. Result of that study revealed that a single injection of α-GalCer induced significantly higher IL-4 and IFN-γ levels in the serum of wildtype mice than $HDC^{-/-}$ mice. On the contrary this cytokine producing capacity of iNKT cells was restored in $HDC^{-/-}$ mice when they were treated with HA 1 hr before α-GalCer stimulation. The reduced function of iNKT cells in $HDC^{-/-}$ mice could result either from a lower incidence or a functional defect of iNKT cells. Further, CD1d/α-GalCer tetramer positive cells were effectively reduced in spleen and liver of $HDC^{-/-}$ mice, both in terms of cell counts and percentage. It turned out that among gated iNKT cells, the percentage of cells that were actually positive for IL-4 and IFN-γ after injection of α-GalCer was strikingly reduced in $HDC^{-/-}$mice compared with controls. Even though HA treatment did not enhance the percentage or the absolute number of iNKT cells significantly, but it did increase the proportion of IL-4 and IFN-γ positive cells among gated iNKT lymphocytes, consistent with the restored serum cytokine levels (Leite-de-Moraes et al. 2009)

The contribution of iNKT cells to immune responses is complex because of their capacity to rapidly produce both Th1 (IFNγ) and Th2-cytokines (IL-4, IL-13 etc.), rapidly upon activation, thereby supporting Th1 or Th2 responses, respectively. The inflammatory nature of asthma is characterized by massive infiltration of eosinophils, lymphocytes, and mast cells in the airway mucosa leading to airway hyperreactivity (AHR), goblet cell hyperplasia and mucus overproduction (Matangkasombut et al. 2008, 2009). iNKT cells in a CD1d-dependent manner skew adaptive immunity towards Th2 responses, or can act directly as effector cells at mucosal surfaces, and they have been confirmed to play pivotal roles in regulating the development of asthma and allergy (Lisbonne et al. 2003, Matangkasombut et al. 2008, 2009, Meyer et al. 2007). NKT cells are remarkably conserved in sequence and function across species (Barral and Brenner 2007, Bendelac et al. 2007, Brutkiewicz 2006, Brutkiewicz and Sriram 2002, Godfrey and Kronenberg 2004, Godfrey et al. 2000). Asthma and chronic obstructive pulmonary disease following chronic viral infections is driven by IL-13, secreted upon CD1d-mediated interaction of macrophages and iNKT cells (Holtzman et al. 2009). This in turn, suggests an additional means for HA to enhance the severity of asthma by promoting optimal IL-4 production by iNKT cells. Consistent with this assumption, recently it has been reported that asthmatic mice treated with the drug JNJ7777120 (Histamine H4 antagonist) developed less airway inflammation than untreated controls (Dunford et al. 2006).

5.6 Concluding Remarks

Histamine is synthesized in all tissues, but particularly abundant in skin, lung and gastrointestinal tract. Mast cells are present in many tissues, and are the main source of histamine. In addition, histamine is also secreted by other immune cells in the body. Histamine has many pivotal roles in different types of allergic and inflammatory reactions. In addition to frank allergic reactions, histamine has significant effects on many aspects of immune reaction by binding to its diverse group of receptors expressed on B and T lymphocytes, dendritic cells, macrophages and a variety of hematopoietic cells. Among other things, histamine influences immune cell maturation and activation, secretion of several cytokines and chemo-tactic responses of cells. In this chapter, we tried to explain the significance of histamine in context with T-regulatory cells and NKT cells. Available literature reveals a new role of histamine through H4R activation in the functional modulation of the immunoregulatory invariant NKT cell population, and thus provides an additional evidence for the complex influence on iNKT cell functions. We discussed how iNKT cells can exacerbate asthma symptoms through Th2 cytokines (IL-4 and IL-13). Similarly, histamine plays a major role in allergic asthma, because its secretion in to the airways triggers a cascade of events, including airway constriction, mucus secretion, vascular leak, and recruitment of immune cells. Importantly, histamine has been found to play a major role in modulation of the immune responses through differential expression and activation of specific histamine receptors. For example, the net effect of signaling via the histamine H2 receptor on cells of hematopoietic origin, including both Th1- and Th2- type immune cells. These effects are attributed to stimulation of regulatory dendritic cells and Th2 cells to produce IL-10, which augments the immunosuppressive activity of TGF-b on T cells.

References

Agea E, Russano A, Bistoni O et al (2005) Human CD1-restricted T cell recognition of lipids from pollens. J Exp Med 202:295–308

Apostolou I, Cumano A, Gachelin G et al (2000) Evidence for two subgroups of CD4-CD8- NKT cells with distinct TCR alpha beta repertoires and differential distribution in lymphoid tissues. J Immunol 165:2481–2490

Apostolou I, Takahama Y, Belmant C et al (1999) Murine natural killer T(NKT) cells [correction of natural killer cells] contribute to the granulomatous reaction caused by mycobacterial cell walls. Proc Natl Acad Sci USA 96:5141–5146

Arad G, Nussinovich R, Na'amad M et al (1996) Dual control of human interleukin-2 and interferon-gamma gene expression by histamine: activation and suppression. Cell Immunol 170:149–155

Arase H, Arase N, Nakagawa K et al (1993) NK1.1+ CD4+ CD8- thymocytes with specific lymphokine secretion. Eur J Immunol 23:307–310

Arase H, Arase N, Ogasawara K et al (1992) An NK1.1+ CD4+8- single-positive thymocyte subpopulation that expresses a highly skewed T-cell antigen receptor V beta family. Proc Natl Acad Sci USA 89:6506–6510

Arrang JM, Drutel G, Garbarg M et al (1995) Molecular and functional diversity of histamine receptor subtypes. Ann N Y Acad Sci 757:314–323

Askenasy N, Kaminitz A, Yarkoni S (2008) Mechanisms of T regulatory cell function. Autoimmun Rev 7:370–375

Bachmann MF, Kohler G, Ecabert B et al (1999) Cutting edge: lymphoproliferative disease in the absence of CTLA-4 is not T cell autonomous. J Immunol 163:1128–1131

Baecher-Allan C, Hafler DA (2004) Suppressor T cells in human diseases. J Exp Med 200:273–276

Banu Y, Watanabe T (1999) Augmentation of antigen receptor-mediated responses by histamine H1 receptor signaling. J Exp Med 189:673–682

Barral DC, Brenner MB (2007) CD1 antigen presentation: how it works. Nat Rev Immunol 7: 929–941

Battistini L, Fischer FR, Raine CS et al (1996) CD1b is expressed in multiple sclerosis lesions. J Neuroimmunol 67:145–151

Bayram H, Devalia JL, Khair OA et al (1999) Effect of loratadine on nitrogen dioxide-induced changes in electrical resistance and release of inflammatory mediators from cultured human bronchial epithelial cells. J Allergy Clin Immunol 104:93–99

Bendelac A (1995) Mouse NK1^{+} T cells. Curr Opin Immunol 7:367–374

Bendelac A, Hunziker RD, Lantz O (1996) Increased interleukin 4 and immunoglobulin E production in transgenic mice overexpressing NK1 T cells. J Exp Med 184:1285–1293

Bendelac A, Killeen N, Littman DR et al (1994) A subset of CD4+ thymocytes selected by MHC class I molecules. Science 263:1774–1778

Bendelac A, Matzinger P, Seder RA et al (1992) Activation events during thymic selection. J Exp Med 175:731–742

Bendelac A, Rivera MN, Park SH et al (1997) Mouse CD1-specific NK1 T cells: development, specificity, and function. Annu Rev Immunol 15:535–562

Bendelac A, Savage PB, Teyton L (2007) The biology of NKT cells. Annu Rev Immunol 25: 297–336

Bendelac A, Schwartz RH (1991) CD4+ and CD8+ T cells acquire specific lymphokine secretion potentials during thymic maturation. Nature 353:68–71

Benlagha K, Weiss A, Beavis A et al (2000) In vivo identification of glycolipid antigen-specific T cells using fluorescent CD1d tetramers. J Exp Med 191:1895–1903

Bennett CL, Christie J, Ramsdell F et al (2001) The immune dysregulation, polyendocrinopathy, enteropathy, X-linked syndrome (IPEX) is caused by mutations of FOXP3. Nat Genet 27: 20–21

Bischoff SC (2007) Role of mast cells in allergic and non-allergic immune responses: comparison of human and murine data. Nat Rev Immunol 7:93–104

Blumberg RS, Terhorst C, Bleicher P et al (1991) Expression of a nonpolymorphic MHC class I-like molecule, CD1D, by human intestinal epithelial cells. J Immunol 147:2518–2524

Bonish B, Jullien D, Dutronc Y et al (2000) Overexpression of CD1d by keratinocytes in psoriasis and CD1d-dependent IFN-gamma production by NK-T cells. J Immunol 165:4076–4085

Broxmeyer HE, Dent A, Cooper S et al (2007) A role for natural killer T cells and CD1d molecules in counteracting suppression of hematopoiesis in mice induced by infection with murine cytomegalovirus. Exp Hematol 35:87–93

Brunkow ME, Jeffery EW, Hjerrild KA et al (2001) Disruption of a new forkhead/winged-helix protein, scurfin, results in the fatal lymphoproliferative disorder of the scurfy mouse. Nat Genet 27:68–73

Brutkiewicz RR (2006) CD1d ligands: the good, the bad, and the ugly. J Immunol 177:769–775
Brutkiewicz RR, Sriram V (2002) Natural killer T (NKT) cells and their role in antitumor immunity. Crit Rev Oncol Hematol 41:287–298
Burdin N, Brossay L, Koezuka Y et al (1998) Selective ability of mouse CD1 to present glycolipids: alpha-galactosylceramide specifically stimulates V alpha 14+ NK T lymphocytes. J Immunol 161:3271–3281
Burdin N, Brossay L, Kronenberg M (1999) Immunization with alpha-galactosylceramide polarizes CD1-reactive NK T cells towards Th2 cytokine synthesis. Eur J Immunol 29:2014–2025
Burdin N, Kronenberg M (1999) CD1-mediated immune responses to glycolipids. Curr Opin Immunol 11:326–331
Carlsson R, Dohlsten M, Sjogren HO (1985) Histamine modulates the production of interferon-gamma and interleukin-2 by mitogen-activated human mononuclear blood cells. Cell Immunol 96:104–112
Caron G, Delneste Y, Roelandts E et al (2001a) Histamine polarizes human dendritic cells into Th2 cell-promoting effector dendritic cells. J Immunol 167:3682–3686
Caron G, Delneste Y, Roelandts E et al (2001b) Histamine induces CD86 expression and chemokine production by human immature dendritic cells. J Immunol 166:6000–6006
Chatila TA, Blaeser F, Ho N et al (2000) JM2, encoding a fork head-related protein, is mutated in X-linked autoimmunity-allergic disregulation syndrome. J Clin Invest 106:R75–81
Chen H, Huang H, Paul WE (1997) NK1.1$^+$ CD4$^+$ T cells lose NK1.1 expression upon in vitro activation. J Immunol 158:5112–5119
Chen H, Paul WE (1998) A population of CD62Llow Nk1.1- CD4+ T cells that resembles NK1.1$^+$ CD4$^+$ T cells. Eur J Immunol 28:3172–3182
Chen Z, Herman AE, Matos M et al (2005) Where CD4+CD25+ T reg cells impinge on autoimmune diabetes. J Exp Med 202:1387–1397
Coutinho A, Hori S, Carvalho T et al (2001) Regulatory T cells: the physiology of autoreactivity in dominant tolerance and "quality control" of immune responses. Immunol Rev 182:89–98
Davodeau F, Peyrat MA, Necker A et al (1997) Close phenotypic and functional similarities between human and murine alphabeta T cells expressing invariant TCR alpha-chains. J Immunol 158:5603–5611
Dellabona P, Padovan E, Casorati G et al (1994) An invariant V alpha 24-J alpha Q/V beta 11 T cell receptor is expressed in all individuals by clonally expanded CD4–8- T cells. J Exp Med 180:1171–1176
Dohlsten M, Sjogren HO, Carlsson R (1986) Histamine inhibits interferon-gamma production via suppression of interleukin 2 synthesis. Cell Immunol 101:493–501
Dunford PJ, O'Donnell N, Riley JP et al (2006) The histamine H4 receptor mediates allergic airway inflammation by regulating the activation of CD4+ T cells. J Immunol 176:7062–7070
Dy M, Arnould A, Lemoine FM et al (1996) Hematopoietic progenitors and interleukin-3-dependent cell lines synthesize histamine in response to calcium ionophore. Blood 87: 3161–3169
Eberl G, Fehling HJ, von Boehmer H et al (1999a) Absolute requirement for the pre-T cell receptor alpha chain during NK1.1+ TCR alphabeta cell development. Eur J Immunol 29: 1966–1971
Eberl G, Lees R, Smiley ST et al (1999b) Tissue-specific segregation of CD1d-dependent and CD1d-independent NK T cells. J Immunol 162:6410–6419
Eberl G, Lowin-Kropf B, MacDonald HR (1999c) Cutting edge: NKT cell development is selectively impaired in Fyn- deficient mice. J Immunol 163:4091–4094
Eguchi-Ogawa T, Morozumi T, Tanaka M et al (2007) Analysis of the genomic structure of the porcine CD1 gene cluster. Genomics 89:248–261
Elenkov IJ, Webster E, Papanicolaou DA et al (1998) Histamine potently suppresses human IL-12 and stimulates IL-10 production via H2 receptors. J Immunol 161:2586–2593
Elewaut D, Brossay L, Santee SM et al (2000) Membrane lymphotoxin is required for the development of different subpopulations of NKT cells. J Immunol 165:671–679

Elliott KA, Osna NA, Scofield MA et al (2001) Regulation of IL-13 production by histamine in cloned murine T helper type 2 cells. Int Immunopharmacol 1:1923–1937

Exley M, Garcia J, Balk SP et al (1997) Requirements for CD1d recognition by human invariant Valpha24+ CD4-CD8- T cells. J Exp Med 186:109–120

Exley M, Garcia J, Wilson SB et al (2000) CD1d structure and regulation on human thymocytes, peripheral blood T cells, B cells and monocytes. Immunology 100:37–47

Fallarino F, Grohmann U, Hwang KW et al (2003) Modulation of tryptophan catabolism by regulatory T cells. Nat Immunol 4:1206–1212

Fehervari Z, Yamaguchi T, Sakaguchi S (2006) The dichotomous role of IL-2: tolerance versus immunity. Trends Immunol 27:109–111

Fontenot JD, Gavin MA, Rudensky AY (2003) Foxp3 programs the development and function of CD4+CD25+ regulatory T cells. Nat Immunol 4:330–336

Gadue P, Morton N, Stein PL (1999) The Src family tyrosine kinase Fyn regulates natural killer T cell development. J Exp Med 190:1189–1196

Galili U, Swanson K (1991) Gene sequences suggest inactivation of alpha-1,3-galactosyltransferase in catarrhines after the divergence of apes from monkeys. Proc Natl Acad Sci USA 88:7401–7404

Galli SJ, Nakae S, Tsai M (2005) Mast cells in the development of adaptive immune responses. Nat Immunol 6:135–142

Gambineri E, Torgerson TR, Ochs HD (2003) Immune dysregulation, polyendocrinopathy, enteropathy, and X-linked inheritance (IPEX), a syndrome of systemic autoimmunity caused by mutations of FOXP3, a critical regulator of T-cell homeostasis. Curr Opin Rheumatol 15:430–435

Gavin MA, Clarke SR, Negrou E et al (2002) Homeostasis and anergy of CD4(+)CD25(+) suppressor T cells in vivo. Nat Immunol 3:33–41

Godfrey DI, Hammond KJ, Poulton LD et al (2000) NKT cells: facts, functions and fallacies. Immunol Today 21:573–583

Godfrey DI, Kronenberg M (2004) Going both ways: immune regulation via CD1d-dependent NKT cells. J Clin Invest 114:1379–1388

Green EA, Choi Y, Flavell RA (2002) Pancreatic lymph node-derived CD4(+)CD25(+) Treg cells: highly potent regulators of diabetes that require TRANCE-RANK signals. Immunity 16: 183–191

Gumperz JE, Roy C, Makowska A et al (2000) Murine CD1d-restricted T cell recognition of cellular lipids. Immunity 12:211–221

Gutzmer R, Langer K, Lisewski M et al (2002) Expression and function of histamine receptors 1 and 2 on human monocyte-derived dendritic cells. J Allergy Clin Immunol 109:524–531

Hameg A, Gouarin C, Gombert JM et al (1999) IL-7 up-regulates IL-4 production by splenic NK1.1+ and NK1.1- MHC class I-like/CD1-dependent CD4+ T cells. J Immunol 162: 7067–7074

Hammond K, Cain W, van Driel I et al (1998a) Three day neonatal thymectomy selectively depletes NK1.1+ T cells. Int Immunol 10:1491–1499

Hammond KJ, Pelikan SB, Crowe NY et al (1999) NKT cells are phenotypically and functionally diverse. Eur J Immunol 29:3768–3781

Hammond KJ, Poulton LD, Palmisano LJ et al (1998b) alpha/beta-T cell receptor (TCR)+CD4-CD8- (NKT) thymocytes prevent insulin-dependent diabetes mellitus in nonobese diabetic (NOD)/Lt mice by the influence of interleukin (IL)-4 and/or IL-10. J Exp Med 187: 1047–1056

Hayakawa K, Lin BT, Hardy RR (1992) Murine thymic CD4+ T cell subsets: a subset (Thy0) that secretes diverse cytokines and overexpresses the V beta 8 T cell receptor gene family. J Exp Med 176:269–274

Heuer JG, Zhang T, Zhao J et al (2005) Adoptive transfer of in vitro-stimulated CD4+CD25+ regulatory T cells increases bacterial clearance and improves survival in polymicrobial sepsis. J Immunol 174:7141–7146

Holden CA, Chan SC, Norris S et al (1987) Histamine induced elevation of cyclic AMP phosphodiesterase activity in human monocytes. Agents Actions 22:36–42
Holtzman MJ, Byers DE, Benoit LA et al (2009) Immune pathways for translating viral infection into chronic airway disease. Adv Immunol 102:245–276
Hong S, Scherer DC, Singh N et al (1999) Lipid antigen presentation in the immune system: lessons learned from CD1d knockout mice. Immunol Rev 169:31–44
Hori S, Nomura T, Sakaguchi S (2003) Control of regulatory T cell development by the transcription factor Foxp3. Science 299:1057–1061
Hotermans G, Bury T, Radermecker MF (1991) Effect of histamine on tumor necrosis factor production by human monocytes. Int Arch Allergy Appl Immunol 95:278–281
Huber S, Sartini D, Exley M (2003) Role of CD1d in coxsackievirus B3-induced myocarditis. J Immunol 170:3147–3153
Idzko M, la Sala A, Ferrari D et al (2002) Expression and function of histamine receptors in human monocyte-derived dendritic cells. J Allergy Clin Immunol 109:839–846
Iizuka K, Chaplin DD, Wang Y et al (1999) Requirement for membrane lymphotoxin in natural killer cell development. Proc Natl Acad Sci USA 96:6336–6340
Jeannin P, Delneste Y, Gosset P et al (1994) Histamine induces interleukin-8 secretion by endothelial cells. Blood 84:2229–2233
Johnson TR, Hong S, Van Kaer L et al (2002) NKT cells contribute to expansion of CD8(+) T cells and amplification of antiviral immune responses to respiratory syncytial virus. J Virol 76:4294–4303
Joyce S, Woods AS, Yewdell JW et al (1998) Natural ligand of mouse CD1d1: cellular glycosylphosphatidylinositol. Science 279:1541–1544
Jutel M, Watanabe T, Klunker S et al (2001) Histamine regulates T-cell and antibody responses by differential expression of H1 and H2 receptors. Nature 413:420–425
Kapsenberg ML, Jansen HM, Bos JD et al (1992) Role of type 1 and type 2 T helper cells in allergic diseases. Curr Opin Immunol 4:788–793
Kashyap M, Thornton AM, Norton SK et al (2008) Cutting edge: CD4 T cell-mast cell interactions alter IgE receptor expression and signaling. J Immunol 180:2039–2043
Kawano T, Cui J, Koezuka Y et al (1997) CD1d-restricted and TCR-mediated activation of valpha14 NKT cells by glycosylceramides. Science 278:1626–1629
Khan MM, Sansoni P, Engleman EG et al (1985) Pharmacologic effects of autacoids on subsets of T cells. Regulation of expression/function of histamine-2 receptors by a subset of suppressor cells. J Clin Invest 75:1578–1583
Khattri R, Cox T, Yasayko SA et al (2003) An essential role for Scurfin in CD4+CD25+ T regulatory cells. Nat Immunol 4:337–342
Kitamura H, Ohta A, Sekimoto M et al (2000) Alpha-galactosylceramide induces early B-cell activation through IL-4 production by NKT cells. Cell Immunol 199:37–42
Koyasu S (1994) CD3+CD16+NK1.1+B220+ large granular lymphocytes arise from both alpha-beta TCR+CD4-CD8- and gamma-delta TCR+CD4-CD8- cells. J Exp Med 179:1957–1972
Krouwels FH, Hol BE, Lutter R et al (1998) Histamine affects interleukin-4, interleukin-5, and interferon-gamma production by human T cell clones from the airways and blood. Am J Respir Cell Mol Biol 18:721–730
Lalazar G, Preston S, Zigmond E et al (2006) Glycolipids as immune modulatory tools. Mini Rev Med Chem 6:1249–1253
Lantz O, Bendelac A (1994) An invariant T cell receptor alpha chain is used by a unique subset of major histocompatibility complex class I-specific CD4+ and CD4–8- T cells in mice and humans. J Exp Med 180:1097–1106
Lantz O, Sharara LI, Tilloy F et al (1997) Lineage relationships and differentiation of natural killer (NK) T cells: intrathymic selection and interleukin (IL)-4 production in the absence of NKR-P1 and Ly49 molecules. J Exp Med 185:1395–1401
Larsen RD, Rivera-Marrero CA, Ernst LK et al (1990) Frameshift and nonsense mutations in a human genomic sequence homologous to a murine UDP-Gal:beta-D-Gal(1,4)-D-GlcNAc alpha(1,3)-galactosyltransferase cDNA. J Biol Chem 265:7055–7061

Lee GK, Park HJ, Macleod M et al (2002) Tryptophan deprivation sensitizes activated T cells to apoptosis prior to cell division. Immunology 107:452–460

Leite-de-Moraes MC, Diem S, Michel ML et al (2009) Cutting edge: histamine receptor H4 activation positively regulates in vivo IL-4 and IFN-gamma production by invariant NKT cells. J Immunol 182:1233–1236

Leurs R, Vollinga RC, Timmerman H (1995) The medicinal chemistry and therapeutic potentials of ligands of the histamine H3 receptor. Prog Drug Res 45:107–165

Lim HW, Broxmeyer HE, Kim CH (2006) Regulation of trafficking receptor expression in human forkhead box P3+ regulatory T cells. J Immunol 177:840–851

Lisbonne M, Diem S, de Castro Keller A et al (2003) Cutting edge: invariant V alpha 14 NKT cells are required for allergen-induced airway inflammation and hyperreactivity in an experimental asthma model. J Immunol 171:1637–1641

Looringh van Beeck FA, Reinink P, Hermsen R et al (2009) Functional CD1d and/or NKT cell invariant chain transcript in horse, pig, African elephant and guinea pig, but not in ruminants. Mol Immunol 46:1424–1431

Lu LF, Lind EF, Gondek DC et al (2006) Mast cells are essential intermediaries in regulatory T-cell tolerance. Nature 442:997–1002

MacDonald HR (1995) NK1.1+ T cell receptor-alpha/beta+ cells: new clues to their origin, specificity, and function. J Exp Med 182:633–638

Makino Y, Yamagata N, Sasho T et al (1993) Extrathymic development of V alpha 14-positive T cells. J Exp Med 177:1399–1408

Malaviya R, Ross E, Jakschik BA et al (1994) Mast cell degranulation induced by type 1 fimbriated Escherichia coli in mice. J Clin Invest 93:1645–1653

Malek TR, Bayer AL (2004) Tolerance, not immunity, crucially depends on IL-2. Nat Rev Immunol 4:665–674

Maloy KJ, Powrie F (2001) Regulatory T cells in the control of immune pathology. Nat Immunol 2:816–822

Manzotti CN, Tipping H, Perry LC et al (2002) Inhibition of human T cell proliferation by CTLA-4 utilizes CD80 and requires CD25+ regulatory T cells. Eur J Immunol 32:2888–2896

Marshall JS (2004) Mast-cell responses to pathogens. Nat Rev Immunol 4:787–799

Matangkasombut P, Pichavant M, Dekruyff RH et al (2009) Natural killer T cells and the regulation of asthma. Mucosal Immunol 2:383–392

Matangkasombut P, Pichavant M, Yasumi T et al (2008) Direct activation of natural killer T cells induces airway hyperreactivity in nonhuman primates. J Allergy Clin Immunol 121:1287–1289

Mazzoni A, Young HA, Spitzer JH et al (2001) Histamine regulates cytokine production in maturing dendritic cells, resulting in altered T cell polarization. J Clin Invest 108:1865–1873

Meretey K, Falus A, Taga T et al (1991) Histamine influences the expression of the interleukin-6 receptor on human lymphoid, monocytoid and hepatoma cell lines. Agents Actions 33:189–191

Mesples B, Fontaine RH, Lelievre V et al (2005) Neuronal TGF-beta1 mediates IL-9/mast cell interaction and exacerbates excitotoxicity in newborn mice. Neurobiol Dis 18:193–205

Metelitsa LS, Naidenko OV, Kant A et al (2001) Human NKT cells mediate antitumor cytotoxicity directly by recognizing target cell CD1d with bound ligand or indirectly by producing IL-2 to activate NK cells. J Immunol 167:3114–3122

Meyer EH, DeKruyff RH, Umetsu DT (2007) iNKT cells in allergic disease. Curr Top Microbiol Immunol 314:269–291

Miyara M, Sakaguchi S (2007) Natural regulatory T cells: mechanisms of suppression. Trends Mol Med 13:108–116

Mochizuki T, Okakura-Mochizuki K, Horii A et al (1994) Histaminergic modulation of hippocampal acetylcholine release in vivo. J Neurochem 62:2275–2282

Molano A, Park SH, Chiu YH et al (2000) Cutting edge: the IgG response to the circumsporozoite protein is MHC class II-dependent and CD1d-independent: exploring the role of GPIs in NK T cell activation and antimalarial responses. J Immunol 164:5005–5009

Moodycliffe AM, Maiti S, Ullrich SE (1999) Splenic NK1.1-negative, TCR alpha beta intermediate CD4+ T cells exist in naive NK1.1 allelic positive and negative mice, with the capacity to rapidly secrete large amounts of IL-4 and IFN-gamma upon primary TCR stimulation. J Immunol 162:5156–5163

Morgan RK, McAllister B, Cross L et al (2007) Histamine 4 receptor activation induces recruitment of FoxP3+ T cells and inhibits allergic asthma in a murine model. J Immunol 178:8081–8089

Mosmann TR (1994) Cytokine patterns during the progression to AIDS. Science 265:193–194

Motoki K, Morita M, Kobayashi E et al (1995) Immunostimulatory and antitumor activities of monoglycosylceramides having various sugar moieties. Biol Pharm Bull 18:1487–1491

Mozes E, Kohn LD, Hakim F et al (1993) Resistance of MHC class I-deficient mice to experimental systemic lupus erythematosus. Science 261:91–93

Munn DH, Sharma MD, Mellor AL (2004) Ligation of B7–1/B7–2 by human CD4+ T cells triggers indoleamine 2,3-dioxygenase activity in dendritic cells. J Immunol 172:4100–4110

Nakagawa K, Iwabuchi K, Ogasawara K et al (1997) Generation of NK1.1+ T cell antigen receptor alpha/beta+ thymocytes associated with intact thymic structure. Proc Natl Acad Sci USA 94:2472–2477

Nakagawa R, Motoki K, Ueno H et al (1998) Treatment of hepatic metastasis of the colon26 adenocarcinoma with an alpha-galactosylceramide, KRN7000. Cancer Res 58:1202–1207

Nelson BH (2004) IL-2, regulatory T cells, and tolerance. J Immunol 172:3983–3988

Nieda M, Nicol A, Koezuka Y et al (2001) TRAIL expression by activated human CD4(+)V alpha 24NKT cells induces in vitro and in vivo apoptosis of human acute myeloid leukemia cells. Blood 97:2067–2074

O'Garra A, Murphy K (1993) T-cell subsets in autoimmunity. Curr Opin Immunol 5:880–886

Ohteki T, Ho S, Suzuki H et al (1997) Role for IL-15/IL-15 receptor beta-chain in natural killer 1.1+ T cell receptor-alpha beta+ cell development. J Immunol 159:5931–5935

Ohteki T, MacDonald HR (1994) Major histocompatibility complex class I related molecules control the development of CD4+8- and CD4–8- subsets of natural killer 1.1+ T cell receptor-alpha/beta+ cells in the liver of mice. J Exp Med 180:699–704

Osna N, Elliott K, Khan MM (2001a) The effects of histamine on interferon gamma production are dependent on the stimulatory signals. Int Immunopharmacol 1:135–145

Osna N, Elliott K, Khan MM (2001b) Regulation of interleukin-10 secretion by histamine in TH2 cells and splenocytes. Int Immunopharmacol 1:85–96

Palathumpat V, Dejbakhsh-Jones S, Holm B et al (1992) Different subsets of T cells in the adult mouse bone marrow and spleen induce or suppress acute graft-versus-host disease. J Immunol 149:808–817

Paust S, Lu L, McCarty N et al (2004) Engagement of B7 on effector T cells by regulatory T cells prevents autoimmune disease. Proc Natl Acad Sci USA 101:10398–10403

Piccirillo CA, Letterio JJ, Thornton AM et al (2002) CD4(+)CD25(+) regulatory T cells can mediate suppressor function in the absence of transforming growth factor beta1 production and responsiveness. J Exp Med 196:237–246

Poluektova LY, Khan MM (1998) Protein kinase A inhibitors reverse histamine-mediated regulation of IL-5 secretion. Immunopharmacology 39:9–19

Porcelli S, Morita CT, Brenner MB (1992) CD1b restricts the response of human CD4–8- T lymphocytes to a microbial antigen. Nature 360:593–597

Porcelli SA (1995) The CD1 family: a third lineage of antigen-presenting molecules. Adv Immunol 59:1–98

Porcelli SA, Modlin RL (1999) The CD1 system: antigen-presenting molecules for T cell recognition of lipids and glycolipids. Annu Rev Immunol 17:297–329

Quezada SA, Bennett K, Blazar BR et al (2005) Analysis of the underlying cellular mechanisms of anti-CD154-induced graft tolerance: the interplay of clonal anergy and immune regulation. J Immunol 175:771–779

Rapoport MJ, Jaramillo A, Zipris D et al (1993) Interleukin-4 reverses T cell unresponsiveness and prevents the onset of diabetes in nonobese diabetic mice. J Exp Med 87–99

Read S, Malmstrom V, Powrie F (2000) Cytotoxic T lymphocyte-associated antigen 4 plays an essential role in the function of CD25(+)CD4(+) regulatory cells that control intestinal inflammation. J Exp Med 192:295–302

Renukaradhya GJ, Khan MA, Shaji D et al (2008a) Vesicular stomatitis virus matrix protein impairs CD1d-mediated antigen presentation through activation of the p38 MAPK pathway. J Virol 82:12535–12542

Renukaradhya GJ, Khan MA, Vieira M et al (2008b) Type I NKT cells protect (and type II NKT cells suppress) the host's innate antitumor immune response to a B-cell lymphoma. Blood 111:5637–5645

Renukaradhya GJ, Sriram V, Du W et al (2006) Inhibition of antitumor immunity by invariant natural killer T cells in a T-cell lymphoma model in vivo. Int J Cancer 118:3045–3053

Renukaradhya GJ, Webb TJ, Khan MA et al (2005) Virus-induced inhibition of CD1d1-mediated antigen presentation: reciprocal regulation by p38 and ERK. J Immunol 175:4301–4308

Robson MacDonald H, Lees RK, Held W (1998) Developmentally regulated extinction of Ly-49 receptor expression permits maturation and selection of NK1.1+ T cells. J Exp Med 187: 2109–2114

Russano AM, Bassotti G, Agea E et al (2007) CD1-restricted recognition of exogenous and self-lipid antigens by duodenal gammadelta+ T lymphocytes. J Immunol 178:3620–3626

Sakaguchi S (2004) Naturally arising CD4+ regulatory t cells for immunologic self-tolerance and negative control of immune responses. Annu Rev Immunol 22:531–562

Sakaguchi S (2005) Naturally arising Foxp3-expressing CD25+CD4+ regulatory T cells in immunological tolerance to self and non-self. Nat Immunol 6:345–352

Sakaguchi S, Sakaguchi N, Asano M et al (1995) Immunologic self-tolerance maintained by activated T cells expressing IL-2 receptor alpha-chains (CD25). Breakdown of a single mechanism of self-tolerance causes various autoimmune diseases. J Immunol 155:1151–1164

Salomon B, Lenschow DJ, Rhee L et al (2000) B7/CD28 costimulation is essential for the homeostasis of the CD4+CD25+ immunoregulatory T cells that control autoimmune diabetes. Immunity 12:431–440

Sato H, Nakayama T, Tanaka Y et al (1999) Induction of differentiation of pre-NKT cells to mature Valpha14 NKT cells by granulocyte/macrophage colony-stimulating factor. Proc Natl Acad Sci USA 96:7439–7444

Schlicker E, Fink K, Hinterthaner M et al (1989) Inhibition of noradrenaline release in the rat brain cortex via presynaptic H3 receptors. Naunyn Schmiedebergs Arch Pharmacol 340: 633–638

Schlicker E, Malinowska B, Kathmann M et al (1994) Modulation of neurotransmitter release via histamine H3 heteroreceptors. Fundam Clin Pharmacol 8:128–137

Schmidt J, Fleissner S, Heimann-Weitschat I et al (1994) Histamine increases anti-CD3 induced IL-5 production of TH2-type T cells via histamine H2-receptors. Agents Actions 42:81–85

Schofield L, McConville MJ, Hansen D et al (1999) CD1d-restricted immunoglobulin G formation to GPI-anchored antigens mediated by NKT cells. Science 283:225–229

Seder RA, Paul WE (1994) Acquisition of lymphokine-producing phenotype by CD4+ T cells. Annu Rev Immunol 12:635–673

Shevach EM (2000) Regulatory T cells in autoimmmunity. Annu Rev Immunol 18:423–449

Siegmund K, Feuerer M, Siewert C et al (2005) Migration matters: regulatory T-cell compartmentalization determines suppressive activity in vivo. Blood 106:3097–3104

Singh N, Hong S, Scherer DC et al (1999) Cutting edge: activation of NKT cells by CD1d and alpha-galactosylceramide directs conventional T cells to the acquisition of a Th2 phenotype. J Immunol 163:2373–2377

Sirois J, Menard G, Moses AS et al (2000) Importance of histamine in the cytokine network in the lung through H2 and H3 receptors: stimulation of IL-10 production. J Immunol 164: 2964–2970

Soga F, Katoh N, Kishimoto S (2007) Histamine prevents apoptosis in human monocytes. Clin Exp Allergy 37:323–330

Sonoda KH, Exley M, Snapper S et al (1999) CD1-reactive natural killer T cells are required for development of systemic tolerance through an immune-privileged site. J Exp Med 190: 1215–1226

Spada FM, Koezuka Y, Porcelli SA (1998) CD1d-restricted recognition of synthetic glycolipid antigens by human natural killer T cells. J Exp Med 188:1529–1534

Stark H (2007) Histamine receptors. Biotrends Rev 1: 2–9. http: //www.biotrend.com

Sykes M (1990) Unusual T cell populations in adult murine bone marrow. Prevalence of CD3+CD4-CD8- and alpha beta TCR+NK1.1+ cells. J Immunol 145:3209–3215

Szeberenyi JB, Pallinger E, Zsinko M et al (2001) Inhibition of effects of endogenously synthesized histamine disturbs in vitro human dendritic cell differentiation. Immunol Lett 76:175–182

Takahama Y, Sharrow SO, Singer A (1991) Expression of an unusual T cell receptor (TCR)-V beta repertoire by Ly-6C+ subpopulations of CD4+ and/or CD8+ thymocytes. Evidence for a developmental relationship between Ly-6C+ thymocytes and CD4-CD8-TCR-alpha beta+ thymocytes. J Immunol 147:2883–2891

Takahashi T, Nieda M, Koezuka Y et al (2000a) Analysis of human V alpha 24+ CD4+ NKT cells activated by alpha-glycosylceramide-pulsed monocyte-derived dendritic cells. J Immunol 164:4458–4464

Takahashi T, Tagami T, Yamazaki S et al (2000b) Immunologic self-tolerance maintained by CD25(+)CD4(+) regulatory T cells constitutively expressing cytotoxic T lymphocyte-associated antigen 4. J Exp Med 192:303–310

Takeda K, Dennert G (1993) The development of autoimmunily in C57BL/6 lpr mice correlates with the disappearance of natural killer type 1-posltive cells: evidence for their suppressive action on bone marrow stem cell proliferation, B cell immunoglobulin secretion, and autoimmune symptoms. J Exp Med 177:155–164

Tang Q, Boden EK, Henriksen KJ et al (2004) Distinct roles of CTLA-4 and TGF-beta in CD4+CD25+ regulatory T cell function. Eur J Immunol 34:2996–3005

Tang Q, Henriksen KJ, Boden EK et al (2003) Cutting edge: CD28 controls peripheral homeostasis of CD4+CD25+ regulatory T cells. J Immunol 171:3348–3352

Taylor PA, Noelle RJ, Blazar BR (2001) CD4(+)CD25(+) immune regulatory cells are required for induction of tolerance to alloantigen via costimulatory blockade. J Exp Med 193: 1311–1318

Terabe M, Berzofsky JA (2007) NKT cells in immunoregulation of tumor immunity: a new immunoregulatory axis. Trends Immunol 28:491–496

Theoharides TC, Conti P (2004) Mast cells: the Jekyll and Hyde of tumor growth. Trends Immunol 25:235–241

Tran DQ, Ramsey H, Shevach EM (2007) Induction of FOXP3 expression in naive human CD4+FOXP3 T cells by T-cell receptor stimulation is transforming growth factor-beta dependent but does not confer a regulatory phenotype. Blood 110:2983–2990

van der Pouw Kraan TC, Snijders A, Boeije LC et al (1998) Histamine inhibits the production of interleukin-12 through interaction with H2 receptors. J Clin Invest 102:1866–1873

Van Rhijn I, Koets AP, Im JS et al (2006) The bovine CD1 family contains group 1 CD1 proteins, but no functional CD1d. J Immunol 176:4888–4893

Vannier E, Dinarello CA (1993) Histamine enhances interleukin (IL)-1-induced IL-1 gene expression and protein synthesis via H2 receptors in peripheral blood mononuclear cells. Comparison with IL-1 receptor antagonist. J Clin Invest 92:281–287

Vannier E, Miller LC, Dinarello CA (1991) Histamine suppresses gene expression and synthesis of tumor necrosis factor alpha via histamine H2 receptors. J Exp Med 174:281–284

Vicari AP, Herbelin A, Leite-de-Moraes MC et al (1996) NK1.1+ T cells from IL-7-deficient mice have a normal distribution and selection but exhibit impaired cytokine production. Int Immunol 8:1759–1766

Wang Y, Goldschneider I, Foss D et al (1997) Direct thymic involvement in anterior chamber-associated immune deviation: evidence for a nondeletional mechanism of centrally induced tolerance to extrathymic antigens in adult mice. J Immunol 158:2150–2155

Watanabe Y, Todome Y, Ohkuni H et al (2002) Cysteine protease activity and histamine release from the human mast cell line HMC-1 stimulated by recombinant streptococcal pyrogenic exotoxin B/streptococcal cysteine protease. Infect Immun 70:3944–3947

Wedemeyer J, Galli SJ (2005) Decreased susceptibility of mast cell-deficient Kit(W)/Kit(W-v) mice to the development of 1, 2-dimethylhydrazine-induced intestinal tumors. Lab Invest 85:388–396

Weltman JK (2000) Update on histamine as a mediator of inflammation. Allergy Asthma Proc 21:125–128

Wildin RS, Ramsdell F, Peake J et al (2001) X-linked neonatal diabetes mellitus, enteropathy and endocrinopathy syndrome is the human equivalent of mouse scurfy. Nat Genet 27:18–20

Yamaguchi Y, Motoki K, Ueno H et al (1996) Enhancing effects of (2S,3S,4R)-1-O-(alpha-D-galactopyranosyl)-2-(N-hexacosanoylamino)-1,3,4-octadecanetriol (KRN7000) on antigen-presenting function of antigen-presenting cells and antimetastatic activity of KRN7000-pretreated antigen-presenting cells. Oncol Res 8:399–407

Yankelevich B, Knobloch C, Nowicki M et al (1989) A novel cell type responsible for marrow graft rejection in mice. T cells with NK phenotype cause acute rejection of marrow grafts. J Immunol 142:3423–3430

Yoshimoto T, Paul WE (1994) CD4pos NK1.1pos T cells promptly produce interleukin 4 in response to in vivo challenge with anti-CD3. J Exp Med 179:1285–1295

Zelenika D, Adams E, Humm S et al (2001) The role of CD4+ T-cell subsets in determining transplantation rejection or tolerance. Immunol Rev 182:164–179

Zeng D, Lewis D, Dejbakhsh-Jones S et al (1999) Bone marrow NK1.1(–) and NK1.1(+) T cells reciprocally regulate acute graft versus host disease. J Exp Med 189:1073–1081

Chapter 6
Immune Regulation by Various Facets of Histamine in Immunomodulation and Allergic Disorders

Trivendra Tripathi, Mohammed Shahid, Farrukh Sobia, Anuradha Singh, Haris M. Khan, Rahat Ali Khan, and Mashiatullah Siddiqui

Abstract Histamine has tremendous biological role, mediated by four types of histamine receptors (H1R–H4R) on secretion by effector cells (mast cells and basophils) through various immunological and non-immunological stimuli. Their patho-physiological implication in all facets of biomedical areas have been reported extensively. It shows proinflammatory or anti-inflammatory effects, depending on the predominance of the types of histamine receptors. It had proinflammatory activity through the H1R, and is involved in the development of various aspects of antigen-specific immune response including the maturation of dendritic cells and the modulation of the balance of type 1 helper (Th1) T cells and type 2 helper (Th2) T cells. Histamine blocks humoral immune responses by means of a specific mechanism in which it induces an increase in the proliferation of Th1 cells and in the production of interferon-γ. Histamine stimulates the release of proinflammatory cytokines and lysosomal enzymes from human macrophages and shows the capacity to influence the activity of immune cells including mast cells, basophils, eosinophils, fibroblasts, lymphocytes, neutrophils, epithelial and endothelial cells, and plays a pivotal role in allergic inflammation which is a complex network of cellular events and involves redundant mediators and signals. In this chapter, we tried to elaborate the newer discoveries of histamine H1–H4-receptors in immunomodulation and allergic conditions, and effect of histamine in immune cells with respect to allergic diseases. We hope that this article would stimulate discussions and active research on this important aspect.

Keywords Histamine · Immunomodulation · Immune cells

M. Shahid (✉)
Department of Microbiology, Jawaharlal Nehru Medical College and Hospital, Aligarh Muslim University, Aligarh, 202002, UP, India
e-mail: shahidsahar@yahoo.co.in

M. Shahid et al. (eds.), *Biomedical Aspects of Histamine*,
DOI 10.1007/978-90-481-9349-3_6,

Contents

6.1 Introduction

Histamine (2-{1H-imidazol-4-yl}ethanamine) is known as biogenic amine, was characterized nearly a century ago by Barger and Dale. Dale later reported histamine ability to mimic anaphylaxis (Akdis and Simons 2006). Histamine is an important chemical mediator and neuron-transmitter on a broad spectrum of physiological and patho-physiological condition in central and peripheral tissues (Stark 2007). It is synthesized and released by basophils, mast cells, lymphocytes, gastric enterochromaffin-like cells and neurons (Akdis and Simons 2006). Histamine was first synthesized by A. Windaus and W. Vogt, its anaphylactic reaction was characterized by H.H. Dale and P.P. Laidlaw and the histamine antagonist activity was detected by D. Bovet and A.M. Staub (Parsons and Ganellin 2006). Thus, different advances in histamine receptors ligands have ever attracted pharmaceutical developments and are still highly topical (Stark 2007). While H1Rs and H2Rs have been successful targets of block-buster drugs for treating allergic diseases and gastric ulcer, respectively, the developments of H3R and H4R receptor ligands are still on their way to market (Stark 2003). Extensive evidence has been accumulated about histamine synthesis, metabolism, receptors, signal transduction, physiological and pathological effects. Despite this, the complex interrelationships and crosstalk by histamine and its receptors in immune cells with respect to allergic conditions and immunomodulation remain to be elucidated.

In this chapter, we tried to elaborate the newer discoveries of histamine H1, H2, H3 and H4-receptors in immunomodulation and allergic conditions, and effect of histamine in immune cells with respect to allergic diseases.

6.2 Histamine in Immunomodulation and Allergic Inflammation

Histamine exerts a very important immunomodulatory effect via H1-, H2-, H3-, and H4-receptors (Shahid et al. 2009, Triggiani et al. 2001; Table 6.1). According to the

Table 6.1 Immunopharmacological profiles of histamine receptor subtypes

Characteristics	Histamine H1R	Histamine H2R	Histamine H3R	Histamine H4R
General function[a,b]	Increased pruritus, pain, vasodilation, vascular permeability, hypotension; flushing, headache, tachycardia, bronchoconstriction, stimulation of airways, vagal stimulation of airway vagal receptors; decreased atrio-ventricular-node conduction time.	Increased gastric acid secretion, vascular permeability, hypotension, flushing, headache, tachycardia, chronotropic and inotropic activity, bronchodilatation, mucus production (airway).	Prevents excessive bronchoconstriction; mediates pruritus (no mast-cell involvement).	Differentiation of myeloblasts and promyelocytes.
Function in immune modulation and allergic inflammation[a,b]	Increases release of histamine and other mediators; increases cellular adhesion molecule expression and chemotaxis of eosinophils and neutrophils; increases antigen-presenting cell capacity, co-stimulatory activity on B cells; increases cellular immunity (Th1), IFN-γ, autoimmunity. Decreases humoral immunity and IgE production.	Decreased eosinophil and neutrophil chemotaxis; induction of interleukin-10, suppression of interleukin-12 by dendritic cells; development of Th2 or tolerance inducing dendritic cells; induction of humoral immunity; suppression of Th2 cells and cytokines; indirect role in allergy, autoimmunity, malignant disease, and graft rejection.	Probably involved in control of neurogenic inflammation through local neuron-mast cell feedback loops; proinflammatory activity; increased APC (antigen-presenting cell) capacity.	Increased Ca^{2+} flux in human eosinophils; increased eosinophil chemotaxis; increases IL-16 production (H2-receptor also involved).
Physiological relevance[b,c]	Cycle of sleeping and waking, food intake, thermal regulation, emotions and aggressive behavior, locomotion, memory, and learning, contraction of smooth muscles.	Neuroendocrine, gastric acid secretion.	Presynaptic heteroreceptor; decreased histamine, dopamine, serotonin, noradrenaline and acetylcholine release; sleep, food intake.	Chemotaxis.
Pathophysiological relevance[b,c]	Allergic reaction.	Gastric ulcer.	Cognitive impairment, seizure, metabolic syndrome	Inflammation, immune reaction.
Antagonists[a,b,c]	*Clinically usable* (Mepyramine, chlorpheniramine, astemizole, terfenadine, loratidine, triprolidine, diphenhy dramine, cetirizine, desloratidine, fexofenadine)	*Clinically usable* (Cimetidine, zolantidine, tiotidine, femotidine, nizatidine, and ranitidine)	Clobenpropit, Iodophenpropit, Thioperamide	JNJ 7777120, JNJ 10191584

[a]Simon (2004), [b]Shahid et al. (2009), [c]Stark (2007)

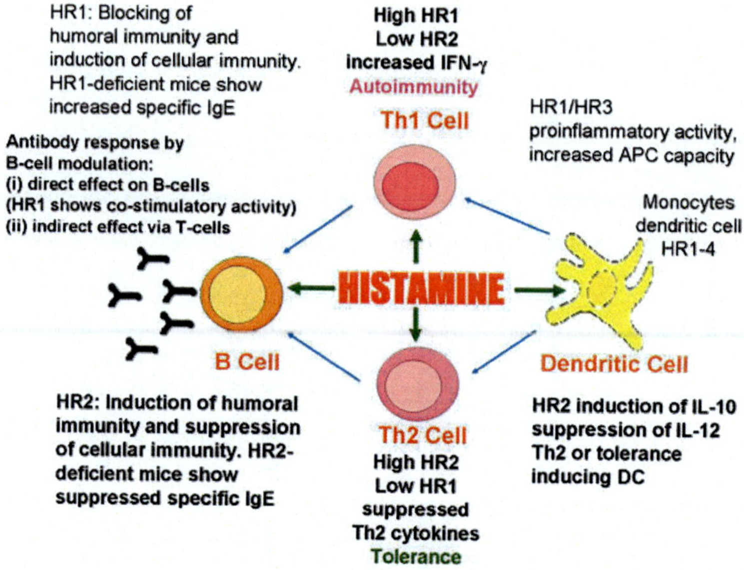

Fig. 6.1 Histamine regulates monocytes, dendritic cells, T cells and B cells in lymphatic organs and subepithelial tissues in allergic inflammation. Monocytes and dendritic cells express all four known histamine receptors (HR1, HR2, H3R and HR4). HR1 and HR2 induce proinflammatory activity and enhanced antigen presenting cell capacity, whereas HR2 plays an important suppressive role on monocytes and monocyte-derived dendritic cells. (Adapted from Shahid et al. 2009)

cell differentiation stage and microenvironment influences, the receptors expression changes. Histamine shows proinflammatory or anti-inflammatory effects, depending on the predominance of the type of histamine receptor (H1R, H2R, H3R and H4R) and on the experimental system studied. Histamine had proinflammatory activity through the H1R, and is involved in the development of various aspects of antigen-specific immune response including the maturation of dendritic cells (DCs) and the modulation of the balance of type 1 helper (Th1) T cells and type 2 helper (Th2) T cells (Shahid et al. 2009). Histamine blocks humoral immune responses by means of a specific mechanism in which it induces an increase in the proliferation of Th1 cells and in the production of interferon γ (IFN-γ) (Shahid et al. 2009, Fig. 6.1). Histamine also stimulates the release of proinflammatory cytokines and lysosomal enzymes from human macrophages and shows the capacity to influence the activity of immune cells including mast cells, basophils, eosinophils, fibroblasts, lymphocytes, neutrophils, epithelial and endothelial cells. The role of histamine in autoimmunity and malignant disease through the H1R was well documented (Akdis and Blaser 2003, Ma et al. 2002). Histamine also plays a pivotal role in allergic inflammation which is a complex network of cellular events and involves redundant mediators and signals. Histamine is released from the granules of mast cells and basophils (FcεRI$^+$ cells) along with several mediators such as tryptase, leukotrienes, prostaglandins, and other newly generated mediators (Shahid et al. 2009). Histamine was found in relatively large (μg) quantities per 1 million cells, in contrast to leukotrienes and other mediators (which are present in picograms), after allergen challenge in sensitized persons (Shahid et al. 2009). Most of the potent effects of histamine in allergic inflammation occur through H1Rs (Akdis and Blaser 2003, MacGlashan 2003, Shahid et al. 2009, Schneider et al. 2002; Table 6.1), while hypotension, flushing, headache, and tachycardia occurred via both the H1- and H2-receptors in the vasculature (Spitaler et al. 2002), whereas nasal congestion and cutaneous itch occurs by both the H1- and H3- receptors (McLeod et al. 1999, Sugimoto et al. 2004). Histamine also acts as a contributor to the late allergic response by generating a stimulatory signal for the production of cytokines, the expression of cell adhesion molecules and class II antigens (Shahid et al. 2009).

6.3 Effect of Histamine in Immune Cells with Respect to Allergic Diseases

Histamine's classical effects, expressed at the organ level, have been documented and were highly emphasized in allergies and autoimmune diseases. Histamine directly or indirectly influences the activity of various inflammatory/effector/immunologic cell types involved in the pathogenesis of several diseases. Indeed, several studies have suggested that histamine receptors (HRs) are expressed on mast cell and basophils; lymphocytes; neutrophils; monocytes, macrophages and dendritic cells (DCs); eosinophils; epithelial cells; endothelial cells, and therefore modulate the function of these cells in immune system (Shahid et al. 2009).

6.3.1 Mast Cells and Basophils

Recent studies shed light on the potent role of histamine in mast cells and basophils, both types of cells can themselves be modulated by histamine as they express H1-, H2- and H4-receptors (Godot et al. 2007, Lippert et al. 2004). The peritoneal and skin mast cells exhibited aberrant granules with very low electron density, in HDC-deficient mice, which indicated the drastic decrease in the granule contents including granule proteases and sulfated proteoglycans (Ohtsu et al. 2001). The critical roles of histamine in cutaneous and systemic anaphylaxis have been suggested by using the HDC-deleted mice (Makabe-Kobayashi et al. 2002, Ohtsu et al. 2002) and it remained a possibility that diminished granule constituents, such as proteases, make contribution to the relief of anaphylaxis in the mutant mice. How histamine regulates allergic responses by maturation of tissue mast cells requires comprehending detailed studies on the effect of absence of histamine on mast cell function. Impact of histamine was also demonstrated in the migration of mast cells which was mediated exclusively through the H4R (Hofstra et al. 2003). It has been shown that histamine acting through H4Rs can stimulate chemotaxis of murine mast cells in vitro (Hofstra et al. 2003) and leads to changes in tissue localization in vivo (Thurmond et al. 2004). A hematopoietic organ, bone marrow, contains certain types of cells which can produce histamine in response to IL-3 (Schneider et al. 1999, Shahid et al. 2009). The role of IL-3-sensitized histamine synthesis in bone marrow remains to be clarified (Shahid et al. 2009), however, a study suggested a unique circuit of newly synthesized histamine and its implication in basophil precursors (Schneider et al. 2005). It has been documented that bidirectional transport of histamine is facilitated largely through organic cation transporter 3 (OCT3) in the plasma membranes of the FcεRI$^+$, c-kit$^-$ bone marrow cells. It had been demonstrated that intracellularly stimulated histamine in the organic cation transporter 3 (OCT3)-deleted cells has suppressive impacts on expression of HDC, IL-4, and IL-6. This suggests not only the feedback inhibition of histamine synthesis but also the suppression of Th2 cytokine production through immature basophils (Gründemann et al. 1999, Tanaka et al. 2003). In addition, histamine receptor binding studies with specific receptor antagonists have suggested that basophils express predominantly H2R, and these were involved in the regulation of IgE-stimulated histamine release, as demonstrated through increased histamine release in the presence of anti-IgE and cimetidine (a H2R antagonist) but not in the presence of anti-IgE and thioperamide (a H3R antagonist) (Bull et al. 1993, Kleine-Tebbe et al. 1990, Tedeschi et al. 1991). H2Rs in mast cells show various effects such as inhibition of histamine release and modulation of cytokine production (Lippert et al. 2000). It has been suggested that H3R functions on mast cells but many of these properties may be attributed to the H4R as the ligands used were not specifically selective. H3R expression was not detected in some types of mast cells (Hofstra et al. 2003).

6.3.2 Lymphocytes

The expression of histamine receptors (HRs) on the cell surface of immunocompetent cells, including lymphocytes (B-cells and T-cells) and their effects mediated by HRs have been published in several studies and significantly reviewed (Sachs et al. 2000), see Fig. 6.1. It has been concluded that both histamine receptors (H1 and H2) are present on the lymphocytes but there is only few data available on the functional significance of the H1R and the distribution of H2R on lymphocyte subsets in general, signaling through the H1R was associated with enhancement and signaling through the H2R with inhibition of lymphocyte responses. It has been suggested by several studies that histamine and its derivatives can inhibit the immune response by enhancing the activity of T suppressor cells through H2R and natural suppressor cells via H1R (Khan et al. 1986, Sansoni et al. 1985). The impacts of histamine on T helper lymphocytes are differential and complex; see in Fig. 6.1. T lymphocytes, mainly T helper lymphocytes, play a significant role in the pathogenesis of atopic asthma. Helper T lymphocytes can be divided into two subsets (T helper type 1 cells (Th1) and Th2) based on their cytokine profile and distinct functions and both the subsets play distinctive roles in the development, initiation, and regulation of the immune response. Th1 cells were found to be responsive in delayed type hypersensitivity (DTH) and cytotoxic response, while Th2 cells were involved in allergic disease via activating B-lymphocytes and regulating antibody (IgG and IgE) secretion; see in Fig. 6.1. Th1 cells secrete important cytokines as interleukin (IL)-2, IFN-γ, IL-3, and granulocyte monocyte colony stimulating factor (GM-CSF), while Th2 cells secrete cytokines such as IL-3, IL-4, IL-5, IL-10, IL-13, and GM-CSF. Histamine downregulates the proliferation of Th1 cells (which control cytotoxic response and delayed-type hypersensitivity) and upregulates the proliferation of Th2 cells (which regulate allergic disease and asthma) (Shahid et al. 2009, Weltman 2000).

Histamine also regulates the development of an allergic state by enhancing the secretion of Th2 cytokines such as IL-4, IL-5, IL-10 and IL-13 and by inhibiting the production of Th1 cytokines IL-2 and IFN-γ and monokine IL-12 (Shahid et al. 2009). It had been demonstrated in several studies that histamine dose-dependently upregulates the secretion of Th2 cytokines (IL-5, IL-10, and IL-13) and downregulates the secretion of Th1 cytokines (IL-2 and IFN-γ) in cloned murine T helper cells (Elliott et al. 2001, Osna et al. 2001a, b). It has also been demonstrated that Th1 and Th2 cells express distinct surface histamine receptor (HR) patterns (Th1 cells that express predominantly H1R and Th2 cells express H2R). Histamine increases Th1-type responses by triggering H1R and negatively regulates both Th1 and Th2-type responses by H2R as suggested by enhanced release of tumor necrosis factor (TNF)-α and decreased release of interleukin (IL)-4 and IL-13, respectively (Jutel et al. 2001). The differential expression of these cells to histamine is a result of the type of intracellular signals generated via histamine activation. Notably, H1R signaling involves calcium-dependent phospholipase stimulation and generation of IP3, while H2R signaling involves adenylate cyclase stimulation and cAMP formation (Shahid et al. 2009).

The receptor binding study of human peripheral blood lymphocytes has suggested that histamine trifluoromethyl-toludine (HTMT) derivative leads to a two-phase enhancement in intracellular calcium (Ca^{2+}) and an increase in inositol phosphate (IP3) production. The increase in calcium (Ca^{2+}) was thoroughly antagonized through high concentrations of histamine but not by the classical histamine H1-, H2- or H3- receptor antagonists (Qui et al. 1990). These observations demonstrate that HTMT has a specific binding site on lymphocytes, which is different for three classic histamine receptors. Several functional studies demonstrated that histamine primarily modulates T-suppressor activity including delayed type hypersensitivity (DTH), cytotoxic T-lymphocyte-mediated target cell killing, cell-mediated lympholysis, and natural killer activity by H2R signaling (Rocklin 1990). Although, some studies suggest that activation of the H2Rs indirectly increase the allergic cascade. Suppressor T-cells were found to be more responsive to histamine than T helper cells or cytotoxic T-cells (Khan et al. 1985). Likewise, the response to histamine in T helper cells and cytotoxic T-cells was highly enhanced after mitogenic stimulation (Khan et al. 1985). It is more important to note that in humans, histamine suppresses the proliferation of mixed T lymphocytes via H2R (Khan and Melmon 1985, 1988). Further, it had been confirmed that histamine inhibited lipopolysaccharide (LPS)-stimulated IFN-γ-gene expression from human peripheral blood mononuclear cells (PBMC) (Horváth et al. 1999). IFN-γ cytokine releases human $CD4^{+}$ T-cell clones, which are classified as either Th0, Th1 or Th2 based on their cytokines (IL-4 and IFN-γ) secretion patterns (Lagier et al. 1997). Notably, histamine-induced inhibition of IFN-γ secretion was seen in Th1 clones but not Th2 clones and the effect was reversed by H2R and not H1- or H3-receptor antagonists. Histamine has been demonstrated to directly enhance the synthesis of the proinflammatory cytokines (IL-1b and IL-6) through lymphocytes, anti-CD23- and anti-CD28-stimulated release of IL-4 and IL-5 (but not IL-2) or IFN from T lymphocytes can be inhibited by terfenadine treatment (Sachs et al. 2000). Similarly, several other studies have suggested that histamine leads to synthesis and release of a lymphocyte chemo-attractant factor (LCF) from H2R bearing lymphocytes and also results in release of two different types of lymphocyte migration inhibitory factors (LyMIFs) from only a subset of H2R bearing lymphocytes (Berman et al. 1984, Center et al. 1983).

6.3.3 Neutrophils

Neutrophils have been demonstrated to express H1R and H2R, and it had been suggested that the impacts of histamine on neutrophils are inhibitory via H2R (Gespach and Abita 1982, Westcott and Kaliner 1983). In vitro studies showed the autologous serum-sensitized chemotaxis of neutrophils both in normal, atopic subjects which is abolished by histamine in a dose-dependent manner, and this inhibition was more effective in atopic individuals (Radermecker and Maldague 1981). It is more important to note that incubation of neutrophils from these individuals with cimetidine, but not promethazine, causes reversal of the histamine-sensitized inhibition of neutrophil chemotaxis (Shahid et al. 2009). In vivo study has demonstrated that the histamine administration by either infusion and subcutaneous injection or inhalation diminished neutrophil chemotaxis in healthy volunteers (Bury et al. 1992). Several studies have suggested that histamine inhibits the activation of neutrophils as demonstrated by inhibition of fMet-Leu-Phe induced superoxide (O^{2-}) formation, degranulation and membrane potential changes acting by H2R signaling (Burde et al. 1983, Seligmann et al. 1983).

6.3.4 Monocytes, Macrophages and Dendritic Cells

The presence of histamine receptors (H1R and H2R) on human monocytes and macrophages (Shahid et al. 2009, Wang et al. 2000) indicate that in allergic disease histamine also modulate the activity of these cells. Differentiation of monocytes into macrophages cause switching over from H2R to H1R (Wang et al. 2000). Several other recent studies have suggested (investigations which were performed with exogenously added histamine) that it has a potential role in modulating maturation and function of monocytes, and dendritic cells. Activated monocytes and dendritic cells have a significant potential role in release of histamine, which acts in autocrine and paracrine fashion and modifies dendritic cell markers. Histamine was found to inhibit the production of TNF-α and IL-12, and to augment the production of IL-10 in response to Toll-like receptor ligands by acting on the H2R, in human monocytes (Atkins et al. 1990a, b), while, in human monocyte-derived dendritic cells similar inhibition of IL-12 and enhancement of IL-10 production was investigated. Recently, H4R involvement in suppression of IL-12 was observed (Marmy et al. 1993, Shahid et al. 2009). In the *P. acnes*-primed and LPS-stimulated hepatitis model, endogenous histamine production via macrophages and Kupffer cells was reported to play a protective role through acting on the H2R (Jarjour et al. 1991). This study was performed with attention to endogenous histamine synthesis in macrophages and Kupffer cells. Furthermore, it has been documented that dendritic cells (DC) are especially antigen-presenting cells, which mature from monocytic and lymphoid precursors and lead to acquisition of DC1 and DC2 phenotypes that drives the development of Th1 and Th2 cells, respectively. Histamine potentially participates in functions and activity of DC precursors as well as their immature and mature forms. It is important to note that immature and mature dendritic cells (DCs) express all four histamine receptors (Gutzmer et al. 2002, Idzko et al. 2002) see in Fig. 6.1 for more details. Furthermore, in the differentiation process of DC1 from monocytes, H1R and H3R act as positive stimulants that enhance antigen-presentation capacity and proinflammatory cytokine production and also Th1 priming activity. H2R acts as a suppressive molecule and enhances IL-10 production, and stimulates IL-10 producing T-lymphocytes (Th2 cells) for antigen-presentation (Mazzoni et al. 2001). The suppressive impact of histamine by H2R seems through the regulation of ICAM-1 and B7.1 expression facilitating the reduction of innate immune responses activated by LPS (Morichika et al. 2003). Indeed, histamine stimulates intracellular Ca^{2+} flux, chemotaxis, and actin polymerization in immature dendritic cells due to activation of H1R and H3R subtypes. Notably, in maturation of dendritic cells (DCs) results in loss of these responses. However, histamine dose dependently augments intracellular cAMP levels and stimulates IL-10 secretion in maturing dendritic cells, while inhibiting production of IL-12 through H2R (Mazzoni et al. 2001). Human monocyte-derived dendritic cells express both histamine receptors (H1R and H2R) and can stimulate CD86 expression via histamine, while human epidermal Langerhans cells express neither H1R nor H2R due to effect of transforming growth factor (TGF)-β (Ohtani et al. 2003).

6.3.5 Eosinophils

Eosinophils express both histamine H1- and H2-receptors. The effect of histamine on eosinophils is stimulatory at lower concentrations. It had been suggested that preincubation of eosinophils with 10^{-5} M or higher concentrations of histamine suppressed the chemotactic response of eosinophils to endotoxin-activated serum (C5a) while preincubation of eosinophils with a lower concentration of 10^{-6} M histamine had the inverse effect, enhancing the C5a-activated eosinophil chemotaxis. Furthermore, H2R- and H1R-antagonists, respectively, inhibited these impacts. The expression of a novel H3R mediates the direct eosinophil chemotactic response towards histamine (Raible et al. 1994, Shahid et al. 2009). It has also been observed that this receptor seems to have similar antagonist binding activities to those reported for the H3R observed in the CNS, although it does not bind *R*-α-methylhistamine or *N*-α-methylhistamine with similar potency as histamine suggesting differences between the activities and function of H3Rs expressed in CNS and on the eosinophil. Histamine acting via the H1R also augments eosinophil C3b receptor expression (Anwar and Kay 1980), and it was considered as an important mechanism that was found to be involved in the amplification of complement-dependent parasite killing. However, 0.1–50 mM histamine was demonstrated to block eosinophil degranulation, as shown by diminished release of C5a-mediated eosinophil peroxidase (Ezeamuzie and Philips 2000). It has been suggested that selective H2R agonists produced an impact similar to that shown by histamine and that cimetidine (H2R-antagonist) reversed this inhibitory impact of histamine. Furthermore, in contrast, treatment with neither mepyramine (H1R-antagonist) nor thioperamide (H3R-antagonist) significantly inhibited the C5a-induced release of eosinophil peroxidase from eosinophils suggesting the significant role of H2R in same respect. An important relation between histamine and eosinophil in allergic disease has been documented in vivo in patients with allergic rhinitis undergoing segmental allergen challenge, and followed by airway sampling via bronchoalveolar lavage (BAL) after 5 min and 48 h (Jarjour et al. 1997). While in response to in vitro antigen challenge, maximal blood histamine release was determined in each patient before segmental bronchoprovocation. The number of eosinophils in BAL samples collected after 48 hr were significantly enhanced and correlated with the maximal basophil histamine release noted for each individual suggesting a direct causal relationship between basophilic mediator release and airway eosinophilia (Shahid et al. 2009).

6.3.6 Epithelial Cells

The implications of histamine have been observed in cultured human bronchial epithelial cells that demonstrate functionally active H1R and H2R as demonstrated by histamine-induced generation of cGMP for H1R and cAMP for H2R and blockage of cGMP release by treatment with pyrilamine and cAMP release by treatment with titotidine (Devalia and Davies 1991). Recently, the expression of H1-receptor on cultured human ocular and nasal epithelial cells indicates that histamine may potently influence the property of these cells (Hamano et al. 1998, Sharif et al. 1996). It has been demonstrated that nasal and bronchial epithelial cells synthesize and release distinct biologically active mediators including cell adhesion molecules, endothelin, cytokines, arachidonic acid metabolites, major histocompatibility complex class (MHC) II antigens, neuropeptide degrading enzymes and nitric oxide that influence the migration, activation and also function of both structural and inflammatory cells involved in the pathophysiology of allergic rhinitis and asthma (Devalia et al. 2000a, b). Notably, the implications of histamine on mediator release from human bronchial epithelial cells demonstrated that H1R modulation with 2 mM histamine led to induction of cytoplasmic phospholipase A2 mRNA, activation of the transcription factor NF-kβ, production of leukotriene B4, and expression of IL-8 (Aoki et al. 1998). It has been shown that histamine-induced enhancement in leukotriene B4 was inhibited by incubation of the cells with specific 5-lipoxygenase activating protein inhibitors and Zileuton, and expression of IL-8 was blocked by diphenhydramine, and 5-lipoxygenase activating protein inhibitors and Zileuton indicating an important network of histamine-modulated inflammatory mechanisms within the airways. Similarly, histamine induced the release of IL-6, IL-8 and GM-CSF from human corneal and conjunctival epithelial cells in a dose-dependent manner at physiologically or pathologically relevant concentrations and several H1R-antagonists, but not H2R-antagonist (ranitidine) or H3R-antagonist (thioperamide) blocked this cytokine release (Yanni et al. 1999). Indeed, the role of epithelial cells as modulators of inflammation, mainly in allergic diseases has been an important subject of much discussion for future prospects (Shahid et al. 2009).

6.3.7 Endothelial Cells

The contribution of endothelial cells to the pathophysiology of allergic disorder has mainly been investigated. The significant effect of histamine on vascular permeability has well been demonstrated and is a consequence of H1R signaling that results in the contraction of F-actin fibres of the endothelial cytoskeleton and formation of gaps in the post capillary venules and extravasation of macromolecules (Burke-Gaffney and Hellewell 2000). The functionally potent H1R and/or H2R is expressed on human endothelial cells present in distinct tissues (the airway mucosa, eye, skin, brain and umbilical vein) (Koizumi and Ohkawara 1999). Human umbilical vein endothelial cells have been the most investigated in mechanistic studies, because of comparatively easier and greater access to these cells. Currently, in a recent study it has been suggested that histamine itself regulates the expression of histamine receptor (HR) subtypes on endothelial cells and influences the overall significant role in inflammatory response in allergic disease (Schaefer et al. 1999). It has been documented that the levels of mRNA for both the receptors (H1R and H2R) were down regulated by histamine, of which the effect on H2R-mRNA was rapid and long lasting, compared with a less pronounced, transient and shorter lasting impact on the H1R-mRNA. Furthermore, the H2R-mRNA was exclusively down regulated as a result of H1R protein activation. Histamine-induced receptor signaling on the endothelial cells directly modulates inflammatory changes in these cells. Therefore, treatment of human umbilical vein endothelial cell cultures with 10^{-4} M or 10^{-5} M histamine resulted in the release of lipophilic neutrophil chemoattractant activity from endothelial cells, an effect inhibited by cimetidine but not by diphenhydramine (Farber et al. 1986). Histamine or H1R- or H2R-agonist stimulated adhesion of neutrophils to endothelial cells, participated in activation of phospholipase C, guanylate cyclase and nitric oxide synthase isozymes as inhibition of these enzymes with specific inhibitors decreases this adhesion (Farber et al. 1986). The impact of histamine was found to be mediated by both H1-receptor and H2-receptor signaling and modulation of P-selectin on endothelial cells in the mesentery. Thus, histamine receptors are involved in significant implications in the field of histamine research in endothelial cells (Shahid et al. 2009).

6.4 Concluding Remarks

Histamine through its receptors comprises a complex system with distinct functions by their differential expression, which changes according to the stage of cell differentiation and microenvironmental influences. Although contrasting findings have been showed, H1R stimulates the immune system cells by potentiating their proinflammatory activity for increased migration to the area of inflammation as well as increased effector functions. H2R on the other hand appears to be a potent suppressor of inflammatory and effector functions. The data on the role of H3R and H4R in immune regulation are limited. The observation that H4R activation promotes the accumulation of inflammatory cells at sites of allergic inflammation opens a new way of therapeutic opportunity based on concurrent histamine H1R- and H4R-antagonist administration, or development of selective dual H1R and H4R-antagonists. H3Rs and H4Rs have led to a strong renewal of the interest in histamine as well as to intensified research on the ligands and the potential therapeutic indications. It is assumed that within the next few years the first histamine H3R-antagonist will go into market and developments on H4R-antagonists will quickly follow. Reports on further details on this important aspect are enthusiastically awaited.

Acknowledgments Trivendra Tripathi acknowledges University Grants Commission, New Delhi, India for providing UGC Fellowship [UGC letter DON F. 19-33/2006 (CU)] and M. Shahid is grateful to Department of Science and Technology, Ministry of Science and Technology, Government of India for awarding "Young Scientist Project Award" (FT/SR-L-111/2006).

References

Akdis CA, Blaser K (2003) Histamine in the immune regulation of allergic inflammation. J Allergy Clin Immunol 112:15–22

Akdis CA, Simons FER (2006) Histamine receptors are hot in immunopharmacology. European J Pharmacol 533:69–76

Anwar AR, Kay AB (1980) H1-receptor dependence of histamine-induced enhancement of human eosinophil C3b rosettes. Clin Exp Immunol 42:196–199

Aoki Y, Qiu D, Zhao GH et al (1998) Leukotriene B4 mediates histamine induction of NF-kB and IL-8 in human bronchial epithelial cells. Am J Physiol-Lung Cell Mol Physiol 2746: L1030-L1039

Atkins PC, Schwartz LB, Adkinson NF et al (1990a) *In vivo* antigen-induced cutaneous mediator release. Simultaneous comparisons of histamine, tryptase and prostaglandin D2 release and the effect of oral corticosteroid administration. J Allergy Clin Immunol 86:360–370

Atkins PC, Von Allmen C, Valenzano M et al (1990b) Determinants of *in vivo* histamine release in cutaneous allergic reactions in humans. J Allergy Clin Immunol 86:371–379

Berman JS, Mcfadden RG, Cruikshank WW et al (1984) Functional characteristics of histamine receptor-bearing mononuclear cells. II. Identification and characterization of two histamine induced lymphokines that inhibit lymphocyte migration. J Immunol 133:1495–1504

Bull HA, Courtney PF, Bunker CB et al (1993) Basophil mediator release in atopic dermatitis. J Invest Dermatol 100:305–309

Burde R, Seifert R, Buschauer A et al (1983) Histamine inhibits activation of human neutrophils and HL-60 leukemic cells via H2-receptors. Naunyn-Schmiedebergs Arch Pharmacol 340: 671–678

Burke-Gaffney A, Hellewell PG (2000) Contribution of endothelial cells to airway inflammation. In: Page CP, Banner KH, Spina B (eds) Cellular mechanisms in airway inflammation. Birkhäuser, Basel, pp 223–244

Bury TB, Corhay JL, Radermecker MP (1992) Histamine-induced inhibition of neutrophil chemotaxis and T lymphocyte proliferation in man. Allergy 47:624–629

Center DM, Cruikshank WW, Berman JS et al (1983) Functional characteristics of histamine receptor-bearing mononuclear cells. I. Selective production of lymphocyte chemoattractant lymphokines with histamine as a ligand. J Immunol 131:1854–1859

Devalia JL, Davies RJ (1991) Human nasal and bronchial epithelial cells in culture. An overview of their characteristics and function. Allergy Proc12:71–79

Devalia JL, Wang JH, Davies RJ (2000a) Airway epithelial cells. In: Page CP, Banner KH, Spina D (eds) Cellular mechanisms in airway inflammation. Birkhäuser, Basel, pp 245–262

Devalia JL, Rusznak C, Davies RJ (2000b) Epithelial cell dysfunction in rhinitis. In: Busse WW, Holgate ST (eds) Asthma and rhinitis. Blackwell Science, London, pp 841–854

Elliott K, Osna N, Scofield M et al (2001) Regulation of IL-13 production by histamine in cloned murine T helper type 2 cells. Int Immunopharmacol 1:1923–1937

Ezeamuzie CI, Philips E (2000) Histamine H (2) receptors mediate the inhibitory effect of histamine on human eosinophil degranulation. Br J Pharmacol 131:482–488

Farber HW, Weller PF, Rounds S et al (1986) Generation of lipid neutrophil chemoattractant activity by histamine-stimulated cultured endothelial cells. J Immunol 137:2918–2924

Gespach C, Abita JP (1982) Human polymorphonuclear neutrophils. Pharmacological characterisation of histamine receptors mediating the elevation of cyclic AMP. Mol Pharmacol 21:78–85

Godot V, Arock M, Garcia G et al (2007) H4 Histamine receptor mediates optimal migration of mast cell precursors to CXCL12. J Allergy Clin Immunol 120:827–843

Gründemann D, Liebich G, Kiefer N et al (1999) Selective substrates for non-neuronal monoamine transporters. Mol Pharmacol 56:1–10

Gutzmer R, Langer K, Lisewski M et al (2002) Expression and function of histamine receptors 1 and 2 on human monocyte-derived dendritic cells. J Allergy Clin Immunol 109:524–531

Hamano N, Terada N, Maesako K et al (1998) Expression of histamine receptors in nasal epithelial cells and endothelial cells-the effects of sex hormones. Int Arch Allergy Immunol 115: 220–227

Hofstra CL, Desai PJ, Thurmond RL et al (2003) Histamine H4 receptor mediates chemotaxis and calcium mobilization of mast cells. J Pharmacol Exp Ther 305:1212–1221

Horváth BV, Szalai C, Mándi Y et al (1999) Histamine and histamine-receptor antagonists modify gene expression and biosynthesis of interferon gamma in peripheral human blood mononuclear cells and in CD19-depleted cell subsets. Immunol Lett 70:95–99

Idzko M, La Sala A, Ferrari D et al (2002) Expression and function of histamine receptors in human monocyte-derived dendritic cells. J Allergy Clin Immunol 109:839–846

Jarjour NN, Calhoun WJ, Schwartz LB et al (1991) Elevated bronchoalveolar lavage fluid histamine levels in allergic asthmatics are associated with increased airway obstruction. Am Rev Respir Dis 144:83–87

Jarjour NN, Sedgwick JB, Swensen CA et al (1997) Late allergic airway response to segmental bronchopulmonary provocation in allergic subjects is related to blood basophil histamine release. J Allergy Clin Immunol 99:87–93

Jutel M, Klunker S, Akdis M et al (2001) Histamine upregulates Th1 and downregulates Th2 responses due to different patterns of surface histamine 1 and 2 receptor expression. Int Arch Allergy Immunol 124:190–192

Khan MM, Melmon KL (1985) Are autocoids more than theoretic modulators of immunity? Clin Immunol Rev 4:1–30
Khan MM, Melmon KL (1988) Selected autacoids as modulators of lymphocyte function. In: Handbook of experimental pharmacology. Springer, Berlin, pp 363–383
Khan MM, Sansoni P, Engleman EG et al (1985) Pharmacological effects of autacoids on subsets of T cells: regulation of expression/function of histamine-2 receptors by a subset of suppressor cells. J Clin Invest 75:1578–1583
Khan MM, Marr-Leisy D, Verlander MS et al (1986) The effects of derivatives of histamine on natural suppressor cells. J Immunol 137:308–314
Kleine-Tebbe J, Schramm J, Bolz M et al (1990) Influence of histamine H3-anatgonists on human leukocytes. Agents Actions 30:137–139
Koizumi H, Ohkawara A (1999) H2 histamine receptor-mediated increase in cultured human keratinocytes. J Dermatol Sci 21:127–132
Lagier B, Lebel B, Bousquet J et al (1997) Different modulation by histamine of IL-4 and interferon-gamma (IFN-γ) release according to the phenotype of human Th0, Th1 and Th2 clones. Clin Exp Immunol 108:545–551
Lippert U, Artuc M, Grützkau A et al (2004) Human skin mast cells express H2 and H4, but not H3 receptors. J Invest Dermatol 123:116–123
Lippert U, Moller A, Welker P et al (2000) Inhibition of cytokine secretion from human leukemic mast cells and basophils by H1- and H2-receptor antagonists. Exp Dermatol 9:118–124
Ma RZ, Gao J, Meeker ND et al (2002) Identification of Bphs, an autoimmune disease locus, as histamine receptor H1. Science 297:620–623
MacGlashan D Jr (2003) Histamine: a mediator of inflammation. J Allergy Clin Immunol 112: S53-S59
Makabe-Kobayashi Y, Hori Y, Adachi T et al (2002) The control effect of histamine on body temperature and respiratory function in IgE-dependent systemic anaphylaxis. J Allergy Clin Immunol 110:298–303
Marmy N, Mottas J, Durand J (1993) Signal transduction in smooth muscle cells from human airways. Respir Physiol 91:295–306
Mazzoni A, Young HA, Spitzer JH et al (2001) Histamine regulates cytokine production in maturing dendritic cells, resulting in altered T cell polarization. J Clin Invest 108:1865–1873
McLeod RL, Mingo GG, Herczku C et al (1999) Combined histamine H1 and H3 receptor blockade produces nasal decongestion in an experimental model of nasal congestion. Am J Rhinol 13:391–399
Morichika T, Takahashi HK, Iwagaki H et al (2003) Histamine inhibits lipopolysaccharide-induced tumor necrosis factor-alpha production in an intercellular adhesion molecule-1- and B7.1-dependent manner. J Pharmacol Exp Ther 304:624–633
Ohtani T, Aiba S, Mizuashi M et al (2003) H1 and H2 histamine receptors are absent on Langerhans cells and present on dermal dendritic cells. J Invest Dermatol 121:1073–1079
Ohtsu H, Kuramasu A, Tanaka S et al (2002) Plasma extravasation induced by dietary supplemented histamine in histamine-free mice. Eur J Immunol 32:1698–1708
Ohtsu H, Tanaka S, Terui T et al (2001) Mice lacking histidine decarboxylase exhibit abnormal mast cells. FEBS Lett 502:53–56
Osna N, Elliott K, Khan MM (2001a) Regulation of interleukin-10 secretion by histamine in Th2 cells and splenocytes. Int Immunopharmacol 1:85–86
Osna N, Elliott K, Khan MM (2001b) The effects of histamine on interferon gamma production are dependent on the stimulatory signals. Int Immunopharmacol 1:125–145
Parsons ME, Ganellin CR (2006) Histamine and its receptors. Br J Pharmacology 147:S127-S135
Qui R, Melmon KL, Khan MM (1990) Effects of histamine trifluoromethyl-toludine (HTMT) on intracellular calcium in human lymphocytes. J Pharmacol Exp Therap 253:1245–1252
Radermecker M, Maldague MP (1981) Depression of neutrophil chemotaxis in atopic individuals. An H2 histamine receptor response. Int Arch allergy Appl Immunol 65:144–152
Raible DG, Lenahan T, Fayvilevich Y et al (1994) Pharmacological characterization of a novel histamine receptor on human eosinophils. Am J Respir Crit Care Med 149:1506–1511

Rocklin RE (1990) Histamine and H2 antagonists in inflammation and immunodeficiency. Marcel Dekker, New York

Sachs B, Hertl M, Merk HF (2000) Histamine receptors on lymphocytes: distribution and functional significance. Skin Pharmacol Appl Skin Physiol 13:313–323

Sansoni P, Silverman ED, Khan MM et al (1985) Immunoregulatory T cells in man: histamine-induced suppressor T cells are derived from Leu 21 (T1) subpopulation distinct from that, which gives rise to cytotoxic T cells. J Clin Invest 75:650–656

Schaefer U, Schmitz V, Schneider A et al (1999) Histamine-induced homologous and heterologous regulation of histamine receptor subtype mRNA in cultured endothelial cells. Shock 12: 309–315

Schneider E, Lemoine FM, Breton-Gorius J et al (1999) IL-3-induced coexpression of histidine decarboxylase, IL-4, and IL-6 mRNA by murine basophil precursors. Exp Hematol 27: 1010–1018

Schneider E, Machavoine F, Pléau JM et al (2005) Organic cation transporter 3 modulates murine basophil functions by controlling intracellular histamine levels. J Exp Med 202:387–393

Schneider E, Rolli-Derkinderen M, Arock M et al (2002) Trends in histamine research: new functions during immune responses and hematopoiesis. Trends Immunol 23:255–263

Seligmann BE, Fletcher MP, Gallin JI (1983) Histamine modulation of human neutrophil oxidative metabolism, locomotion, degranulation, and membrane potential changes. J Immunol 130:1902–1909

Shahid M, Tripathi T, Sobia F et al (2009) Histamine, histamine receptors and their role in immunomodulation: an updated systematic review. Open Immunol J 2:9–41

Sharif NA, Xu SX, Magnino PE et al (1996) Human conjunctival epithelial cells express Histamine-1 receptors coupled to phosphoinositide turnover and intracellular calcium mobilisation. Role in ocular allergic and inflammatory diseases. Exp Eye Res 63:169–178

Spitaler MM, Hammer A, Malli R et al (2002) Functional analysis of histamine receptor subtypes involved in endotheliummediated relaxation of the human uterine artery. Clin Exp Pharmacol Physiol 29:711–716

Stark H (2003) Recent advances in histamine H3/H4 receptor ligands Exp Opin Ther Pat 13: 851–865

Stark H (2007) Histamine receptors. Biotrends Reviews 1:2–9. http://www.biotrend.com. Assessed Sept 2009

Sugimoto Y, Iba Y, Nakamura Y et al (2004) Pruritus-associated response mediated by cutaneous H3 receptors. Clin Exp Allergy 34:456–459

Tanaka S, Deai K, Inagaki M et al (2003) Uptake of histamine by mouse peritoneal macrophages and a macrophage cell line, RAW264.7. Am J Physiol Cell Physiol 285:C592-C598

Tedeschi A, Lorine M, Arquati M et al (1991) Regulation of histamine release from human basophil leukocytes role of H1, H2 and H3 receptors. Allergy 46:626–631

Thurmond RL, Desai PJ, Dunford PJ et al (2004) A potent and selective histamine H4 receptor antagonist with anti-inflammatory properties. J Pharmacol Exp Ther 309:404–413

Triggiani M, Gentile M, Secondo A et al (2001) Histamine induces exocytosis and IL-6 production from human lung macrophages through interaction with H1 receptors. J Immunol 166: 4083–4091

Wang KY, Arima N, Higuchi S et al (2000) Switch of histamine receptor expression from H2 to H1 during differentiation of monocytes into macrophages. FEBS Lett 473:345–348

Weltman JK (2000) Update on histamine as a mediator of inflammation. Allergy Asthma Proc 3:125–128

Westcott S, Kaliner M (1983) Histamine H-1 binding site on human polymorphonuclear leukocytes. Inflammation 7:291–300

Yanni JM, Weimer LK, Sharif NA et al (1999) Inhibition of histamine-induced human conjunctival epithelial cell responses by ocular allergy drugs. Arch Opthalmol 117:643–647

Part V
Histamine in Regulation of Cell Proliferation and Differentiation

Chapter 7
Effects of Histamine on Lymphocytes

Manzoor M. Khan

Abstract Histamine originally identified in 1900s is an important mediator of allergic disease, asthma and inflammation. Histamine has modulatory effects on different subpopulations of lymphoid cells. The pharmacologic effects of histamine are mediated through four types of membrane histamine receptors, H1R, H2R, H3R and H4R, which are all heptahelical G-protein-coupled receptors. Histamine receptors possess all structural features of G-protein-coupled receptors, including seven putative transmembrane domain, amino terminal glycosylation sites, and phosphorylation sites for protein kinase A and protein kinase C. Stimulation of H1R and H2R activates G_q and G_s respectively, whereas both H3R and H4R are coupled to $G_{i/o}$. Histamine affects a number of immune processes including regulation of T cells, antibody isotopes, antigen presenting cells and peripheral T cell tolerance. The conventional wisdom regarding the effects of histamine on Th1/Th2 subsets is that it shifts responses from Th1 to Th2 subsets resulting in allergic and asthmatic disease. While expression of H2 receptors on T cells has been well characterized; there is not a consensus on the function and expression of H1 receptors in the regulation of T cells. It has been suggested that Th1 cells may show a dominant expression of H1R and Th2 cells may show increased H2R. The effects of histamine on cytokine release and expression by T cells have been well established. Histamine suppresses the expression of Th1 cytokines and stimulates the secretion of Th2 cytokines via H2R. The recently discovered H4 receptors have drawn considerable interest pertaining to their effects on the regulation of immune response and inflammation. H4 receptor activates dendritic cells, regulates chemotaxis and migration of mast cells and eosinophils, and modulates cytokine release from T cells and dendritic cells. Histamine also regulates cytokine-dependent signal transduction pathways including JAK-STAT pathway. This chapter provides an overview of recent developments in understanding the role of histamine and its receptors in regulating the function of immune effector cells involved in allergic disease and asthma.

M.M. Khan (✉)
Department of Pharmaceutical Sciences, Creighton University Medical Center, Omaha, NE 68178, USA
e-mail: mmkhan@creighton.edu

M. Shahid et al. (eds.), *Biomedical Aspects of Histamine*,
DOI 10.1007/978-90-481-9349-3_7,

Keywords Histamine · Histamine receptors · Mast cell · Immune cells · Allergic inflammation · Cell Proliferation · iNKT

Abbreviations

Th1	T helper type 1 cells
Th2	T helper type 2 cells
Th3	T helper type 3 cells
GPCR	G protein-coupled receptors
IL	interleukin
STAT	signal transduction and activator of transcription
TNF	tumor necrosis factor
IFN	interferon
MAP kinase	mitogen activated protein kinase
Camp	3′-5′-cyclic adenosine monophosphate
cGMP	3′-5′-cyclic guanosine monophosphate
NF-κB	nuclear factor kappa B
JAK	Janus kinase
mDC	myeloid dendritic cells
ICAM-1	intracellular adhesion molecule-1

Contents

7.1 Introduction

Histamine was originally identified by Sir Henry Dale one hundred years ago (Barger and Dale 1910, Dale and Laidlaw 1910). It was characterized as a mediator of allergic reaction after Dale and Laidlaw found that it mimicked the effects of anaphylaxis (Dale and Laidlaw 1910, 1911, Best et al. 1927). Since its discovery histamine has become one of the most investigated compound in medicine and its production, distribution, kinetics, metabolism, receptors, second messengers and physiological and pathological roles have been extensively studied. Histamine is synthesized by a variety of tissues in human and a number of stimuli are responsible for its release. Though mast cells in the immune system are the predominant source of histamine in humans it is present in almost all tissues including basophils, gastric enterochromaffin-like cells, lymphocytes, platelets, macrophages and neurons in concentrations ranging from 1 to 100 μg/g (Beaven 1976). In the mast cells it is stored in large cytoplasmic granules and released by exocytosis (Galli 1993). Both immunological and non-immunological mechanisms including allergens, drugs, endogenous peptides (bradykinin, substance P), cold, and mechanical factors are implicated in histamine's release. While the focal point of this chapter is the effects of histamine on lymphocytes and immune response, it has been long known to play a role in nervous, cardiovascular and gastrointestinal systems as well as in inflammation and anaphylaxis. Thus, it was not surprising when this mediator of inflammation was found to modulate immune response. In the immune system histamine is an important mediator of allergic disease, asthma and inflammation, where it exerts its effects via specific receptors on the cell surface of immunocompetent cells. The effects of histamine on immune response vary widely based on the receptor expression/distribution of this amine and the physiological/pathological environment of immune cells. As a result there is ample conflicting data regarding the effects of histamine on lymphocytes. This chapter describes the latest developments in the state of histamine effects on Th1/Th2 paradigm as they play a critical role in the development of allergic disease and asthma. In addition to the role of the effects of histamine on T cells, its role in regulating B cells, antigen presenting cells specifically the dendritic cells and polymorphonuclear leukocytes is also discussed as they relate to the modulation of immune response and allergic inflammation.

7.2 Histamine and Immune Response

The first report that histamine played a role in immune response was published by Pepys (1955), who observed that histamine injection in combination with an antigen administered into the site of a tuberculin skin test suppressed the delayed hypersensitivity reactions in human. This finding was unexpected from a mediator of inflammation and indeed the observation was not appreciated until many years later. The initial studies exploring the role of histamine as immune modulator focused on the modulation of function/expression of histamine receptors in response to commitment to physiological function and exposure to antigen. The receptors for histamine on selected leukocytes were reported by Melmon et al. (1972). Affinity chromatographic techniques were used to delineate cells which expressed histamine receptors. Furthermore, the role of cAMP in the modulation of inflammation and immunity was described (Bourne et al. 1974). It was observed that precursor B cells do not express histamine receptors but the cells which are committed to synthesize antibodies respond to histamine (Melmon et al. 1974, Shearer et al. 1974). The allogeneic exposure of effector T cells makes them increasingly responsive to histamine depending on the length of exposure (Lichtenstein 1976). The thymocytes do not respond to histamine but after their exposure to corticosteroids the cells which are resistant to corticosteroid become responsive to histamine (Rozkowski et al. 1977). The original notion about the immunoregulatory effects of this autacoid was that the response to histamine was dependent on the state of activation of lymphocytes. The pioneering research focused on the immunosuppressive effects of histamine and the role of H2 receptors was highlighted (Garovoy et al. 1983, Melmon and Khan 1987, Melmon et al. 1981, Rocklin 1976, Rocklin and Beer 1983, Rocklin and Habarek-davidson 1984). While H2 receptors are involved in the activation of suppressive responses, it was suggested that stimulation of H1 receptors enhanced the suppressive activity of natural suppressor cells (Khan et al. 1985a). Furthermore, the presence of H2 receptors on $CD4^+$ (helper T cells) and $CD8^+$ (cytolytic T cells) subsets by measuring cAMP accumulation in response to histamine was documented (Khan et al. 1985b). The evidence is now compelling that histamine regulates immune response by affecting the function and cell surface expression of lymphocytes, leukocytes, antigen presenting cells, and regulating the secretion of cytokines and chemokines. Histamine affects a variety of cell types involved in immune response including T lymphocytes, B lymphocytes, macrophages, monocytes, mast cells, dendritic cells and endothelial cells. These cells express various histamine receptors and some are capable of synthesizing and secreting histamine. Histamine selectively recruits immune effectors cells and regulate their development, maturation, proliferation, activation, polarization and effector function and may also be implicated in peripheral T cell tolerance (Jutel et al. 2002, 2005, Marone et al. 2003, Packard and Khan 2003).

7.3 Histamine Receptors on Immune Cells

The effects of histamine on immune response are mediated through four pharmacologically distinct receptors, H1, H2, H3, and H4 (Table 7.1). These four receptor subsets are all members of a large superfamily that has seven membrane-spanning regions and are G protein coupled (GPCR) family (Parson and Ganellin 2006). However, no receptor subfamilies have been identified within the four histamine receptor subsets. There is significant difference in the structure of H1 and H2 receptors. H1 receptor seems to be more closely related to muscarinic receptor and H2 receptor appears to be related to 5-HT1 receptors. The H4 receptor exhibits 40% homology to the H3 receptor but is vastly different from H1 and H2 receptors.

Table 7.1 Distribution and function of histamine receptors in immune system

Receptor subset	Distribution	Responses and function
Histamine- H1 receptor	Lymphocytes, T and B cells, Monocytes, eosinophils, neutrophils, Smooth muscle, Endothelial cells	Immune regulation, Increase release of histamine, increased expression of adhesion molecules, Increased capacity of antigen presenting cells, Chemotaxis of eosinophils and neutrophils, Increased Th1 function
Histamine H2 receptor	Lymphocytes, T cells, B cells, Monocytes, Eosinophils, neutrophils, Dendritic cells, neutrophils, vascular smooth muscles	Activation of Th2 lymphocytes, Cytokine release or inhibition, Decreased neutrophil and eosinophil chemotaxis, regulation of humoral response, stimulation of adenylate cyclase
Histamine H3 receptor	Monocytes, Dendritic cells, Eosinophils, endothelium	Regulation of antigen presenting cells, Enhanced proinflammatory activity, Regulation of neurogenic inflammation, Modulation of histamine release, inhibition of cAMP
Histamine H4 receptor	Bone marrow, Helper T cells, thymus, neutrophils, eosionophils, dendritic cells, mast cells, basophils, splenocytes	Antigen uptake and cross presentation, Regulation of cytokine and chemokine secretion, Recruitment and activation of inflammatory cells (eosinophils, mast cells, neutrophils, T lymphocytes, dendritic cells), Mast cell chemotaxis, immune modulator, increased cytokine (IL-16) production, inhibition of cAMP

All four types of histamine receptors possess constitutive activity (Leurs et al. 2002). Similar to most other G-protein-coupled receptors, histamine receptors exist as equilibrium between their inactive and active conformations. Agonists stimulate the active and inverse agonists the inactive conformation. An agonist has a preferential affinity for the active state of receptor which results in the stabilization of the receptor in its active conformation. This leads to continued activation signal initiating from histamine receptor. The inverse agonists have a preferential affinity for the inactive state. The binding of the inverse agonist to the receptor results in an inactive state since the receptor is stabilized in this state thus leading to an inhibition of signal transduction emanating from histamine receptors (Leurs et al. 2002).

The H1 receptors are coupled to Gq/ii and activates a number of intracellular signals including Ca^{2+}, cGMP, phospholipase A2, phopholipase D and NFκB. Histamine via H1 receptors causes its classical symptoms of immediate hypersensitivity reaction in nose, skin and lungs. The role of H1 receptors in anaphylaxis is well established and H1 antagonists are widely used as therapeutic agents (Simons 2002, 2003a, b, Simons and Simons 1994). The demonstration of the presence of H1 receptors on lymphocytes, mast cells, antigen presenting cells and endothelial cells expanded our understanding of the crucial role they play in regulating immune response and specifically T lymphocytes (Khan et al. 1987, 1989). The H2 receptors are linked to Gαs and activate a number of signals including adenylate cyclase, cAMP, c-Jun, c-Fos, p70S6K, and PKC. Osband et al. (1981) directly demonstrated the presence of H2 receptors on lymphocytes. The effects of H2 receptors on lymphocytes and immune response are inhibitory and dependent on the accumulation of cAMP. The role of H2 receptors in immunoregulatory mechanisms has been well established. The H3 receptors are linked to Gi/o, activate several intracellular signals including Ca^{2+} and MAP kinases, and inhibit cAMP formation (Schwartz and Arrang 2002). They control histamine release in addition to other CNS functions. Histamine controls mast cells via its effects on H3 receptors which may regulate neuropeptide containing neurons. This function may be related to a local neuron-mast cell feedback loop controlling neurogenic inflammation. Excessive inflammatory responses result after the dysregulation of this feedback loop. The H4 receptors are linked to Gi/os and cause intracellular Ca^{2+} flux and inhibit cAMP accumulation. These receptors are expressed on immune cells including the bone marrow, spleen, thymus, mast cells, monocytes, natural killer cells, neutrophils, eosinophils, T cells and some other tissues. In response to inflammatory signals the expression of H4 receptors is induced or modified in peripheral tissues including spleen, thymus, bone marrow and leukocytes (Akdis et al. 2006, Hill et al. 1997, Jutel and Akdis 2007, Parsons and Ganellin 2006). The distribution and functions of different histamine receptor subsets are shown in Table 7.1.

7.4 Effects of Histamine on T Lymphocytes

7.4.1 Helper T Cells

T lymphocytes develop in thymus and as a result are called T cells. The presence of the T cell receptor differentiates T cells from other lymphocytes. One subset of T cell, helper T cells, is identified by the presence of $CD4^+$ receptors on their cell surface. The helper T cells could also be divided on the basis of cytokines they secrete (Romagnani 1992). $CD4^+$ Helper T cells are diverse and consistently-expanding group of lymphocytes that now include Th0, Th1, Th2, Th3, Th17 and regulatory T cells. Th1 and Th2 cells were originally identified by Mosmann et al. (1986) and have been the focus of intensive investigation for their role in infection, autoimmunity, allergic disease and asthma. The classification of Th0, Th1 and Th2 cells is based on their cytokine secretion profiles. Cytokines are small glycoproteins synthesized and secreted by a variety of cells but predominantly leukocytes. T cells communicate with other cells either by cell–cell interaction or through release of soluble factors including cytokines. The cytokines play a crucial role in a number of physiological and pathological functions in immune and inflammatory responses. Following activation, naïve helper T cells become Th0 cells and have characteristics of both Th1 and Th2 cells, Th0 cells later differentiate into respective subsets (Kohda et al. 2002). Th1 and Th2 subsets are involved in the development, initiation and regulation of adaptive immunity. The role of

Th1 cells in delayed type hypersensitivity and cytotoxicity and Th2 cells in regulating IgG and IgE synthesis has been well established. Th1 cells secrete IL-2, IL-3, IFN-γ, TNF-α, TNF-β and GM-CSF. Since all helper T cells secrete IL-2 the classification of IL-2 as a Th1 cytokine is misleading. Th2 cells secrete IL-4, IL-5, IL-6, IL-9, IL-10, IL-13, TNF-β and GM-CSF (Fig. 7.1) The Th17 lineage is an additional effector CD4 T cell arm recently identified, since the discovery of Th1 and Th2 subsets. Th17 cells have a distinct cytokine secretion pattern as they release IL-17, IL17F and IL-6. They develop from pathways distinct from Th1 and Th2 cells and do have several notable lineages parallel to Th1 cells and their development depends on TGF-β (Weaver et al. 2006). Consequently, the effects of histamine on helper T cells and cytokines are pivotal in regulating a number of essential human functions in health and disease. The effects of histamine on helper T cells are differential and complex as they relate to the etiology and pathogenesis of allergic disease and asthma. Histamine induces an imbalance in Th1/Th2 ratio which is associated with many disease states. The evidence from many laboratories suggest that histamine increases the secretion of Th2 cytokines

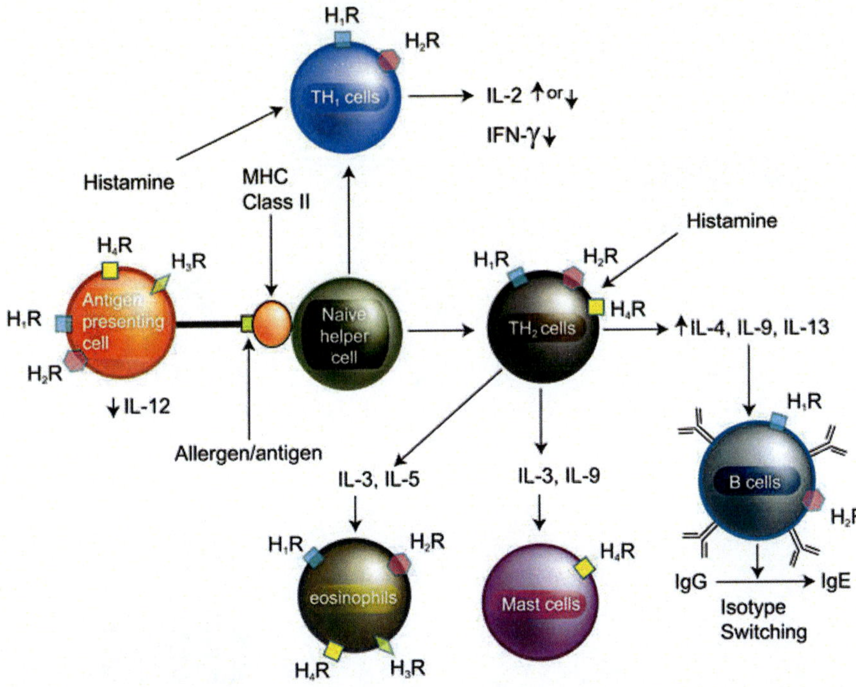

Fig. 7.1 Effects of histamine on Th1/Th2 paradigm. Th1 cells regulate delayed hypersensitivity and cytotoxic response whereas Th2 cells control antibody production and isotype switch as it relates to allergic disease and asthma. In nonatopic individuals there is a balance between Th1 and Th2 cells and the respective cytokine they release. In contrast, in atopic individuals there is an increase in Th2 cells and their cytokines and a decrease in Th1 cells and the cytokines they release. Histamine increase the production of Th2 cytokines which increase the number of Th2 cells and decrease the levels of Th1 cytokines

(IL-5, IL-10, and IL-13) and suppresses the secretion of Th1 cytokines (IL-2, IFN-γ) (Fig. 7.2) (Elenkov et al. 1998, Elliott et al. 2001, Katoh et al. 2005, Kohka et al. 2000, Marone et al. 2003, Osna et al. 2001a, b, Poluektova and Khan 1998, Packard and Khan 2003, Schneider et al. 2002, Takahashi et al. 2004, Van der Pouw Kraan et al. 1998). The effect of histamine favoring Th2 responses has been well established (Packard and Khan 2003). Histamine inhibits IL-12 synthesis while augmenting IL-10 production thus providing favorable conditions for the differentiation and development of Th2 cells (Elenkov et al. 1998). However, this understanding was questioned by the observations that histamine could either augment or suppress IFN-γ secretion based on the type of the involvement of histamine receptor (Akdis and Simons 2006, Jutel et al. 2001). In their studies H1 receptors enhanced and H2 receptors suppressed IFN-γ production in H1 and H2 receptor knockout mice. This could be attributed to the differential expression of histamine receptors or unique pharmacological activity of the agonists. Alternatively, the use of H1R and H2R KO mice may have attributed to this discrepancy. Of importance is the observation that in wildtype mice the use of respective receptor antagonists does not produce the

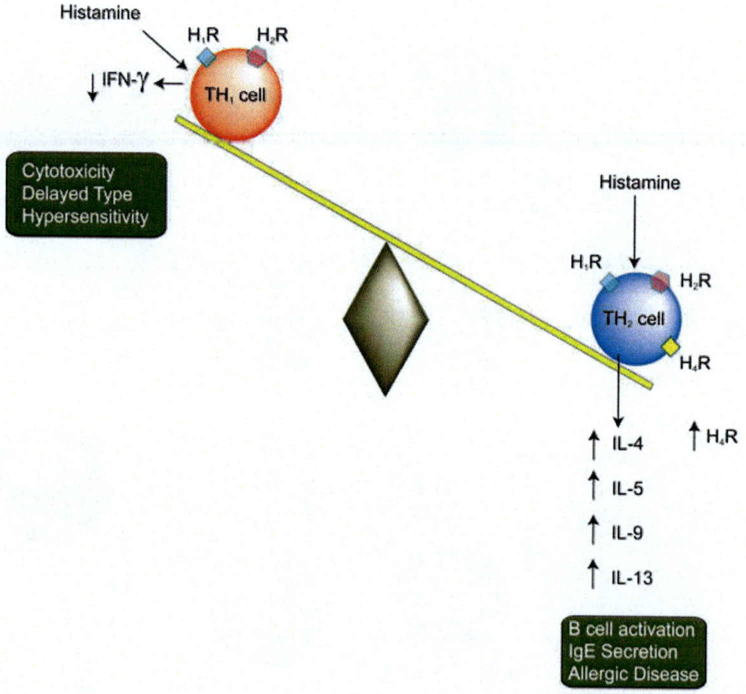

Fig. 7.2 Helper T cell subsets and immune effector cells; Th1 and Th2 subset are implicated in the etiology/pathogenesis of allergic disease and asthma. Both of the subsets are derived from naïve T helper cells and their development and differentiation is dependent on various cytokines. The stimulation of Th1 and Th2 subsets results in the secretion of other cytokines which provide support for the proliferation of mast cells, eosinophils and B cells. This figure depicts the cytokines which result in the development of the components of allergic inflammation

same results, suggesting that the complete deletion of the receptor is necessary to produce these unique results.

Jutel et al. (2001) have reported that Th1 cells richly express H1 receptors while Th2 cells predominantly express H2 receptors. However, H2 receptors are also expressed on Th1 cells and H1 receptors on Th2 cells. Using H1 and H2 receptor KO mice they found that H1 receptors are involved in promoting Th1 responses whereas, H2 receptors play a role in suppressing both Th1 and Th2 responses. They observed that H1 receptor KO mice exhibited enhanced secretion of Th2 cytokines, IL-4 and IL-13, and a decrease in the levels of Th1 cytokine, IFN-γ. However, augmented secretion of both Th1 and Th2 cytokines was reported in H2 receptor KO mice. As previously pointed out, these observations differ from the conventional wisdom regarding the effects of histamine on Th1/Th2 paradigm.

Jutel et al. (2001) have further suggested that in some circumstances histamine inhibits Th2 cell proliferation and induces Th1 cells resulting in a negative feedback to the allergic response. This process is augmented by IL-3 which is a mast cell and basophil growth factor. In addition, IL-3 also induces histamine decarboxylase activity in hematopoietic cells. It has been reported that IL-3 induces the expression of H1 receptors on Th1 cells but not Th2 cells. Higher levels of Th2 cytokines and lower levels of Th1 cytokines have been observed in asthmatic children when compared with controls. The imbalance is attributed to the levels of IL-5, IL-12, IL-13 and IFN-γ. Consequently, histamine plays a significant role in regulating the Th1/Th2 levels as histamine is capable of promoting the differentiation of $CD4^+$ T cells into a Th2 profile (Caron et al. 2001a, Dunford et al. 2006, Mazzoni et al. 2001).

It has been suggested that H4 receptors play a role in the activation of T cells. The H4 receptors are expressed on $CD4^+$ T cells and are upregulated on Th2 cells when they are stimulated with IL4, a Th2 cytokine (Gutzmer et al. 2009). The patients with atopic dermatitis have an augmented expression of H4 receptors on peripheral $CD4^+$ T cells. Histamine via H4 receptors inhibits IL12 which is a Th1 priming cytokine and activates AP-1 which is an important mediator in Th2 cells and is needed for the synthesis of IL-4, IL-5 and IL-13. While there is an induction of the transduction factor AP-1 as a result of stimulation of H4 receptors, there is no effect on the secretion of AP-1-associated cytokines. However, stimulation of AP-1 results in enhanced secretion of IL-31 via H4 receptors. IL-31 is synthesized by activated Th2 cells, and plays a role in atopic dermatitis but not in psoriasis (Gutzmer et al. 2009).

Other evidence for supporting a role of H4 receptors in immunomodulation comes from the observation that histamine causes the release of IL-16 from T cells (Gantner et al. 2002). IL-16 is a $CD4^+$ cells chemoattractant which mediates inflammation. The effects of histamine on IL-16 are mediated via H2 and H4 receptors (Gantner et al. 2002). Histamine serves as a lymphocyte chemoattractant factor and mediates migration either via H1 or H4 receptors but not through H2 receptors. Both H1 and H4 receptors can produce a migratory signal, however, the responding cell populations for the two receptors differ. In this process histamine via H4 receptors enrich regulatory T cell population (later described) which expresses high levels of

CD25 and the transcription factor, Fox P3. The suppressive function of these cells is dependent on IL-10 and not on TGF-β or IL-16 (Morgan et al. 2007).

The observations that the H4 receptor antagonists, when administered during sensitization, inhibit inflammatory and T cell responses after antigen challenge suggest a role of H4 receptors in initial priming of T cells. Activation of H4 receptors by histamine inhibits Th2 responses including a decrease in the production of IL-4, IL-5 and IL-13 (Dunford et al. 2006). However, there is no increase in the production of Th1 cytokines, as the levels of IFN-γ are not altered, and there is no increase in the synthesis of antigen-specific IgG2a. Furthermore, when H4 receptors are blocked there is suppression in the production of IL-6 and IL-17A by T cells. This data suggests that the H4 receptors activate T cells via dendritic cells but the source of histamine is not mast cells. Rather dendritic cells are capable of synthesizing their own histamine under various conditions. Of interest is the observation that Toll Like Receptor (TLR) ligands which generally stimulate Th1 responses provide a signal to the dendritic cells for the synthesis of histamine (Dunford et al. 2006). Based on these observations, it is becoming increasingly evident that H4 receptors play an important role in histamine-induced etiology and pathogenesis of asthma. A defect in H4 receptor function results in reduced production of Th2 cytokines IL-4, IL-5 and IL-13. Furthermore, absence of H4 receptors results in the suppression of the production of the inflammatory cytokines IL-6 and IL-17A by T cells. Both of these cytokines play an important role in the disease progression of asthma. However, this defect does not result in an increased Th1 response as levels of INF-γ are not affected. Based on the role of H4 receptors, it is evident that H4 antagonists may serve as potential clinical agents for the treatment of asthmatic disease as there is a correlation between levels of histamine and severity of asthmatic disease (Gutzmer et al. 2005, Thurmond et al. 2008, Zampeli and Tiligada 2009).

7.4.2 Regulatory T Cells

Regulatory T cells play an important role in modulating immune responses to both self and foreign agents. (Beisset et al. 2006) There are several classifications of regulatory T cells but they could be divided into two general classes: naturally occurring and antigen specific (Bluestone and Abbas 2003, Lohr et al. 2006). The naturally occurring $CD4^+$CD25+FoxP3 regulatory T cells are derived from the thymus, whereas antigen-specific CD25+ regulatory T cells have various phenotypes and are produced in the periphery and secrete IL-10 and/or TGF-β. Histamine blocks the suppressive ability of $CD4^+$CD25+ regulatory T cells. This effect is mediated via H1 receptors and H2 receptor agonists and antagonists have no effect on this function. While both $CD4^+$CD25+ regulatory T cells and $CD4^+$CD25+ responder T cells express H1 receptors, histamine acts only on regulatory T cells and not on responder T cells. The suppressor function of regulatory T cells is programmed by the transcription factor, Foxp3. In the presence of histamine the Foxp3 expression is abolished in regulatory T cells. Foxp3 levels correlate with the suppressive activity of $CD4^+$CD25+ regulatory T cells and the maintenance of Foxp3 expression in regulatory T cells is dependent on IL-2. As histamine suppresses the expression of CD25 on regulatory T cells it is possible that that the maintenance of Foxp3 expression in regulatory T cells may be due to its effects on the consumption of IL-2. Alternatively histamine may directly inhibit Foxp3 expression instead of inhibiting constitutive regulatory T cell expression of CD25 resulting in a decrease in Foxp3 (Forward et al. 2009). Histamine via H4 receptors causes the recruitment of inducible regulatory T cells as intratracheal administration of the H4 receptor agonist causes the accumulation of Foxp3+ T cells in mouse lungs (Morgan et al. 2007). This suggests a role for histamine via H4 receptors in recruiting regulatory T cells to resolve acute inflammation. According to Jutel et al. (2005), regulatory T cells-induced peripheral tolerance, control immune responses after immunotherapy, based on the administration of the allergens. Both contact dependent and independent mechanisms are involved in this regulation. An essential role in this tolerance is demonstrated by the production of IL-10 and TGF-β secreted by allergen-specific T cells. The peripheral tolerance resulting from specific immunotherapy is inhibited by histamine which via H2 receptors enhances the production of IL-10 by dendritic cells and Th2 cells, and the suppressive activity of TGF-β on T cells (Jutel et al. 2005). These observations suggest a role of H2 receptors in peripheral tolerance as well.

7.4.3 Invariant Natural Killer Cells (iNKT)

Histamine regulates the development of invariant natural killer T (iNKT) cells. iNKT cells play a role in the regulation of various immune responses because of their ability to produce multiple cytokines. However, their role is intriguing since they produce IL-4 and IFN-γ, the two cytokines which are associated with Th2 and Th1 responses, respectively. Histamine free histidine decarboxylase knockout mice have a deficiency in the numbers and function of iNKT cells resulting in suppression of IL-4 and IFN-γ production. The administration of histamine in these mice restores normal levels of IL-4 and IFN-γ. These mechanisms are associated with H4 receptors, as the reversal by the administration of histamine is antagonized by H4R antagonists. H4R knockout mice exhibit iNKT cells deficiency, suggesting that histamine via H4 receptors may play a role in their development (Leite-de-Moraes et al. 2009)

7.5 Effects of Histamine on B Lymphocytes

The presence of histamine receptors on B cells was first reported by Melmon et al. (1974). They found that the precursors of B cells did not possess histamine receptors, but immunologically committed B cells secreting antibodies exhibited these receptors. Rocklin et al. (1979) reported that histamine decreases the activation of antigen-induced suppressor cells which regulate antibody production. The effect is mediated by H1 receptors and generally results in enhanced antibody production when B cells are stimulated with specific antigens.

Histamine via H1 receptors induces IgM-dependent B cell proliferation which is not observed in H1 receptor KO mice. In response to thymus independent antigens H1 receptor KO mice exhibit a decrease in antibody production (Banu and Watanabe 1999). Thus histamine via H1 receptors plays a role in the activation/suppression of B cell activity. The effects of histamine on antibody production differ in responses to T-cell independent and dependent antigens. Higher levels of IgG1 and IgE are produced in response to ovalbumin in H1 receptor KO mice. (Jutel et al. 2001) However, less IgE is produced by ovalbumin in H2 receptor KO mice. Increased levels of IL-4 and IL-13 are observed in H2 receptor KO mice but IgE levels in response to ovalbumin are decreased as the levels of IFN-γ are high. As previously pointed out H2 receptors are associated with increased IL-4 and IL-13 production, generally. These intriguing observations suggest a role of H1 receptor in Th1-mediated humoral responses.

7.6 Effects of Histamine on Lymphocyte Transcription Factors

Cytokine-induced signal transduction is mediated by several transcription factors. The TCR activation results in cytokine production which binds to its receptors and exerts their effects through various signaling proteins including Signal of Transducer and Activator of Transcription-1, 4 and 6 (STAT-1, STAT-4, STAT-6). After phosphorylation, these factors are translocated from the cytoplasm to nucleus and bind to the cytokine responsive element of DNA. The phosphorylation of STAT factors and their translocation to nucleus plays an important role in the regulation of Th1/Th2 cytokine balance. STAT4 deficient mice do not generate Th1 cells and STAT6 deficient mice do not generate Th2 cells. STAT-1 mediates the effects of IFN-γ, IL-5, IL-6 and IL-13. Histamine upregulates IFN-γ-induced phosphorylation of STAT-1 (Osna et al. 2001c). This hyperphosphorylation of STAT1 by histamine is mediated via both H1 and H2 receptors (Sakhalkar et al. 2005). Furthermore, there is a convergent crosstalk between H1 and H2 receptor pathways, Ca2+-PKC and cAMP-PKA, respectively. Accordingly, Ca2+-PKC induced STAT-1 phosphorylation is completely dependent on PKA. In another study histamine acting on H4 receptors suppressed the mitogen induced STAT1 phosphorylation and its interaction with DNA in peripheral blood lymphocytes from nonatopic individuals (Horr et al. 2006). A role for STAT1 in asthmatic disease has been suggested, since spontaneous phosphorylation of STAT1 is observed in asthmatic airways and not in the nonasthmatic subjects, thus providing histamine an additional mechanism for affecting the etiology/pathogenesis of asthmatic disease via both H1 and H2 receptors.

STAT gene family plays a critical role in the differentiation of helper T cell subsets. STAT-4 has a crucial role in the development of Th1, Th2 subsets balance. STAT-4 is activated by IL-12 which is a prominent cytokine in relation to the development of Th1 subset, production of IFN-γ and cell-mediated immunity. It augments Th1 cytokine production and inhibits Th2 cytokine production. The activation of STAT-4 in helper T cells causes the development of IFN-γ secreting Th1 cells and inhibits the differentiation of IL-4 secreting Th2 cells. Histamine hyper-phosphorylates STAT-4 via H1 receptors and Ca2+-PKC pathway is involved in this process (Liu et al. 2006). While H1 receptor and H2 receptor antagonists exhibit inverse agonism, when their effects are examined on the hyper-phosphorylation of STAT-1, they do not exhibit similar responses on the hyper-phosphorylation of STAT-4.

Conversely, STAT-6 is a transcription factor which is mainly activated by IL-4 and IL-13 and leads to the differentiation of Th2 cells. Histamine augments IL-4-induced phosphorylation of STAT-6 via H1 receptors (Kharmate et al. 2007). Histamine does not affect STAT-6 phosphorylation in IL-4 KO splenocytes in the presence of anti-IL-13 suggesting that the effects of histamine on STAT-6 phosphoryaltion are mediated via IL-4 secretion, which causes the hyper-phosphorylation of STAT-6. It is feasible that H1 receptors-induced secretion of IL-4 utilizing PKC-Ca2+ pathway and tyrosine kinase provides a signal to PKC to activate STAT-6, a mechanism also involved in tumor promoting genes. In another study an H4 receptor antagonist inhibited STAT6 DNA binding in peripheral blood lymphocytes from atopic individuals (Michel et al. 2008). These observations provide evidence regarding the role of H1, H2 and H4 receptors in regulating the phosphorylation of cytokine-induced transcription factors.

7.7 Regulation of Dendritic Cells by Histamine

Dendritic cells are professional antigen presenting cells and are important in the control of developing immune responses, since they regulate both the initiation and polarization of acquired immune response (Banchereau et al. 2000). The dendritic cells have monocytic (myeloid dendritic cells) or lymphoid (plasmacytoid dendritic cells) lineage; myeloid dendritic cells acquire mDC1 and mDC2 phenotypes. The mDC1 are major stimulator of T cells and the mDC2 may fight wound infection. The precursors for dendritic cells reside in bone marrow and these progenitor cells initially transform into immature dendritic cells which have a low potential for the activation of T cells. After the immature dendritic cells contact pathogens via Toll-like receptors they are activated to mature dendritic cells and migrate to lymphoid organs.

The hall mark of dendritic cells is the expression of molecules on their cell surface and the cytokines they secrete depending on their environment. They mature in response to inflammatory signals and ingress into the secondary lymphoid organs, where they stimulate naïve T cell precursors. While macrophages and B cells can only activate memory T cells, the dendritic cells could activate both the memory and Naïve T cells. The mechanisms of the development of Th1 responses to the dendritic cells as they pertain to their induction, development, maintenance, effector function and memory function are better known than for Th2 cells. Th1 cells play a role in the pathology of a number of serious debilitating diseases whereas Th2 cells are involved in protection against helminthes and the allergic disease is their unfortunate side effect (MacDonald and Maizels 2008). Nonetheless, Th2 cells counterregulate the development of Th1 responses. Dendritic cells regulate the development of both Th1 cells and Th2 cells. However, the mechanisms by which dendritic cells are involved in the development of Th2 cells are not well understood. The dendritic cells which result in the development of Th2 cells develop not only in response to infection but also to allergens (Lambrecht and Hammmad 2003). Our current understanding is that naïve Th cells are activated by dendritic cells after they bind to a ligand of the innate Toll-like receptors such as lipopolysaccharides or CpG. After these ligands bind to their receptors there is signal transduction through the adopter MyD88 which results in the recognition of MHC class II molecules on dendritic cells by the TCR (T cell receptor). A different signal causes the upregulation of costimulatory molecules CD40, CD80 and CD86. The generation of Th1 response also requires the production of IL-12 from dendritic cells. For the production of Th2 cells the dendritic cells need to express MHC class II molecules, CD40, CD80 and CD86 but the Th2-specific drivers have not been identified (MacDonald and Maizels 2008). All four histamine receptors are expressed on both immature and mature dendritic cells. Histamine modulates the function and development of dendritic cells and is involved in the normal differentiation of human dendritic cells (Szeberenyi et al. 2001). It increases the expression of costimulatory molecule CD86 and regulates chemokine secretion (Caron et al. 2001), and causes the differentiation of meyloid DCs toward the DC2 type by inhibiting IL-12 synthesis via both H1 and H2 receptors. Activation of H4 receptors by histamine causes chemoattraction in myeloid dendritic cells and activation of H4 receptors suppresses IL-12p70 secretion (Gutzmer et al. 2005). The stimulation of H4 receptors is also required for antigen-specific induction of CD+ T cells by dendritic cells (Gutzmer et al. 2005).

Histamine could act as an autocrine factor in the differentiation of dendritic cells, since during their differentiation by cytokines endogenous histamine is synthesized. Szeberenyi et al. (2001) have suggested that histamine regulates the expression of dendritic cell receptors during their differentiation. The role of histamine receptors is diverse on the dendritic cells: H1 and H3 receptors provide a positive stimulus during their development and differentiation of the dendritic cells from monocytes. This stimulus also includes augmented antigen presentation ability, production of proinflammatory cytokines and priming activity for Th1 cells. However, the effects of H2 receptors are suppressive on antigen presentation. Histamine via H2 receptors on dendritic cells increases IL-10 production and promotes the development of Th2 cells (Caron et al. 2001, Mazzoni et al. 2001). Chemokine production is also enhanced by histamine from dendritic cells. In immature dendritic cells H1 and H3 receptors are involved in histamine-mediated intracellular Ca2+ flux, actin polymerization and chemotaxis.

Histamine also helps in cross presentation of soluble allergens by dendritic cells and as a consequence activate allergen-specific $CD8^+$ T cells (Amaral et al. 2007). The etiology and pathogenesis of allergic response in the airway involves a prominent role of $CD8^+$ T cells (Gelfand and Dakhama 2006), in addition to $CD4^+$ T cells. These cells exhibit a Tc2 phenotype, secrete IL-4, IL-5 and IL-13, while

Table 7.2 Beneficial and harmful effects of dendritic cells

Effects on cell type	Protective effects	Deleterious effects
Th1 cells	Anti bacterial, antiviral and antitumor responses	Rheumatoid arthritis, Experimental allergic encephalitis, Multiple sclerosis, Experimental collagen-induced arthritis
Th2 cells	Immunity against helminthes	Allergic disease and asthma
Th17 cells	Beneficial in candida and pnemocystis carinii	Chronic inflammatory bowel disease, Psoriasis, Experimental allergic encephalitis, Collagen-induced arthritis, Experimental autoimmune uveitis, Fungal infections
Regulatory T cells	Tolerance to auto antigens Suppression of inflammatory response	Suppression of anti-tumor responses Inhibition of anti-microbial responses

Source: Schakel (2009)

expressing high affinity leukotriene B4 receptors. Consequently, the effects of histamine on dendritic cells play a crucial role in the development of both CD+ and $CD8^+$ helper T cells. Since dendritic cells play a dual role; while protecting us by inducing acquired immune responses, and harming us as they stimulate autoimmunity or inhibit immune response against cancer (Table 7.2) (Schakel 2009), their regulation by histamine receptor-specific agonists and antagonists may have clinical applications.

7.8 Histamine Receptors and Allergic Inflammation

Histamine acts as a mediator of both acute and chronic phases of allergic inflammation. The role of histamine in cellular immunity through regulation of T cells and the control of cytokine production has already been discussed. Histamine also plays a role in chemokine production and migration of inflammatory cells, which is in addition to its conventional role in immediate hyper-responsiveness. The role of histamine in mediating inflammatory responses through H1 receptors has been well understood. The anaphylactic symptoms are long known to be associated with H1 receptors resulting in the development of several generations of H1 receptor antagonists. In addition to anaphylaxis histamine also plays a role in other inflammatory states including the autoimmune disease. Histamine via H1 receptors regulates early T cell receptor signals which lead to Th1 cells differentiation and autoimmune disease. H1 receptors on $CD4^+$ cells and not on antigen presenting cells (APC) are responsible for the activation of p38 Mitogen activated Protein Kinase (MAPK) and IFN-γ production from helper T cells

(Noubade et al. 2007). The deletion of H1 receptor on helper T cells results in an increase in resistance to autoimmune encephalomyelitis (EAE). Th1 cells and IFN-γ play an important role in the development of EAE. H1 receptor is expressed on unstimulated $CD4^+$ T cells but its activation results in the down-regulation of H1 receptors. H2, H3 and H4 receptors also play a role in affecting susceptibility to EAE and influence $CD4^+$ T cells. All four subtypes of histamine receptors are present on unstimulated $CD4^+$ T cells and are down regulated in both Th1 and Th2 polarized cells. However, memory $CD4^+$ T cells selectively express H3 receptors. This suggests a regulated expression of T cells during the transition of naïve to memory T cells. The effects of histamine on allergic inflammation are mediated through its effects on proinflammatory cytokines. It induces the synthesis and secretion of IL-1α, IL-1β, IL-6 and several chemokines including IL-8 (Caron et al. 2001, Jutel et al. 2005, Triggiani et al. 2001, Vannier and Dinarello 1993). The effects of histamine on IL-8 (RANTES), monocyte chemotactic protein 1 and 3, eotaxin, increased expression of adhesion molecules including ICAM-1, VCAM-1 and P-selectin on endothelial cells are all mediated via H1 receptors. (Kubes and Kanwar 1994, Lo and Fan 1987, Yamaki et al. 1998). Histamine is a leukocyte chemoattractant, and is involved in calcium influx, actin polymerization, altering cell shape, and upregulation of adhesion molecules. It regulates cytokine production from both the mononuclear and polymorphonuclear leukocytes. NF-κB is a transcription factor responsible for the initiation of inflammatory response and H1 antagonists inhibit NF-κB expression which may suggest that some H1 antagonists may inhibit allergic inflammation (Holden et al. 2007).

7.8.1 Monocytes

Histamine inhibits IL-1, TNF-α, IL-12 and IL-18 production by human monocytes but induces IL-10 synthesis. The activation of monocyte/macrophage and the cytokine environment play a role in switching T cell responses from Th1 to Th2 cells by histamine. It inhibits the expression of intercellular adhesion molecule-1 (ICAM- 1) on monocytes when induced by IL-18. While histamine inhibits IL-18-induced IL-12, interferon-gamma, and TNF-alpha responses, it reverses inhibition of IL-10 production by IL-18. The inhibition of INF-γ by IL-18 results from the suppression of IL-12 production in response to histamine. Histamine provides its negative feedback on IL-18-activated cytokine cascade through its inhibitory effect on ICAM-1 expression and IL-12 production in monocytes (Takahashi et al. 2002). Therefore, it is evident that the effects of histamine on different subsets of immune cells are differential and often confusing.

H4 receptors are expressed on monocytes which are upregulated by IFN-γ (Dijkstra et al. 2007). They induce calcium influx in monocytes as reported in other tissues. In addition, there is inhibition of intracellular CCL2 levels by histamine via H4 receptors. CCL2 is a chemokine, which plays an important role in allergic inflammation.

7.8.2 Eosinophils

Histamine has long been known as a selective chemoattractant for eosinophils. It was believed that H1 receptors caused allergen-induced accumulation of eosinophils in a variety of tissues including nose, airways and skin. The regulation of eosinophil migration by histamine was dose dependent. High concentrations of histamine suppressed eosinophil chemotaxis which was mediated via H2 receptors and at low concentrations increased eosinophil chemotaxis which appeared to be mediated by H1 receptors. However, the true receptor which causes histamine-induced chemotaxis of eosinophils is H4 (Zampeli and Tiligada 2009). H4 receptors are expressed on eosinophils where they play a role in their selective recruitment in allergic responses. Histamine itself is not a powerful chemoattractant for eosinophils but induction of H4 receptors augments eosinophil migration toward eotaxins (Buckland et al. 2003). Furthermore, IL-5 enhances the chemoattractive activity of histamine for eosinophils (Ling et al. 2004). Histamine via H4 receptors affects eosinophil migration which augments histamine-mediated immune responses culminating in inflammation. This information and other observations led to the evidence that H4 receptors control leukocyte traffic and pro-inflammatory responses. Furthermore, cytoskeletal changes are also induced by histamine in eosinophils via H4 receptors (Buckland et al. 2003). Histamine provides a negative feedback on eosinophils where it reverses IL-5-induced human eosinophil survival by increasing apoptosis (Hasala et al. 2008). In this pathway histamine does not employ the standard intracellular second-messenger pathways including cyclic AMP, protein kinase A or phospholipase C. Instead histamine utilizes some alternate mechanisms in inducing apoptosis of human eosinophils.

7.8.3 Mast Cells

H4 receptors are constitutively expressed on human mast cells and regulate autocrine and paracrine histamine-mediated responses. It is known that H4 receptors are responsible for the redistribution and recruitment of mast cells in the mucosal epithelium when responding to an allergen which causes an augmentation of allergic symptoms and contributes to allergic inflammation. The activation of H4 receptors on murine mast cells causes chemotaxis and intracellular Ca2+ flux but does not result in their degranulation (Hofstra et al. 2003, Nakayama et al. 2004). This results in the selective recruitment of immune effector cells and the development of chronic allergic inflammation.

Histamine acts in synergy with CXCL12 to induce precursor mast cells migration. CXCL12, a constitutive chemokine, is a potent chemoattractant for both precursor and mature mast cells and plays a key role in inflammatory allergic airways The effects are specific for the migration of precursor mast cells, since histamine does not affect the CXC12-mediated migration of monocytes or $CD4^{+}$

Table 7.3 Role of H4 receptors in inflammatory diseases

Allergy
Asthma
Acute Inflammation
Chronic Puritis
Autoimmune Disease- rheumatoid Arthritis
Cancer
Colitis
Pain
Ischemia
Psoriasis?

Source: Zampeli and Tiligada (2009)

T cells. This effect of histamine is mediated via H4 receptors; whereas H1 receptors provide a negative feedback on CXCL12-induced migration of precursor mast cells. Histamine has no effect on CXCR7 expression which is a novel receptor for CXCL12 (Godot et al. 2007) H4 receptors not only play a crucial role in allergic inflammation but as shown in Table 7.3 are also involved in other disease states.

7.8.4 Suppression of Allergic Inflammation

The net effect of signaling via the histamine H2 receptor on cells of hemopoietic origin, including both Th1 and Th2 subsets, is suppression of inflammation. These effects result from the stimulation of regulatory dendritic and Th2 cells to produce IL-10, which enhances the suppressive activity of TGF-β on T cells (Morgan et al. 2007). There is also a reciprocal cross talk between histamine and cytokines/chemokines which involves H4 receptors. The expression of H4 receptors is unregulated by IFN-γ in human CD14+ monocytes and inflammatory dendritic cells. The H4 receptor –induced Ca2+ mobilization and suppression of Th2 chemokine CCL2 from monocytes, suggest a negative homeostatic mechanism to shift Th1/Th2 paradigm from a Th2 to Th1 state. This is the result of high histamine levels in allergic inflammation (Zampeli and Tiligada 2009).

7.9 Histamine and Cytokine Regulation of Immediate Hypersensitivity

The main sources of histamine for immediate hypersensitivity reactions are mast cells and basophils (Schwartz 1994). Immunoglobulin E (IgE) antibodies are generated in an allergic response to an allergen and bind to the mast cell and basophil surfaces through high-affinity F_c receptors specific for IgE. The synthesis of IgE is regulated by helper T cells and cytokines. The mechanisms related to Th1/Th2 balance are pivotal in the regulation of IgE synthesis and allergen-induced histamine release. The cytokines which play a critical role in this regulation include IL-4, IL-9,

IL-12 and IL-13, as IL-12 drives Th1 mediated responses and IL-4, IL-9 and IL-13 drive Th2 mediated responses. The transcription factors, STAT-6 and NF-κB, which require costimulatory molecule CD40 and its ligand CD154 are needed for the synthesis of IgE. Furthermore, the transcription factors GATA-3 and c-maf favor IgE synthesis. Besides isotype switching the terminal differentiation of B lymphocytes affects serum IgE levels and is regulated by IL-6. Furthermore, regulatory T cells and dendritic cells play a role in IgE synthesis and secretion, indirectly. As already discussed, histamine regulates the function of T cells and dendritic cells and the synthesis of cytokines, thus providing a negative feedback and perhaps affecting B cell function as it relates to the synthesis of IgE. According to Jutel et al. (2001) $H1R^{-/-}$ mice exhibit elevated antigen-specific serum IgE, IgG_1, IgG_{2b}, and IgG_3 levels suggesting a role for H1 receptors in regulating antibody synthesis. Bryce et al. (2006) have suggested that H1 receptors are essential for the generation of allergic lung responses. Despite the augmentation of Th2 responses to antigen in the absence of H1 receptors they are required by T cells for migration toward histamine and for recruitment to the sites of allergen challenge.

7.10 Concluding Remarks

Until a few decades ago, histamine was not considered as even a minor contributor in the regulation of immune response. When it appeared that the release of histamine could be initiated by immune-related events, investigators accepted the role of histamine as contributor to inflammation associated with the immune response. Yet, at that time little consideration was given to the possibility that histamine a mediator and modulator of inflammation could substantially affect the immune response itself.

The possibility that histamine could regulate immunity gained credence when it was discovered that lymphocytes expressed H2 receptors and their distribution was not random. The presence of histamine H1 and H2 receptors was then demonstrated on different subsets of lymphocytes followed by the discovery that histamine via these two receptors regulated the secretion of various cytokines both from immune and non-immune cells. At the same time it also became apparent that many cell types which were the target of histamine's effects and were present at the sites of the generation of immune response such as lymph nodes, thymus and sites of graft and tumor rejection, also synthesized and secreted histamine. The discovery of H4 receptors which are primarily expressed on T cells, dendritic cells, eosinophils, mast cells, neutrophils and basophlis, cell types intimately involved in the immune response, expanded our understanding of the immunomodulatory role of histamine beyond what was traditionally known. Specifically, the effects of histamine on the maturation of dendritic cells, the regulation of Th1/Th2 paradigm and chemotaxis of mono-and polymorphonuclear leukocytes guide us to the clinical applications for a variety of disease states including allergic inflammation and asthma. Nonetheless, the complexity of immune response and diversity of the effects exerted by histamine in different environment makes it very challenging to determine the total effects of histamine when simultaneously acting on all receptors and when studied in isolation. The results obtained with histamine receptor subset knockout mice have made these interpretations even more challenging. Despite all the contradictory data and confusion in the state of histamine's effects on lymphocytes immune regulation, it may not be too long before we see novel histamine receptor agonists and antagonists used as immune modulators.

References

Akdis CA, Estelle F, Simons R (2006) Histamine receptors are hot in immunopharmacology. Eur J Pharmacol 533:69–76

Akdis CA, Simons FER (2006) Histamine receptors are hot in immunopharmacology. Eur J Pharmacol 533:69–76

Amaral MM, Davio C, Ceballos A et al (2007) Histamine improves antigen uptake and cross presentation by dendritic cells. J Immunol 179:3425–3433

Banchereau J, Biere F, Caux C et al (2000) Immunobiology of dendritic cells. Annu Rev Immunol 18:767–811

Banu Y, Watanabe T (1999) Augmentation of antigen receptor- mediated responses by histamine H1 receptor signaling. J Exp Med 189:673–682

Barger G, Dale HH (1910) The presence in ergot and physiological activity of β-iminazolylethylamine. J Physiol 40:38–40

Beaven MA (1976) Histamine. N Engl J Med 294:30–36

Beisset S, Schwartz A, Schwarz T (2006) Regulatory T cells. J Inv Dermatol 126:16–24

Bluestone JA, Abbas AK (2003) Natural versus adaptive regulatory T cells. Nat Rev Immunol 3:253–257

Best CH, Dale HH, Dudley JW et al (1927) The nature of the vasodilator constituents of certain tissue extracts. J Physiol (London) 62:397–417

Bourne HR, Lichtenstein LM, Melmon KL et al (1974) Modulation of inflammation and immunity by cyclic AMP. Science 184(132):19–28

Buckland KF, Williams TJ, Conroy DM (2003) Histamine induces cytoskeletal changes in human eosinophils via the H_4 receptor. Br J Pharmacol 140:1117–1127

Bryce PJ, Mathias CB, Harrison KL et al (2006) The H1 histamine receptor regulates allergic lung responses. J Clin Inv 116:11624–1632

Caron G, Delneste Y, Roelandts E et al (2001) Histamine induces CD86 expression and chemokine production by human immature dendritic cells. J Immunol 166:6000–6006

Caron G, Delneste Y, Roelants E et al (2001a) Histamine polarizes dendritic cells into Th2 cell-promoting effector dendritic cells. J Immunol 167:3682–3686

Dale HH, Laidlaw PP (1910) The physiological action of β-imidazolylethyamine. J Physiol (London) 41:318–344

Dale HH, Laidlaw PP (1911) Further observations on the action of β-imidazolylethyamine. J Physiol (London) 43:182–195

Dijkstra D, Leurs R, Chazot P et al (2007) Histamine downregulates monocyte CCL2 production through the histamine H4 receptor. J Allergy Clin Immunol 120:300–307

Dunford PJ, O'Donnell NO, Riley JP et al (2006) The histamine H4 receptor mediates allergic airway inflammation by regulating the activation of $CD4^+$ T cells. J Immunol 176:7062–7070

Elenkov IJ, Webster E, Papanicolaou DA et al (1998) Histamine potentially suppress human IL-12 and stimulates IL-10 production via H2 receptors. J Immunol 161:2586–2593

Elliott K, Osna N, Khan MM (2001) Regulation of IL-13 production by histamine in cloned murine T helper type 2 cells. Int Immunopharmacol 1:1923–37

Forward NA, Furlong SJ, Yang Y et al (2009) Mast cells down-regulate $CD4^+CD25+$ T regulatory suppressor function via histamine H1 receptor interaction. J Immunol 183:3014–3022

Galli SJ (1993) New concepts about the mast cell. N Engl J Med 328:257–265

Gantner F, Sakai K, Tusche MW et al (2002) Histamine H4 and H2 receptor control histamine-induced interleukin -16 release from human from human $CD8^+$ T cells. J Pharmacol Exp Ther 303:300–307

Garovoy MR, Reddish MA, Rocklin RE (1983) Histamine induced suppressor factor (HSF): inhibition of helper T cells generation and function. J Immunol 130:357–361

Gelfand EW, Dakhama A (2006) $CD8^+$ T lymphocytes and leukotriene B4: novel interactions in the persistence and progression of asthma. J Allergy Clin Immunol 117:577–582

Godot V, Arock M, Garcia G et al (2007) H4 histamine receptor mediates optimal migration of mast cell precursors to CXCL12. J allergy Clin Immunol 120:927–931

Gutzmer R, Mommert S, Gschwandtner M et al (2009) The histamine H4 receptor in functionally expressed on Th2 cells. J Allergy Clin Immunol 123:619–625

Gutzmer R, Diestel C, Mommert S et al (2005) Histamine H4 receptor stimulation suppresses IL-12p70 production and mediates chemotaxis in human monocyte-derived dendritic cells. J Immunol 174:5224–5232

Hasala H, Giembycz M A, Janka-Junttila M et al (2008) Histamine reverses IL-5-afforded human eosinophil survival by inducing apoptosis: pharmacological evidence for a novel mechanism of action of histamine. Pulm Pharmacol Ther 21:222–233

Hill S J, Ganellin C R, Timmerman H et al (1997) International classification of pharmacology XIII. Classification of histamine receptors. Pharmacol Rev 49:253–278

Hofstra CL, Desai PJ, Thurmond RL et al (2003) Histamine H4 receptor mediates chemotaxis and calcium mobilization of mast cells. J Pharm Exp Ther 305:1212–1221

Holden NS, Gong W, King EM et al (2007) Potentiation of NF-κB dependent transcription and inflammatory mediator release by histamine in human airway epithelial cells. Br J Pharmacol 152:891–902

Horr B, Borck H, Thurmond RL et al (2006) STAT1 phosphorylation and cleavage is regulated by the histamine H4 receptor in human atopic and nonatopic individuals. Int Immunopharmacol 6:1577–11585

Jutel M, Akdis CA (2007) Histamine as an immune modulator in chronic inflammatory responses. Clin Exp Allergy 37:308–310

Jutel M, Blaser K, Akdis CA (2005) Histamine in allergic inflammation and immune modulation. Int Arch Allergy Immunol 137:82–92

Jutel M, Watanabe T, Akdis M, et al (2002) Immune regulation by histamine. Curr Opin Immunol 14:735–740

Jutel M, Watanabe T, Klunker S et al (2001) Histamine regulates T-cells and antibody responses by differential expression of H1 and H2 receptors. Nature 413:420–425

Katoh N, Soga F, Nara T et al (2005) Histamine induces the generation of monocyte derived dendritic cells that express CD14 but not CD1a. J Inv Derm 125:753–760

Khan MM, Sansoni P, Engleman et al (1985b) Pharmacologic effects of autacoids on subsets of T cells: regulation of expression/function of histamine-2 receptors by a subset of suppressor cells. J Clin Inv 75:1578–1583

Khan MM, Melmon KL, Fathman CG et al (1985a) The effects of autacoids on cloned murine lymphoid cells: modulation of IL-2 secretion and the activity of natural suppressor cells. J Immun 134:4100–4106

Khan MM, Wilson AL, Melmon KL (1987) Characterization of histamine type I (H_1) receptors on natural supressor lymphoid cells. Biochem Pharm 36:3867–3871

Khan MM, Keaney KM, Melmon KL et al (1989) Histamine modulates the activity of antigen specific cytolytic T-cell by impairing the effector target recognition. Cellular Immunol 52: 147–159

Kharmate G, Liu Z, Patterson E et al (2007) Histamine affects STAT6 phosphorylation via its effects on IL-secretion: role of H1 receptors in the regulation of Il-4 production. Int Immunopharmacol 7:277–286

Kohda F, Koga T, Uchi H et al (2002) Histamine-induced IL-6 and IL-8 production are differentially modulated by IFN-γ and IL-4 in human keratinocytes. J Dermatological Sci 28:34–41

Kohka H, Nishibori M, Iwagaki H (2000) Histamine is a potent inducer of IL-18 and IFN-γ in human peripheral blood mononuclear cells. J Immunol 164:6640–6646

Kubes P, Kanwar S (1994) Histamine induces leukocyte rolling in post-capillary venules. A P-selectin-mediated event. J Immunol 152:3570–3577

Lambrecht BN, Hammmad H (2003) Taking our nreath away: dendritic cells in the pathogenesis of asthma. Nat Rev Immunol 3:994–1003

Leite-de-Moraes MC, Diem S, Michel M-L et al (2009) Histamine receptor H4 activation positively regulates in vivo IL-4 and IFN-γ production by invariant NKT cells. J Immunol 182:1233–1236

Leurs R, Church MK, Taglialatela M (2002) H1-antihistamines: inverse agonism, anti-inflammatory actions and cardiac effects. Clin Exp Allergy 32:489–498

Lichtenstein LM (1976) The interdependence of allergic and inflammatory process. In: Johansson SGO, Strandberg K, Uvnas B (eds) Molecular and Biological aspects of the acute allergic reaction, Plenum Press, NY, pp 233–254

Ling P, Ngo K, Nguyen S et al (2004) Histamine H4 receptor mediates eosinophil chemotaxis with cell shape change and adhesion molecule upregulation. Br J Pharmacol 142:161–171

Liu Z, Kharmate G, Patterson E et al (2006) Histamine regulates phosphorylation of STAT-4 via H1 receptors. Int Immunopharmacol 6:485–493

Lo WW, Fan TP (1987) Histamine stimulates inositol phosphate accumulation via the H1 receptors in cultured human endothelial cells. Biochem Biophys Res Commun 148:47–53

Lohr J, Knowchel B, Abbas AK (2006) Regulatory T cells in periphery. Immunol Rev 212:149–162

MacDonald AS, Maizels RM (2008) Alarming dendritic cells for Th2 induction. J Exp Med 205:13–17

Marone G, Granata F, Spadaro G et al (2003) The histamine-cytokine network in allergic inflammation. J Allergy Clin Immunol 112:S83-S88

Mazzoni A, Young HA, Spitzer JH et al (2001) Histamine regulates cytokine production in maturing dendritic cells, resulting in altered T cell polarization. J Clin Inv 108:1865–1873

Melmon KL, Khan MM (1987) Histamine as immune modulator. Trends Pharm Sci 8:437–441

Melmon KL, Bourne HR, Weinstein J et al (1972) Receptors for histamine can be detected on the surface of selected leukocytes. Science 177:707–709

Melmon KL, Rocklin RE, Rosenkranz RP (1981) Autacoids as modulators of inflammatory and immune response. Am J Med 71:100–106

Melmon KL, Weinstein Y, Shearer GM et al (1974) Separation of specific antibody-forming mouse cells by their adherence to insolubilized endogenous hormones. J Clin Inv 53:22–30

Michel I, Borck H, McElligott et al (2008) Histamine receptor H4 selective ligands influence the STAT6 transcription activation domain (TAD) and the DNA binding. Inflamm Res 57: S47-S48

Morgan RK, McAllister B, Cross L et al (2007) Histamine 4 receptors activation induces recruitment of FoxP3+ T cells and inhibit allergic asthma in a murine model. J Immunol 178: 8081–8089

Mosmann TR, Cherwinski H, Bomd MW et al (1986) Two types of murine helper T cell clones. I. Definition according to profiles of lymphokine activities and secreted proteins. J Immunol 136: 2348–2357

Nakayama T, Kato Y, Hieshiema K et al (2004) Liver expressed chemokine/cc chemokine ligand 16 attracts eosinophils by interacting with histamine H4 receptors. J Immunol 173:2073–2083

Noubade R, Rincon M, Teuscher C (2007) IFN-gamma production by CD4 T cells requires histamine H1 receptor during their initial phase of activation. J Immunol 178:87.25

Osband ME, Cohen EB, Miller BR et al (1981) Biochemical analysis of specific histamine H1 and H2 receptors on lymphocytes. Blood 58:87–90

Osna N, Elliott K, Khan MM (2001a) Protein Kinase A is involved in histamine-mediated inhibition of IFNγ depending on the stimulatory signal. Immunopharmacol 1:125–145

Osna N, Elliott K, Khan MM (2001b) Regulation of interleukin-10 secretion by histamine in Th2 cells and splenocytes. Int Immunopharmacol 1:85–86

Osna N, Elliott K, Lewis R et al (2001c) Histamine utilizes JAK-STAT pathway in regulating cytokine production. Int Immunopharmcol 1:759–762

Pepys J (1955) Fixation of tuberculin in skin in skin of tuberculin sensitive human subjects. Clin Sci 14:253–265

Poluektova LY, Khan MM (1998) PKA inhibitors reverse histamine-mediated regulation of IL-5 secretion. Immunopharmacology 39:9–19

Packard KA, Khan MM (2003) Effects of histamine on Thl/Th2 cytokine balance. Int Immunopharmacol 3:909–920

Parsons M, Ganellin CR (2006) Histamine and its receptors. Br J Pharmacol 147:S127–S135

Rocklin RE (1976) Mondulation of cellular-immune responses in vivo and in vitro by histamine receptor bearing lymphocytes. J Clin Inv 56:1051–1058

Rocklin RE, Beer DJ (1983) Histamine and immune modulation. Adv Intern Med 28:225–235

Rocklin RE, Habarek-Davidson A (1984) Pharmacol modulation in vitro of human histamine-induced suppressor cell activity. Int J Immunopharmacol 6:179–186

Rocklin RE, Greineder DK, Melmon KL (1979) Histamine induced suppressor factor (HSF): further studies on the nature of the stimulus and the cell which produces it. Cell Immunol 44: 404–415

Romagnani S (1992) Human Thl and Th2 subsets: regulation of differentiation and role in protection and immunopathology. Int Arch Allergy Immunol 98:279–285

Roszkowski KM, Plaut M, Lichtenstein LM (1977) Selective display of histamine receptors on lymphocytes. Science 195:683–685

Sakhalkar S, Patterson E, Khan MM (2005) Inverse agonism exhibited by histamine H1 and H2 receptor antagonists in histamine-induced STAT-1 phosphorylation. Int Immunopharmacol 5:1200–1209

Schakel K (2009) Dendritic cells – why can they help and hurt us. Exp Dermatol 18:264–273

Shearer GM, Weinstein Y, Melmon KL (1974) Enhancement of immune response potential of mouse lymphoid cells fractionated over insolubilized conjugated histamine columns. J Immunol 113:597–607

Schneider E, Rolli-Derkinderen M, Arock M et al (2002) Trends in histamine reaserch: new functions during immune responses and hematopoiesis. Trends Immunol 23:255–263

Schwartz JC, Arrang JM (2002) Histamine. In: Davis KL, Charney D, Coyle JT et al (eds) Neuropsychopharmacology: the fifth generation of progress. Lippincott Williams and Wilkins, Philadelphia, pp 179–190

Schwartz LB (1994) Mast cells: function and contents. Curr Opin Immunol 6:91–97

Simons FE (2003) H_1-antihistamines: more relevant than ever in the treatment of allergic disorders. J Allergy Clin Immunol 112:S42–S52

Simons FE, Simons KJ (1994) The pharmacology and use of H_1-receptor-antagonist drugs. N Engl J Med 330:1663–1670

Simons SER (2003b) Antihistamines. In: Adkinson J, Franklin N, Younginger JW et al (eds) Middelton's allergy: principles and practice, 6th edn. Mosby, Philadelphia, PA, pp 834–869

Simons FE (2002) Comparative pharmacology of H1 antihistamines: clinical relevance. Am J Med 113:38s-46s

Szeberenyi JB, Pallinger E, Zsinko M et al (2001) Inhibition of the effects of endogenously synthesized histamine disturbs in vitro human dendritic cell differentiation. Immunol Lett 76: 175–182

Takahashi HK, Yoshida A, Iwagaki H et al (2002) Histamine regulation of interleukin-18-initiating cytokine cascade is associated with down-regulation of intercellular adhesion molecule-1 expression in human peripheral blood mononuclear cells. J Pharmacol Exp Ther 300: 227–235

Takahashi HK, Iwagaki H, Mori S et al (2004) Histamine inhibits lipopolysaccharides-induced interleukin (IL)-18 production in human monocytes. Clin Immunol 112:30–34

Thurmond RL, Gelfand EW, Dunford PJ (2008) The role of histamine H1 and H4 receptors in allergic inflammation. Nat Rev 7:41–53
Triggiani M, Gentile M, Secondo A et al (2001) Histamine induces exocytosis and IL-6 production from human lung macrophages through interaction with H_1 receptors. J Immunol 166: 4083–4091
Van der Pouw Kraan TC, Snijiders A, Boeije LC et al (1998) Histamine inhibits the production of interleukin -12 through interaction via H2 receptors. J Clin Inv 102:1866–1873
Vannier E, Dinarello CA (1993) Histamine enhances interleukin-1-induced IL-1 gene expression and protein synthesis via H2 receptors in peripheral blood mononuclear cells. Comparison with Il-1 receptor antagonists. J Clin Inv 92:281–287
Weaver CT, Harrington LE, Mangan PR et al (2006) Th17, an effector CDT cell lineage with regulatory T cell ties. Immunity 24:677–688
Yamaki K, Thorlacius II, Xie X et al (1998) Characteristics of histamine-induced leukocyte rolling in the undisturbed microcirculation of the rat mesentry. Br J Pharmacol 123:390–399
Zampeli E, Tiligada E (2009) The role of histamine H4 receptors in immune and inflammatory disorders. Br J Pharmacol 157:24–33

Chapter 8
Histamine Aspects in Acid Peptic Diseases and Cell Proliferation

Jameel Ahmad, Monika Misra, Waseem Rizvi, and Anil Kumar

Abstract Histamine is a naturally occurring imidazole derivative. In human, histamine is present in nearly all tissues of the body. Four different histamine receptors subtypes have been cloned and designated as H1 to H4 receptors. H1 and H2 receptors have wide distribution in comparison to H3 and H4 receptors. H1 antihistamines (H1 receptor blockers) are among the most widely used drugs. H2 receptor activation is a strong stimulant for gastric acid secretion. Hence, histamine H2 receptors (H2R) antagonist has been used for the treatment of peptic ulcer and other gastric hypersecretory states such as Zollinger-Ellison syndrome. The H3 receptors have also been cloned and their receptor ligands are in early clinical phase trials for obesity and other disorders like memory, learning deficit and epilepsy. The most recently discovered H4 receptor antagonists are being investigated for their use in inflammatory conditions such as asthma and rheumatoid diseases. Histamine is also involved in other functions, such as the cell proliferation and differentiation. Therefore its role is also defined in embryogenesis, organogenesis and tumorigenesis. In this chapter, we review H2 receptor antagonist, their present status in acid-peptic diseases and the emerging role of histamine in cell proliferation and differentiation with special reference to tumorigenesis.

Keywords Histamine · Acid-peptic Disease · Cell proliferation · Tumorigenesis

Abbreviations

AML	acute myeloid leukemia
ASO	antisense oligonucleotides
CCK	cholecystokinin
CSF	cerebrospinal fluid
CNS	central nervous system

J. Ahmad (✉)
Department of pharmacology, Jawaharlal Nehru Medical College and Hospital, Aligarh Muslim University, Aligarh 202002, UP, India
e-mail: ahmad.drjameel@gmail.com

M. Shahid et al. (eds.), *Biomedical Aspects of Histamine*,
DOI 10.1007/978-90-481-9349-3_8,

DAG diacylglycerole
DAO diamine oxidase
HDC histidine decarboxylase
H1R histamine H1 receptor
H2R histamine H2 receptor
H3R histamine H3 receptor
H4R histamine H4 receptor
HMT histamine *N*-methyl transferase
IL-2 inteleukin-2
MAO-B mono amine oxidase-B
PLP pyridoxal 5-phosphate
SERM selective estrogen receptor modulator
STAT5 signal transducer and activator of transcription

Contents

8.1 Introduction

Histamine was first time isolated from mammalian liver and lung by Best et al. (1927). It was so named histamine after the Greek word for tissue, *histos*. It is now well established that histamine plays a key role in gastric acid secretion and type 1 hypersensitivity reaction. Histamine is stored in mast cells, basophils and also in neurons (Haas et al. 2008, Parsons and Ganellin 2006, Schwartz and Haas 1992). The concentration of histamine is directly proportional to numbers of mast cells. The skin, gastric and intestinal mucosa, mucosa of bronchial tree, liver and placenta are rich in histamine. Non-mast cell histamine containing tissues are brain and gastric mucosa. Almost all tissues of human body contain histamine ranging from less than 1 μg/g to more than 100 μg/g. In mast cells and basophils, the concentration of histamine approximated is 0.1–0.2 pmol/cell and 0.01 pmol/cell, respectively (Rang et al. 2007, Skidgel and Erdos 2006). Human cerebrospinal fluid (CSF) also contains histamine (Khandewal et al. 1982). In brain it serves as neurotransmitter. Histamine exerts its effect through four receptors designated as histamine receptor H1 (H1R), H2R, H3R, and H4R, according to the chronological order of their discovery (Hill et al. 1997, Parsons and Ganellin 2006, Shahid et al. 2009). These all receptors belong to 7-transmembrane G protein-coupled receptor family. Histaminergic system is one of most productive area of clinical pharmacology. H1 antihistamines (e.g., cetirizine) and H2 blockers (e.g., ranitidine) are frequently used drugs for the treatment of allergic conditions and acid peptic diseases, respectively and have reached blockbuster status (Chazot 2009, Kaufman et al. 2002). Recently, role of histamine has been addressed in cell proliferation and differentiation (Davenas et al. 2008, Schneider et al. 2002, Tutton 2007). The tumorigenesis (Haak-Frendscho et al. 2000, Rivera et al. 2000) and hematopoiesis (Liu et al. 2001, Schneider et al. 2002) are newly described functions of histamine.

In this chapter, we initially describe the different histamine receptors with emphasis on H2 receptor antagonists in acid peptic diseases and later part of this chapter has been focused on the effects of histamine in cell proliferation and differentiation. We have also discussed the therapeutic potential of histamine, its agonists and antagonists in different tumor conditions.

8.2 Biosynthesis and Metabolism of Histamine

Histamine is synthesized from histidine by the action of enzyme histidine decarboxylase (E.C.4.1.1.22). Histidine decarboxylase (HDC) is a pyridoxal 5-phosphate (PLP)-dependent homodimeric enzyme which catalyzes the decarboxylation of histidine to histamine (Wu et al. 2008). HDC is a rate limiting enzyme which itself undergoes post-translational processing for histamine synthesis. Histamine synthesis is regulated by the post-translational processing of histidine decarboxylase (Furuta et al. 2007, Tanaka 2003). The enzyme histidine decarboxylase is expressed only in histamine releasing cells. It is present in mast cells, neurons of posterior hypothalamus and enterochromaffin-like cells, basophils and macrophages etc. (Medina et al. 2003, 2005, Watanabe and Ohtsu 2002). L histidine is also partly decarboxylated to histamine by the enzyme L-amino acid decarboxylase. Only a small amount of released histamine is excreted unchanged (2–3%) in urine and the metabolism of remaining histamine (more than 97%) occurs through two major pathways. It is inactivated by two major enzymes: histamine *N*-methyltransferase (HMT, EC 2.1.1.8) via methylation (brain and periphery) and diamine oxidase (DAO, EC 1.4.3.6) via oxidative deamination (peripheral tissues only). *N*-methytransferase (E.C. 2.1.1.8) is ubiquitously found whereas diamine oxidase (E.C. 1.4.3.6) is mainly located in the periphery. Histamine *N*-methyltransferase catalyzes the conversion of histamine to *N*-methyl histamine (Katzung 2007). *N*-methyl histamine so formed is acted upon by monoaminase oxidase (MAO) to form *N*-methyl imidazole acetic acid. In the other pathway, histamine undergoes oxidative deamination by diamine oxidase (also known as histaminase) to form imidazole acetic acid (Fig. 8.1).

HDC can be targeted for certain pathological conditions where histamine production is the cause of disease and may be future strategy for new drug development (Moya-Garcia et al. 2005). The characterization of HDC is difficult at present due to its instability and also because of its post-translation maturation to attain active form in mammals (Moya-Gracia et al. 2009). Certain substances have been found to inhibit HDC; these are alpha-fluromethylhistidine and histidine methyl ester (DeGraw et al. 1977, Moya-Gracia et al. 2009). Alpha-fluromethylhistidine and histidine methyl ester are the substrates analogues of HDC and they react with PLP.

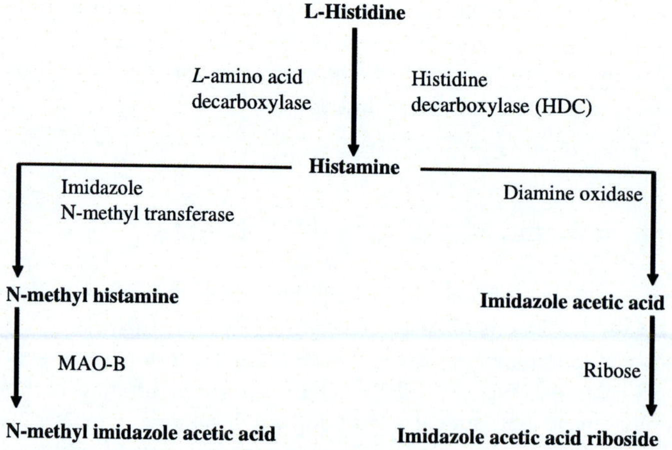

Fig. 8.1 Biosynthesis and metabolism of histamine

8.3 Histamine Release by Different Agents

Histamine as preformed mediator is stored in mast cells. The storage of histamine in mast cells was established by Riley and West (1952). It is released from mast cells by exocytosis during inflammatory or allergic reactions. Initial studies were done on histamine release by using compound 48/80 (Feldberg and Mongar 1954). Replenishment of the histamine after secretion from mast cell or basophil is a slow process and may take days or weeks. However, turnover of histamine is fast in non-mast cell because of its continuous release. Release of histamine becomes of clinical importance for those who develop anaphylactic reaction by certain drugs. It can be released by any of the following mechanisms.

8.3.1 Immunologic Release

In immunological process, the interaction of antigen to IgE antibodies present on mast cell surface can cause histamine release. This release is a mediator of immediate type of hypersensitivity reaction and allergic responses.

8.3.2 Chemical and Mechanical Release

In chemical or mechanical injury of mast cell histamine can be released by degranulation of mast cells. Certain drugs can stimulate histamine release without prior sensitization. Some basic drugs e.g. Morphine, D-tubocurarine can release histamine by non receptor action (Rang et al. 2007). Pentamidine, trimethaphan, succinylcholine, dextran, hydralazine, bile salts, detergents, radiocontrast media and compound 48/80 etc. are other agents which can cause histamine release. The venoms of wasp may contain potent histamine-releasing peptides (Johnson and Erdos 1973). Histamine release may be responsible for vancomycin-induced red-man syndrome and hypotension (Levy et al. 1987). Histamine liberators do not deplete tissues of non-mast cell histamine. There are also agents which cause inhibition of histamine release like $beta_2$ agonists, e.g., adrenaline, ephedrine, isoproterenol and mast cell membrane stabilizers e.g., ketotifen, pizotifen, disodium cromoglycate.

8.4 Histamine Receptors

Histamine mediates it physiological effects through four receptors which are G protein coupled receptors (Hough 2001, Leurs et al. 2001, Thurmond et al. 2008) meaning that these receptors signal through coupling with and activating specific G-proteins. Histamine has multiple and variable effects. The diversity in physiological action of histamine may be due to differential expression and regulation of H1 to H4 receptors and their distinct intracellular signals (Akdis 2008, Akdis and Simons

2006). Histamine receptors are designated H1 by Ash and Schild (1966) (based on the pharmacological effects of known pharmacological ligands); H2 by Black et al. (1972), H3 by Arrang et al. (1987) and H4 receptors by Hough (2001).

8.4.1 Histamine H1 Receptors

H1 histamine receptors couple to Gq/11 and lead phospholipase C activation. This causes the production of ionositol-1, 4, 5-triphosphate (IP3) and diacylglycerol (DAG) from cell membrane phospholipids. These increase intracellular calcium, activating Ca^{++}/calmodulin-dependant protein kinase and phospholipase A2. In 1940s, H1 receptor antagonists (H1 antihistamines) were developed. These agents have been widely used for allergic and other conditions. However, H1 antihistaminic like terfenadine and astemizole were found to be associated with cardiac side effects and no longer used (Estelle and Simons 2004). With increasing molecular knowledge of histamine, the new antihistamines with good efficacy and safety are being synthesized. The further discussion of H1 antihistaminic agents is beyond the scope of this chapter.

8.4.2 Histamine H2 Receptors

The most prominent effect of H2 receptors is the stimulation of gastric acid secretion apart from positive inotropic and chronotropic effects on heart. Histamine stimulates the parietal cell directly by binding to H2 receptors coupled to activation of adenylate cyclase and generation of adenosine 3′, 5′-cyclic monophosphate (cAMP) (Hill et al. 1997, Soll and Walsh 1979). However, recent studies with the cloned receptor have shown that they can also activate the phosphoinositide signaling cascade through G protein independent mechanisms (Valle and Gantz 1997). In addition to the above effects, the H2 receptors are also involved in the regulation of gastrointestinal motility, intestinal secretion, regulation of cell growth and differentiation (Valle and Gantz 1997). In late 1970s and 1980s, H2 receptor antagonists revolutionized the treatment of acid peptic disease and other gastric hypersecretory states such as Zollinger-Ellison syndrome caused by gastrinoma, a gastrin producing tumor (Hung et al. 2003, Jensen et al. 2006). These receptors have been discussed in this chapter in details.

8.4.3 Histamine H3 Receptors

H3 receptors were described as presynaptic autoreceptors. H3 receptors couple to $G_{i/o}$ to inhibit adenylyl cyclase (Hough 2001, Leurs et al. 2001). They mediate synthesis of histamine and inhibition of histamine release from histaminergic neurons in the rat brain (Arrang et al. 1987). The activation of H3 autoreceptors can inhibit histamine synthesis and also release while H3 receptor blockers can enhance the release of neurotransmitter (Fox et al. 2005, Medthurst et al. 2007,

2009). Histaminergic dysregulation has been found in different CNS disorders. Hence, H3 ligands are being investigated for their clinical utility particularly in CNS disorder. H3 receptor agonists developed so far are N^{α}-methylhistamine, (*R*)-α-methylhistamine and imetit (Leurs et al. 2009, Lovenberg et al. 1999). Nonimidazole H3R inverse agonists e.g. tiprolisant, ABT-239 and GSK189254 etc. have also been developed for certain disorders (Sander et al. 2008). Many H3 receptor ligands are in early phase clinical trials for obesity, memory disorder, learning deficit and epilepsy (Parsons and Ganellin 2006).

8.4.4 Histamine H4 Receptors

H4 receptors are expressed in bone marrow, spleen, peripheral blood, small intestine, heart, colon, lung etc. In hematopoietic cells, they are present in neutrophils, mast cells, eosinophils, basophils, monocytes, T cells and dendritic cells (Leurs et al. 2009). H4 receptor reveals about 40% homology with H3 receptor (Katzung 2007, Oda and Matsumoto 2001, Oda et al. 2000). However, the homology of H4R to the H1R and H2R is approximately 19%. This may be the reason for delay in the identification of H4R (Sander et al. 2008). Similar to H3, H4 receptors are also coupled to $G_{i/o}$ and inhibit adenylyl cyclase (Hough 2001, Leurs et al. 2001). The development of the H4R antagonist JNJ-7777120 for asthma and allergic rhinitis has opened the door for targeting H4R. Many H4 receptor antagonists are in clinical phase trials for inflammatory conditions such as asthma and rheumatoid disease (Engelhardt et al. 2009, Jablonowski et al. 2003, Parsons and Ganellin 2006, Tiligada et al. 2009). Some antihistamines previously considered as antagonists may have action of inverse agonists. Clobenpropit which have agonistic action at H4 receptors is also an antagonist or inverse agonist at H3 receptors (Estelle and Simons 2004, Katzung 2007, Parsons and Ganellin 2006, Skidgel and Erdos 2006).

As far as gene cloning of these receptors is concerned, the gene for H1 and H2 were cloned in 1991 (Gantz et al. 1991, Yamashita et al. 1991). The gene for H3 was cloned by J and J researchers team led by Lovenberg et al. 1999 and different research groups led to the identification of H4 gene in 1999/2000 (Leurs et al. 2009). Table 8.1 shows histamine receptor subtypes, distribution, ligands, receptor coupling mechanism and their functions (Shahid et al. 2009, Simons 2004).

The cellular expressions of histamine receptor can predict the response of cell to histamine. However the interpretation of the overall response of a tissue is not easy task.

8.5 Physiology of Gastric Acid

Activation of proton pump (H^+K^+ATPase) causes the gastric acid (HCl) secretions. The secretion of gastric acid is regulated by many factors. At the parietal cell level these factors are paracrine (histamine), endocrine (gastrin) and neurocrine (acetylcholine).

Table 8.1 Characteristics of histamine receptors

Characteristic	H1 receptor	H2 receptor	H3 receptor	H4 receptor
Receptor described, human gene cloned (year)	1966, 1991	1972, 1991	1983, 1999	1994, 2000/2001
Chromosomal location in humans	3p25, 3p14–21	5q35.3	20q13.33	18q11.2
Receptor expression	Widespread including neurons, smooth muscle, endothelium	Widespread including gastric mucosal parietal cells, smooth muscles, heart , neurons	High expression in histaminergic neurons , presynaptic location	High expression in bone marrow and peripheral hematopoietic cells
G receptor coupling	Gαq11: ↑IP3, DAG, ↑intracellular calcium, calcium calmoudlin e NOS, Protein kinase C, phospholipase A2 , cGMP,	Gαs: ↑cyclic AMP, Ca2+, protein kinase C, c-fos, phos-pholipase C	Gi/o: ↓ cyclic AMP	Gi/o: ↓cyclic AMP, Mitogen activated protein kinase
Representative agonist	2CH3-histamine	Dimaprit	(r)- α CH3 histamine	Clobenprit
Representative inverse agonist	Chlorphenramine	Ranitidine	Thioperamide, clobenprit	JNJ7777120, Thioperamide
Function	Mediates allergic response,↑ pruritis, pain, vasodilation, vascular permeability, hypotension; flushing, bronchoconstriction, stimulation of airway vagal afferents and cough receptors; stimulation of emesis, cycle of sleep-wake, decreased atrioventricular-node conduction time.	Increased gastric acid secretion, ↑ vascular permeability, hypotension, ↑chronotropic and ionotropic activity, bronchodilatation, mucus production (airway).	Presynaptic autoreceptor and hetroreceptor: decreased histamine, dopamine, serotonin, noradrenaline, acetylcholine, Prevents excessive bronchoconstriction; mediates pruritus (no mast-cell involvement).	Differentiation of myeloblasts and promyelocytes

8.5.1 Gastric acid Secretion

In the process of hydrochloric acid formation, chloride ions are transported from parietal cell cytoplasm into lumen of canaliculus and sodium ions are transported out of canaliculus into the parietal cell cytoplasm. This results in negative potential of –40 to –70 millivolts in the canaliculus. Due to this, the potassium ion (K^+) and small number of sodium (Na^+) ion from cell cytoplasm diffuse into the canaliculus. The water present in the parietal cell gets dissociated into H^+ and OH^- (hydroxyl ion). The H^+ are actively secreted into the canaliculus in exchange for K^+ (potassium ion). This H^+K^+ exchange is catalyzed by an enzyme known as H^+K^+ATPase or proton pump (Guyton and Hall 2006). Activation of proton pump causes gastric acid secretion (Fig. 8.2) and the secretion of gastric acid can be inhibited by class of drugs known as proton pump inhibitors.

8.5.2 Regulation of Gastric Acid Secretion

Gastric acid secretion at the level of the parietal cell is regulated by paracrine, endocrine and neurocrine factors (Guyton and Hall 2006). Stimuli for the activation of gastric acid can originate in brain or in stomach. According to Single-cell hypothesis all three secretagogues viz acetylcholine, histamine and gastrin act directly on the parietal cell and in Two-cell hypothesis the gastrin and acetylcholine act either

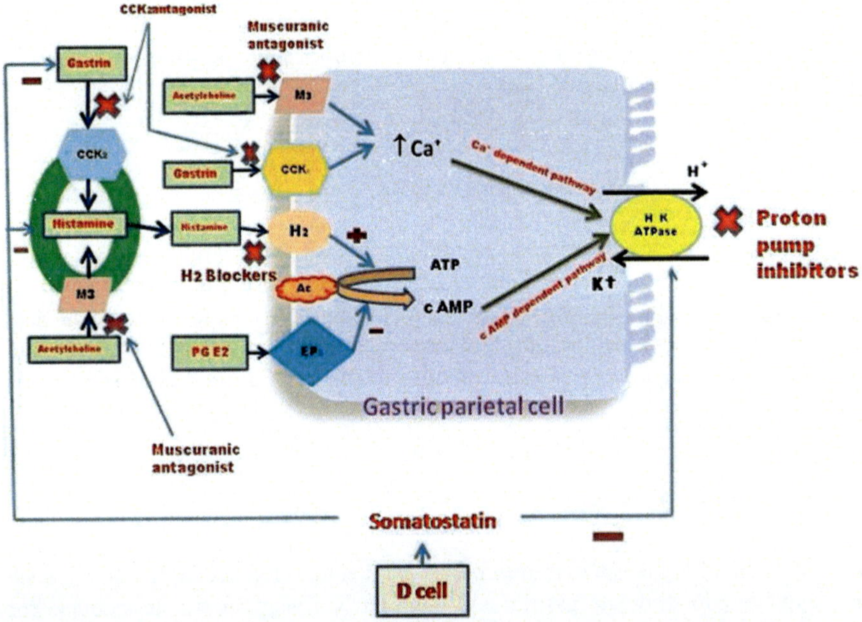

Fig. 8.2 Mechanism of histamine in gastric acid secretion

only by releasing histamine, or partly by releasing histamine and partly by direct action on their respective receptors on the parietal cell (Black and Shankley 1987, Rang et al. 2007, Soll and Berglindh 1987).

Stomach mucosa contains two important types of tubular glands. These are oxyntic glands (gastric glands or acid-forming glands), the hallmark of which is parietal cells and pyloric glands, the hallmark of which is the gastrin or G cell (Ganong 2005). The oxyntic glands secretions include hydrochloric acid, pepsinogen, intrinsic factor and mucus while pyloric glands secrete are mucus, hormone gastrin, and also small amount of pepsinogen.

8.5.2.1 Paracrine: Histamine

Histamine released from ECL (enterochromaffin-like) cells acts as a paracrine mediator. It diffuses from its site of release to nearby parietal cells to cause the activation of H2 receptors.

8.5.2.2 Endocrine: Gastrin

Gastrin, a peptide hormone is synthesized in endocrine cells of the mucosa of the gastric antrum and duodenum and causes stimulation of the secretion of acid by the parietal cells. For gastrin secretion, the important stimuli are amino acids and small peptides, which act directly on the gastrin-secreting cells.

8.5.2.3 Neuronal: Acetylcholine

Acetylcholine released from postganglionic enteric neurons stimulates specific muscarinic receptors of parietal cells.

8.6 Phases of Gastric Acid Secretion

Acid secretion occurs under basal condition, follows the cicardian pattern (highest levels occurring during the night and lowest levels during the morning hours). Cholinergic input via the vagus nerve and histaminergic input from local gastric sources are major factors to basal acid secretion. Stimulation of gastric acid secretion occurs in three phases depending on the sites from where signals are originating.

8.6.1 Cephalic Phase

It occurs when food is eaten or even before food enters stomach. Sight, smell, taste and appetite can stimulate gastric acid secretion via vagus nerve. It accounts for 20% of gastric secretion. Acetylcholine can also increase the release of histamine from the ECL cells in the fundus of the stomach and that of gastrin from G cells in the gastric antrum. So it is an indirect effect of Ach on parietal cells to release histamine.

8.6.2 Gastric Phase

This phase of secretion accounts for 70% of gastric acid secretion. The gastric phase is activated once food enters the stomach. The nutrients like amino acids and amines directly stimulate the G cell to release gastrin which in turn activates the parietal cell via direct and indirect mechanisms. Distension of the stomach wall also gives rise to gastrin release and acid production.

8.6.3 Intestinal Phase

Intestinal and also the last phase of gastric acid secretion is initiated due to presence of food in the upper portion of the small intestine. The duodenal mucosa also release small amount of gastrin. Somatostatin, the gastrointestinal hormone is released from D cells of gastric mucosa in response to HCl. It inhibit acid production by both direct (parietal cell) and can also by indirect mechanisms i.e. decreased histamine release from enterochromaffin-like cells and gastrin release from G cells. There are four important cells, G cells (for gastrin secretion), D (for somatostatin secretion), enterochromaffin-like (ECL) cells and parietal cells. G and ECL cell products stimulate acid secretion (positive feedback) while D cells inhibit acid release through negative feedback (Joseph et al. 2003). However among the different stimuli, the histamine is the powerful stimulant of gastric acid secretion and is also considered as an essential for gastric acid secretion (Moessner 2005).

The ECL cells, called histaminocytes are located in the oxyntic glands. The receptors for acetylcholine, histamine and gastrin are M_3, H2, and CCK_2 respectively, located on basolateral membrane of parietal cells in the body and fundus of the stomach.

The histamine binding to its receptor causes activation of H2 receptors and gastric acid secretion. The binding of the acetylcholine and gastrin to their respective receptors, (M3 and CCK2) causes an increase in intracellular calcium concentration which in turn stimulate protein kinase that stimulate H^+K^+ ATPase and resulting in acid secretion on the canalicular surface (H^+K^+ ATPase stimulation causes H^+ ion secretion in the apical canaliculi of parietal cells). Although, the a H^+K^+ ATPase (proton pump) can be activated by histamine, acetylcholine (Ach) and gastrin, yet H2 receptor have dominant role because acetylcholine and gastrin exert their effect partly directly by stimulating the parietal cell (M3 and CCK_2 receptors) and to a greater extent indirectly by releasing histamine from histaminocytes. Histamine also stimulates secretions in small and large intestine (Katzung 2007).

8.7 Parietal Cells and Signaling Pathways

In the parietal cells, the two major signaling pathways are present (Fig. 8.2).

8.7.1 Cyclic AMP Dependent Pathway: for Histamine

The H2 receptors activate H^+/K^+ ATPase by generating cAMP through the activation of G_s-adenylylcyclase-cyclic AMP-PKA pathway.

8.7.2 Ca^{2+}-Dependent Pathway: for ACh and Gastrin

The gastrin and muscarinic receptors function through G_q-PLC-IP_3-Ca^{2+} pathway in parietal cells by increasing cytosolic Ca^{2+}. Each of these signaling pathway, the cyclic AMP and the Ca^{2+}-dependent pathways, in turn regulates a series of downstream kinase cascades, which activate H^+K^+ATPase exchanges of hydrogen and potassium ions across the parietal cell membrane and creating the largest known ion gradient in vertebrates, generated with an intracellular pH of about 7.3 and an intra-canalicular pH of about 0.8. The H^+/K^+-ATPase is a membrane-bound protein and is composed of two subunits: the larger alpha-subunit couples the ion transport to hydrolysis of ATP, the smaller beta-subunit is required for appropriate assembly of the holoenzyme. The alpha-subunit gene expression occurs via activation of the H2 receptors (Tari et al. 1994). The alpha-subunit has active catalytic site and uses the chemical energy of ATP to transfer H^+ ions from parietal cell cytoplasm to the secretory canaliculi in exchange for K^+. Both the membrane and extracytoplasmic domain contain the ion transport pathway, and therefore, this region is the target for the antisecretory drugs (proton pump inhibitors).

8.8 Acid Peptic Diseases

The ulcers usually occur within the stomach and/or duodenum. In the United States, 4 million individuals (new cases and recurrences) are affected per year with acid peptic disorders and the lifetime prevalence of peptic ulcer disease in the United States is ~12% in men and 10% in women (Vall 2008). Although acid peptic disorders occur due to the result of distinctive mechanism, yet they have common pathogenic mechanisms i.e. either excessive acid secretion or diminished mucosal defense. An ulcer occurs when levels of acid (and pepsin) overwhelm mucosal defense mechanisms and is defined as disruption of the mucosal integrity of the stomach and/or duodenum leading to a local defect or excavation due to active inflammation. The recent knowledge in gastric acid secretion and drug therapy for acid-peptic disease include:

(1) H2 receptor antagonists
(2) H^+K^+ATPase (proton pump) inhibitors and
(3) Identification of Helicobacter pylori as the major causative agent for duodenal ulcer.

The histamine H2 receptor blockade has revolutionized the treatment of acid-peptic disease. Before the availability of the H2 receptor antagonists, the standard of care was simply acid neutralization in the stomach lumen, generally with inadequate results. The long history of safety and efficacy with the H2 receptor antagonists eventually led to their availability without a prescription. The proton-pump inhibitors (PPIs) represent a further therapeutic advance due to more potent inhibition of acid secretion. PPIs are replacing the H2 receptor antagonists in clinical practice.

8.9 H2 Receptor Antagonist in Acid Peptic Disease

The H2 receptor blockers inhibit acid production by reversibly competing with histamine for binding to H2 receptors present on parietal cells. The first H2 blocker, burimamide was developed by Black et al. (1972) but this was having insufficient oral activity (Parsons and Ganellin 2006). The next was metiamide and proved to be effective in duodenal ulcer. However, its use was associated with reversible granulocytopenia in humans (Parsons and Ganellin 2006). The thiourea group in the side chain of metiamide was the cause of this toxicity. The new molecule was developed in which thiourea group was replaced with a cyanoguanidine group. This was found to be devoid of metiamide toxicity. Cimetidine is the prototypical of histamine H2 receptor blocker from which the later members of the class were developed. The cimetidine was the culmination of a project at Smith, Kline and French (SK and F, now GlaxoSmithKline) by Black et al. 1972 (Parsons and Ganellin 2006). This was one of the first drug discovered using rational drug design approach, starting from the structure of histamine receptor molecule. Sir James W. Black shared the 1988 Nobel Prize in Physiology or Medicine for the discovery of cimetidine and propranolol. The discovery of H2R antagonists and their usefulness in control of gastric acid secretion and ulcer healing was considered as real breakthrough both in elucidation of gastric acid secretory mechanisms and ulcer therapy.

Cimetidine which is introduced in 1977 has gained wide popularity for acid peptic diseases. Later on many H2 receptors blockers were discovered in particular, ranitidine (Bradshaw et al. 1979) and many are in market for peptic ulcer diseases. The ranitidine was lacking the propensity to cause drug interaction as seen with cimetidine because it does not affect cytochrome *P*450 enzymes (Fig. 8.3).

The pharmacological actions of H2 receptors and their pathophysiological role are discussed briefly to understand the therapeutic basis of the uses of H2 antagonist in acid peptic ulcer disease.

These different H2 receptor antagonists (cimetidine, ranitidine, famotidine and nizatidine etc) differ mainly in their pharmacokinetic properties. They are less

Fig. 8.3 Molecular structure of histamine H2 receptor antagonists

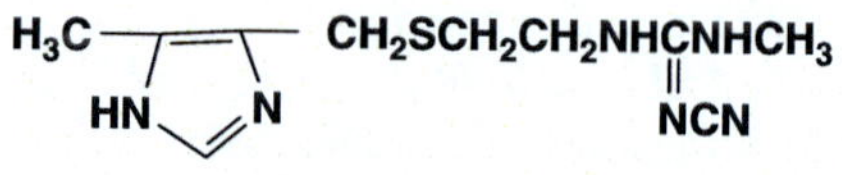

Cimetidine

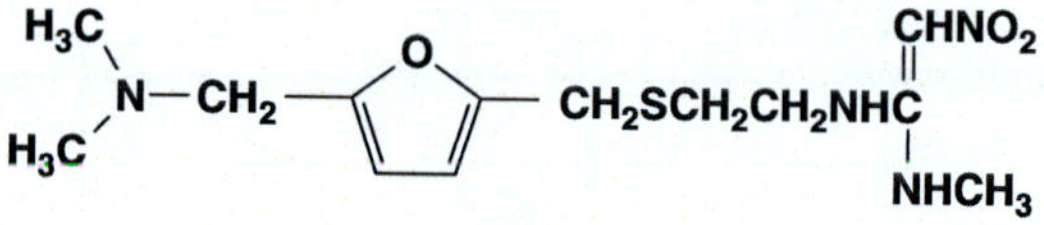

Ranitidine

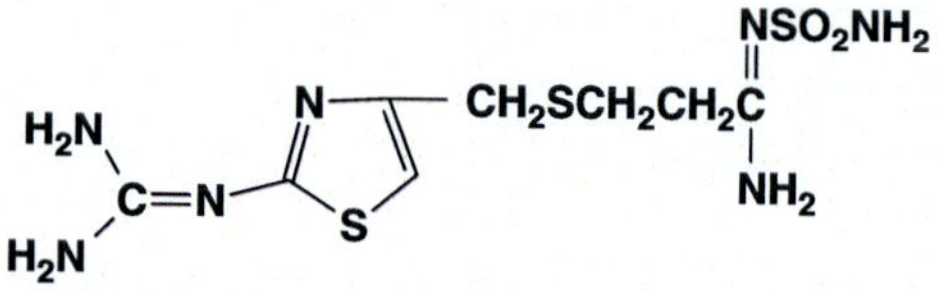

Famotidine

potent than proton pump inhibitors (e.g. omeprazole) but still suppress 24 h gastric acid secretion by about 70%.

The H2 receptor blockers inhibit basal acid secretion predominantly, which accounts for their efficacy in suppressing nocturnal acid secretion because acid secretion follows the cicardian pattern (highest levels occurring during the night and lowest levels during the morning hours. The most important determinant of duodenal ulcer healing is the level of nocturnal acidity, evening dosing of H2 receptor antagonists is adequate therapy in most instances.

The H2 receptors are associated with a wide range of physiological actions extending from gastric acid secretion to cell differentiation and cell proliferation. Histamine level and histamine receptors particularly H2 receptors expressions have been found to be associated with cell proliferation and tumor production (Hegyesi et al. 2001, Tasaka et al. 1993). Now we review histamine function in relation to cell proliferation, differentiation and tumor production. The prospects of histamine or histamine receptor ligands in treatment of different tumor will also be discussed.

8.10 Histamine in Cell Proliferation, Differentiation and Tumorigenesis

Histamine has well recognized role in the allergic reactions (H1 receptors), gastric acid secretion (H2 receptors) and as a neurotransmitter (H3 receptor). Besides these well-known effects of histamine, it is also involved in embryogenesis and organogenesis (Wagner et al. 2003). Association of histamine in cell differentiation and proliferation has been shown in many studies (Davenas et al. 2008, Schneider et al. 2005, Tutton 2007). There are increasing evidences now that histamine is associated with hematopoiesis (Dy and Schneider 2002, Pallinger et al. 2001, Schneider et al. 1990). The expression of H4 receptors in the bone marrow during hematopoiesis (Petit-Betron et al. 2009) and the requirement of histamine for successful extramedullary and splenic hematopoiesis further ascertain role of histamine in the hematopoiesis (Horvath et al. 2010). The effects of histamine are multiple and variable or sometimes even counteracting effects are observed. This variability in effects may be due to the different histamine tissue concentrations, receptor types which are activated and differential expression of the histamine receptors. Even the during the cell differentiation and development the histamine receptor expression can be changed (Thurmond et al. 2008, Triggiani et al. 2007). The noteworthy aspect of histamine is its association with tumor production. Increase levels of mRNA encoding enzyme HDC, HDC protein and histamine production are reported in many cancers including colorectal, glial tumors and prostatic adenomas (Haak-Frendscho et al. 2000, Rivera et al. 2000). However, this is not the end of list but there are so many other tumors whose production have been linked with histamine e.g., colorectal and colon cancer (Cianchi et al. 2005, Reynolds et al. 1996, Verga et al. 2005). The administration of histamine dihydrochloride along with IL-2 can inhibit the growth of malignant melanoma and therefore it is employed as therapy for this tumor (Falus et al. 2001).

8.10.1 Histamine and Hematopoiesis

In past, histamine was related with the regulation of hematopoietic progenitor cells (Byron 1977, Schneider et al. 1990) based on H2 receptors. The H2 receptor agonists such as 4-methylhistamine and dimaprit could increase the number of granulocyte colony-forming units (G-CFU) in a culture medium meaning their role in proliferation and differentiation of neutrophils (Tasaka et al. 1993). However, it is now known that the H4 receptors are preferentially expressed in the hematopoietic cells and are involved in the hematopoeisis (Liu et al. 2001, Schneider et al. 2002). H4 receptors have been identified in peripheral blood leukocytes, thymus, spleen, small intestine, colon and bone marrow (Oda and Matsumoto 2001).

The elevated levels of histamine receptors in hematopoietic progenitors suggest the role of histamine in bone marrow regeneration (Horvath et al. 2006). The enzyme HDC is responsible for the synthesis of histamine, so the proliferative capacity and interleukin-3 signaling of stem cells are affected in HDC knocked out mice as compared to wild-type mice and STAT5 mRNA expression has also been decreased in granulocyte-myeloid colonies of HDC knocked out mice. The STAT5 proteins are transcription factors and have been suggested to play an important role in hematopoiesis. These observations have again supported the histamine role in hematopoiesis (Horvath et al. 2010). However, the role of H4R in hematopoeisis has not been fully addressed till now.

The important cells of hematopoietic lineage on which H4 receptors expressed are mast cells, basophils and eosinophils (Liu et al. 2001, Oda et al. 2000). In case of eosinophils, the H4 receptors are involved in changing the shape of eosinophils, eosinophil chemotaxis, and also in upregulation of adhesion molecules. It is known now that the eosinophils, mast cells, neutrophils and dendritic cells play their role in inflammatory responses and H4 receptors are involved in the recruitment and activation of these cells (Buckland et al. 2003, Gutzmer et al. 2005, Hofstra et al. 2003, Leurs et al. 2009, Ling et al. 2004, Takeshita et al. 2003). The interactions of H4R with eosinophils suggest the potential therapeutic use of H4 receptor for the treatment of allergic disorder. (Ling et al. 2004).

In the patients of acute myeloid leukemia (AML) the complete remission is difficult to achieve and relapses are often seen in these patients after the present day available chemotherapy. Recently phase III clinical study has shown that post-consolidation treatment with the combination of histamine dihydrochloride and IL-2 can prevent relapse in patients of AML (Romero et al. 2009).

8.10.2 *Histamine in Melanoma*

Melanoma is a malignant tumor of melanocytes. Most of melanomas arise predominantly from skin but they can also arise from other sites as well. The tumor has a high rate of metastasis with poor prognosis. The epidemiologic data has documented an increase incidence as well as mortality rate of malignant melanoma, causing 67% of the deaths attributable to skin cancer (Callen et al. 1978).

Histidine decarboxylase (HDC) is the key enzyme for the production of histamine and it is considered as a specific marker for the biosynthesis of histamine. It has already been reported that the level of mRNA encoding HDC, HDC protein and histamine production are increased significantly in many human tumors (Haak-Frendscho et al. 2000, Rivera et al. 2000). The melanoma tissue and cell lines also have elevated levels of enzyme HDC, gene expression and histamine (Haak-Frendscho et al. 2000, Tilly et al. 1990). Considering these findings, the HDC-specific antisense oligonucleotides (ASO) was given in vitro to see the antiproliferative effect of HDC-specific ASO. The results showed the decrease in metastatic melanoma growth. It is now clear that the metastatic melanoma cells are having elevated H2 receptors expression and translational block of HDC may be responsible for antiproliferative effect of HDC-specific ASO (Hegyesi et al. 2001). These results may suggest a possible application of ASO for the therapy of melanoma in future.

The presence of melanoma-derived histamine can affect the growth of melanoma either by direct stimulation or suppression of melanoma growth (Falus et al. 2001). In the melanoma cells, the proliferation can decrease if histamine acts via H1 receptors or increase, where histamine acts via H2 receptors i.e. stimulation or suppression of melanoma growth depends on the types of histamine receptors predominance in the local tissue (Reynolds et al. 1996).

In advance melanoma (or stage IV melanoma), no single agent in form of chemotherapy or immunotherapy has shown significant survival of patients. Interleukin-2 (IL-2) are effective activator of tumor-specific cytotoxic T cells and natural killer (NK) cells in vitro, but only small number of melanoma patients are benefited with the administration of IL-2. However, histamine in combination of IL-2 improves the duration of survival of melanoma patients with liver metastases. This increase in survival of melanoma patients may be by increasing type 1 T-cell responses and also by promoting induction of melanoma-specific T cells (Asemissen et al. 2005).

The possible explanation offered for the compromised efficacy of IL-2 is the presence of an immunosuppressive environment within tumors (Asemissen et al. 2005, Hellstrand 2002, Whiteside 2002). The increased numbers of monocytes are found in and close to the tumor and their rising number can cause a less favorable prognosis for patients of melanomas (Hellstrand and Hermodsson 2006). The monocytes and macrophages are the important phagocytic cells and contribute to the immunosuppressive effect of tumor via production of reactive oxygen metabolites (ROM). The monocyte/macrophage-derived ROM can inhibit cytotoxicity of tumor-reactive T cells and also NK cells by making alterations in signal transducing molecules. The death of lymphocytes cell may occur by the process of apoptosis (Hansson et al. 1996, Hellstrand et al. 1994, Kono et al. 1996). Therefore, it has been hypothesized that phagocyte-derived reactive oxygen metabolites (ROM) play significant role and can down regulate the intratumoral lymphocytes. This can also render lymphocytes unresponsive to cytokines. Histamine dihydrochloride has been used to check the synthesis of reactive oxygen species in monocytes and thereby protect NK and T cells. It also synergize with IL-2 in inducing NK and T-cell activation (Hellstrand and Hermodsson 1991).

Unlike the growth of melanocytes, the growth of melanoma cells does not depend upon exogenous mitogens but these cells have acquired the benefits of expressing growth factor and cytokines themselves (Moretti et al. 1999). This has provided an escape mechanism for the melanoma cells to regulate cell proliferation. There is other mechanism for the help of these melanoma cells in which local T-cells polarization get shifted towards the T-helper 2 (Th2) cells. So there are many factors which influence the growth of melanoma. These are autocrine and paracrine factors (Falus et al. 2001).

8.10.3 Histamine in Breast Cancer

Histamine was found to be associated with proliferative activity in breast cancer. An embryo synthesizes histamine on the fourth day of pregnancy in mouse (Dey and Johnson 1980). The role histamine in cell proliferation and in breast development has already been reported (Cricco et al. 1994, Davio et al. 1994, Wagner et al. 2003). The human mammary glands have binding sites for both the H1 and H2 receptors and 75% malignant carcinomas express H2 receptors. The H2R agonists were found to increase the cell growth while H1 receptors agonist caused dose dependant inhibition of cell growth (Lemos et al. 1995). In woman suffering from ductal breast cancer have elevated level of histamine in plasma as well as in tissue of breast cancer (Mach-Szczypiński et al. 2009). Several clinical trials have now been carried out with H2R antagonists in breast cancer but the use of these H2R antagonists have not shown significant benefits in patients of breast cancer (Bolton et al. 2000, Bowrey et al. 2000). Even the ranitidine, H2R antagonists have been linked with increased risk of hormone estrogen receptor-positive or progesterone receptor-positive ductal carcinoma (Mathes et al. 2008). However, use of H2 blockers in general is not associated with any increase risk of breast cancer.

These observations that H2 receptors are expressed in malignant carcinoma of breast but H2R antagonists like cimetidine has no effect on tumor cell proliferation (Bowrey et al. 2000) invite many possible explanations. In some studies, the proliferation of the malignant cell line mediated via H3 receptors and H2 receptor may not have their involvement (Vesuna and Raman 2006). We know that the four histamine receptors differ in binding affinities, expression, regulation and intracellular mechanism of signal generation are also involved in cross talk between the ligand and receptors (Banu and Watanabe 1999, Jutel et al. 2009). There is also important finding about the histamine receptors that they are differentially expressed in different cancer types e.g., those of the brain, colon and breast. The cimetidine has been found to have effect on the tumor infiltrating lymphocytes in colorectal cancer (Adams and Morris 1997, Adams et al. 1994) but no such effects were seen in breast cancer. Selective estrogen receptor modulator (e.g. tamoxifen) can bind to histamine-like receptors and have antihistamine effect to reduce proliferation (Kroeger and Brandes 1985). Now question arises that whether histamine receptor expression in cancer cells contributes to tumorigenesis or is such expression pattern a consequence of cellular transformation (Vesuna and Raman 2006).

The H3R level of expression was significantly higher in carcinomas than the non-tumoral breast tissue surrounding carcinomas. Similarly benign lesions expressed low level of H4R (13%) as compared to carcinomas (44%). The H3R expression was also found to be correlated in carcinomas with the expression of HDC and histamine content (Medina et al. 2008) suggesting a novel molecular target for new therapeutic approach.

These are the few examples of histamine association with tumors. There are so many tumors in which histamine has its role. The cell proliferation has also been linked with H1R e.g. human pancreatic carcinoma cell line PANC-1 (Cricco et al. 2004). The H2/H4 receptors were found to have proliferative and proangigenic effects (Cianchi et al. 2005).

8.11 Final Remark

Histamine has key role in many physiological processes including inflammation and gastric acid secretion. Hence, H1 and H2 receptor antagonists have been successfully used for allergic and acid peptic diseases, respectively. Nowadays H2 receptor antagonists (e.g. ranitidine) are available as over the counter drugs in many countries. However, H2 receptor antagonists have largely been superseded by proton pump inhibitors e.g. lansoprazole, omeprazole, pantoprazole and rabeprazole etc.

Proton pump inhibitors are well tolerated and relatively free of side effects. They are most potent inhibitors of gastric acid secretion available today.

H3 receptor antagonists particularly nonimidazole derivatives are in clinical trials for obesity and a variety of central nervous system disorders, such as cognitive dysfunction, memory performance, attention deficit hyperactivity disorder and epilepsy. The most recently discovered H4 receptors promise the potential to provide drugs acting on the immunological system with possible applications in allergy, inflammation, pruritus and autoimmune diseases and asthma. The possibility of synergy between H1 and H4 receptors can suggest benefit of blocking both the receptors in allergic diseases. The proliferation and differentiation of cells are the other function of histamine. Histamine receptors and HDC expression is increased many tumors. The results of clinical trials in patients of metastatic melanoma suggest that the addition of histamine dihydrochloride to the patients receiving IL-2 and IFN-α therapy prolongs survival time and induces regression of tumor. Similarly, histamine along with IL-2 prevents the relapses of acute myeloid leukemia (AML). Therefore more work is needed to confirm the putative benefit of histamine in neoplastic diseases.

References

Adams WJ, Lawson JA, Morris DL (1994) Cimetidine inhibits in vivo growth of human colon cancer and reverses histamine stimulated in vitro and in vivo growth. Gut 35:1632–1636

Adams WJ, Morris DL (1997) Pilot study–cimetidine enhances lymphocyte infiltration of human colorectal carcinoma: results of a small randomized control trial. Cancer 80(1):15–21

Akdis CA (2008) Immune regulation by histamine H_4 receptors in skin. J Invest Dermatol 128:1615–1616

Akdis CA, Simons FE (2006) Histamine receptors are hot in immunopharmacology. Eur J Pharmacol 533:69–76

Arrang JM, Garbarg M, Lancelot JC et al (1987) Highly potent and selective ligands for histamine H_3 receptors. Nature 327:117–123

Asemissen AM, Scheibenbogen C, Letsch A et al (2005) Addition of histamine to interleukin 2 treatment augments type 1 T-cell responses in patients with melanoma in vivo: immunologic results from a randomized clinical trial of interleukin 2 with or without histamine (MP 104). Clin Cancer Res 11:290–297

Ash ASF, Schild HO (1966) Receptors mediating some actions of histamine. Br J Pharmacol 27:427–439

Banu Y, Watanabe T (1999) Augmentation of antigen receptor–mediated responses by histamine H1 receptor signaling. J Exp Med 189:673–682

Best CH, Dale HH, Dudley JW et al (1927) The nature of the vasodilator constituents of certain tissue extract. J Physiol 62:397–417

Black JW, Shankley NP (1987) How does gastrin act to stimulate oxyntic cell secretion. Trends Pharmacol Sci 8:486–490

Black JW, Duncan WAM, Durant GJ et al (1972) Definition and antagonism of histamine H_2 receptors. Nature 236:385–390

Bolton E, King J, Morris DL (2000) H2 antagonists in the treatment of colon and breast cancer. Semin Cancer Biol 10:3–10

Bowrey PF, King J, Magarey C et al (2000) Histamine, mast cells and tumour cell proliferation in breast cancer: does preoperative cimetidine administration have an effect. Br J Cancer 82: 167–170

Bradshaw J, Brittain RT, Clitherow JW et al (1979) Ranitidine (AM 19065), a new potent, selective histamine H_2-receptors antagonist. Br J Pharmacol 66:464
Buckland KF, Williams TJ, Conroy DM (2003). Histamine induces cytoskeletal changes in human eosinophils via the H4 receptor. Br J Pharmacol 140:1117–1127
Byron JW (1977) Mechanism for histamine H2-receptor induced cell-cycle changes in the bone marrow stem cell. Agents Actions 7:209–213
Callen PJ, Chanda JJ, Stawiski MA et al (1978) Malignant melanoma. Arch Dermatol 114:369–370
Chazot PL (2009) Advance in histamine pharmacology reveal new drug targets. Br J Pharmacol 157:1–3
Cianchi F, Cortesini C, Schiavone N et al (2005) The role of cyclooxygenase-2 in mediating the effects of histamine on cell proliferation and vascular endothelial growth factor production in colorectal cancer. Clin Cancer Res 11:6807–6815
Cricco G, Martin G, Medina V et al (2004) Histamine regulates the MAPK pathway via the H_2 receptors in PANC-1 human cells. Inflamm Res 53:S65-S66
Cricco GP, Davio CA, Martin G et al (1994) Histamine as an autocrine growth factor in experimental mammary carcinomas. Inflammation Res 43:17–20
Davenas E, Rouleau A, Morisset S et al (2008) Autoregulation of McA-RH7777 hepatoma cell proliferation by histamine H3 receptors. J Pharmacol Exp Ther 326:406–413
Davio CA, Cricco GP, Martin G et al (1994) Effect of histamine on growth and differentiation of the rat mammary gland. Agents Actions 41:C115–117
DeGraw JI, Engstrom J, Ellis M et al (1997) Potential histadine decarboxylase inhibitor. 1.alpha and β-beta substituted histidine analogs. J Med Chem 20:1671–1674
Dey SK, Johnson DC (1980) Histamine formation by mouse preimplantation embryos. J Reprod Fertil 60:457–460
Dy M, Schneider E (2004) Histamine-cytokine connection in immunity and hematopoiesis. Cytokine Growth Factor Rev 15:393–410
Engelhardt H, Smits RA, Leurs R et al (2009) A new generation of anti-histamines: histamine H4 receptor antagonists on their way to the clinic. Curr Opin Drug Discov Develop 12:628–643
Estelle F, Simons R (2004) Advances in H1 antihistamines. N Engl J Med 351:2203–2217
Falus A, Hargita H, Eszter L et al (2001) Paracrine and autocrine interactions in melanoma: histamine is a relevant player in local regulation. Trends Immunol 22:648–652
Feldberg W, Mongar JL (1954) Comparison of histamine release by compound 48/80 and octylamine in perfused tissues. Br J Pharmacol 9:197–201
Fox GB, Esbenshade TA, Pan JB et al (2005) Pharmacological properties of ABT-239[4-(2-{2-[2R)-2-Methylpyrrolidinyl]ethyl}-benzofuran-5-yl)benzonitrile]:II.Neuro-physiological charecterization and broad preclinical efficacy in cognition and schizophrenia of a potent and selective histamine H3 receptor antagonist. J Pharmacol Exp Ther 333:176–190
Furuta K, Nakayama K, Sugimoto Y (2007) Activation of histidine decarboxylase through post-translational cleavage by Caspase-9 in a mouse mastocytoma P-815. J Biol Chem 282: 13438–13446
Ganong WF (2005) Review of medical physiology. In: Ganong WF (ed) Regulation of gastrointestinal function, 22nd edn. McGraw-Hill, Philadelphia
Gantz I, Munzert G, Tashiro T et al (1991) Molecular cloning of the human histamine H_2 receptors. Biochem Biophys Res Commun 178:1386–1392
Gutzmer R, Diestel C, Mommert S et al (2005) Histamine H4 receptor stimulation suppresses IL-12p70 production and mediates chemotaxis in human monocyte-derived dendritic cells. J Immunol 174:5224–5232
Guyton AC, Hall JE (2006) Secretory functions of ailmentary tract. In: Guyton AC, Hall JE (eds) Textbook of medical physiology, 11th edn. Elsevier. Philadelphia, Pennsylvania. pp 794–799
Haak-Frendscho M, Darvas ZS, Hegyesi H et al (2000) Histidine decarboxylase immunoreactivity in human melanoma. J Invest Dermatol 115:345–352
Haas HL, Sergeeva OA, Selbach O (2008) Histamine in the nervous system. Physiol Rev 88: 1183–1241

Hansson M, Asea A, Ersson U et al (1996) Induction of apoptosis in NK cells by monocyte-derived reactive oxygen metabolites. J Immunol 156:42–47

Hegyesi H, Somlai B, Varga VL et al (2001) Suppression of melanoma cell proliferation by histidine decarboxylase specific antisense oligonucleotides. J Invest Dermatol 117:151–153

Hellstrand K (2002) Histamine in cancer immunotherapy: a preclinical background. Semin Oncol 29:35–40

Hellstrand K, Hermodsson S (1991) Cell-to-cell mediated inhibition of natural killer cell proliferation by monocytes and its regulation by histamine H_2-receptors. Scand J Immunol 34(6):741–52

Hellstrand K, Hermodsson S (2006) Cell-to-Cell mediated inhibition of natural killer cell proliferation by monocytes and its regulation by histamine H_2-receptors. Scand J Immunol 34:741–752

Hellstrand K, Asea A, Dahlgren C et al (1994) Histaminergic regulation of NK cells. Role of monocyte-derived reactive oxygen metabolites. J Immunol 153:4940–4947

Hill SJ, Ganellin CR, Timmerman H et al (1997) International Union of Pharmacology. XIII. Classification of histamine receptors. Pharmacol Rev 49:253–278

Hofstra CL, Desai PJ, Thurmond RL et al (2003) Histamine H4 receptor mediates chemotaxis and calcium mobilization of mast cells. J Pharmacol Exp Ther 305:1212–1221

Horvath Z, Pallinger E, Horvath G et al (2006) Histamine H1 and H2 receptors but not H4 receptors are upregulated during bone marrow regeneration. Cell Immunol 244:110–115

Horvath Z, Pallinger E, Horvath G et al (2010) Extramedullary hematopoiesis is dysregulated in histamine-free histidine decarboxylase knockout ($HDC^{-/-}$) mice. Inflamm Res 59(6):429–436

Hough LB (2001) Genomics meets histamine receptors: new subtypes, new receptors. Mol Pharmacol 59:415–419

Hung PD, Schubert ML, Mihas AA (2003) Zollinger-Ellison syndrome. Curr Treat Options Gastroenterol 6:163–170

Jablonowski JA, Grice CA, Chai W et al (2003) The first potent and selective non-imidazole human histamine H_4 receptor antagonists. J Med Chem 46:3957–3960

Jensen RT, Niederle B, Mitry E et al (2006) Gastrinoma (duodenal and pancreatic). Neuroendocrinology 84:173–182

Johnson AR, Erdos EG (1973) Release of histamine from mast cells by vasoactive peptides. Proc Soc Exp Biol Med 142:1252–1256

Joseph IMP, Zavros Y, Merchant JL et al (2003) A model for integrative study of human gastric acid secretion. J Appl Physiol 94:1602–1618

Jutel M, Akdis M, Akdis CA (2009) Histamine, histamine receptors and their role in immune pathology. Clin Exp Allergy 39:1786–1800

Katzung BG (2007) Histamine, serotonin and the ergot alkaloids. In: Katzung BG (ed) Basic clinical pharmacology, 10th edn. McGraw-Hill, Medical Publishing Division, New York

Kaufman DW, Kelly JP, Rosenberg L et al (2002) Recent patterns of medication use in the ambulatory adult population of the United States: the Slone survey. JAMA 287:337–344

Khandewal JK, Hough LB, Morrishow AM et al (1982) Measurement of tele-methyl histamine and histamine in human cerebrospinal fluid, urine, plasma. Agents Action 12:583–587

Kono K, Salazar-Onfray F, Petersson M et al (1996) Hydrogen peroxide secreted by tumor-derived macrophages down-modulates signal-transducing zeta molecules and inhibits tumor-specific T cell and natural killer cell-mediated cytotoxicity. Eur J Immunol 26:1308–13013

Kroeger EA, Brandes LJ (1985) Evidence that tamoxifen is a histamine antagonist. Biochem Biophys Res Commun 131:750–755

Lemos B, Davio C, Gass H et al (1995) Histamine receptors in human mammary gland, different benign lesions and mammary carcinomas. Inflamm Res 44(Suppl 1):S68–S69

Leurs R, Wantanabe T, Timmerman H (2001) Histamine receptors are finally “coming out”. Trends Pharmacol Sci 22:337–339

Leurs RL, Chazot PL, Shenton FC et al (2009) Molecular and biochemical pharmacology of the histamine H_4 receptors. Br J Pharmacol 157:14–23

Levy JH, Kettlekamp N, Goertz P et al (1987) Histamine release by vancomycin: a mechanism for hypotension in man. Anesthesiology 67:122–125

Ling P, Ngo K, Nguyen S et al (2004) Histamine H_4 receptor mediates eosinophil chemotaxis with cell shape change and adhesion molecule upregulation. Br J Pharmacol 142:161–171

Liu C, Jiang X, Wilson SJ et al (2001) Cloning and pharmacological characterization of a fourth histamine receptor (H_4) expressed in bone marrow. Mol Pharmacol 59:420–426

Lovenberg TW, Roland BL, Wilson SJ et al (1999) Cloning and functional expression of the human histamine H_3 receptor. Mol Pharmacol 55:1101–1107

Mach-Szczypiński JV, Stanosz S, Sieja K et al (2009) Metabolism of histamine in tissues of primary ductal breast cancer 58:867–870

Mathes RW, Malone KE, Daling JR et al (2008) Relationship between histamine H_2-receptor antagonist medications and risk of invasive breast cancer. Cancer Epidemiol Biomarkers Prev 17:67–72

Medthurst AD, Atkins AR, Beresoford IJ et al (2007) GSK 189254, a nobel H_3 receptor antagonist that bind to histamine H_3 receptors in Alzheimer's disease brain and improves cognitive performance in preclinical models. J Pharmacol Exp Ther 321:1032–1045

Medthurst AD, Roberts JC, Lee J et al (2009) Characterization of histamine H_3 receptors in Alzheimer's Disease brain and amyloid over-expressing TASTPM mice Br J Pharmacol 157:130–138

Medina MA, Correa-Fiz F, Rodrigeuez-Caso C et al (2005) A comprehensive view of polyene and histamine metabolism to the light of new technologies. J Cell Mol Med 9:854–864

Medina MA, Urdilates JL, Rodrigeuez-Caso C et al (2003) Biogenic amine and polyamines: similar bio-chemistry for different physiological mission and biomedical application. Crit Rev Biochem Mol Biol 38:23–59

Medina V, Croci M, Crescenti E et al (2008) The role of histamine in human mammary carcinogenesis: H3 and H4 receptors as potential therapeutic targets for breast cancer treatment. Cancer Biol Ther 7:28–35

Moessner J (2005) Developments in the inhibition of gastric acid secretion. Eur J Clin Invest 35:469–475

Moretti S, Pinzi C, Spallanzani A et al (1999) Immunohistochemical evidence of cytokine networks during progression of human melanocytic lesions. Int J Cancer 84:160–168

Moya-Garcia AA, Medina MA, Sanchez-Jimenez F (2005) Mammalian histidine decarboxylase: from structure to function. Bioessays 27:57–63

Moya-García AA, Pino-Angeles A, Gil-Redondo R, et al (2009) Structural features of mammalian histidine decarboxylase reveal the basis for specific inhibition. Br J Pharmacol. 157(1): 4–13

Oda T, Matsumoto S (2001) Identification and characterization of histamine H4 receptor. Nippon Yakurigaku Zasshi 118:36–42

Oda T, Morika WAN, Saito Y et al (2000) Molecular cloning and characterization of a novel type of histamine receptor preferentially expressed in leukocytes. J Biol Chem 275: 36781–36786

Pallinger E, Buzas E, Laszlo V (2001) Characterization of flow cytometry of hematopoietic progenitors in bone marrow of histadine decarboxylase knock out and wild type of mice. Inflamm Res 50:S89–S90

Parsons ME, Ganellin CR (2006) Histamine and its receptors. Br J Pharmacol 147:S127–S135

Petit-Betron AF, Machavoine F, Defresne MP et al (2009) H4 histamine receptors mediate cell cycle arrest in growth factor-induced murine and human hematopoietic progenitor cells. PLos One 7:e6504

Rang HP, Dale MM, Ritter JM et al (2007) Local hormone, inflammation, and immune reaction. In: Rang et al (eds.) Rang and Dale's pharmacology, 6th edn. Churchill Livingstone Elsevier, London

Reynolds JL, Akhter J, Morris DL (1996) In vitro effect of histamine and histamine H1 and H2 receptor antagonists on cellular proliferation of human malignant melanoma cell lines. Melanoma Res 6:95–99

Riley JF, West GB (1952) Histamine in tissue mast cells. J Physiol 117:72–73

Rivera SE, Cricco GP, Engel NI et al (2000) Histamine as an autocrine growth factor: an unusual role for a widespread mediator. Semin Cancer Biol 10:15–24

Romero AI, Thoren FB, Aurelius J et al (2009) Post-consolidation immunotherapy with histamine dihydrochloride and interleukin-2 in AML. Scand J Immunol 70:194–205

Sander K, Kottke T, Star H (2008) Histamine H_3 receptor antagonists Go to clinics. Biol Pharm Bull 1:2163–2183

Schneider E, Piquet-Pellorce C, Dy M (1990) New role for histamine in interleukin-3 induced proliferation of hematopoietic stem cells. J Cell Physiol 143:337–343

Schneider E, Rolli Dorkinderen M, Arock M et al (2002) Trends in histamine research: new functions during immune responses and hematopoiesis. Trends Immunol 23:255–263

Schwartz JC, Haas HL (1992) The histamine receptor. Wiley-Liss, New York

Shahid M, Tripathi T, Sobia F et al (2009) Histamine, histamine receptors, and their role in immunomodulation: an updated systematic review. Open Immunol J 2:9–41

Simons FE (2004) Advances in H1-antihistamines. N Engl J Med 351:2203–2217

Skidgel RA, Erdos EG (2006) Histamine, bradykinin and their antagonists. In: Bruton LL, Lazo JS, Parker KL (eds) Goodman & Gillman's the pharmacological basis of therapeutics, 11th edn. Mc Graw Hill Medical Publishing Divison, New York

Soll AH, Berglindh T (1987) Physiology of isolated gastric glands and parietal cells: receptors and effectors regulating function. In: Johnson LR (ed) Physiology of the gastrointestinal tract, 2nd edn. Raven, New York

Soll AH, Walsh JH (1979) Regulation of gastric acid secretion. Annu Rev Physiol 41:35–53

Takeshita K, Sakai K, Bacon KB et al (2003) Critical role of histamine H4 receptor in leukotriene B4 production and mast cell-dependent neutrophil recruitment induced by zymosan in vivo. J Pharmacol Exp Ther 307:1072–1080

Tanaka S (2003) Physiological function mediated by histamine synthesis. Yakugaku Zasshi 123:547–559

Tari A, Yamamoto G, Yonei Y et al (1994) Effect of histamine on rat gastric H(+)K(+) ATPase alpha-subunit expression. Am J Physiol Gastrointest Liver Physiol 266:G444–G450

Tasaka K, Mio M, Shimazawa M et al (1993) Histamine-induced production of interleukin-1 alpha from murine bone marrow stromal cells and its inhibition by H2 blockers. Mol pharmacol 43:365–371

Thurmond RL, Gelfand EW, Dunford PJ (2008) The role of histamine H1 and H4 receptors in allergic inflammation: the search for new antihistaminic. Nat Rev Drug Discov 7: 41–53

Tiligada E, Zampeli E, Sander K et al (2009) Histamine H3 and H4 receptors as novel drug targets. Expert Opin Investig Drugs 18:1519–1531

Tilly BC, Tertoolen LG, Remorie R et al (1990) Histamine as a growth factor and chemoattractant for human carcinoma and melanoma cells: action through Ca2(+)-mobilizing H1 receptors. J Cell Biol 110:1211–1215

Triggiani M, Petraroli A, Loffredo S et al (2007) Differentiation of monocytes into macrophages induces the upregulation of histamine H1 receptor. J Allergy Clin Immunol 119:472–481

Tutton PJM (2007) The influence of histamine on epithelial cell proliferation in the jejunum of the rat. Clin Exp Pharmacol Physiol 3:369–373

Vall JD (2008) Peptic ulcer disease and related disorders. In: Fauci AS, Kasper DL, Longo DL et al (eds) Harrison's principles of internal medicine, 17th edn. McGraw Hill Medical Publishing Division, New York

Valle JD, Gantz I (1997) Novel insights into histamine H2 receptor biology. Am J Physiol Gastrointest Liver Physiol 273:G987–G996

Verga C, Horvath K, Berko A et al (2005) Inhibitory effects of histamine H_4 receptors antagonists on experimental colitis in rat. Eur J Pharmacol 522:130–138

Vesuna F, Raman V (2006) Histamine a potential therapeutic agent for breast cancer treatment. Cancer Biol Ther 5:1472–1473

Wagner W, Ichikawa A, Tanaka S et al (2003) Mouse mammary epithelial histamine system. J Physiol Pharmacol 54:211–213

Watanabe T, Ohtsu H (2002) L-Histidine decarboxylase as a probe in studies on histamine. Chem Rec 2:369–376

Whiteside TL (2002) Tumor-induced death of immune cells: its mechanisms and consequences. Semin Cancer Biol 12:43–50

Wu F, Yu J, Gehring H (2008) Inhibitory and structural studies of novel coenzyme-substrate analogs of human histidine decarboxylase. FASEB J 22:890–897

Yamashita M, Fukui H, Sugama K et al (1991) Expression cloning of a cDNA encoding the bovine histamine H_1 receptors. Proc Natl Acad Sci USA 88:11515–11519

Part VI
Histamine Role in Pathogenesis and Diagnosis of Allergic, Inflammatory, Autoimmune and Cancer Diseases

Chapter 9
Histamine: Role in Pathogenesis of Autoimmune, Allergic, Inflammatory and Malignant Diseases

Trivendra Tripathi, Mohammed Shahid, Haris M. Khan, Mashiatullah Siddiqui, Aijaz Ahmed Khan, and Rahat Ali Khan

Abstract Recent years have witnessed importance of histamine in immunopathophysiological implications in several diseases. Moreover, its role in development of disease pathology is still being elucidated. Accumulating evidences have highlighted that histamine has the possible role in pathology of autoimmunity by modulating the cytokine network and influence T-lymphocytes (Th1 and Th2) balance, and antibody isotype switching. Hence, there is a real need to search for newer role of histamine in disease development. In this review, we will highlight histamine role in pathology of autoimmunity and its mechanism, and also histamine role in pathogenesis of autoimmune, allergic, inflammatory and malignant diseases such as chronic urticaria (CU), atopic dermatitis (AD), autoimmune myocardium (AM) and multiple sclerosis (MS) & experimental autoimmune encephalomyelitis (EAE); allergic rhinitis, anaphylaxis (acute) and asthma; atherosclerosis; and malignant melanoma, respectively. There are several steps in the autoimmune attack/allergic march where histamine might play an important role.

Keywords Histamine · Autoimmune · Allergic · Inflammatory · Malignant melanoma

Abbreviations

HDC	histidine decarboxylase enzyme
IL	interleukin
GM-CSF	granulocyte-monocyte colony stimulating factor
CU	chronic urticaria
CAU	chronic autoimmune urticaria
AD	atopic dermatitis
AM	autoimmune myocardium

M. Shahid (✉)
Department of Microbiology, Jawaharlal Nehru Medical College and Hospital, Aligarh Muslim University, Aligarh, 202002, UP, India
e-mail: shahidsahar@yahoo.co.in

M. Shahid et al. (eds.), *Biomedical Aspects of Histamine*,
DOI 10.1007/978-90-481-9349-3_9,

MS	multiple sclerosis
EAE	experimental autoimmune encephalomyelitis
MHC	major histocompatibility complex
H1R	histamine receptor 1
H2R	histamine receptor 2
H3R	histamine receptor 3
H4R	histamine receptor 4
EAO	experimental autoimmune orchitis
Th1	T helper 1
Th2	T helper 2
SPZ	streptozotocin
TNF	tumor necrosis factor
IgG	immunoglobulin-G
IgE	immunoglobulin-E
ThEA	2-thiazolylethylamine
CNS	central nervous system
MBP	myelin basic protein
HRs	histamine receptors
MOG	myelin oligodendrocyte glycoprotein
cGMP	cyclic guanosine monophosphate
SCID	severe combined immunodeficient

Contents

9.1 Introduction

Histamine is probably one of the most important ancient mediator of biological functions. It is synthesized and stored in cytoplasmic granules within mast cells and basophils by decarboxylation of L-histidine using the pyridoxal-5′-phosphate-dependent L-histidine decarboxylase enzyme (HDC) via a histidine-PLP schiff – base intermediate (Finch and Hicks 1976). Histamine was synthesized for the first time in 1907 and characterized in 1910 as a substance "beta-1" (Barger and Dale 1910). The relation between histamine and anaphylactic reactions was made rapidly in 1929, and was identified as a mediator of anaphylactic reactions in 1932 (Dale 1929, Steinhoff et al. 2004). During inflammation, various immunological and non-immunological stimuli stimulate histamine release from basophils and mast cells (FcεRI$^+$ cells) (Marone et al. 1997, Patella et al. 1998). However, several myeloid and lymphoid cell types (dendritic cells (DCs) and T cells), which do not store histamine, show high HDC activity and are capable of producing high amounts of histamine (Szeberényi et al. 2001). In vitro HDC activity is modulated by cytokines such as interleukin (IL)-1, IL-3, IL-12, IL-18, granulocyte-monocyte colony stimulating factor (GM-CSF), macrophage-colony stimulating factor, tumor necrosis factor (TNF-α) and calcium ionophore. However, HDC activity has been shown in vivo in conditions such as lipopolysaccharides (LPS) stimulation, infection, inflammation, and graft rejection (MacGlashan 2003, Schneider et al. 2002). The drugs targeting its receptors have been in clinical use for more than 60 years. It was being documented that histamine played an important role as a mediator of allergic reactions and exerts a range of effects on many physiological and pathological processes. It is being demonstrated that antihistamines became widely used in the treatment of various allergic diseases, however, the exact roles of histamine for pathogenesis of allergic and autoimmune diseases are still being elucidated. Histamine was coined after the Greek word for tissue "histos". It acts as a mediator for broader spectrum of activities in various physio-pathological conditions including cell proliferation, differentiation, hematopoiesis, embryonic development, regeneration, wound healing, aminergic neurotransmission and numerous other brain functions such as sleep/nociception, food intake and aggressive behavior, secretion of pituitary hormones, regulation of gastrointestinal and circulatory functions, cardiovascular system (vasodilatation and blood pressure reduction), as well as inflammatory reactions, modulation of the immune response, endocrine functioning and homeostasis (Dy and Schneider 2004, Fumagalli et al. 2004, Jutel et al. 2002, MacGlashan 2003, Schneider et al. 2002, Shahid et al. 2009). It is also responsible for the pathogenesis of autoimmune/allergic/inflammatory/cancer diseases such as chronic urticaria (CU), atopic dermatitis (AD), autoimmune myocardium (AM), multiple sclerosis (MS), experimental autoimmune encephalomyelitis (EAE), allergic rhinitis, anaphylaxis, asthma, atherosclerosis and malignant melanoma. An increase in the histamine levels in skin and plasma of patients of AD, CU, MS, and in psoriatic skin and also in bronchoalveolar lavage fluid from patients with allergic asthma have been postulated to play a possible role in pathogenesis of these diseases (Thurmond et al. 2008), however the exact role of histamine in these allergic and autoimmune diseases are still being elucidated. The biological pleiotropic effects of histamine are mediated by four subtypes of histamine receptors (H1R, H2R, H3R and H4R) transducing extracellular signals through different G-proteins: $G_{q/11}$ for H1, $G_{\alpha s}$ for H2, $G_{i/o}$ for H3 and H4-receptors. Specific activation or blockade of histamine receptors has led to a tremendous increase in the knowledge of the roles of histamine in physiology and pathology of disease conditions (Jutel et al. 2005).

Thus, after a century of histamine discovery, the exact mechanism for the potential role in pathogenesis of autoimmune diseases is still to be answered. However, the complex interrelationship and cross talk by histamine and its receptors in allergic and autoimmune diseases have opened a new concepts for comprehend its pathophysio-mechanism in these diseases. Recently, a research article describing the paracrine and autocrine interaction in melanoma revealed that histamine is a relevant player in local regulation in melanoma cells (Falus et al. 2001). In this chapter, we will discuss and highlight the possible role of histamine in the pathogenesis some of the autoimmune, allergic, inflammatory, and malignant diseases.

9.2 Histamine Receptors in Autoimmunity

Bordetella pertussis-induced histamine sensitization (Bphs) is one of the first non-major histocompatibility complex (MHC)-linked genes demonstrated to be involved in the susceptibility to multiple autoimmune diseases. It is located on mouse chromosome 6 and has been identified as histamine receptor 1 (H1R) gene (Dy and Schneider 2004, Ma et al. 2002). In experimental autoimmune orchitis (EAO) and experimental allergic encephalomyelitis (EAE) models, deletion of H1R gene leads to a delay in disease onset and a decrease in the severity of clinical signs when compared to wild type mice. Studies on T lymphocyte parameters show that EAE antigen-stimulated proliferation as well as antibody production is not affected in H1R-deleted mice. The key observation when comparing these mice with the wild type was a striking decrease in the production of IFN-γ, while IL-4 was increased. These data were consistent with the involvement of H1R in antigen-induced EAE, in which the T cell response in H1R-deleted mice is biased towards T helper 2 (Th2), which could be associated with a less severe pathology (Dy and Schneider 2004). Analysis of mRNA from MS lesions revealed increased amounts of H1R transcripts and its blockade by H1R-antagonists diminished EAE induction (Pedotti et al. 2003a). Several experimental data support the notion that proinflammatory reactions are preferentially increased or induced via the H1R, while inflammatory and immune responses are downregulated through the histamine receptor 2 (H2R). Even though this paradigm is still a matter of debate, it might be relevant to EAE since H2R-agonists, such as dimaprit, reduced clinical signs compared to vehicle in EAE mice (Emerson et al. 2002). However, paradoxically, H2R-deleted mice are also less sensitive to EAE induction because of their low T helper 1 (Th1) effector cell response that results from a dysregulation of cytokine production by antigen-presenting cells. The latter produce less IL-12 and IL-6 and more MCP1 than their wild type or H1R-deleted counterpart (Teuscher et al. 2004). Further researches are needed to understand in more detail how the interaction between H1R and H2R influence T cell polarization, the histamine-cytokine/histamine-antibody connection in autoimmunity has to be considered and provides new approaches of learning how pathogenic effector T cells emerge (Dy and Schneider 2004). Histamine levels are increased in plasma and tissues of streptozotocin (SPZ)-induced diabetic rats as well as in patients with diabetes mellitus. Recent studies in the mouse model have demonstrated that hyperglycemia itself or hyperglycemia initiated events are responsible both for enhancing HDC activity and for sensitizing to the action of LPS as HDC inducer (Oguri et al. 2003).

9.3 Autoimmunity and its Possible Mechanism Induced by Histamine

More than a century ago, autoimmune diseases were recognized and researchers began to associate them with viral and bacterial infections. Autoimmune diseases tend to cluster in families and in individuals, which demonstrate that common mechanism is involved in disease susceptibility. Genetic as well as environmental factors (such as infections) are responsible to develop autoimmune diseases (Rose 2002). Genetic factors are imperative in the progress of autoimmune disease, since such diseases develop in certain strains of mice (systemic lupus erythematosus or lupus in MRL mice) without any apparent infectious environmental trigger (Fairweather and Rose 2004). However, environmental factors (such as infections) also are responsible for progress of autoimmune diseases such as diabetes, multiple sclerosis, myocarditis, lyme arthritis, rheumatoid arthritis, lupus erythematosis, rheumatic fever, chagas' disease, myasthenia gravis and Guillain-Barré syndrome (Fairweather and Rose 2004).

Thus, an autoimmune disease occurs when a response against a self-antigen(s) involving T cells, B cells, or autoantibodies induces injury systemically or against a particular organ (Rose 2002). Autoimmune diseases can affect virtually every site in the body, including the endocrine system, connective tissue, gastrointestinal tract, heart, skin, and kidneys (Rose 2001, 2002). It has been documented that at least 15 diseases are known to be the direct result of an autoimmune response, while circumstantial evidence implicates >80 conditions with autoimmunity (Rose 2001, 2002). In some instances, such as myocarditis, multiple sclerosis and rheumatoid arthritis, the autoimmune disease can be induced experimentally by administering self-antigen in the presence of adjuvant (cardiac myosin, myelin basic protein and collagen, respectively) (Rose 1997). There are two mechanisms related to infections induce autoimmunity:

"Molecular mimicry", an important mechanism often called to explain the association of infection with autoimmune disease that antigens (or more properly epitopes) of the microorganism closely resemble with self-antigens. The induction of an immune response to the microbial antigen results in cross-reaction with self antigens and induction of autoimmunity (Wucherpfennig 2001). Molecular mimicry (epitope-specific cross-reactivity between microbes and self-tissues) has successfully been shown in animal models, while it has not been clearly demonstrated to occur in human diseases (Olson et al. 2001, Rose and Mackay 2000).

"Bystander effect", another important mechanism stated that microorganisms expose self-antigens to the immune system by directly damaging tissues during an active infection (Horwitz et al. 1998, Tough et al. 1996). Nonetheless, whether pathogens mimic self-antigens, release sequestered self-antigens (or both), is still difficult to determine. Thus, antigen-specific mechanisms, nonspecific mechanisms could also lead to autoimmunity after infection (Fairweather et al. 2001, 2004).

The role of histamine in pathogenesis of autoimmune diseases was often questioned in the existing literature (Nielsen and Hammer 1992). In addition, also the mechanisms of histamine in induction of autoimmunity remain unclear, because of inadequate model systems and reagents. Recently, the gene encoding histamine receptor 1 (H1R) was identified as Bphs, which represents an autoimmune disease locus (Dy and Schneider 2004, Ma et al. 2002). H1R differs at 3 amino acid residues in autoimmune orchitis- and allergic encephalomyelitis-susceptible and resistant mice. Histamine induces increased proliferation and IFN-γ production in Th1 cells. Th2 cells express predominantly H2R, which acts as the negative regulator of proliferation and IL-4 and IL-13 production. Histamine enhances Th1-type responses by triggering H1R. T-cells from H1R-deficient mice produce significantly less severe autoimmune disease. Apparently, the IFN-γ inducing capacity of H1R on T-cells might play a role in tissue injury mechanisms of several other diseases of allergic, infectious, and autoimmune origin, as well as allograft rejection, whereas both Th1- and Th2-type responses are negatively regulated by H2R and suggests its role for peripheral tolerance (Akdis and Blaser 2003) (for more description kindly see Fig. 9.1).

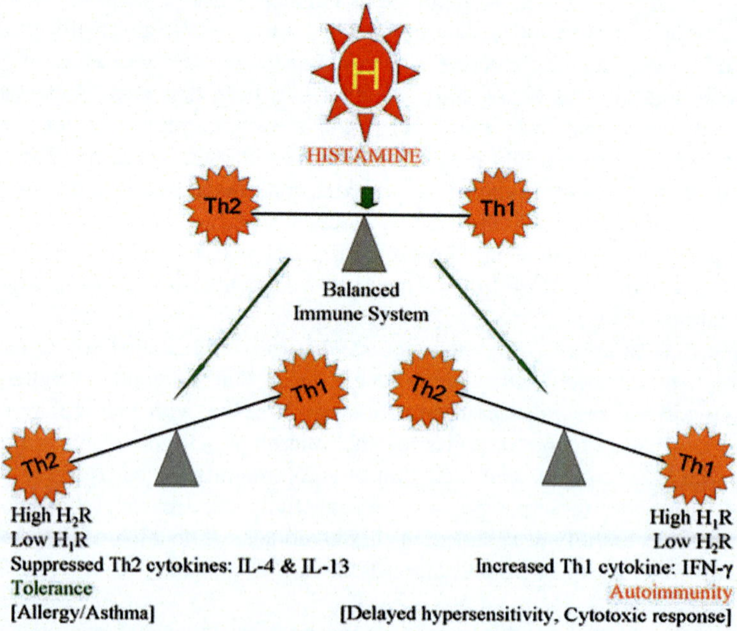

Fig. 9.1 Possible role of histamine in pathogenesis of autoimmune, allergic and infectious diseases as well as allograft rejection and peripheral tolerance

9.4 Immunobiological Role of Histamine in Life Threatening Diseases

9.4.1 Autoimmune Disorders

9.4.1.1 Chronic Urticaria

Urticaria (from latin urtica disica = stinging nettle) is the medical word for hives (pale red swellings of skin "wheals" that occur in groups on any part of the skin) (Sharma et al. 2004). A wheal consists of three features: (a) a central swelling of variable size, almost invariably surrounded by a reflex erythema, (b) associated itching or sometimes burning, (c) its fleeting nature with the skin returning to its normal appearance usually within 1–24 h (Zuberbier et al. 2001). Urticaria affects up to 25–30% of people at some time in their lives. However, being labeled as chronic urticaria (CU), if attacks occur at least twice a week for six weeks. It affects people of all races and is about twice as common in women as in men (Clive et al. 2002, Katelaris and Peake 2006, Sharma et al. 2004). Hives in urticaria are formed by blood plasma, causing the release of histamine from "mast cell" lie along the blood vessels in the skin (Sheikh 2005).

Urticaria is classified, based on its temporal evolution as acute (less than 6 weeks) or chronic (more than 6 weeks) for more details see Fig. 9.2. Urticaria

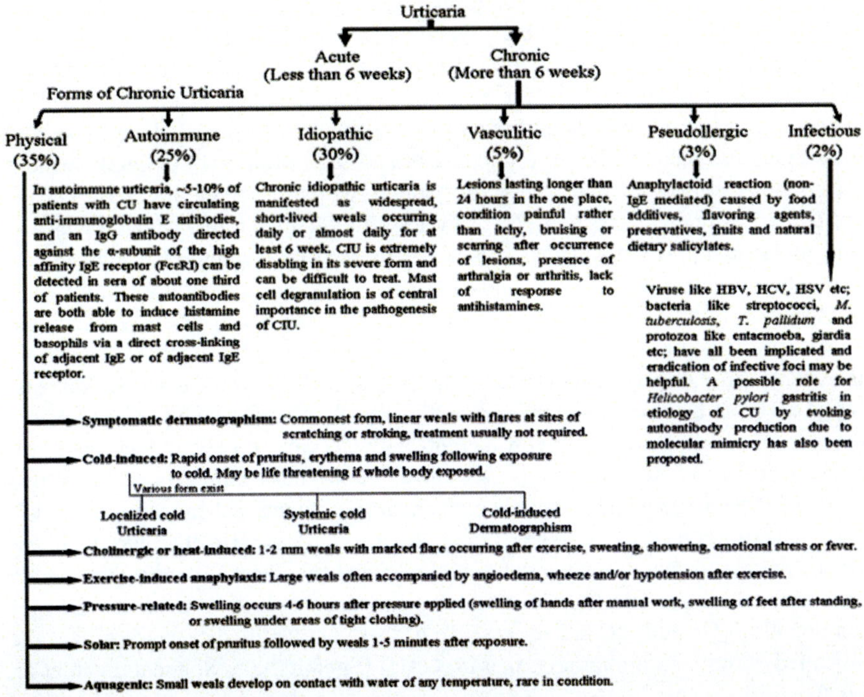

Fig. 9.2 Classification of urticaria

is often transient but can be chronic; there is no identifiable exogenous allergen in most forms of chronic urticaria (Champion 1990). It has been noted that intradermal injection of autologous serum elicits an immediate weal and flare response and mast cell degranulation in the majority of patients with CU (Grattan et al. 1990). It has been demonstrated that implicate an autoimmune mechanism (anti-IgE antibody) as the precipitating event in CU. IgM anti-IgE antibodies are found in cold urticaria, which suggests a pathogenic role for IgG (Hide et al. 1993, Lee et al. 2002). Recently, an increased incidence of anti-IgE and/or specific autoantibodies against the high affinity of IgE receptor (FcεRI) on mast cells has been demonstrated in the serum of patients with CU that mediate histamine release in vitro and in vivo (Grattan et al. 1991, Niimi et al. 1996), and suggest that anti-FcεRIα-antibody is relevant to the pathogenesis in some cases of severe CU (Sabroe and Greaves 1997, Tong et al. 1997).

Notably, it has been described that histamine-releasing autoantibodies are found in chronic idiopathic urticaria and suggested that these autoantibodies are important in the pathogenesis of CU by stimulating or facilitating degranulation of basophils and cutaneous mast cells through cross-linking cell surface IgE receptors (Grattan et al. 1991) in the existing literature. It is further reported that serum histamine releasing activity from patients with CU appears in an IgG-containing fraction of the serum, which may contain IgE in some cases, while another study noted that a large fraction of patients with CU have antibodies directed to functional FcεRIα and suggested that CU may be autoimmune in origin. It is also reported that histamine release from mast cells in CU is complement dependent (Ferrer et al. 1999, Riboldi et al. 2002, Tong et al. 1997). Thus; mast cells are considered to be the primary effector cells in CU by releasing a variety of inflammatory mediators, such as histamine, prostaglandins, leukotriene, tryptase, interleukin (IL)-1, IL-6, IL-8, and tumor necrosis factor (TNF)-α (Bradding et al. 1992, Moller et al. 1993). A more recent study suggested that sera from patients with CU containing anti-FcεRIα-antibody release mediators and TNF-α by activating human foreskin mast cells, and this release can play a pathogenic role in CU by activating endothelial cells, in part due to the actions of tumor necrosis factor-α from mast cells (Lee et al. 2002).

Recently, the frequency of autoantibodies to FcεRIα in CU has been estimated at 30–50% (Sheikh 2005). Autoantibodies to FcεRIα can be functional, meaning that, they can cause histamine release from basophils in vitro, evidence increasingly suggests that such autoantibodies are also functional in vivo. Considerable evidence that the serum from many patients with CU can cause an immediate autologous wheal and flare response (i.e. a positive autologous serum skin test), and that many of these patients have evidence of circulating functional immunoglobulin-G (IgG) autoantibodies to the high affinity IgE receptor, FcεRIα, the current mainstream thought is that in such patients the IgG autoantibodies are causing the visible urticarial skin lesions. In CU the autoantibodies, causing histamine release are predominantly IgG1 and IgG3. The presence of these autoantibodies characterizes the so-called chronic autoimmune urticaria (CAU) (Sheikh 2005, Soundararajan et al. 2005).

Drug Treatment of Chronic Urticaria

1st line treatment: Antihistamine, H1R and H2R blockers, depending on severity of the urticaria.
2nd line treatment: Corticosteroids and Anti-leukotrienes.
3rd line treatment: Immunomodulators (cyclosporine, methotrixate) (Muller 2004). Kindly see Fig. 9.3 for more details.

9.4.1.2 Atopic Dermatitis

Atopic dermatitis (AD) or atopic eczema is a chronic relapsing pruritic skin disease with a high incidence in the first year of life. AD can persist into childhood, symptoms usually remit by puberty. AD is characterized by two phases:1st phase with

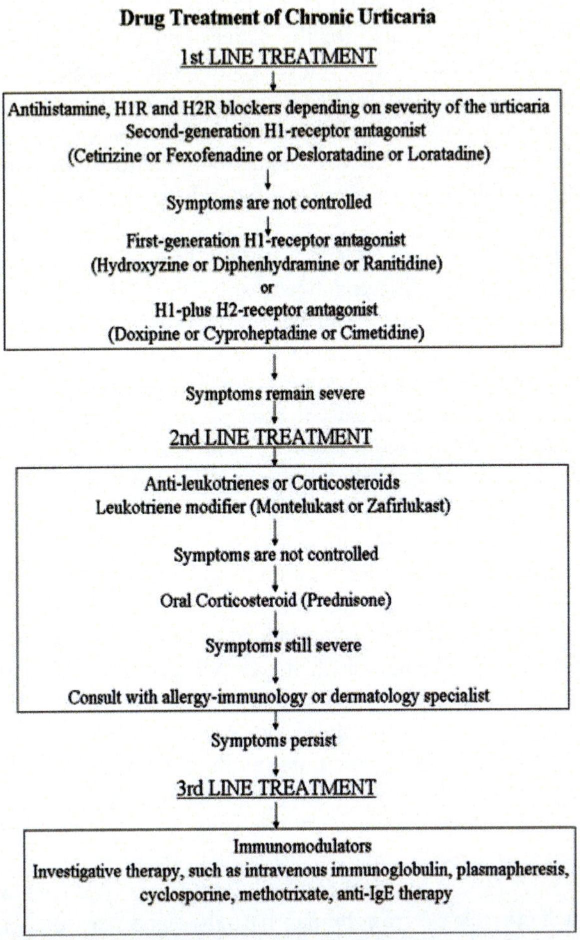

Fig. 9.3 Diagnosis of chronic urticaria

acute lesions predominated by Th2 cytokines (IL-4, IL-5 and IL-13), 2nd phase that is associated with eczematous chronic atopic dermatitis lesions by Th1 cytokine (INF-γ and IL-12). AD can also be present in adults and affects more than 10% of the total population, with 80–90% of those affected being children under 5 years of age in Western population (Sehra et al. 2008). AD often regarded as a cutaneous form of atopy, as a result 50–80% of children with AD will develop asthma or allergic rhinitis by 5 years of age later in life and the high serous concentration of IgE (Di Tullio 2001). This temporal progression of atopic symptoms from AD to allergic sensitization of the skin, food allergy, hay fever (allergic rhinitis) and later airway hyperresponsiveness and airway inflammation or asthma, has been named the "allergic march" (Gustafsson et al. 2000, Spergel and Paller 2003).

In AD, the skin becomes extremely itchy. Scratching leads to redness, swelling, cracking, "weeping" clear fluid, and finally crusting and scaling. It is frequently perceived as a minor dermatological disorder. However, the high prevalence of this condition carries financial and social cost not only for the community, regarding medical and hospital cost but also for the patient and the patient's family (Kemp 2003). In AD, inflammation results from interactions of immune cells (T cells [Th1 and Th2], dendritic cells (langerhans dendritic cells and inflammatory dendritic epidermal cells), mast cells and eosinophils) and kerotinocytes. The complex picture of the AD lesion is aggravated by environmental and genetic factors that increase the difficulty of understanding the mechanisms behind this complex pathology (Sehra et al. 2008).

It has been documented that patients suffering from AD exhibit IgE autoreactivity to human patients. These autoantigens are expressed in a variety of cell and tissue types. The increasing evidence showed that IgE autoreactivity, as well as other autoimmune phenomena frequently occur in atopic dermatitis and may be associated with severity of disease. Moreover, it has been shown that autosensitization can induce a mixed Th2/Th1 autoimmunity in mice similar to that observed in AD. All these findings points to a possible role for IgE autoreactivity in the pathogenesis of AD. Several mechanisms of IgE autoimmunity may contribute to the pathogenesis of AD (Mittermann et al. 2004).

Histamine released primarily from mast cells, has been implicated as an important mediator in immediate allergic inflammatory reactions. However, its role in chronic inflammatory dermatoses such as pathogens of AD is much less clear. Marone et al. (1987) showed that basophils from children with AD were hyperreactive and release more histamine than basophils from unaffected individuals. However, in adults the evidence is less conclusive (Stephan et al. 1989). Bull et al. (1993) showed that basophils from adults with AD release the same amount of histamine as, but less leukotriene C4 than, basophils of unaffected adults and further demonstrated that increased basophil release of histamine do not play a role for itch and erythema of atopic dermatitis in adults. However, anti-IgE antibodies have been detected in serum of patients with atopic dermatitis (Quinti et al. 1986). In addition to this, Marone et al. (1989) has documented that IgG anti-IgE from a patient with AD induced mediator release from human basophils and mast cells isolated from skin and lung parenchyma, and provided evidence that the releasing activity of IgG anti-IgE autoantibody in patients with AD resides in the IgG fraction and is directed against epitope(s) present on human IgE. However, these observations showed an excellent correlation between the histamine releasing activity of rabbit anti-IgE and naturally occurring human IgG anti-IgE that might have a clinical relevance in some patients with AD.

Drug Treatment of Atopic Dermatitis

Multifunctional antihistamines or 3rd generation "antiallergic" drugs appear to offer a variety of advantages beyond their ability to inhibit histamine release, such as inhibition of mediator release and interference with eosinophil migration (Hanifin 1990).

9.4.1.3 Autoimmune Myocardium

It is well known that histamine is a mediator of the immediate hypersensitivity reaction of the heart and plays an important role as a modulator of immune. The contribution of anaphylactic reaction of the heart has been documented and during immunologic reaction endogenous histamine is released from the heart. The heart exposed during the immune response to low concentration of histamine showed modification in automaticity and contractility. The contractile effect of histamine, as well as the H1R population and H2R-mediated cAMP production were measured in cardiac tissue from control normal and autoimmune myocarditis mice (Goren et al. 1994).

The histaminergic H1Rs with distinct high and low affinity binding sites were characterized by the specific H1R-antagonist [3H]mepyramine in autoimmune myocardium and notably demonstrated that no saturable binding of the radiolabelled H1R-antagonist was observed in normal myocardium. Furthermore, it has been reported that the reaction of autoimmune myocardium with specific H1R-agonist [2-thiazolylethylamine (ThEA)] triggered positive inotropy and negative chronotropy, which were inhibited by mepyramine. Inhibitors of phospholipase C and protein kinase C attenuated both the inotropic and chronotropic effects of ThEA, suggesting the participation of phosphoinositide hydrolysis in this phenomenon, and it was verified by measurement of polyphosphoinositide hydrolysis in autoimmune myocardium following the reaction of ThEA with histaminergic H1Rs. Thus, it has concluded that functional H1Rs could involve a distinctive mechanism operating in autoimmune myocardium as a result of cardiac antigen immunization (Goren et al. 1993).

Histamine triggered positive chronotropy and negative inotropy at high concentrations in both control and autoimmune auricles, H2Rs being the most important mediator of these responses. In contrast, in atria from autoimmune myocarditis mice, histamine at lower concentrations caused positive inotropy and negative chronotropy. These effects, not verified in the normal control atria, are mediated by H1Rs (Goren et al. 1994). The expression of H2Rs and H1Rs mediating the cardiac response to histamine was evaluated through histamine-stimulated cAMP level and binding of [3H]mephyramine respectively, and both control and autoimmune myocardium were able to increase cAMP levels, an effect that was inhibited by H2R-antagonist drug. The amount of cAMP was significantly higher in control myocardium than in those from autoimmune myocardium with distinct high and low affinity binding sites. In control myocardium non-saturable binding was detected. These results are suggested that H1Rs and H2Rs coexist in heart from autoimmune myocarditis mice, whereas only H2Rs are present in myocardium from control mice and the presence of H1Rs in autoimmune myocardium could be important factor in the regulation of its physiological behavior (Goren et al. 1994).

9.4.1.4 Multiple Sclerosis and Experimental Autoimmune Encephalomyelitis

Multiple sclerosis (MS) is an incurable chronic inflammatory disease of the central nervous system (CNS) that predominantly affects young adults, has a high socio-economic impact, which increases as disability progresses. Experimental autoimmune encephalomyelitis (EAE) and its human disease counterpart, MS, are considered to be $CD4^+$ T-cell mediated autoimmune diseases affecting the CNS. EAE can be induced in many species by active immunization with myelin antigen. The classic encephalitogenic antigen is myelin basic protein (MBP), the first to be identified. Other myelin and non-myelin antigen were also shown to induce EAE. Several lines of indirect evidence suggest that mast cells could also play a role in the pathogenesis of both MS and EAE. Mast cell-derived histamine, serotonine, kallikreins and TNF-α can enhance micro-vascular permeability, leukocyte rolling, adhesion and extravasation of inflammatory cells into the brain and spinal cord. In the animal model of MS, EAE, mediated by Th1 cells, histamine receptor 1 and 2 (H1R and H2R) are present on inflammatory cells in brain lesions. Th1 cells reactive to myelin proteolipid protein expressed more H1R and less H2R compared with Th2 cells (Musio et al. 2006, Steinman and Zamvil 2003, Zamvil and Steinman 2003, Lock et al. 2002).

$CD4^+$ T helper cells reactive to myelin, which produce proinflammatory cytokines, such as IFN-γ, osteopontin, and TNF, are known to play a key role in pathogenesis and progression (Steinman 2003). $CD4^+$ Th1 cells mediate demyelination in MS, but how they become sensitized and enter the brain to induce brain inflammation remains obscure. Recent observations suggest that EAE elicit, in the same subjects, not only Th1- but also Th2-associated immune responses (Pedotti et al. 2001, 2003a, b). Th2 cytokines associated with allergic disorders have recently been implicated in MS, while genes upregulated in MS plaques include the mast cell-specific tryptase, the IgE receptor (FcεRI), and H1R. Histamine has been shown to influence T cell polarization by having effects that favor the development of a Th2 response (Idzko et al. 2002), whereas in polarized T cells, depending on the receptor engaged, histamine can promote Th1 responses through H1R and downregulate both Th1 and Th2 responses through H2R (Jutel et al. 2001). These evidences suggest that histamine influences the development of EAE. Blockade of histamine with H1R antagonists has been shown to reduce the pathological change associated with EAE (Dimitriadou et al. 2000), and inhibition of early-phase EAE has been reported in either H1R or H2R knockout mice (Ma et al. 2002, Teuscher et al. 2004). Histamine receptors were shown to be expressed in EAE. H1R and H2R are expressed on mononuclear cells within the inflammatory foci in the brains of mice with EAE (Pedotti et al. 2003a). The H1R gene was over expressed in the chronic plaques of MS patients at autopsy (Dimitriadou et al. 2000). Interestingly Bphs, a gene controlling the susceptibility to EAE and other autoimmune diseases, has been recently reported to be H1R (Ma et al. 2002). These evidences show that histamine has significant role in the development of EAE and that blockade of specific histamine receptors (HRs), such as H1R or H2R, can ameliorate EAE. However, the influence of histamine on EAE during the chronic phase has not yet been established. Recently, Ohtsu (2008) has used $HDC^{-/-}$ mice to investigate the role of endogenous histamine in the development and progression of EAE and demonstrated that myelin oligodendrocyte glycoprotein- (MOG) 35–55-induced chronic EAE is more severe in a setting of profound histamine deficiency. MOG 35-55-reactive T cells from $HDC^{-/-}$ mice produced more IFN-γ, TNF, MCP-1, and leptin compared with $HDC^{+/+}$ mice. The CNS inflammatory infiltrates that develop in the brain parenchyma in $HDC^{-/-}$ mice are more diffuse, with a large component of polymorphonuclear leukocytes and eosinophils.

9.4.2 Allergic Disorders

9.4.2.1 Allergic Rhinitis

Allergic rhinitis has been characterized by itching, sneezing, rhinorrhea, and nasal obstruction. Perennial allergic rhinitis can be distinguished from non-allergic, non-infectious forms of rhinitis [idiopathic (vasomotor) rhinitis, non-allergic rhinitis with eosinophilia syndrome, hormonal rhinitis, drug-stimulated rhinitis, and food-induced rhinitis]. The treatment of allergic diseases (allergic rhinitis) consists of allergen avoidance, anti allergic medication, and immunotherapy for specific allergens which is known as desensitization or hyposensitization. Recently, the drugs commonly used to treat allergic rhinitis are antihistamines (histamine antagonists) and anticholinergic agents for the relief of symptoms and corticosteroids to suppress allergic inflammation. H1R-antagonists (loratadine, cetirizine, and fexofenadine) are less sedating and more pharmacologically selective than earlier antihistamines. Some H1R-antagonists (cetirizine) block allergen-sensitized infiltration of tissue by eosinophils, an influence that may be independent of their impacts on H1R (Slater et al. 1999).

Specific immunotherapy, which has been used for the treatment of allergic diseases for nearly 100 years, consists of administering increasing concentrations of extracts of allergen over a long period. The mode of action of specific immunotherapy is complex. IgG "blocking" antibodies compete with IgE for allergen. They may also prevent the aggregation of complexes of IgE and the α chain of the high affinity IgE receptor (FcεRIα) on mast cells by altering the steric conformation. In addition, they may interfere with antigen trapping by IgE bound to antigen-presenting cells. Several studies have shown that specific immunotherapy inhibits the release of pharmacologic mediators (histamine) from mast cells and basophils, prevents infiltration of allergic lesions by inflammatory cells, and decreases the number of mast cells in tissue (Kay 2001).

9.4.2.2 Anaphylaxis (Acute)

Anaphylaxis is a severe, systemic allergic reaction caused by the systemic release of histamine and other pharmacologic mediators. It comprises a constellation of symptoms, of which the most serious are laryngeal edema, lower-airway obstruction, and hypotension. The common causes of anaphylaxis are IgE mediated sensitivity to foods (e.g., peanuts, nuts, fish, shellfish, and dairy products), bee and wasp stings, drugs, and latex. Treatment of anaphylaxis involves prompt administration of epinephrine, repeated if necessary, since epinephrine reverses the actions of histamine within minutes. This treatment can be followed by an H1R-antagonist and corticosteroids. Preloaded epinephrine syringes are available for self-administration (Kay 2001).

9.4.2.3 Asthma

Asthma comprises episodes of wheezy breathlessness due to airway narrowing, which is partially or totally reversible. Airway hyperresponsiveness is almost invariably an accompanying feature. Causes of asthma depend on the interplay between genetic factors, the environment, and several specific and nonspecific triggers (Kay 2001). Nevertheless, most patients with asthma are atopic, although a minority has intrinsic, nonatopic asthma that often has a later onset and a more protracted course than atopic asthma. Recent studies indicate that there are more similarities than differences in the airway abnormalities of atopic and nonatopic asthma (Humbert et al. 1999). Both variants are characterized by tissue infiltration by eosinophils and activated T cells and increased production of interleukin-4, interleukin-5, interleukin-13, and CC chemokines. In both types, there are similar numbers of bronchial mucosal cells that contain messenger RNA for the ε germ-line transcript (Iε) and ε heavy chain of IgE (Cε) (Humbert et al. 1999). This suggests that intrinsic asthma may be associated with local production of IgE antibodies against unknown antigens and that immunologic triggers have a role in both nonatopic and atopic asthma (Kay 2001).

Inhaled and intravenous histamine cause bronchoconstriction as one of the first recognized properties of histamine, which is inhibited by H1R antagonists. Antigen induced IgE-mediated mast cell degranulation in the lung causes an increase in both cAMP and cyclic guanosine monophosphate (cGMP) (Platshon and Kaliner 1978). The rise in cGMP is blocked by H1R-antihistamines, suggesting that this effect is mediated by H1R. Histamine stimulates phosphoinositide hydrolysis (Grandordy and Barnes 1987), increases the concentration of inositol-1,4,5-triphosphate, and increases intracellular Ca^{2+} (Hardy et al. 1996). Histamine contracts both the central and peripheral airways in vitro, with a more potent effect on peripheral airways. As a manifestation of airway hyper reactivity, asthmatic individuals are more sensitive to the bronchoconstrictor effect of histamine than normal individuals. Although several studies suggested a basal tone of smooth muscle mediated by histamine binding to H1R, currently constitutive intrinsic activity of H1R without any occupation by histamine could be more relevant. Histamine induces proliferation of cultured airway smooth muscle cells (Panettieri et al. 1990). A difference in histamine response between species has been reported and indicating a role for H2R-mediated bronchodilatation in cats, rats, rabbits, sheep, and horses (Chand and Eyre 1975). However, in human subjects H2R-antihistamines, such as cimetidine and ranitidine, do not cause bronchoconstriction in normal or asthmatic individuals (Thomson and Kerr 1980, White et al. 1987). Although there is no direct evidence that it plays a role in disease pathogenesis, H2R-mediated gastric secretion is impaired in asthma (Gonzales and Ahmed 1986). Rather, a beneficial effect of H2R-antihistamines given for the treatment of gastritis was observed in asthma (Field and Sutherland 1998). Recent studies suggested that histamine might play significant role in the modulation of the cytokine network in the lung through H2R, H3R and H4R, which are expressed in distinct cells and cell subsets (Sirois et al. 2000). Apparently, in the same signaling patterns, β2-adrenergic receptors might function similar to H2R in human subjects (Benovic 2002). Recently discovered, H4R has given new tools to several researchers to further address the function of histamine and its receptors in asthma. H4R expression and function on mast cells, eosinophils, basophils, dendritic cells and T cells, all suggest its role in the asthmatic response (Benovic 2002). As the clinically used H1R-antagonists have little, if any, affinity for the H4R, clinical information obtained using these compounds would not be predictive of the role for H4R in asthma (Venable and Thurmond 2006). Indeed, the circumstantial evidence for a role of histamine in asthma, along with the general lack of clinical efficacy of H1R ligands in the disease may suggest involvement of the H4R. Although there are no reports of human studies with H4R antagonists, the receptor does appear to play a role in a mouse model of asthma. As for H1R, H4R-knock-out mice or those given H4R antagonists during sensitization have reduced lung inflammation and a reduction in Th2 and inflammatory cytokines (Dunford et al. 2006). There is a reduction in antigen-specific antibody responses, which suggests a role for H4Rs in the initial priming of the immune system. However, in contrast to some of the H1R antagonists, H4R antagonists given during the allergen challenge phase of the model are equally effective to those given during sensitization (Dunford et al. 2006). The effect was seen at both the sensitization and challenge phase of the model appear to be due to a crucial role for H4Rs on dendritic cells in the proper education or priming of Th2-type T cells. Restimulation of splenocytes or lymphocytes showed a reduction in Th2 and inflammatory cytokines upon blocking H4R activation, but no effect on proliferation (Dunford et al. 2006). In vivo effects of H4R antagonists were independent of mast cells, showing that these cells were not the source of histamine in this model (Benovic 2002). In vitro data were suggested that histamine production by dendritic cells may be important in activating H4Rs; however recent data have also suggested that neutrophils may be a major source of histamine in lung (Xu et al. 2006). The dual H4R/H2R agonist, 4-methylhistamine, has been demonstrated to reduce airway hyperreactivity and inflammation when given by an inhaled route in a similar mouse model of asthma, which is thought to be due to the recruitment of regulatory T cells (Benovic 2002).

Although evidence exists for a role of histamine in driving asthmatic responses, there is little evidence for clinical efficacy of H1R antagonists in the management of the disease. However, their use at high doses or early in the disease history to prevent progression is supported by recent animal data and may be warranted. Furthermore, H4Rs may account for other functions of histamine that are not blocked by H1Rs. H4R antagonists may prove beneficial for the relief of asthma symptoms and could perhaps work in synergy with H1R antagonists (Benovic 2002). The role of histamine and other redundant G-protein-coupled receptors in the regulation of immune-inflammatory pathways in the lung remain to be intensely focused in future studies.

9.4.3 Inflammatory Disease

9.4.3.1 Atherosclerosis

Macrophages, which are present in all stages of atherosclerosis, increase in number during the disease progression. The number of macrophages located in atheromatous plaque is much greater than that of mast cells, especially at the shoulder region of the lipid core. Recently it has been demonstrated that a histamine-producing enzyme HDC, is highly expressed macrophages in human atherosclerotic lesion (Higuchi et al. 2001, Sasaguri and Tanimoto 2004). The mode of secretion of histamine from monocytes/macrophages is not only by degranulation, the regional histamine derived from macrophages may be relatively low in concentration but longer lasting in duration. Macrophage-derived histamine chronically participates in the pathogenesis of atherosclerosis. While mast cells are known as a source of histamine, monocytes/macrophages also express histamine receptors (Higuchi et al. 2001, Tanimoto et al. 2001), and suggesting the presence of an auto-and/or paracrine network in relation to the monocytic function. Futhermore, HDC is a rate-limiting enzyme and histamine production from macrophages is mainly regulated by HDC expression (Zwadlo-Klarwasser et al. 1998). The difference in histamine biology between mast cells and macrophages stimulate several investigators to research the molecular mechanisms of the gene regulation of HDC and HRs in monocytes/macrophages and role of histamine in atherosclerosis.

Histamine functions via its noble receptors, determining the expression of receptors in atherosclerotic lesion is important for understanding the histamine role in atherogenesis. Histological localization of H1R in human atherogenesis lesion has shown that human H1R mRNA is located in atherosclerosis (Takagishi et al. 1995). Human H1R-mRNA was expressed in the macrophages, smooth muscle cells (SMCs) and endothelial cells (ECs) in atheromatous plaque, demonstrated by using the in situ hybridization technique. Human monocytes/macrophages, in in vitro experiments, express both human H1R- and H2R-mRNA, and the expression profile of HRs has been shown to be switched from H2R to H1R during macrophages differentiation (Tanimoto et al. 2001). On the contrary, SMCs express only human H1R, which is up-regulated by platelet-derived growth factor-BB (Takagishi et al. 1995, Tanimoto et al. 2001). Since monocytes/macrophages produce histamine through increased expression of HDC, the auto/paracrine pathway of histamine in monocytes/macrophages may be able to have a central role in the histamine contribution to atherosclerosis (Sasaguri and Tanimoto 2004).

Antihistamine drugs (histamine-antagonists) could be used as therapeutic agents for atherosclerosis and several evidences as support this expectation.

(a) HDC deficient mice showing reduced intimal thickening after ligation and cuffing experiments (Sasaguri et al. 2005).
(b) H1R-antagonist mepylamine inhibiting calcium influx induced by histamine in vascular smooth muscular cells (Satoh et al. 1994).
(c) H1R and H2R antagonist preventing the intimal thickening in the femoral arteries of mice, which have been induced by a photochemical reaction between localized irradiation by green light and intravenously administered rose bengal (Miyazawa et al. 1998).

Although a variety of antihistamine drugs are already available on the market, while using such drugs for the treatment of atherosclerosis is feasible. Selective histidine decarboxylase inhibitors (e.g., α-fluoromethylhistidine) might be useful agents for the preventive and/or treatment of atherosclerosis, because both H1R and H2R antagonists act to prevent the thickening of intima (Miyazawa et al. 1998). Newly identified histamine receptors (H3R and H4R) might be potential targets for the treatment of atherosclerotic diseases in future, and may attract several investigators for potential research in atherosclerotic diseases.

9.4.4 Malignant Diseases

9.4.4.1 Allergy-Cancer an Important Relation and Role of Allergic Agent "Histamine" in Cancer

The relation of allergy and cancer has enhanced the interest in immunology of cancer (Carrozzi and Viegi 2005). An association between allergic-related disorder and cancer development has been the subject of epidemiological studies. Both positive and negative associations have been observed and two contradictory hypotheses have been proposed to explain the relationship between allergic conditions and malignancies. First, *the immune surveillance hypothesis*, which proposes that allergic conditions may lead to a decreased risk of malignancy by enhancing the ability of the immune system to detect and eliminate malignant cells, and second *the antigenic stimulation hypothesis*, states that immune-stimulating conditions lead to an increased risk of malignancy (Carrozzi and Viegi 2005, Söderberg et al.

2004). Previous studies (all are concerned asthma only) lend support to the antigenic stimulation hypothesis for hematological malignancies, as increased risk, or tendencies toward increased risks, were found for a history of allergy (Eriksson et al. 1995, Kallen et al. 1993, Mills et al. 1992, Talbot-Smith et al. 2003), whereas some of them support the immune surveillance hypothesis by showing decreased risks (Kallen et al. 1993, Vesterinen et al. 1993). Söderberg et al. (2004) demonstrated that allergic conditions, like asthma and hay fever, are increasing and it is of great importance to clarify if and how they are connected to hematological malignancies. The contradictory findings may have many explanations, e.g. that different immunological mechanisms may be involved in different types of asthma, that the pathogenesis is likely to be different even in seemingly similar hematological malignancies, and that new forms of pharmacological therapy may influence not only the outcome of asthma but also the risk of developing cancer. To solve these problems, large prospective epidemiological studies on individuals with clinically strictly defined allergic conditions, including data on pharmacological treatment and severity of disease, need to be combined with information about morphologically defined hematological malignancies, including subtyping with techniques from modern molecular biology. In their recent findings, they have demonstrated that chronic antigenic stimulation from allergic conditions might increase the risk of some hematological malignancies (Söderberg et al. 2004). However, there is an important main question-is allergy a "risk" or a "protective" factor for cancer?-appears now well outlined, but far to be solved (Carrozzi and Viegi 2005). As the immune system may be the last line of defense against cancer development (as defense mechanisms existing in different stages of carcinogenesis- such as detoxification of metabolites coming from environmental carcinogens, trapping or decomposition of reactive oxygen species, DNA repair enzymes, natural inhibitors of proliferating initiated cells, etc.) (Carrozzi and Viegi 2005). The association between allergic conditions and cancer risk is in all probability complex and the risk of developing a neoplasm could depend both on the type of allergic condition and on the type of tumor (Carrozzi and Viegi 2005). Results from the existing literature still appear inconsistent or contradictory. Cancer immuno-epidemiology will hopefully clarify the role of immunity in protecting the host from nascent transformed cells and in regulating inflammatory response to pathogens, and it will provide reliable estimation of cancer risk for individuals with different immunological competences (Carrozzi and Viegi 2005).

Histamine has been implicated as one of the mediators involved in regulation of proliferation in both normal and neoplastic tissue (Haak-Frendscho et al. 2000). The concentration of local histamine in proliferating tissues compared with that in immediate hypersensitivity ("allergic") reaction is relatively low, its effectiveness acting on the autocrine and paracrine way is strongly implicated and a growth-factor-like activity of histamine (malignant growth with the level of histamine production) has been described (Tilly et al. 1990). Exogenously added histamine not only stimulates DNA synthesis and cell division but also evokes a chemotactic response in human Hela and A431 carcinoma cells and A875 melanoma cells. These novel actions of histamine are mediated by the H1R that triggers the hydrolysis of phosphoinositides with consequent formation of various second messengers, and suggests that histamine may have a novel role in the migration and proliferation of H1R-bearing (tumor) cells (Tilly et al. 1990). Highly increased histamine biosynthesis and content has been reported in different human and experimental neoplasias, such as in breast carcinomas and adenocarcinomas (Haak-Frendscho et al. 2000). In vitro and in vivo experiments using histamine receptor-antagonists (Van der van et al. 1993, Watson et al. 1993) have demonstrated that histamine acts through the specific histamine membrane receptors (H1-, H2-, and H3-) and may regulate tumor growth and development (Cricco et al. 1993) in a paracrine or autocrine manner. Moreover, the most compelling evidence supporting a significant role for histamine in gastric and colorectal carcinomas are the results of clinical trials showing increased survival of gastric cancer patients after treatment with cimetidine, H2R-antagonist (Haak-Frendscho et al. 2000). In addition to promoting the proliferation of tumor cells, increased histamine levels have potent immunosuppressive effects that favor tumor cell growth by blunting natural killer activity and activating the suppressor function of T cells (Haak-Frendscho et al. 2000). Expression of the HDC gene in melanoma cell lines is approximately one-tenth that of the basophilic cell line KU-812F as determined by competitive RT-PCR (Haak-Frendscho et al. 2000). An increased HDC activity has been measured in human colorectal tumor specimens and the inhibitory effects of α-fluoromethyl-histidine, a suicide inhibitor of HDC has been demonstrated in tumor models (Garcia-Caballero et al. 1988, Haak-Frendscho et al. 2000). However, in human melanoma, histamine level as detected by high performance liquid chromatography, was elevated (Reynolds et al. 1996). Recently, it has been demonstrated that HDC immunoreactivity in all of the melanoma cell lines were tested. This immunoreactivity was corresponded to the presence of HDC m-RNA, as assessed by RT-PCR and neucleotide sequencing, as well as by in situ hybridization. These findings demonstrated that human primary and metastatic melanoma tissues from surgical samples was HDC immunoreactive, and further suggested that HDC immunoreactivity (indicating local (autocrine or paracrine rather than type I like “allergic”) action of histamine) may be useful as clinical correlate for melanoma staging (Haak-Frendscho et al. 2000).

A very recent study, examined the effect of H2R-antagonists and exogenous histamine on growth of malignant melanoma implant in mice, and they administered H2R-antagonists to B16BL6 malignant-melanoma-implanted syngeneic mice, and measured the tumor volume. Their results demonstrated that both roxatidine and cimetidine (H2R-antagonist) suppressed growth of B16BL6 implant compared with control (Tomita et al. 2005). On the other hand, systemically administered histamine stimulated growth of B16BL6 implants. Furthermore, they demonstrated that the histamine-stimulated B16BL6 implant growth was suppressed by co-administration of cimetidine (H2R-antagonist) in a dose-dependent manner. However, H2R-antagonists were not responsible to affect in vitro proliferation of B16BL6 cells. They suggested that both endogenous and exogenous histamine have ability to stimulate growth of malignant melanoma implants *via* H2Rs expressed in host cells (Söderberg et al. 2004).

9.4.4.2 Malignant Melanoma

Malignant melanoma is a well-known life-threatening tumor (with a high rate of metastasis and strong malignant potential). Recently, the immune response against melanoma was compromised through multiple escape mechanisms of the tumor, which have been uncovered partially via thorough immunological and molecular analyses. These analyses were documented by gene-expression profiling. It has been suggested that melanoma-derived histamine should be included as a significant factor participated in bi-directional interactions between the tumor tissue and infiltrating immune cells. Notably, the presence and activity of histamine has been demonstrated to be relevant by directly stimulating or suppressing growth of the melanoma (i.e. depending on the local histamine receptor balance) and indirectly shifting the local T-cell polarization towards a predominance of Th2 cells (Falus et al. 2001).

Surprisingly, an ambivalent, double-faced nature of histamine on the growth of melanoma is shown by the contrasting effect of signals through H1- and H2-receptors. The net outcome of direct effects (mediated by histamine + H1- or H2-receptor-specific antagonists, or receptor-selective agonists) suggests that in melanoma cells, histamine acting through the H1R decreases cell proliferation, whereas it enhances growth when acting through H2Rs (Brandes et al. 1991, Hegyesi et al. 2001, Reynolds et al. 1996). In vitro, a strong antiproliferative effect of HDC-specific antisense oligonucleotides on metastatic melanoma cell lines expressing elevated numbers of H2Rs has been detected (Hegyesi et al. 2001), simultaneous with the decreased amount of immunopositive HDC protein. The results suggest that translational blockade of HDC, mediated by antisense oligonucleotides, inhibits the otherwise stimulatory capacity of locally produced histamine. A similar conclusion is drawn when the enzymatic activity of HDC is inhibited by irreversible binding of α fluoro-methyl histidine. This suggests that the actual number and availability of H1Rs and H2Rs, their relative ratio and actual local balance are key factors that determine whether local histamine stimulates or suppresses growth of the melanoma. Various antihistamines might shift this local balance and enhance or impair the local efficacy of endogenous histamine on the growth of melanoma and its malignant phenotype (Falus et al. 2001). This fact suggests a possible, newly recognized role for histamine receptor antagonists in the treatment of melanoma. The investigation is necessary to reveal or exclude unexpected side-effects of HRs-antagonists on melanoma growth. After xenotransplantation of a human melanoma-cell line into severe combined immunodeficient (SCID) mice, growth of the tumor was prevented by the systemic application of H2R antagonist, resulting in a significantly elevated survival rate of melanoma grafted mice (Falus et al. 2001). The histological analysis of melanoma grafts in antihistamine-treated mice revealed massive infiltration of interferon (IFN)-producing host (murine) macrophages into the human melanoma xenograft. It has suggested that, in addition to the direct effect of histamine on tumor growth (depending on the type and balance of HRs on melanoma cells), histamine influences locally the competent immune cells (Falus et al. 2001). The newly discovered, HRs (H3R and H4R) might be potential tool for further investigation the pathology of malignant melanoma.

9.5 Conclusions and Future Prospects

Histamine receptors have been an important drug targets for many years to regulate several diseases. Their physiological and pathological relevance and distribution in various tissues are being documented, while the exact role of histamine receptors in immunobiology is still unclear. Histamine role in cytokines and antibodies generation profile over a span of time are still unclear or lacking in existing literatures in several chronic diseases. The scope of histamine research has been implicated in immune responses of both the Th1 and Th2 lymphocytes. The newly discovered H4-receptor, play an important role in inflammation and has opened a new way for the functions of histamine in inflammation, allergy and autoimmune diseases. The data on the role of H3- and H4-receptors on immune regulation are limited. Due to lack of immunomodulatory researches on H3- and H4-receptors, we planned ongoing studies to find out immunomodulatory and immunoregulatory role using specific histamine receptors (H1, H2, H3 and H4)-antagonists and agonists that showing T cell and B cell activation. Thus, there is indeed urgent need to redouble efforts both in vivo and in vitro study on histamine, histamine receptors and their role in immunoregulation and immunomodulation on cytokines and antibodies network in immune response that are potentially harmful to generate allergic/autoimmune diseases and to search for important beneficial role to pursue novel strategies to cope with diagnosis and treatment of allergies and autoimmune diseases.

Acknowledgments Trivendra Tripathi acknowledges University Grants Commission, New Delhi, India for providing UGC Fellowship [UGC letter DON F. 19-33/2006 (CU)] and M. Shahid is grateful to Department of Science and Technology, Ministry of Science and Technology, Government of India for awarding "Young Scientist Project Award" (FT/SR-L-111/2006).

References

Akdis CA, Blaser K (2003) Histamine in the immune regulation of allergic inflammation. J Allergy Clin Immunol 112:15–22

Barger G, Dale HH (1910) The presence in ergot and physiological activity of B-iminazoylethylamine. J Physiol Paris 40:38–40

Benovic J (2002) Novel β2-adrenergic receptor signaling pathways. J Allergy Clin Immunol 110:S229–S235

Bradding P, Feather IH, Howarth PH et al (1992) Interleukin 4 is localized to and released by human mast cells. J Exp Med 176:1381–1386

Brandes LJ et al (1991) Enhanced cancer growth in mice administered daily human equivalent doses of some H1-antihistamines: predictive *in vitro* correlates. J Natl Cancer Inst 86: 770–775

Bull HA, Courtney PF, Bunker CB et al (1993) Basophil mediator release in atopic dermatitis. J Invest Dermatol 100:305–309

Carrozzi L, Viegi G (2005) Allergy and cancer: a biological and epidemiological rebus. Allergy 60:1095–1097

Champion RH (1990) A practical approach to urticarial syndromes dermatologist's view. Clin Exp Allergy 20:221–224

Chand N, Eyre P (1975) Classification and biological distribution of histamine receptor sub-types. Agents Actions 5:277–295

Clive EH, Ruth A, Malcom W (2002) Chronic urticaria. J Am Acad Dermatol 46:645–657

Cricco GP, Davio CA, Bergoc RM (1993) Inhibition of tumor growth induced by histamine: in vivo and in vitro studies. Agents Actions 38:175–177

Dale HH (1929) Some chemical factors in the control of the circulation: lecture 3. Lancet 1: 167–223

Di Tullio G (2001) Il Ruolo delle intolleranze alimentary nella etiopatogenesi della dermatite atopica. La Med Biol 103–110

Dimitriadou V, Pang X, Theoharides TC (2000) Hydroxyzine inhibits experimental allergic encephalomyelitis (EAE) and associated brain mast cell activation. Int J Immunopharmacol 22:673–684

Dunford PJ, O'Donnell N, Riley JP et al (2006) The histamine H4 receptor mediates allergic airway inflammation by regulating the activation of CD^{4+} T cells. J Immunol 176:7062–7070

Dy M, Schneider E (2004) Histamine-cytokine connection in immunity and hematopoiesis. Cytokin Grow Fact Rev 15:393–410

Emerson MR, Orentas DM, Lynch SG et al (2002) Activation of histamine H2 receptors ameliorates experimental allergic encephalomyelitis. NeuroReport 13:1407–1410

Eriksson NE, Holmen A, Hogstedt B et al (1995) A prospective study of cancer incidence in a cohort examined for allergy. Allergy 50:718–722

Fairweather D, Kaya Z, Shellam GR et al (2001) From infection to autoimmunity. J Autoimmun 6:175–86

Fairweather I, McGlone F, Reilly D et al (2004) Controlled dermal cell damage as human *in vivo* model for localised pain and inflammation. Inflamm Res 53:118–123

Fairweather D, Rose NR (2004) Women and autoimmune diseases. Emerging Infect Dis 10: 2005–2011

Falus A, Hegyesi H, Lázár-Molnár E et al (2001) Paracrine and autocrine interactions in melanoma: histamine is a relevant player in local regulation. TRENDS Immunol 22:648–652

Ferrer M, Nakazawa K, Kaplan AP (1999) Complement dependence of histamine release in chronic urticaria. J Allergy Clin Immunol 104:169–172

Field SK, Sutherland LR (1998) Does medical antireflux therapy improve asthma in asthmatics with gastroesophageal reflux? a critical review of the literature. Chest 114:275–283

Finch L, Hicks PE (1976) The cardiovascular effects of intraventricularly administered histamine in the anaesthetized rat. Naunyn Schmiedebergs Arch Pharmacol 293:151–157

Fumagalli F, Baiardini I, Pasquali M et al (2004) Antihistamines: do they work? Further well-controlled trials involving larger samples are needed. Allergy 59:74–77

Garcia-Caballero M, Neugebauer E, Campos R (1988) Increased histidine decarboxylase (HDC) activity in human colorectal cancer: results of a study on ten patients. Agents Actions 23: 357–360

Gonzales H, Ahmed T (1986) Suppression of gastric H2-receptor-mediated function in patients with bronchial asthma and ragweed allergy. Chest 89:491–496

Goren N, Perez Leiros C, Sterin-Borda L et al (1993) Expression of histamine H1 receptors in autoimmune myocarditis mice. Can J Physiol Pharmacol 71:639–644

Goren N, Perez Leiros C, Sterin-Borda L et al (1994) Effect of histamine in autoimmune myocarditis mice. Int J Immunopharmacol 16:737–745

Grandordy BM, Barnes PJ (1987) Airway smooth muscle and disease workshop: phosphoinositide turnover. Am Rev Respir Dis 36:S17-S20

Grattan CEH, Boon AP, Eady RAJ et al (1990) The pathology of the autologous serum skin test response in chronic urticaria resembles IgE mediated late-phase reactions. Int Arch Allergy Immunol 93:198–240

Grattan CEH, Francis DM, Hide M et al (1991) Detection of circulating histamine releasing autoantibodies with functional properties of anti-IgE in chronic urticaria. Clin Exp Allergy 21:695–704

Gustafsson D, Sjoberg O, Foucard T (2000) Development of allergies and asthma in infants and young children with atopic dermatitis-a prospective follow-up to 7 years of age. Allergy 55:240–245

Haak-Frendscho M, Darvas Z, Hegyesi H et al (2000) Histidine decarboxylase expression in human melanoma. J Invest Dermatol 115:345–352.

Hanifin JM (1990) The role of antihistamines in atopic dermatitis. J Allergy Clin Immunol 86: 666–669

Hardy E, Farahani M, Hall IP (1996) Regulation of histamine H1 receptor coupling by dexamethasone in human cultured airway smooth muscle. Br J Pharmacol 118:1079–1084

Hegyesi H, Somlai B, Varga VL et al (2001) Suppression of melanoma-cell proliferation by histidinedecarboxylase-specific antisense oligonucleotides. J Invest Dermatol 117: 151–153

Hide M, Francis DM, Grattan CEH et al (1993) Autoantibodies against the high-affinity IgE receptor as a cause of histamine release in chronic urticaria. N Engl J Med 328: 1599–1604

Higuchi S, Tanimoto A, Arima N et al (2001) Effects of histamine and interleukin-4 synthesized in arterial intima on phagocytosis by monocytes/macrophages in relation to atherosclerosis. FEBS Lett 505:217–222

Horwitz MS, Bradley LM, Harbertson J et al (1998) Diabetes induced by coxsackievirus: initiation by bystander damage and not molecular mimicry. Nat Med 4:781–785

Humbert M, Menz G, Ying S et al (1999) The immunopathology of extrinsic (atopic) and intrinsic (non-atopic) asthma: more similarities than differences. Immunol Today 20:528–533

Idzko M, la Sala A, Ferrari D et al (2002) Expression and function of histamine receptors in human monocyte-derived dendritic cells. J Allergy Clin Immunol 109:839–846

Jutel M, Blaser K, Akdis CA (2005) Histamine in chronic allergic responses. J Invest Allergol Clin Immunol 15:1–8

Jutel M, Watanabe T, Akdis M et al (2002) Immune regulation by histamine. Curr Opin Immunol 14:735–740

Jutel M, Watanabe T, Klunker S et al (2001) Histamine regulates T-cell and antibody responses by differential expression of H1 and H2 receptors. Nature 413:420–425

Kallen B, Gunnarskog J, Conradson TB (1993) Cancer risk in asthmatic subjects selected from hospital discharge registry. Eur Respir J 6:694–697

Katelaris CH, Peake JE (2006) Allergy and the skin: eczema and chronic urticaria. MJA 185: 517–522

Kay AB (2001) Allergy and allergic diseases. Second of two parts. N Engl J Med 344:109–113

Kemp AS (2003) Cost of illness of atopic dermatitis in children: a societal perspective. Pharmacoeconomics 21:105–113

Lee KH, Kim JY, Kang DS et al (2002) Increased expression of endothelial cell adhesion molecules due to mediator release from human foreskin mast cells stimulated by autoantibodies in chronic urticaria sera. J Invest Dermatol 118:658–663

Lock C, Hermans G, Pedotti R (2002) Gene-microarray analysis of multiple sclerosis lesions yields new targets validated in autoimmune encephalomyelitis. Nat Med 8:500–508

Ma RZ, Gao J, Meeker ND et al (2002) Identification of Bphs, an autoimmune disease locus, as histamine receptor H1. Science 297:620–623

MacGlashan D Jr (2003) Histamine: a mediator of inflammation. J Allergy Clin Immunol 112: S53-S59

Marone G, Casolaro V, Paganelli R et al (1989) IgG anti-IgE from atopic dermatitis induces mediator release from basophils and mast cells. J Invest Dermatol 93:246–252

Marone G, Casolaro V, Patella V et al (1997) Molecular and cellular biology of mast cells and basophils. Int Arch Allergy Immunol 114:207–217

Marone G, Giugliano R, Lembo G et al (1987) Human basophil releasability. II. Changes in basophil releasability in patients with atopic dermatitis. J Invest Dermatol 87:19–23

Mills PK, Beeson WL, Fraser GE et al (1992) Allergy and cancer: organ site-specific results from the adventist health study. Am J Epidemiol 136:287–295

Mittermann I, Aichberger KJ, Bünder R et al (2004) Autoimmunity and atopic dermatitis. Curr Opin Allergy Clin Immunol 4:367–371

Miyazawa N, Watanabe S, Matsuda A et al (1998) Role of histamine H1 and H2 receptor antagonists in the prevention of intimal thickening. Eur J Pharmacol 362:53–59

Moller A, Lippert U, Lessmann D et al (1993) Human mast cells produce IL-8. J Immunol 151:3261–3266

Muller BA (2004) Urticaria and angioedema: a practical approach. Am Family Physician 69: 1123–1128

Musio S, Gallo B, Scabeni S et al (2006) A key regulatory role for histamine in experimental autoimmune encephalomyelitis: disease exacerbation in histidine decarboxylase-deficient mice. The J Immunol 176:17–26

Nielsen HJ, Hammer JH (1992) Possible role of histamine in pathogenesis of autoimmune diseases: implications for immunotherapy with histamine-2 receptor antagonists. Med Hypotheses 39:349–355

Niimi N, David M, Kermani FF et al (1996) Dermal mast cell activation by autoantibodies against the high affinity IgE receptor in chronic urticaria. J Invest Dermatol 106:1001–1006

Oguri S, Motegi K, Endo Y (2003) Augmented lipopolysaccharide induction of the histamine-forming enzyme in streptozotocin-induced diabetic mice. Biochim Biophys Acta 1637:83–90

Ohtsu H (2008) Progress in allergy signal research on mast cells: the role of histamine in immunological and cardiovascular disease and the transporting system of histamine in the cell. J Pharmacol Sci 106:347–353

Olson JK, Croxford JL, Calenoff MA et al (2001) A virus-induced molecular mimicry model of multiple sclerosis. J Clin Invest 108:311–318

Panettieri RA, Yadvish PA, Kelly AM et al (1990) Histamine stimulates proliferation of airway smooth muscle and induces cfos expression. Am J Physiol 259:L365–L371

Patella V, Giuliano A, Bouvet JP et al (1998) Endogenous superallergen protein Fv induces IL-4 secretion from human $Fc\varepsilon RI^+$ cells through interaction with the V_H3 region of IgE. J Immunol 161:5647–5655

Pedotti R, Devoss JJ, Youssef S et al (2003a) Multiple elements of the allergic arm of the immune response modulate autoimmune demyelination. Proc Natl Acad Sci USA 100:1867–1872

Pedotti R, Mitchell D, Wedemeyer J et al (2001) An unexpected version of horror autotoxicus: anaphylactic shock to a self-peptide. Nat Immunol 2:216–222

Pedotti R, Sanna M, Tsai M et al (2003b) Severe anaphylactic reactions to glutamic acid decarboxylase (GAD) self peptides in NOD mice that spontaneously develop autoimmune type 1 diabetes mellitus. BMC Immunol 4:2

Platshon LF, Kaliner M (1978) The effects of the immunologic release of histamine upon human lung cyclic nucleotide levels and prostaglandin generation. J Clin Invest 62:1113–1121

Quinti I, Brozek C, Wood N et al (1986) Circulating IgG autoantibodies to IgE in atopic syndromes. J Allergy Clin Immnol 77:586–594

Reynolds JL, Akhter J, Morris DL (1996) In vitro effect of histamine and histamine H1 and H2 receptor antagonists on cellular proliferation of human malignant melanoma cell lines. Melanoma Res 6:95–99

Riboldi P, Asero R, Tedeschi A (2002) Chronic urticaria: new immunologic aspects. IMAJ 4: 872–873

Rose NR (1997) Autoimmune diseases: tracing the shared threads. Hosp Pract 15:147–154

Rose NR (2001, 2000) An immunology primer. In: Morton CC, Fagan T (eds) Proceedings from sex differences in immunology and autoimmunity, Society for Women's Health Research, Washington, Boston, MA, pp 7–9

Rose NR (2002) Mechanisms of autoimmunity. Semin Liver Dis 22:387–394

Rose NR, Mackay IR (2000) Molecular mimicry: a critical look at exemplary instances in human diseases. Cell Mol Life Sci 57:542–551

Sabroe RA, Greaves MW (1997) The pathogenesis of chronic idiopathic urticaria. Arch Dermatol 133:1003–1008

Sasaguri Y, Tanimoto A (2004) Role of macrophage-derived histamine in atherosclerosis-chronic participation in the inflammatory response. J Atherosclerosis Thrombosis 11:122–130

Sasaguri Y, Wang KY, Tanimoto A et al (2005) Role of histamine produced by bone marrow-derived vascular cells in pathogenesis of atherosclerosis. Circ Res 96:974–981

Satoh T, Sugama K, Matsuo A et al (1994) Histamine as an activator of cell growth and extracellular matrix reconstruction for human vascular smooth muscle cells. Atherosclerosis 110:53–61

Schneider E, Rolli-Derkinderen M, Arock M et al (2002) Trends in histamine research: new functions during immune responses and hematopoiesis. Trends Immunol 23:255–263

Sehra S, Barbé-Tuana FM, Holbreich M et al (2008) Clinical correlations of recent developments in the pathogenesis of atopic dermatitis. An Bras Dermatol 83:57–73

Shahid M, Tripathi T, Sobia F et al (2009) Histamine, histamine receptors and their role in immunomodulation: an updated systematic review. Open Immunol J 2:9–41

Sharma BYK, Gera MV, Tiwari LGVD (2004) Chronic urticaria: expanding the autoimmune kaleidoscope. MJAFI 60:372–378

Sheikh J (2005) Autoantibodies to the high-affinity IgE receptor in chronic urticaria: how important are they? Curr Opin Allergy Clin Immunol 5:403–407

Sirois J, Menard G, Moses AS et al (2000) Importance of histamine in the cytokine network in the lung through H2 and H3 receptors: stimulation of IL-10 production. J Immunol 164: 2964–2970

Slater JW, Zechnich AD, Haxby DG (1999) Second-generation antihistamines: a comparative review. Drugs 57:31–47

Söderberg KC, Hagmar L, Schwartzbaum J (2004) Allergic condition and risk of hematological malignancies in adults: a cohort study. BMC Public Health 4:51

Soundararajan S, Kikuchi Y, Joseph K (2005) Functional assessment of pathogenic IgG subclasses in chronic autoinnune urticaria. J Allergy Clin Immunol 115:815–821

Spergel JM, Paller AS (2003) Atopic dermatitis and the atopic march. J Allergy Clin Immunol 112:S118–S127

Steinhoff M, Griffiths C, Church M et al (2004) Histamine. In: Burns T, Breathnach S, Cox N, Griffiths C (eds) Rook's textbook of dermatology. Blackwell Science, Oxford, UK, pp 9.50–2

Steinman L (2003) Optic neuritis, a new variant of experimental encephalomyelitis, a durable model for all seasons, now in its seventieth year. J Exp Med 197:1065–1071

Steinman L, Zamvil S (2003) Transcriptional analysis of targets in multiple sclerosis. Nat Rev Immunol 3:483–492

Stephan V, Kühr J, Urbanck R (1989) Anti-IgE- and complement-induced histamine release from peripheral leukocytes in normals and atopics. Int Arch Allergy Appl Immunol 90:326–330

Szeberenyi JB, Pallinger E, Zsinko M et al (2001) Inhibition of effects of endogenously synthesized histamine disturbs *in vitro* human dendritic cell differentiation. Immunol Lett 76:175–182

Takagishi T, Sasaguri Y, Nakano R et al (1995) Eapression of the histamine H1 receptor gene in relation to atherosclerosis. Am J Pathol 146:981–988

Talbot-Smith A, Fritschi L, Divitini ML et al (2003) Allergy, atopy, and cancer: a prospective study of the 1981 Busselton cohort. Am J Epidemiol 157:606–612

Tanimoto A, Murata Y, Nomaguchi M et al (2001) Histamine increases the expression of LOX-1 via H2 receptor in human monocytic THP-1 cells. FEBS Lett 508:345–349

Teuscher C, Poynter ME, Offner H et al (2004) Attenuation of TH1 effector cell responses and susceptibility to experimental allergic encephalomyelitis in histamine H2 receptor knockout mice is due to dysregulation of cytokine production by antigen-presenting cells. Am J Pathol 164:883–892

Thomson NC, Kerr JW (1980) Effect of inhaled H1 and H2 receptor antagonist in normal and asthmatic subjects. Thorax 35:428–434

Thurmond RL, Gelfand EW, Dunford PJ (2008) The role of histamine H1 and H4 receptor in allergic inflammation: the search for new antihistamines. Nat Rev 7:41–53

Tilly BC, Tertoolen LGJ, Remorie R et al (1990) Histamine as a growth factor and chemoattractant for human carcinoma and melanoma cells: action through Ca^{2+}-mobilizing H1 receptors. J Cell Biol 110:1211–1215

Tomita K, Nakamura E, Okabe S (2005) Histamine regulates growth of malignant melanoma implants via H2 receptors in mice. Inflammopharmacology 13:281–289

Tong LJ, Balakrishnan G, Kochan JP et al (1997) Assessment of autoimmunity in patients with chronic idiopathic urticaria. J Allergy Clin Immunol 99:461–465

Tough DF, Borrow P, Sprent J (1996) Induction of bystander T cell proliferation by viruses and type I interferon in vivo. Science 272:1947–1950

Van der van LTM, Prinsen IM, Jansen GH et al (1993) Growth of cultured human glioma tumour cells can be regulated with histamine and histamine antagonists. Br J Cancer 68:475–483

Venable JD, Thurmond RL (2006) Development and chemistry of histamine H4 receptor ligands as potential modulators of inflammatory and allergic responses. Antiinflamm Antiallergy Agents Med Chem 5:307–322

Vesterinen E, Pukkala E, Timonen T et al (1993) Cancer incidence among 78,000 asthmatic patients. Int J Epidemiol 22:976–982

Watson SA, Wilkinson LJ, Robertson JFR et al (1993) Effect of histamine on the growth of human gastrointestinal tumours: reversal by cimetidine. Gut 34:1091–1096

White JP, Mills J, Eiser NM (1987) Comparison of the effects of histamine H1-and H2-receptor agonists on large and small airways in normal and asthmatic subjects. Br J Dis Chest 81: 155–169

Wucherpfennig KW (2001) Structural basis of molecular mimicry. J Autoimmun 16:293–302

Xu X et al (2006) Neutrophil histamine contributes to inflammation in mycoplasma pneumonia. J Exp Med 203:2907–2917

Zamvil SS, Steinman L (2003) Diverse targets for intervention during inflammatory and neurodegenerative phases of multiple sclerosis. Neuron 38:685–688

Zuberbier T, Greaves MW, Juhlin L et al (2001) Definition, classification, and routine diagnosis of urticaria: a consensus report. J Invest Dermatol Symp Proc 6:123–127

Zwadlo-Klarwasser G, Vogts M, Hamann W et al (1998) Generation and subcellular distribution of histamine in human blood monocytes and monocyte subsets. Inflamm Res 47:434–439

Chapter 10
Biological Characteristics of Histamine Receptors in Airways Disease Management

Rajni Kant Shukla, Priyanka Jain, and Sandeep Bhattacharya

Abstract Histamine, a biogenic amine is an important mediator isolated from ergot extracts and released from activated mast cells provoked by allergen and has a substantial role in the pathophysiology of asthma. It not only mediates multiple biological actions but also play an important role in vascular dilatation and smooth muscles contraction during anaphylaxis. Cell growth and differentiation, a significant event in the biological system have been regulated by its receptors both in normal and transformed tissues. The discovery of noble histamine H4-receptors prompted us to reinvestigate the role of histamine in pulmonary allergic responses. In asthma and other types of allergic inflammation, mast cells and basophils are the postulated major sources of histamine. In this chapter, we would highlight the potential histamine role in airways diseases and try to update the current aspects of histamine in asthma and fill the gap in existing literature.

Keywords Histamine · Histamine receptors · Airways diseases · COPD · COAD · Asthma

Abbreviations

DCs	dendritic cells
Th1	T helper 1 cells
Th2	T helper 2 cells
IFN-γ	interferon gamma
MHC II	major histocompatibility complex class II antigens
GM-CSF	granulocyte macrophage colony-stimulating factor
IL	interleukine
HDC	histidine decarboxylase
IgE	immunoglobulin-E
COAD	chronic obstructive airways disease

S. Bhattacharya (✉)
Department of Physiology, C.S.M. Medical University, Erstwhile King George's Medical University, Lucknow, UP, India
e-mail: dr.sabhattacharya@gmail.com; rickylkw2006@gmail.com

M. Shahid et al. (eds.), *Biomedical Aspects of Histamine*,
DOI 10.1007/978-90-481-9349-3_10, © Springer Science+Business Media B.V. 2010

AHR	airway hyper responsiveness
MCs	mast cells
COPD	chronic obstructive pulmonary disease
ETS	environmental tobacco smoke
HNMT	histamine *N*-methyltransferase
H1	histamine H1-receptor
H2	histamine H2 receptor
H3	histamine H3 receptor
H4	histamine H4 receptor
CXCl12	chemokine (C-X-C motif) ligand 12
OVA	ovalumin

Contents

10.1 Introduction

Histamine is a biogenic amine involved in the local immune responses as well as regulates physiological function in the gut and acting as a neurotransmitter (Marieb 2001). It was first discovered as a contaminant in extracts of ergot resulting from bacterial action. Dale and Laidlaw in 1910 discovered the first pharmacological properties attributed to histamine. They found that histamine stimulate smooth muscles and had potent vasopressor action. They isolated histamine from samples of liver and lung (Babe and Serafin 1996). Histamine exerts important immunomodulatory effect through its four receptors (H1-, H2-, H3- and H4-receptors) (Akdis and Blaser 2003, MacGlashan 2003, Shahid et al. 2009, Triggiani et al. 2001). Many of the study showed that the histamine receptors mediate proinflammatory or anti-inflammatory effects. H1R is involved in proinflammatory activity and also in the development of different aspects of antigen-specific immune response including the maturation of dendritic cells (DCs) and modulation of the balance of T helper 1 (Th1) cells and T helper 2 (Th2) cells (Shahid et al. 2009). Histamine blocks humoral immune responses by means of a specific mechanism in which it induce an increase in the proliferation of Th1 cells and in the production of interferon gamma (IFN-γ) (Diel et al. 1999). Histamine stimulates human macrophages cells to release the proinflammatory cytokines and lysosomal enzymes that show the capacity to influence the activity of immune cells including mast cells, basophils, eosinophils, lymphocytes, neutrophils, epithelial and endothelial cells (Shahid et al. 2009).

Histamine has been observed in cultured human bronchial epithelial cells that demonstrate functionally active H1 and H2 receptor activity (Devalia and Davies 1991). It has been demonstrated that nasal and bronchial epithelial cells synthesize and release biologically active mediators including cell adhesion molecules, endothelin, cytokines, arachidonic acid metabolites, major histocompatibility complex class (MHC) II antigens, neuropeptide degrading enzymes and nitric oxide that influence the migration, activation and also function of both structural and inflammatory cells involved in the pathophysiology of allergic rhinitis and asthma (Devalia et al. 2000a). Histamine has modulated inflammatory mechanisms within the airways. Similarly, histamine induced the release cytokines (IL-6, IL-8 and GM-CSF) from human corneal and conjunctival epithelial cells (Yanni et al. 1999). Certainly, the role of epithelial cells as modulators of inflammation mainly in allergic diseases has been an important subject of much discussion for future prospects.

Epidemiology of a disease helps in determining the prevalence and natural history of the respiratory disease. The pathogenetic mechanisms of the respiratory disease have lot of contradiction. Respiratory diseases are related to respiratory system that includes diseases of the lung, pleural cavity, bronchial tubes, trachea, upper respiratory tract and the nerves and muscles of breathing (Anonymous 1). The respiratory tract is divided into 3 segments: (i) Upper respiratory tract: Nose and nasal passages, paranasal sinuses and throat or pharynx, (ii) Respiratory airways: Voice box or larynx, trachea, bronchi and bronchioles, (iii) Lungs: Respiratory bronchioles, alveolar ducts, alveolar sacs and alveoli (Anonymous 1).

10.2 Histamine Uptake into and Release from Histamine Producing Cells

Histamine was first identified as an autocoid having potent vasoactive properties. It cannot be generated by another enzymatic pathway (Dy and Schneider 2004, Parsons and Ganellin 2006). Histidine decarboxylase (HDC) is an enzyme that is expressed in various cells through out the body including central nervous system, neurons, gastric-mucosa, parietal cells, mast cells and basophils (Akdis and Blaser 2003, MacGlashan 2003, Schneider et al. 2002). Only basophils and mast cells can store the histamine in specific granules is a powerful bronchospastic mediator. Its actions are mediated via membrane, bronchial smooth muscle contraction, increased vascular permeability, increased airways mucus production and production of prostaglandins (Bhatia and Kant 2008). Histamine can also be released in large amounts during degranulation in response to various immunological [immunoglobulin-E (IgE), or cytokines] or non-immunological stimuli (Dy and Schneider 2004, Shahid et al. 2009).

10.3 Role of Histamine in Pathogenesis of Respiratory Diseases

Cerri et al. (2006) reported that histamine induces monocytes to release Macro particle (like cytokine IL-8) capable of modulating airway inflammation. Inflammation has a central role in the pathophysiology of asthma. As noted in the definition of asthma, airway inflammation involves an interaction of many cell types and multiple mediators with the airways that eventually results in the characteristic pathophysiological features of the disease: bronchial inflammation and airflow limitation that result in recurrent episodes of cough, wheeze and shortness of breath. The processes by which these interactive events occur and lead to clinical asthma are still under surveillance. Although distinct phenotypes of asthma exist (e.g., intermittent, persistent, exercise-associated, aspirin-sensitive or severe asthma), airway inflammation remains a consistent pattern. The pattern of airway inflammation in asthma, however, does not necessarily vary depending upon disease severity, persistence and duration of disease. The cellular profile and the response of the structural cells in asthma are quite consistent (Anonymous 2).

10.3.1 Role of Histamine in Obstructive Airways Disease (COAD)

Obstructive lung diseases (COAD) are related to lungs where the bronchial tubes become narrowed making it hard to move air in and especially out of the lungs. The flow of air into and out of the lungs is impaired (Paul 2008). Nonallergic airway hyperresponsiveness to chemical mediators such as histamine or methacholine is a characteristic feature of bronchial asthma. Hyperresponsiveness to these chemicals has also been established in patients with COAD, particularly in those who also have chronic bronchitis (i.e., mucous hyper secretion) (Bahous et al. 1984, Fletcher 1968, MacGlashan 2003, Oppenheimer et al. 1968, Ramsdale et al. 1984, Ramsdell et al. 1982), but in case of asthma, reduced airway caliber is only mildly correlated with hyperresponsiveness (Cockcroft et al. 1977, Ryan et al. 1982) and does not generally occur until the airways are severely hyperresponsive (Ryan et al. 1982). In case of COAD with bronchitis, there is a marked linear correlation between airway hyperresponsiveness and reduced airway caliber (Bahous et al. 1984). The subjects with COAD are not responsive to cold air as opposed to those with asthma and airflow obstruction was clearly differentiated (Bahous et al. 1984). These data have led to the speculation that airways hyperresponsiveness is different in asthma and COAD, being due to airway smooth muscle hyperresponsiveness in the former and reduced airway caliber in the latter (Bahous et al. 1984). Here few studies related to the airways responsiveness in patients whose COAD is predominantly emphysematous, and the cause of intrinsic airways disease, patients with non-emphysematous COAD and chronic bronchitis have more responsive to histamine; in other way those who were with emphysematous non-bronchitis COAD are not responsive with histamine. Studies of non-asthmatic COAD patient revealed the major and minimal clinical evidence of emphysema (Hathirat et al. 1970, Jones and Meade 1961) and little chronic bronchitis (Verma et al. 1988).

10.3.2 Role of Histamine in Bronchial Asthma

Term bronchial asthma was define as breathlessness or shortness of breath, refers to one of the episodic manifestations of obstructive pulmonary disease with episodes of wheeze and dyspnoea. The tracheobronchial tree has hyper-responsiveness to variety of stimuli manifesting physiologically by generalized airways obstruction, responding either to some primary treatment or spontaneously over a short period of time and clinically by paroxysmal attacks of cough, wheeze, dyspnoea, heavy chest etc (Anonymous 3). It is an important cause of pulmonary disability, which affects the both sexes and age is no bar to this. It is considered as a disease of T cell origin and an end result of interaction between host genetics and environmental factor. Allergic asthma is a complex disease associated with airway hyper responsiveness (AHR) and chronic airway inflammation (Anonymous 4). It is a complex disorder involving heterogeneous group of patients where airways hyper-responsiveness occurs due to airways inflammation, leading to airways obstruction. In response to varied assortment of exogenous and endogenous stimuli, airways get narrowing which is reversible. With respect of inflammation neuro-immunochemical also stimulate the airways smooth muscles and inflammation that leading to mucosal cellular infiltration, mucosal oedema and accumulation of mucus because of excessive bronchial secretions and their impaired clearance, epithelial damage and basement membrane thickening (Bhatia 2006). This mechanism has important role to play immediate response to allergens and late response of bronchial hyperresponsiveness, macrophages and eosinophils.

Allergies are caused by an immune response to a normally innocuous substances (i.e. pollen and dust), which comes in contact with lymphocytes specific for that substances or antigen. In several cases the lymphocytes triggers to respond mast cells and than a free-floating IgE (an immunoglobulin associated with allergic response) molecule to bind specific antigen on cell surface receptors of mast cells, and then mast cells trigger the histamine release (Janeway et al. 1999).

At the time of immediate airway response aerosol antigen challenge of sensitized guinea pigs, there is an increase in airway epithelial permeability to large molecules (Goto et al. 2000, Ranga et al. 1983). This increase in epithelial permeability is reproduced by aerosol challenge with histamine (Boucher et al. 1978). Histamine play important role in immune system and mediator of allergic diseases such as asthma, hay fever etc. The development of some allergic reactions, infections and tumors are associated with excessive histamine production (Elenkov et al. 1998). Histamine is released from activated mast cells provoked by allergen, and has a substantial role in the pathophysiology of asthma through its ability to stimulate smooth muscle cell contraction, vasodilatation, increased venular permeability and further mucus secretion. Plasma histamine concentrations are elevated during the early and late responses to inhaled allergens, and may also increase during spontaneous acute asthma episodes (Hart 2001).

Pathogenesis of the bronchial asthma was remained unclear in most of the studies in vitro as well as in vivo (Bhat et al. 1976, Schild et al. 1951). Plasma histamine levels were increase in asthmatic patients that promote asthma attacks (Bruce et al. 1976, Simon et al. 1977). The H1 receptor of histamine have very important role in the pathogenesis of asthma attack, however in comparison of H1 the role of H2 receptor is less clear in pathogenesis of asthma. Bourne et al. (1971) demonstrated when histamine adds to leukocyte preparations, it inhibits mediator release induced by antigen exposure (Bourne et al. 1971). In vitro, histamine causes bronchial smooth muscle contraction but in the presence of H1 receptor blockade, histamine causes dose related smooth muscle relaxation, which is abolished by H2 receptor blockade (Dunlop and Smith 1977), and further suggested that H2 receptor stimulation by histamine released from mast cells may limit the severity of asthmatic reactions both by a direct effect on bronchial smooth muscle and by limitation of further mediator release. Conversely H2 receptor blockade might enhance asthmatic attacks or lead to increased bronchial hyperreactivity (Stick 2002), while therapeutically useful in the reduction of gastric acid secretion. In vitro studies suggest that the H2 receptor has a role in the modulation of mechanisms involved in asthmatic attacks. Exogenous histamine has been shown to inhibit the release of histamine from leucocytes and this effect is blocked by H2 receptor blockade with antihistamine drugs (Lichtenstein and Gillespie 1975).

Histamine has been well known to mediate inflammatory and allergic responses acting predominately through H1 receptors. H1 receptor antagonists have been used to treat allergies for many years (Hill et al. 1997). Several in vivo and in vitro studies build up an evidence (uses animal models disease and human biological samples) that the fundamental role of the H4 receptor in histamine-induced chemotaxis of mast cells, eosinophils and other immune cells (Dunford et al. 2006, Ikawa et al. 2005, Thurmond et al. 2004). In murine mast cells, H4 receptor was activated to mediate chemotaxis and intracellular Ca^{2+} mobilized without affecting degranulation, and thus providing a mechanism for the selective recruitment of these effector cells into the tissues and the amplification of the histamine mediated reaction eventually leading to chronic allergic inflammation (Hofstra et al. 2003). Accommodating evidence for an autoregulatory function of the MC-expressed H4 receptor comes from its critical role in zymosan-induced recruitment of neutrophils in vivo possibly via regulation of leukotriene B4 release from MCs (Takeshita et al. 2003, Thurmond et al. 2004). The H4 receptor mediates redistribution and recruitment of MCs in the mucosal epithelium in response to allergens, thus amplifying allergic symptoms and maintaining chronic inflammation (Takeshita et al. 2003). Recently, a study was conducted on mice, and showed that H4 receptor deficient mice have reduced lung inflammation due to decrease Th2 response and upon oral gavage administration of selective antagonists in a Murine model of allergic airway inflammation documented the role of the H4 receptor in modulating Th2 allergic responses by influencing $CD4^+$ T cell activation attributed to decreased cytokine and chemokine production by DCs (Dunford et al. 2007); both H4 agonists and antagonists have observed beneficial actions in asthmatic mice were attributed to the local versus systemic administration of the compounds respectively (Morgan et al. 2007). Moreover, it characterized the role of H4 receptor in the modulation of the asthmatic response revealed the inhibitory effect of H4 receptor agonists on antigen specific responses in human peripheral blood mononuclear cells and T cell lines. However, that was not reversed by the H3/H4 receptor antagonist thioperamide (Sugata et al. 2007). Additional data are providing important conclusive evidence concerning the optimal therapeutic exploitation of H4 receptor ligands in chronic airways disease (Daugherty 2004).

10.3.3 Role of Histamine in Chronic Obstructive Pulmonary Disease (COPD)

Chronic obstructive pulmonary disease (COPD) is a major cause of chronic morbidity and mortality throughout the world. Many people suffer from this disease for years and die prematurely from it or its complications (Anonymous 5). COPD often develops in long-time smokers in middle age; patients often have a variety of other diseases related to either smoking or aging (Soriano et al. 2005). Only 15–20% of smokers develop clinically significant COPD is misleading (Rennard and Vestbo 2006). A much higher proportion may develop abnormal lung function at some point if they continue to smoke (Lokke et al. 2006). Smoking is the best-studied risk factor in COPD, it is not the only one and there is consistent evidence from epidemiologic studies that nonsmokers may also develop chronic airflow obstruction (Behrendt 2005, Celli et al. 2005). Age at starting to smoke, total pack-years smoked, and current smoking status are predictive of COPD mortality. But study showed that not all smokers develop clinically significant COPD, which suggests that any other factors are responsible for modify the biology of each individuals risk like genetic factors (Smith and Harrison 1997). Passive exposure of the cigarette smoke (also known as environmental tobacco smoke or ETS) may also have respiratory symptoms (Anonymous 6) and COPD (Eisner et al. 2005) by increasing the lungs total burden of inhaled particles and gases (Leuenberger et al. 1994).

Pathological changes characteristic of COPD are found in the proximal airways, peripheral airways, lung parenchyma and pulmonary vasculature (Dayal et al. 1994, Hogg 2004). The pathological changes include chronic inflammation with increased numbers of specific inflammatory cell types in different parts of the lung and structural changes resulting from repeated injury and repair. Some patients develop COPD without smoking, but the nature of the inflammatory response in these patients is unknown (Birring et al. 2002).

This abnormal inflammatory response may induce parenchymal tissue destruction (resulting in emphysema), and disrupt normal repair and defense mechanisms (resulting in small airway fibrosis). These pathological changes lead to air trapping and progressive airflow limitation during the time of smoking neutrophils macrophages and lymphocytes release inflammatory mediator. They interact with structural cells of airways and lung parenchyma (Barnes et al. 2003). In inflammatory lung disorders, histamine acts as a mediator of both acute and chronic phases. Accumulating data support the function of histamine in cellular immunity through control of cytokine and chemokine production and migration of inflammatory cells, beyond its traditional role in mediating immediate airway hyperresponsiveness (Barnes et al. 1998). Many cells of airways involved in inflammatory responses and provide signaling for the expression of H1, H2 and H4 receptors, which regulate the chronic conditions in humans. Histamine receptors activation can have varying form concentration to concentration and sometime counteracting effects of particular cell. Also, receptors level may change under the pathophysiological conditions or different stages of cell development and could vary among species. Like, H1 receptor expression increases on in vitro differentiation of monocytes into macrophages and inflammatory stimuli can upregulate the expression of H4 receptors in monocytes (Dijkstra et al. 2007, Triggiani et al. 2007). Level of H4 receptor in lung is low, where its expression in bronchial epithelial, smooth muscle cells and microvascular endothelial cells may contribute to the airway disease phenotypes in various ways (Gantner et al. 2002). The H4 receptor mediates redistribution and recruitment of MCs in the mucosal epithelium in response to allergens, thus amplifying allergic symptoms and maintaining chronic inflammation. Many studies were done over animal model (Guinea pigs) showed airways hyperrespnsiveness in those who were exposed to cigarette smoke to different stimuli (Dusser et al. 1989, Han-Pin and Ling-Chung 1995, Hulbert et al. 1985, James et al. 1987, Lee et al. 1995). The histopathological findings in animal exposed to cigarette smoke showed increased intra-alveolar sputum, increased lymphatic tissue, destruction alveolar wall and intracellular bleeding, which pathological changes similar to the COPD patient (Boskabady and Snashall 1997, Jeffery 1997, Rennard 1997, Saetta et al. 1998).

10.4 Association Between COPD and Asthma

Although both COPD and asthma are associated with chronic inflammation of the respiratory tract, there are discernible differences in the inflammatory cells and mediators involved in the two diseases, which in turn account for differences in physiological effects, symptoms and response to therapy. However, there are greater similarities between the lung inflammation in severe asthma and COPD (Thomson et al. 2004).

COPD can coexist with asthma, the other major chronic obstructive airway disease characterized by an underlying airway inflammation. However, individuals with asthma who are exposed to noxious agents, particularly cigarette smoke

(Thomson et al. 2004), may also develop fixed airflow limitation and a mixture of "asthma-like" and "COPD-like" inflammation (Lange et al. 1998).

During the time of inflammation, histamine is released from preformed stores in mast cells and basophils. Histamine leads to vasodilatation and increase permeability in vascular permeability in smooth muscles cells or bronchoalveolar lavage fluid and endothelial cells; this negatively correlates with airway function (Broide et al. 1991, Casale et al. 1987, Jarjour et al. 1991, Liu et al. 1990, Wardlaw et al. 1988, Wenzel et al. 1988).

10.5 Histamine Receptors and Airways

During ingestion of histamine-rich food or alcohol, rhinorrea or nasal obstruction may occur in patients with histamine intolerance; in extreme cases, attacks of asthma may also occur. Reduced HNMT activity has been shown for patients with food allergy (Kuefner et al. 2004) and asthma (Preuss et al. 1998). Important functions of histamine receptors in airways were described as: (a) bronchoconstriction by stimulation of H1 receptors on smooth muscles, (b) mucosal edema from increased microvascular permeability (H1) leading to transudation of fluid and macromolecules through wide intercellular gaps (>12 nm). In addition, perfusion of previously non-perfused capillary beds may contribute to mucosal edema, (c) stimulation of lung irritant receptors can induce airway smooth muscle contraction through vagal (cholinergic) pathways, (d) direct stimulation of vagal (cholinergic) nerves can induce airway smooth muscle contraction, (e) vagal postganglionic receptors can induce airway smooth muscle contraction, (f) stimulation of H1 receptors increases mucus secretions, and stimulation of H2 receptors increases mucus viscosity. Histamine is metabolized within minutes and therefore by itself does not accumulate. However, an effect of inhaled histamine on airway diameter in usual dosages may be detectable for up to 70 min. Therefore, when subsequent doses are inhaled a small cumulative effect is to be expected (Anonymous 7).

10.5.1 Mast Cells Put in the Development of Allergic Airway Disease

The role of mast cells for the development of allergic airway disease is critically dependent on the sensitization and allergen exposure procedure. Several mice studies have observed the airways inflammation with systemic sensitization with adjuvant hyperrespossivenss (Mehlhop et al. 1997, Nogami et al. 1990, Takeda et al. 1997). Mast cells and basophils are generally thought to be the major sources of histamine and can themselves be modulated by histamine as they express H1, H2 and H4 receptors, although how this varies between different mast cell types is not yet clear (Godot et al. 2007, Hofstra et al. 2003, Lippert et al. 2004). Activation of H4 receptors in human mast cell precursors can synergize with other chemoattractants such as CXCl12 (Daugherty 2004). Histamine does not appear to have any direct effect on mast cell degranulation (Garcia-Martin et al. 2006, Morgan et al. 2007). H1 receptor antagonist on mast cell was reported by several studies, but these results may be due to off target effects. In case of H2 receptors, mast cells can have various effects including inhibition of histamine release and modulation of cytokine production (Bissonnette 1996, Lichtenstein and Gillespie 1975, Lippert et al. 2000). There are also reports of H3 receptor function on mast cells, but many of these activities may be attributed to the H4 receptor, as the ligands used are not particularly selective, and studies have reported that H3 receptor expression is not detected in some types of mast cells (Lippert et al. 2004, Morgan et al. 2007).

10.5.2 Histamine and Allergic Bronchial Asthma

Histamine is a major mediator that elicits a number of the acute physiologic responses in allergic asthma (Koarai et al. 2003). The role in asthma is supported by many lines of evidence, including the release of histamine from cells participating in allergic responses, reproduction of features of allergic inflammation by application of histamine, reduction of allergic inflammation by histamine receptor antagonists, and recently hampered eosinophilia in mice genetically modified not to synthesize histamine (Morrow et al. 1991). Mast cells and basophils in hematopoietic cells, enterochromaffin-like cells in gastric wall, and neurons in tuberomammillary nucleus in the hypothalamus are major sources of histamine in the cellular level. Some foods contain high histamine, occasionally in amounts sufficient to cause histamine poisoning, which resembles the conventional anaphylaxis. For instance, absorbed histamine is the causative toxin of scombroid-fish poisoning (Gutzmer et al. 2002). Mast cells and basophils are the postulated major sources of histamine in allergic reaction. Histamine release from these cells is triggered by the interaction of an allergen with specific immunoglobulin E (IgE) bound to the high-affinity IgE receptor on the cell membrane or by nonspecific stimuli, including exercise or cold and dry air. It acts not simply but in a rather complicated manner in each symptom of allergic asthma. Histamine has not only the direct actions on smooth muscle and sensory nerves but also indirect action on vagal reflexes, causing the cough phenomenon. The actions of histamine are mediated by their receptors, including H1–H4 receptor (Thurmond et al. 2008). The role of histamine in immunology has started to be clarified recently in several reports. Previous studies have suggested that histamine enhances Th2 responses through modulation of dendritic cell (DC) function and regulation of IL-10 and IL-12 production. DCs express H1 receptor and H2 receptor (Caron et al. 2001), and their exposure to histamine induces a shift toward the DC2 phenotype, especially their repertoire of cytokines and chemokines, which promotes Th2 immune responses (Elenkov et al. 1998, Mazzoni et al. 2001). Histamine inhibits IL-12 production, while enhancing IL-10 synthesis in lipopolysaccharide-treated leukocytes (Jutel et al. 2001, van der Pouw Kraan et al. 1998). These observations suggest a Th2-promoting influence of histamine. In contrast, studies with mice bearing a targeted deletion of the H1 receptor show reduced production of IFN-γ and increased IL-4 and IL-13 secretion, results more consistent with the Th1-polarizing function of this receptor (Godot et al. 2007). Recently H4 receptor was shown to play an important role in allergic lung inflammation, especially for their activity for recruitment of lung eosinophils and lymphocytes and Th2 responses (Dunford et al. 2006). Blockade of the H4 receptor on dendritic cells leads to decreases in cytokine and chemokine production and limits their ability to induce Th2 responses in T-cells. Koarai et al. (2003) conducted a study, and found the role of endogenous histamine on eosinophilic recruitment and hyperresponsiveness in an allergic bronchial asthma mouse model using L-histidine dacarboxylase gene knockout mice. Histamine levels of the airways in $HDC^{-/-}$ mice were largely diminished compared with $HDC^{+/+}$ mice. Inhalation challenge with ovalumin (OVA) in OVA-sensitized $HDC^{+/+}$ mice caused eosinophil accumulation in the lung as well as airway hyper-responsiveness to methacholine 3 days after the challenge. The eosinophil recruitment to lung was significantly reduced in $HDC^{-/-}$ mice. In the bone marrow, the proliferation of eosinophils was induced after OVA challenge in $HDC^{+/+}$ mice; however, the proliferation was significantly suppressed in $HDC^{-/-}$ mice. In contrast, airway hyper-responsiveness was not suppressed in $HDC^{-/-}$ mice. These results suggest that endogenous histamine is involved in the accumulation of eosinophils into the airways after allergic challenge, possibly acting in the bone marrow. Since histamine has eosinophil chemotactic activity via H4 receptor, reduced eosinophils in $HDC^{-/-}$ mice could be explained through the activity via H4 receptor (O'Reilly et al. 2002). Allergen-induced airway hyperresponsiveness occurred independently of airway eosinophilia in this model (Ohtsu 2008).

10.6 Role of Histamine in Management of Airways Disease

Airway inflammation is a major factor in the pathogenesis and pathophysiology of asthma. The importance of inflammation to central features of asthma continues to expand and underscore this characteristic as a primary target of treatment. It has also become evident; however, that airway inflammation is variable in many aspects including intensity, cellular/mediator pattern, and response to therapy. Previous study showed various phenotypes of inflammation became an evidence for the better management of asthma. Earlier studies have indicated that although current management is effective in controlling symptoms, reducing airflow limitations, and preventing exacerbations, present treatment does not appear to prevent the underlying severity of asthma. The Expert panel's recommendations for asthma treatment, which are directed by knowledge of basic mechanisms, should result in improved control of asthma and a greater understanding of therapeutic effectiveness (Anonymous 2).

Inhaled histamine is used for during the time of hyper reactivity (Curry 1947) that is prevented by H1 receptor blocking agents given parenterally (Popa 1977) and by inhalation (Nogrady and Bevan 1978). Despite the fact that orally administered H1 blockers are clinically ineffective in asthma, when given by inhalation, such agents are potent bronchodilators (Nogrady et al. 1978).

10.7 Concluding Remarks

The clinical treatment of asthma still poses a major challenge. The clarification of histamine's control over the cytokine network and the Th1/Th2 balance provides a basis for the potential use of antihistamines in the prevention and treatment of atopic asthma. Recently asthma is routinely treated with inhaled histamine receptor agonists and inhaled corticosteroids. H1 and H2 receptor antagonists have the ability to modulate cytokine secretion profiles and the Th1/Th2 balance. Histamine has a key role in many physiological processes including inflammation, and drugs that target H1 receptors have been successful for the treatment of allergy, but not without limitations. Furthermore, the discovery of a H4 receptor and its emerging role in inflammation has spurred new interest for the functions of histamine in inflammation, allergy and autoimmune diseases. Early results in animal models suggest that H4 receptor antagonists may have utility in treating various conditions in humans, in particular in diseases in which histamine is known to be present. Combined H1 and H4 receptor antagonism might bring added benefit over monotherapy. The recent data on the functions of H1 and H4 receptors have given idea for the managements of airways disease. Antihistamines with unique immunomodulating properties were effective in the prevention of atopic asthma.

Acknowledgement This work is supported by the Council of Science and Technology, Uttar Pradesh, Lucknow, India (CST/SEPRD/D-3404).

References

Akdis CA, Blaser K (2003) Histamine in the immune regulation of allergic inflammation. J Allergy Clin Immunol 112:15–22

Anonymous 1: National Institutes of Health – common cold. http://www3.niaid.nih.gov/topics/commonCold/. Retrieved on 2008-05-07

Anonymous 2: http://www.ncbi.nlm.nih.gov/bookshelf/br.fcgi?book=asthma3&part=A39. Accessed Oct 2009

Anonymous 3: American Thoracic Society (1987) Standards for the diagnosis and care of patients with chronic obstructive pulmonary disease (COPD) and asthma. Am Rev Respir Dis 136:225–244

Anonymous 4: The state of asthma in America: asthma in America survey. http://www.asthmainamerica.com. Accessed 9 Feb 2009

Anonymous 5: World Health Report (2000) World Health Organization, Geneva. http://www.who.int/whr/2000/en/statistics.htm. Accessed 12 Nov 2009

Anonymous 6: The health consequences of involuntary exposure to tobacco smoke: a report of the surgeon general, department of health and human services. Washington, DC, US, 2006

Anonymous 7: http://www.spirxpert.com/brrespuk/histamine.htm. Accessed 24 Nov 2009

Babe KS, Serafin WE (1996) Histamine, bradykinin, and their antagonists. Goodman and Gilman's the pharmacological basis of therapeutics. McGraw-Hill, New York, pp 581–593

Bahous J, Cartier A, Ouimet G et al (1984) Nonallergic bronchial hyperexcitability in chronic bronchitis. Am Rev Respir Dis 129:216–220

Barnes PJ, Chung KF, Page CP (1998) Inflammatory mediators of asthma: an update. Pharmacol Rev 50:515–596

Barnes PJ, Shapiro SD, Pauwels RA (2003) Chronic obstructive pulmonary disease: molecular and cellular mechanisms. Eur Respir 22:672–688

Behrendt CE (2005) Mild and moderate to severe COPD in nonsmokers. Distinct demographic profiles. Chest 128:1239–1244

Bhat KN, Arroyave CM, Marney SR et al (1976) Plasma histamine changes during provoked bronchospasm in asthmatic patients. J Allergy Clin Immunol 58:647–656

Bhatia RS (2006) Rising trend in respiratory diseases: reasons and remedies. In: Bhatia RS (ed) Selected topics in chest medicine. Arora, Lucknow, India, pp 23–34

Bhatia RS, Kant S (2008) Bronchial asthma, 1st edn. Peepee, India

Birring SS, Brightling CE, Bradding P et al (2002) Clinical, radiologic, and induced sputum features of chronic obstructive pulmonary disease in nonsmokers: a descriptive study. Am J Respir Crit Care Med 166:1078–1083

Bissonnette EY (1996) Histamine inhibits tumor necrosis factor a release by mast cells through H2 and H3 receptors. Am J Respir Cell Mol Biol 14:620–626

Boskabady MH, Snashall PD (1997) Enhanced histamine H1 receptor blockade with chlorpheniramine in the asthmatic tracheobronchial tree: further evidence for increased drug delivery in asthma. Med JIRI 11:115–122

Boucher RC, Ranga V, Pare PD et al (1978) Effect of histamine and methacholine on guinea pig tracheal permeability to HRP. J Appl Physiol 45:939–948

Bourne HR, Melmon KL, Lichtenstein LM (1971) Histamine augments leukocyte adenosine 3′, 5′-monophosphate and blocks antigenic histamine release. Science 173:743

Broide D, Gleich G, Cuomo A et al (1991) Evidence of ongoing mast cell and eosinophil degranulation in symptomatic asthma airway. J Allergy Clin Immunol 88:637–648

Bruce C, Weatherstone R, Seaton A et al. (1976) Histamine levels in plasma, blood and urine in severe asthma, and the effect of corticosteroid treatment. Thorax 31:724–729

Caron G, Delneste Y, Roelandts E et al (2001) Histamine polarizes human dendritic cells into Th2 cell-promoting effector dendritic cells. J Immunol 167:3682–3686

Casale TB, Wood D, Richardson HB et al (1987) Elevated bronchoalveolar lavage fluid histamine levels in allergic asthmatics are associated with methacholine bronchial hyperresponsiveness. J Clin Invest 79:1197–1203

Celli BR, Halbert RJ, Nordyke RJ et al (2005) Airway obstruction in never smokers: results from the third national health and nutrition examination survey. Am J Med 118:1364–1372

Cerri C, Neri T, Tedone R et al (2006) Histamine-stimulated monocytes release microparticles that upregulate IL-8 synthesis by human alveolar ephitelial cells. (P-1347) http://www.ersnet.org/learning_resources_player/abstract_print_06/files/113.pdf. Accessed 30 Nov 2009

Cockcroft DWE, Killian DN, Mellon JJA et al (1977) Bronchial reactivity to inhaled histamine: a method and clinical survey Clin Allergy 7:235–243

Curry J (1947) Comparative action of acetylbetamethylcholine and histamine on the respiratory tract in normals, patients with hay fever and subjects with bronchial asthma. J Clin Invest 26:430–438

Daugherty BL (2004) Histamine H4 antagonism: a therapy for chronic allergy? Br J Pharmacol 142:5–7

Dayal HH, Khuder S, Sharrar R et al (1994) Passive smoking in obstructive respiratory disease in an industrialized urban population. Environ Res 65:161–171

Devalia JL, Davies RJ (1991) Human nasal and bronchial epithelial cells in culture. An overview of their characteristics and function. Allergy Proc 12:71–79

Devalia JL, Rusznak C, Davies RJ (2000a) Epithelial cell dysfunction in rhinitis, in asthma and rhinitis. In: Busse WW, Holgate ST (eds) Blackwell Science, London, pp 841–854

Devalia JL, Wang JH, Davies RJ (2000b) Airway epithelial cells. In: Page CP, Banner KH, Spina D (eds) Cellular mechanisms in airway inflammation. Birkhäuser, Basel, pp 245–262

Diel F, Horr B, Borck H et al (1999) Pyrethroids and piperonyl-butoxide affect human T-lymphocytes in vitro. Toxicol Lett 107:65–74

Dijkstra D, Leurs R, Chazot P et al (2007) Histamine downregulates monocyte CCL2 production through the histamine H4 receptor. J Allergy Clin Immunol 120:300–307

Dunford PJ, O'Donnell N, Riley JP et al (2006) The histamine H4 receptor mediates allergic airway inflammation by regulating the activation of CD4+ T cells. J Immunol 176:7062–7070
Dunford PJ, Williams KN, Desai PJ et al (2007) Histamine H4 receptor antagonists are superior to traditional antihistamines in the attenuation of experimental pruritus. J Allergy Clin Immunol 119:176–183
Dunlop LS, Smith AP (1977) The effect of histamine antagonists on antigen-induced contraction of sensitized human bronchus in vitro. Br J Pharmacol 59:475P
Dusser DJ, Djokic TD, Borson DB (1989) Cigarette smoke induces bronchoconstrictor hyperresposiveness to substance P and inactivates airways netural endopeptidase in guinea pig. J Clin Invest 84:900–906
Dy M, Schneider E (2004) Histamine-cytokine connection in immunity and hematopoiesis. Cytokine Growth Factor Rev 15:393–410
Eisner MD, Balmes J, Katz BP et al (2005) Life time environmental tobacco smoke exposure and the risk of chronic obstructive pulmonary disease. Environ Health Perspect 4:7–15
Elenkov IJ, Webster E, Papanicolaou DA et al (1998) Histamine potently suppresses human IL-12 and stimulates IL-10 production via H2 receptors. J Immunol 161:2586–2593
Fletcher CM (1968) Bronchial infection and reactivity in chronic bronchitis. J R Coll Physiol (London) 2:183–90
Gantner F, Sakai K, Tusche MW et al (2002) Histamine H4 and H2 receptors control histamine induced interleukin-16 release from human CD8+ T cells. J Pharmacol Exp Ther 303: 300–307
Garcia-Martin E, Mendoza JL, Martinez C et al (2006) Severity of ulcerative colitis is associated with a polymorphism at diamine oxidase gene but not at histamine N-methyltransferase gene. World J Gastroenterol 12:615–620
Godot V, Arock M, Garcia G et al (2007) H4 Histamine receptor mediates optimal migration of mast cell precursors to CXCL12. J Allergy Clin Immunol 120:827–843
Goto Y, Uchida Y, Nomura A et al (2000) Dislocation of E-cadherin in the airway epithelium during an antigen-induced asthmatic response. Am J Respir Cell Mol Biol 23:712–718
Gutzmer R, Langer K, Lisewski M et al (2002) Expression and function of histamine receptors 1 and 2 on human monocyte-derived dendritic cells. J Allergy Clin Immunol 109:524–531
Han-Pin K, Ling-Chung L (1995) Sensory neuropeptides in netural endopeptidase activity in guinea pig aiways. Life Sci 57:2187–2196
Hart PH (2001) Regulation of the inflammatory response in asthma by mast cell products. Immunol Cell Biol 79:149
Hathirat S, Renzetti AD, Mitchell M (1970) Measurement of the total lung capacity by helium dilution in a constant volume system. Am Rev Respir Dis 102:760–770
Hill SJ, Ganellin CR, Timmerman H et al (1997) International union of pharmacology. XIII. Classification of histamine receptors. Pharmacol Rev 49:253–278
Hofstra CL, Desai PJ, Thurmond RL et al (2003) Histamine H4 receptor mediates chemotaxis and calcium mobilization of mast cells. J Pharmacol Exp Ther 305:1212–1221
Hogg JC (2004) Pathophysiology of airflow limitation in chronic obstructive pulmonary disease. Lancet 364:709–721
Hulbert WM, Mclean T, Hogg JC (1985) The effect of acute airways inflammation on bronchial reactivity in guinea pig. Am Rev Respiratory Dis 132:7–11
Ikawa Y, Suzuki M, Shiono S et al (2005) Histamine H4 receptor expression in human synovial cells obtained from patients suffering from rheumatoid arthritis. Biol Pharm Bull 28:2016–2018
James AL, Dirks P, Ohtaka H (1987) Airwaya responsiveness to intravenous and inhaled acetylcholine in the guine pig after cigarette smoke exposure. Am Rev Respiratory Dis 136:1158–1162
Janeway CA, Travers P, Walport M et al (1999) Immunobiology: the immune system in health and disease, 4th edn. Current Biology Publication, London, p 602
Jarjour N, Calhoun W, Schwartz L et al (1991) Elevated bronchoalveolar lavage fluid histamine levels in allergic asthmatics are associated with increased airway obstruction. Am Rev Respir Dis 144:83–87

Jeffery PK (1997) Pathology of asthma and COPD: a synopsis. Eur Resip Rev 7:206–210

Jones RS, Meade F (1961) A theoretical and experimental analysis of anomalies in the estimation of pulmonary diffusing capacity by the single breath method. Q J Exp Physiol 46: 131–143

Jutel M, Klunker S, Akdis M et al (2001) Histamine upregulates Th1 and downregulates Th2 responses due to different patterns of surface histamine 1 and 2 receptor expression. Int Arch Allergy Immunol 124:190–192

Koarai A, Ichinose M, Ishigaki-Suzuki S et al (2003) Disruption of L-histidine decarboxylase reduces airway eosinophilia but not hyperresponsiveness. Am J Respir Crit Care Med 167: 758–763

Kuefner MA, Schwelberger HG, Weidenhiller M et al (2004) Both catabolic pathways of histamine via histamine-N-methyltransferase and diamine oxidase are diminished in the colonic mucosa of patients with food allergy. Inflamm Res 53:S31–S32

Lange P, Parner J, Vestbo J et al (1998) A 15-year follow-up study of ventilatory function in adults with asthma. N Engl J Med 339:1194–1200

Lee LY, Lou YP, Hong JL et al (1995) Cigarette smoke-induced bronchoconstruction and release of tachykinins in guinea pig lungs. Resp Physiol 99:173–181

Leuenberger P, Schwartz J, Ackermann-Liebrich U et al (1994) Passive smoking exposure in adults and chronic respiratory symptoms (SAPALDIA Study). Swiss study on air pollution and lung diseases in adults, SAPALDIA team. Am J Respir Crit Care Med 150:1222–1228

Lichtenstein LM, Gillespie E (1975) Effects of the H1 and H2 antihistamines on allergic histamine release and its inhibition by histamine. J Pharmacol Exp Ther 192:441–450

Lippert U, Artuc M, Grützkau A et al (2004) Human skin mast cells express H2 and H4, but not H3 receptors. J Invest Dermatol 123:116–123

Lippert U, Moller A, Welker P et al (2000) Inhibition of cytokine secretion from human leukemic mast cells and basophils by H1- and H2-receptor antagonists. Exp Dermatol 9:118–124

Liu MC, Bleecker ER, Lichtenstein LM et al (1990) Evidence for elevated levels of histamine, prostaglandin D2, and other bronchoconstricting prostaglandins in the airways of subjects with mild asthma. Am Rev Resp Dis 142:126–132

Lokke A, Lange P, Scharling H et al (2006) Developing COPD – a 25 years follow-up study of the general population. Thorax 61:935–939

MacGlashan D Jr (2003) Histamine: a mediator of inflammation. J Allergy Clin Immunol 112: S53–S59

Marieb E (2001) Human anatomy and physiology. Benjamin Cummings, San Francisco, p 414

Mazzoni A, Young HA, Spitzer JH et al (2001) Histamine regulates cytokine production in maturing dendritic cells, resulting in altered T-cell polarization. J Clin Invest 108:1865–1873

Mehlhop PD, van de Rijn M, Goldberg AB et al (1997) Allergen-induced bronchial hyperreactivity and eosinophilic inflammation occur in the absence of IgE in a mouse model of asthma. Proc Natl Acad Sci USA 94:1344–1349

Morgan RK, McAllister B, Cross L et al (2007) Histamine 4 receptor activation induces recruitment of FoxP3+ T cells and inhibits allergic asthma in a murine model. J Immunol 178:8081–8089

Morrow JD, Margolies GR, Rowland J et al (1991) 2nd evidence that histamine is the causative toxin of scombroid-fish poisoning. N Engl J Med 324:716–720

Nogami M, Suko M, Okudaira H et al (1990) Experimental pulmonary eosinophilia in mice by Ascaris suum extract. Am Rev Respir Dis 141:1289–1295

Nogrady SG, Bevan C (1978) Inhaled antihistamines-bronchodilatation and effects on histamine and methacholine-induced bronchoconstriction. Thorax 33:700–704

Nogrady SG, Hartley JPR, Handslip PJ et al (1978) Bronchodilatation following inhalation of the antihistamine clemastine. Thorax 33:479–482

O'Reilly M, Alpert R, Jenkinson S et al (2002) Identification of a histamine H4 receptor on human eosinophils – role in eosinophil chemotaxis. J Recept Signal Transduct Res 22:431–448

Ohtsu H (2008). Progress in allergy signal research on mast cells: the role of histamine in immunological and cardiovascular disease and the transporting system of histamine in the cell. J Pharmacol Sci 106:347–353

Oppenheimer EA, Rigatto M, Fletcher CM (1968) Airways obstruction before and after isoprenaline, histamine, and prednisolone in patients with chronic obstructive bronchitis. Lancet 1:552–557

Parsons ME, Ganellin CR (2006) Histamine and its receptors. Br J Pharmacol 147:S127–S35

Paul K (2008) Chronic obstructive pulmonary disease and emphysema. Retrieved-04-19. Retrieved April 24, 2008, from http://www.emedicine.com/med/topic857.htm

Popa VT (1977) An H1 blocker chlorpheniramine increase the tolerance to inhaled histamine and allergen in asthmatic subjects. Am Rev Respir Dis 115(Suppl)71.7

Preuss CV, Wood TC, Szumlanski CL et al (1998) Human histamine N-methyltransferase pharmacogenetics: common genetic polymorphisms that alter activity. Mol Pharmacol 53:708–717

Ramsdale EH, Morris MM, Roberts RS et al (1984) Bronchial responsiveness to methacholine in chronic bronchitis: relationship to airflow obstruction and cold air responsiveness. Thorax 39:912–918

Ramsdell JW, Nachtwey FG, Moser KM (1982) Bronchial hyperreactivity in chronic obstructive bronchitis. Am Rev Respir Dis 126:829–832

Ranga V, Powers MA, Padilla M et al (1983) Effect of allergic bronchoconstriction on airways epithelial permeability to large polar solutes in the guinea pig. Am Rev Respir Dis 128:1065–1070

Rennard S (1997) Pathophysilogical mechanism of COPD. Eur Res Rev 7:206–210

Rennard S, Vestbo J (2006) COPD: the dangerous underestimate of 15%. Lancet 367:1216–1219

Ryan G, Latimer KM, Dolovich J et al (1982) Bronchial responsiveness to histamine: relationship to diurnal variation of peak flow rate, improvement after bronchodilator, and airway calibre. Thorax 37:423–429

Saetta M, Timens W, Jeffery PK et al (1998) Management of chronic obstructive pulmonary disease. Eur Resp Monograph 7

Schild HO, Hawkins DF, Mongar JL et al (1951) Reactions of isolated human asthmatic lung and bronchial tissue to a specific antigen. Lancet 2:376–382

Schneider E, Rolli-Derkinderen M, Arock M et al (2002) Trends in histamine research: new functions during immune responses and hematopoiesis. Trends Immunol 23:255–263

Shahid M, Tripathi T, Sobial F et al (2009) Histamine, Histamine Receptors, and their Role in Immunomodulation: An Updated Systematic Review. The Open Immunology Journal 2:9–41

Simon RA, Stevenson DD, Arroyave CM et al (1977) The relationship of plasma histamine to the activity of bronchial asthma. J Allergy Clin Immunol 60:312–316

Smith CA, Harrison DJ (1997) Association between polymorphism in gene for microsomal epoxide hydrolase and susceptibility to emphysema. Lancet 350:630–633

Soriano JB, Visick GT, Muellerova H et al (2005) Patterns of comorbidities in newly diagnosed COPD and asthma in primary care. Chest 128:2099–2107

Stick SM, Pulmonary physiology, airway responsiveness and asthma. MJA Vol 177 16 September 2002

Sugata Y, Okano M, Fujiwara T et al (2007) Histamine H4 receptor agonists have more activities than H4 agonist in antigen-specific human T-cell responses. Immunology 121:266–275

Takeda K, Hamelmann E, Joetham A et al (1997) Development of eosinophilic airway inflammation and airway hyperresponsiveness in mast cell-deficient mice. J Exp Med 186: 449–454

Takeshita K, Sakai K, Bacon KB et al (2003) Critical role of histamine H4 receptor in leukotriene B4 production and mast cell dependent neutrophil recruitment induced by zymosan in vivo. J Pharmacol Exp Ther 307:1072–1078

Thomson NC, Chaudhuri R, Livingston E (2004) Asthma and cigarette smoking. Eur Resp 24:822–833

Thurmond RL, Desai PJ, Dunford PJ et al (2004) A potent and selective histamine H4 receptor antagonist with anti-inflammatory properties. J Pharmacol Exp Ther 309:404–413

Thurmond RL, Gelfand EW, Dunford PJ (2008) The role of histamine H_1 and H_4 receptors in allergic inflammation: the search for new antihistamines. Nat Rev Drug Dis 7:41–53

Triggiani M et al (2007) Differentiation of monocytes into macrophages induces the upregulation of histamine H1 receptor. J Allergy Clin Immunol 119:472–481

Triggiani M, Gentile M, Secondo A et al (2001) Histamine induces exocytosis and IL-6 production from human lung macrophages through interaction with H1 receptors. J Immunol 166:4083–4091

van der Pouw Kraan TC, Snijders A, Boeije LC et al (1998) Histamine inhibits the production of interleukin-12 through interaction with H2 receptors. J Clin Invest 102:1866–1873

Verma VK, Cockcroft DW, Dosman JA (1988) Airway responsiveness to inhaled histamine in chronic obstructive airways disease. Chronic bronchitis vs emphysema. Chest 94:457–461

Wardlaw AJ, Dunnette S, Gleich GJ et al (1988) Eosinophils and mast cells in bronchoalveolar lavage in subjects with mild asthma. Relationship to bronchial hyperreactivity. Am Rev Respir Dis 137:62–69

Wenzel SE, Fowler AA, Schwartz LB (1988) Activation of pulmonary mast cells by bronchoalveolar allergen challenge in vivo release of histamine and tryptase in atopic subjects with and without asthma. Am Rev Respir Dis 137:1002–1008

Yanni JM, Weimer LK, Sharif NA et al (1999) Inhibition of histamine-induced human conjunctival epithelial cell responses by ocular allergy drugs. Arch Opthalmol 117:643–647

Part VII
Histamine Role in Inflammation and Allergy

Chapter 11
Mast Cells as a Source and Target for Histamine

Ewa Brzezińska-Błaszczyk

Abstract Mast cells are distributed throughout the body and without any doubt are a major cellular source of histamine in the organism. Decarboxylation of histidine to form histamine takes place in Golgi apparatus and then this amine is stored in cytoplasmic secretory granules as a complex with proteoglycans at acidic pH. Histamine is released together with other preformed mediators during mast cell degranulation and it dissociates in tissues from the proteoglycan-histamine complex by cation exchange with extracellular sodium and at neutral pH. It is well known that cross-linking of high affinity IgE receptors (FcεRI) stimulates mast cell degranulation and histamine release. However, there is emerging evidence that receptors for IgG (FcγR) can also activate mast cells to histamine release. Moreover, it is now well established that several endogenous factors, such as some proinflammatory molecules, defensins, cathelicidins, neuropeptides, different cytokines and chemokines, as well as other cell-derived peptides induce histamine release from mast cells. Mast cells also degranulate in response to some bacterial cell wall components and bacterial toxins. Nowadays, it is documented that mast cells express specific histamine receptors, such as H1, H2 and H4, thus it can be presumed that histamine, together with other humoral factors might affect tissue mast cells homeostasis and reactivity, and might regulate its own secretion, as well.

Keywords Histamine · Mast cells · Endogenous factors

Abbreviations

bFGF	basic fibroblast growth factor
BMMC	bone marrow-derived mast cell
CBMC	cord blood-derived mast cell
CD	cluster of differentiation

E. Brzezińska-Błaszczyk (✉)
Department of Experimental Immunology, Medical University of Łódź, Pomorska 251, 92–213 Łódź, Poland
e-mail: ewab@csk.umed.lodz.pl

M. Shahid et al. (eds.), *Biomedical Aspects of Histamine*,
DOI 10.1007/978-90-481-9349-3_11, © Springer Science+Business Media B.V. 2010

CGRP	calcitonin gene-related peptide
ConA	concanavalin A
CRH	corticotropin-releasing hormone
CTMC	connective tissue mast cell
ECM	extracellular matrix
ECP	eosinophil cationic protein
EDN	eosinophil-derived neurotoxin
EPO	eosinophil peroxidase
ET	endothelin
FSMC	fetal skin-derived mast cell
GM-CSF	granulocyte-macrophage colony stimulating factor
GRO	growth-related oncogene
HDC	histamine decarboxylase
HMC-1	human mast cell line
IFN	interferon
IL	interleukin
IP-10	interferon inducible protein
ITAM	immunoreceptor tyrosine-based activation motif
LAM	lipoarabinomannan
LPS	lipopolysaccharide
LT	leukotriene
LTA	lipoteichoic acid
MBP	major basic protein
MC_T	tryptase-containing mast cell
MC_{TC}	tryptase- chymase-containing mast cell
MCP	monocyte chemoattractant protein
M-CSF	macrophage colony stimulating factor
MIP	macrophage inflammatory protein
MMC	mucosal mast cell
MMP	metalloproteinase
MPO	myeloperoxidase
NAP	neutrophil activating peptide
NFAT	nuclear factor of activated T cells
NGF	nerve growth factor
NK	neurokinin
NP	natriuretic peptide
NPY	neuropeptide Y
NT	neurotensin
PACAP	pituitary adenylate cyclase activating polypeptide
PAF	platelet activating factor
PAMP	pathogen-associated molecular pattern
PDGF	platelet-derived growth factor
PG	prostaglandin
PGN	peptydoglican
PKC	phospholipase C

PMA	phorbol myristate acetate
RBL-2H3	rat basophilic leukemia 2H3 line
SCF	stem cell factor
SDF	stromal cell-derived factor
sgIGSF	spermatogenic Ig superfamily
SP	substance P
STAT	signal transducers and activator of transcription
TGF	transforming growth factor
TLR	Toll-like receptor
TNF	tumour necrosis factor
VEGF	vascular endothelial growth factor
VIP	vasoactive intestinal peptide

Contents

11.1 Introduction

Histamine was first identified in 1911 owing to its potent vasoactive properties. Following the recognition, histamine has been one of the most studied endogenous substances possessing a wide spectrum of activities. Nowadays, it is well recognized that the fundamental pleiotropic regulatory character of histamine in cellular events is attributed to its binding to four subtypes of G-protein coupled receptors, designated H1, H2, H3, and H4 that are differentially expressed in various cell types. The H1 receptors are mainly involved in the regulation of vascular permeability and smooth muscle contraction. The H2 receptor stimulation evokes an increase of gastric acid secretion, an increase of mucus secretion in bronchi and the relaxation of smooth muscles of small blood vessels. The H3 receptors are classified as presynaptic receptors controlling neurotransmission in the central nervous system.

Growing evidence indicate that the H4 receptor signaling modulates immune system processes and inflammatory reactions (MacGlashan 2003, Repka-Ramirez and Baraniuk 2002, Schneider et al. 2002).

Histamine (2-(4-imidazolyl)-ethylamine) is an endogenous short-acting biogenic amine synthesized from the basic amino acid L-histidine through the catalytic activity of the rate-limiting enzyme L-histidine decarboxylase (HDC). It should be indicated that histamine can be synthesized in several cell types of peripheral and central tissues, because almost every cell populations is endowed with potential ability to express the activity of HDC. The activity of HDC is modulated by various cytokines, such as interleukin (IL)-1, IL-3, IL-12, IL-18, and tumour necrosis factor (TNF), and by some growth factors, such as granulocyte-macrophage colony stimulating factor (GM-CSF) and macrophage colony stimulating factor (M-CSF), as well (Schneider et al. 1987, Yamaguchi et al. 2000a, b, Yoshimoto et al. 1999).

It has been proven, that cells that are able to synthesize histamine de novo, in adequate conditions, include hematopoietic cell populations (Kawaguchi-Nagata et al. 1985, Piquet-Pellorce and Dy 1991), various types of blood cells, such as monocytes (László et al. 2001, Zwadlo-Klarwasser et al. 1998), platelets (Váczi et al. 2001), neutrophils (Shiraishi et al. 2000), and CD4$^+$ T cells and CD8$^+$ T cells (Kubo and Nakano 1999, Sonobe et al. 2004), as well as macrophages (Takamatsu et al. 1996), dendritic cells (Szeberényi et al. 2001a, b), enterochromaffin-like cells (Prinz et al. 2003), neurons (Arrang et al. 1983, Haas et al. 2008), chondrocytes (Maślińska et al. 2004), and tumours (Falus et al. 2001). These cells lack specific cytoplasmic granules for histamine storage, and this is why this amine is released as soon as it is synthesized. For this reason, the cells present the high HDC activity but low intracellular histamine content. To mark histamine distinction from the stored molecule, the histamine thus generated is termed "neosynthesized" or "nascent" (Dy and Lebel 1983, Dy et al. 1981).

The unique body cells that can synthesize and then store histamine within secretory cytoplasmic granules are mast cells in tissues, as well as basophils in the blood. Decarboxylation of histidine to form histamine takes place in the Golgi apparatus of mast cells and basophils. Histamine is then stored associated by ionic linkage with the carboxyl groups of proteins and proteoglycans of the secretory granules at acidic pH. This amine is released, together with other preformed mediators stored within granules, during mast cell degranulation. In tissues, histamine dissociates from the proteglycan-protein complex by cation exchange with extracellular sodium and at neutral pH.

Considering that: (1) mast cells are widely distributed throughout the connective tissue of the body; (2) the number of mast cells in tissues is very high, especially in anatomical sites which interface with the environment, such as skin, airways, and gastrointestinal tract, as well as in close proximity to blood vessels, nerves, smooth muscle cells, epithelial cells, mucus-producing cells, and hair follicles (for example: estimated concentrations of mast cells range from 500 to 4,000 per mm^3 in lungs, from 7,000 to 12,000 per mm^3 in skin, and about 20,000 per mm^3 in gastrointestinal tract); (3) mast cells store histamine in preformed cytoplasmic secretory granules; (4) mast cells can release substantial amounts of preformed histamine in a single stimulatory event through a process termed degranulation; and (5) various triggers, both endogenous and exogenous, can elicit massive and very rapid mast cell degranulation response, it appears to be allowed to claim that mast cells are a major cellular source of histamine in the organism.

11.2 Mast Cells

11.2.1 Origin, Distribution and Heterogeneity

Mast cells are multifunctional long-lived secretory cells, characterized by its content of numerous large cytoplasmic granules. These cells originate from CD (cluster of differentiation) 34^+, $CD13^+$, $CD117^+$ multipotential hematopoietic stem cells in bone marrow (Kirshenbaum et al. 1991, 1999, Rodewald et al. 1996), and circulate in small numbers as agranular committed progenitors. Developing mast cells subsequently migrate to peripheral tissues where they terminate their maturation and differentiation under the influence of various factors in the tissue environment (Hallgren and Gurish 2007, Okayama and Kawakami 2006, Welle 2005).

Mature mast cells have small nucleus and round to oval in shape. Cytoplasm contains filaments, microtubule, rough endoplasmic reticulum, Golgi vesicles, free ribosomes, mitochondria, lysosomes, and lipid bodies. The most characteristic cytoplasmic organelle in mast cells are numerous membrane-bound secretory granules (Kalesnikoff and Galli 2008, Metcalfe et al. 1997).

Mast cells do not represent a homogenous population. In rodents, two mast cell subsets are described: connective tissue mast cells (CTMCs) (typical mast cells) and mucosal mast cells (MMCs) (atypical mast cells). CTMCs are predominantly found in skin and peritoneal cavity, and MMCs are mainly found in mucosal layer of gut and lungs. There are phenotypical differences between these two mast cell subsets, such as size, proteoglycan and neutral protease composition, as well as histamine content. Cytoplasmic granules of typical mast cells contain heparin, carboxypeptidase A and 10–20 pg of histamine per cell, while granules of atypical mast cells contain chondroitin sulphate and only about 1 pg of histamine per cell. In addition, these mast cell subpopulations exhibit functional differences, with MMCs mainly producing leukotriene (LT)C_4 and CTMC mainly producing prostaglandin (PG)D_2 upon IgE-FcεRI activation (Kitamura 1989).

By analogy to rodent mast cells, in humans two analogous subsets of mast cells are described that differ depending on whether their cytoplasmic granules contain the neutral protease tryptase alone (MC_T) or tryptase along with chymase (MC_{TC}) (Irani et al. 1986). MC_{TC} are predominantly found within connective tissues, while MC_T are mainly located at mucosal surfaces. It is now realized that variable amounts of both mast cell subtypes are present within any given tissue; for example, in skin 99% of mast cell population belong to MC_{TC} subset, but 1% of these cells is classified as MC_T type, and in small intestine submucosa 77% of mast cells are categorized as MC_{TC} and 23% as MC_T subtypes. On the contrary, in alveolar tissue 93% of mast cells are recognized as MC_T and 7% as MC_{TC} subsets, and in small intestine mucosa 81% of mast cells belong to MC_T and 19% to MC_{TC} subopulations. Cytoplasmic granules of MC_{TC} subset contain tryptase (about 35 pg per cell), chymase, carboxypeptidase and cathepsin G, while granules of MC_T contain only tryptase (about 10 pg per cell). These two human mast cell populations, MC_{TC} and MC_T, also display functional heterogeneity, with the former producing mainly IL-4, and the latter producing both IL-5 and IL-6 (Bradding et al. 1995).

Mature mast cells express numerous surface receptors (Valent et al. 2001), and thereby their biological and secretory activities can be influenced by a lot of endogenous humoral factors. It is undisputable that mast cells constitutively possess a relatively high level of high affinity receptor for IgE (FcεRI) (Kinet 1999, Metcalfe et al. 1997). What is more, mast cells express several other receptors for the Fc portion of immunoglobulin (FcR), including FcγRI, FcγRII, and FcγRIII (Tkaczyk et al. 2004). Besides FcR receptors these cells have receptors specific for some cytokines and chemokines (Juremalm and Nilsson 2005), for several neuropeptides and hormones, and for certain complement products (Nilsson et al. 1996), as well as for other proinflammatory factors. As it will be discussed later in this chapter, mast cells also express specific receptors for histamine. Finally, it should be emphasized that mast cells have different kinds of Toll-like receptors (TLRs), i.e. specific receptors for pathogen-associated molecular patterns (PAMPs) (Matsushima et al. 2004a, Supajatura et al. 2002, Varadaradjalou et al. 2003).

11.2.2 Mast Cell Mediators

Mast cells have the potential to secrete a wide variety of biologically active mediators, cytokines, and chemokines (Table 11.1). These include: [1] granule-associated mediators, including histamine, neutral proteases and metalloproteinases (MMPs), as well as some preformed cytokines, such as IL-3, -4, -5, -6, and -10, TNF, vascular endothelial growth factor (VEGF), nerve growth factor (NGF), transforming growth factor (TGF)-β, basic fibroblast growth factor (bFGF), and chemokine CXCL8 (IL-8); [2] newly generated arachidonic acid metabolites, including LTs, PGs and platelet activating factor (PAF); and [3] de novo synthesized interleukins, TNF, interferon (IFN)-γ, a lot of growth factors, such as NGF, TGF-β, stem cell factor (SCF), platelet-derived growth factor (PDGF), GM-CSF, and chemokines, such as CXCL8, CCL2 (monocyte chemoattractant protein-1, MCP-1), CCL3 (macrophage inflammatory protein (MIP)-1α), CCL4 (MIP-1β), CCL5 (RANTES), and CCL20 (MIP-3α) (Kalesnikoff and Galli 2008, Krishnaswamy et al. 2001, Metcalfe et al. 1997, Rao and Brown 2008).

Table 11.1 Major mast cell-derived mediators

granule-associated mediators	histamine, heparin/chondroitin sulphate neutral protease (tryptase, chymase, carboxypeptidase A) MMPs (MMP-2, -3, -9) acid hydrolases, peroxidase
granule-associated cytokines/chemokines	IL-3, -4, -5, -6, -10 TNF, VEGF, NGF, TGF-β, bFGF CXCL8
lipid-derived mediators	LTs (LTB_4, LTC_4, LTD_4) PGs (PGD_2, PGE_2) PAF
De novo synthesized cytokines	IL-1, -2, -3, -4, -5, -6, -9, -10, -12, -13, -16, -18, -25 TNF, IFN-γ, NGF, TGF-β, SCF, PGDF, GM-CSF
De novo synthesized chemokines	CCL2, CCL3, CCL4, CCL5, CCL20 CXCL8

There is some data proving that mast cells can also produce and release corticotropin-releasing factor (CRH) and its structurally related urocortin (Kempuraj et al. 2003), as well as endothelin-1 (ET-1) (Liu et al. 1998) and osteopontin (Nagasaka et al. 2008). It is also documented that mast cells can be a source of some antimicrobial peptides, such as human cathelicidin LL-37 or mouse cathelicidin-related CRAMP and β-defensin-4 (Di Nardo et al. 2003), as well as amphiregulin – a member of epidermal growth factor family (Okumura et al. 2005, Wang et al. 2005), CXCL5 (ENA-78) (Lukacs et al. 1998), as well as granzyme B (Pardo et al. 2007).

It should be emphasized that many of mast cell products, for example histamine, LTs, PGs, TNF, IL-1β, IL-6, and chemokines, exert proinflammatory activities. However, some of the products that might be released by mast cells, for example IL-10 and TGF-β, exhibit antiinflammatory or immunosuppressive properties. Mast cell mediators, mainly neutral proteases and MMPs, can promote changes in tissues, including local degradation of extracellular matrix (ECM) proteins and remodeling of structural elements of tissues. It seems important that mast cells produce both Th2-skewing cytokines such as IL-4, IL-5, and IL-13 and Th1-skewing cytokines such as IL-12, IL-18, and IFN-γ. Moreover, mast cells are also an important source of several chemokines, including those associated with Th2 response, such as CCL5, or connected with Th1-type responses, such as CXCL8. Considering this data it is obvious that mast cells take part not only in maintaining homeostasis (Galli and Tsai 2008, Maurer et al. 2003, Metcalfe et al. 1997, Rao and Brown 2008), but also are important players in inflammatory processes (Galli and Tsai 2008, Metz et al. 2007, Theoharides and Kalogeromitros 2006), tissue remodeling (Galli and Tsai 2008), and strongly influence immune responses (Metz and Maurer 2007, Rao and Brown 2008). These cells are also involved in host defense against pathogens (Galli and Tsai 2008, Krishnaswamy et al. 2001).

11.3 Factors Stimulating Mast Cells to Histamine Release

11.3.1 FcR-Dependent Mast Cells Activation

11.3.1.1 FcεRI-Dependent Mast Cell Stimulation

High affinity receptor for IgE FcεRI is predominantly expressed on mast cells and basophils. FcεRI is a heterodimer composed of a ligand-binding α chain, a signal transducting γ chain dimer, and a signal-augmenting β chain. FcεRI can bind IgE in the absence of antigen with high affinity (affinity constant = 10^9–10^{10} M^{-1}), and the binding of IgE stabilizes the receptor at the plasma membrane, with the binding of IgE to the receptor α chain as a minimal requirement (Borkowski et al. 2001, Kubo et al. 2001). On cross-linking of IgE receptor by IgE-multivalent antigen complexes, immunoreceptor tyrosine-based activation motifs (ITAMs) on β and γ chains become phosphorylated and initiate a signaling cascade (Gilfillan and Tkaczyk 2006), resulting in three distinct pathways of mediator production; within seconds to minutes of FcεRI cross-linking cytoplasmic granules fuse with each other and with the cell surface membrane, ejecting their contents into the extracellular milieu; within minutes mast cells start to generate eicosanoids derived from the cleavage of arachidonic acid from membrane phospholipids; and within hours mast cells synthesize cytokines and chemokines (Rivera and Gilfillan 2006).

There is growing evidence that IgE, a natural ligand for FcεRI, has powerful regulatory effect on expression of its receptor. Although mast cells express a relatively high level of FcεRI constitutively, the level of this receptor can be further upregulated by soluble monomeric IgE (Asai et al. 2001, Kawakami and Galli 2002, Kitaura et al. 2004, Yamaguchi et al. 1999). For rat basophilic leukemia (RBL)-2H3 cells which are regarded as a mucosal mast cell line, it is shown that incubation with IgE results in a doubling of IgE receptor expression on the cell surface (Furuichi et al. 1985). For murine bone marrow-derived mast cells (BMMCs), a 6-fold upregulation of receptor density upon prolongated culture with IgE is reported (Hsu and MacGlashan 1996). Yamaguchi et al. (1997) also achieved an increased receptor expression by administration IgE in vivo. It should be stressed that whereas IgE greatly elevates FcεRI expression, IgE cross-linkage with multivalent antigen rapidly decreases FcεRI levels to approximately the baseline expression of cells cultured without IgE. This reduction is mediated by internalization of receptor-IgE-antigen complexes, coupled by degradation of those aggregates containing antigen (Mao et al. 1992, Robertson et al. 1986).

Accumulating evidence has indicated that IgE-mediated activation of mast cells can occur even in the absence of the multivalent antigen. It is documented that IgE alone promotes, via autocrine production of IL-3 (Kohno et al. 2005) or IL-6 (Cruse et al. 2008, Kitaura et al. 2005), the survival of mast cells, and stimulates mast cell adhesion to fibronectin (Kitaura et al. 2005, Lam et al. 2003). Matsuda et al. (2005) observed that exposure of mast cells to IgE significantly enhances production and release of some chemokines, such as CXCL8 and CCL2. Furthermore, binding of IgE to its receptor in the absence of antigen results in de novo synthesis of HDC

(Tanaka et al. 2002). Monomeric IgE stimulates nuclear factor of activated T cells (NFAT) translocation into the nucleus, a rise in cytosol Ca^{2+}, degranulation, and membrane ruffling in the cultured RBL-2H3 cells and BMMCs (Oka et al. 2004, Pandey et al. 2004). Also Cruse et al. (2005) documented that IgE alone induces a rise in cytosolic Ca^{2+} and dose-dependent histamine release, as well as LTC_4 production and CXCL8 synthesis. Oka et al. (2004) indicated that IgE, at concentrations too low to increase either Ca^{2+} rise or degranulation, significantly induces actin assembly, which serves as a negative feedback control in mast cell Ca^{2+} signaling and degranulation. Yamaguchi et al. (1999) stated that IgE-dependent enhancement of FcεRI expression is associated with a significantly enhanced ability of human mast cells to secrete histamine, as well as PGD_2 and LTC_4, upon subsequent passive sensitization with IgE and challenge with anti-IgE.

11.3.1.2 FcγR-Dependent Mast Cell Stimulation

There is emerging evidence that, in addition to FcεRI, receptors for IgG (FcγRs) can also regulate mast cell activation and mediator release. It should be pointed out, however, that FcγRs, under appropriate conditions, may either induce or inhibit stimulation of mast cells.

Okayama et al. (2000, 2001a, 2003) stated that resting human mast cells exhibit minimal message for FcγRI, however pretreatment of these cells with IFN-γ upregulates FcγRI expression; FcεRI, FcγRII and FcγRIII expression is not affected by IFN-γ. Furthermore, aggregation of FcγRI results in significant degranulation and histamine release, in PGD_2 and LTC_4 generation, as well as in upregulation of mRNA expression for specific cytokines including IL-1β, IL-3, IL-5, IL-6, IL-13, TNF, and GM-CSF. Woolhiser et al. (2001) documented that IFN-γ-pretreated human mast cells, sensitized with IgG1 antibodies, both degranulate and generate PGD_2 and LTC_4, and synthesize TNF, as well. What is more, these authors observed that simultaneous activation of mast cells via FcγRI and FcεRI (Woolhiser et al. 2001) or via FcγRI and C3a complement peptide (Woolhiser et al. 2004) leads to additive degranulation.

Low affinity IgG receptors (FcγRIII) are present on mature mast cells, but not on immature cells (Katz et al. 1990, Okayama et al. 2001b), and SCF (Katz and Lobell 1995) and IL-4 (Chong et al. 2003) can induce upregulation of FcγRIII surface expression. Cross-linking of these receptors results in degranulation and generation of various lipid mediators (Chong et al. 2003, Daëron et al. 1992, Katz et al. 1992). Dastych et al. (1997) showed that aggregation of FcγRIII on mast cells leads to mast cell adhesion to fibronectin, as well.

It is established that human resting (Okayama et al. 2001b, Zhao et al. 2006) and mouse mature (Fong et al. 1996, Katz et al. 1990) mast cells express IgG receptors FcγRII. While FcγRI and FcγRIII seem to upregulate mast cell activity, aggregation of FcγRII negatively regulates IgE-induced mast cell response. Coagreggation of FcεRI with FcγRII, with bispecific antibodies, inhibits antigen-induced histamine release by human mast cells (Kepley et al. 2004, Tam et al. 2004), as well as cytokine production and Ca^{2+} mobilization (Kepley et al. 2004). IgE-induced release of mediators and cytokines can be inhibited by cross-linking FcεRI to FcγRII (Daëron et al. 1995).

11.3.2 Endogenous Factors

11.3.2.1 Proinflammatory Factors

Considering that mast cells play a crucial role in the inflammation developed during many pathological processes as well as bacterial infection and tissue damage it is of great importance to understand mast cell activation by proinflammatory factors. Nowadays, it seems that some of the most important proinflammatory factors that can stimulate mast cells to degranulation and histamine release, in a FcR-independent manner, are complement peptides. The activation of complement system cascade results in the cleavage of complement components C3 and C5 and generation of peptides such as C3a and C5a, named anaphylatoxins. It is now well established that C5a peptide triggers mast cell degranulation and histamine release from human skin (el-Lati et al. 1994, Füreder et al. 1995a, Kubota 1992, Oskeritzian et al. 2005) and synovial (Kiener et al. 1998) mast cells. However, C5a fragment does not induce human mast cells isolated from lung, uterus, tonsil, heart or human mast cell (HMC)-1 cell line to degranulation (Füreder et al. 1995a, Schulman et al. 1988). Mast cells degranulation is also observed in response to C3a stimulation (el-Lati et al. 1994, Kubota 1992, Legler et al. 1996, Mousli et al. 1992). el-Lati et al. (1994) indicated that both C3a and C5a can trigger histamine release from mast cells in a dose-dependent manner, with C5a being 40–50 times more potent. C3a and C5a peptides act through specific receptors, such as complement component 3a receptor 1 (C3aR1) and C5aR (CD88), respectively (Füreder et al. 1995a, Kiener et al. 1998, Legler et al. 1996, Oskeritzian et al. 2005). Füreder et al. (1995a) found that C5aR is detectable on human skin and a subset (5–15%) of cardiac mast cells, and on HMC-1 cells, but not on lung, uterus or tonsillar mast cells. Oskeritzian et al. (2005) stated that C5aR is expressed only on connective tissue mast cell subpopulation (MC_{TC}).

It seems very interesting that C3a peptide can inhibit IgE-induced triggering of the mucosal type RBL-2H3 cells (Erdei and Pecht 1996, Erdei et al. 1997). Even more interesting are observations proving that antigen-dependent stimulation of mast cells can induce neoexpression of a functional C5aR (Soruri et al. 2008).

Defensins and cathelicidins are the host defense peptides which act as potent, broad spectrum antibiotics. It is indicated that both β-defensin-2 (Befus et al. 1999, Kase et al. 2009, Niyonsaba et al. 2001) and human cathelicidin LL-37 (Niyonsaba et al. 2001) activate mast cells to degranulation and histamine release, whereby potentiating innate immune response against pathogens. Wojtecka-Łukasik and Maśliński (1992) demonstrated mast cell degranulation in response to fibronectin and fibrinogen degradation products.

11.3.2.2 Neuropeptides

Mast cells are found in close proximity to nerve endings at several anatomical sites such as skin, lungs, intestinal mucosa, and central nervous system, and adhesion molecules such as N-cadherin and spermatogenic Ig superfamily (sgIGSF), recently termed cell adhesion molecule-1 (CADM1) (Ito et al. 2008) have been shown to mediate physical interaction between these cells (Furuno et al. 2005, Suzuki et al. 2004, Watabe et al. 2004). According to electron microscopy, membrane-membrane apposition with a spatial gap of approximately 20 nm or less is detected between nerve and mast cells (Stead et al. 1987, 1989). These anatomical findings indicate that mast cells and neurons interact in a bidirectional manner and represent a functional unit (Bauer and Razin 2000, Suzuki et al. 2001, Van Nassauw et al. 2007).

There is a lot of data suggesting that substance P (SP), neuropeptide that functions as a neurotransmitter and neuromodulator, strongly stimulates mast cell degranulation and histamine release. This peptide induces histamine release from rat, murine and hamster peritoneal mast cells (Ali et al. 1986, Barrocas et al. 1999, Fewtrell et al. 1982, Mousli et al. 1989, Ogawa et al. 1999, Piotrowski and Foreman 1985), from human skin (Brzezińska-Błaszczyk and Zalewska 1998, Columbo et al. 1996, Lowman et al. 1988, Zalewska et al. 1997) and intestinal (Brzezińska-Błaszczyk et al. 1998) mast cells, as well as from dural (Ottosson and Edvinsson 1997) and brain (Cocchiara et al. 1999) mast cells. Other tachykinin neuropeptides, closely SP-related, such as neurokinin A (NKA) and neurokinin B (NKB), stimulate histamine release from rat peritoneal and human skin mast cells (Lowman et al. 1988, Ogawa et al. 1999). van der Kleij et al. (2003) clearly showed functional expression of NK1 receptors on mast cell surface and documented its role in SP-induced histamine release. It is also stated that SP dose-dependently potentiates anti-IgE-induced histamine release from rat peritoneal mast cells at concentrations which alone induced insignificant or low level of histamine release (Lau et al. 2001). Thus, SP can modulate immunologic activation of mast cells.

Calcitonin gene-related peptide (CGRP), a member of the calcitonin family of peptides produced in both peripheral and central neurons, induces human skin (Lowman et al. 1988), rat dural (Ottosson and Edvinsson 1997) and peritoneal (Piotrowski and Foreman 1986) mast cells to degranulation, however CGRP is about fourfold less potent than SP in releasing histamine (Piotrowski and Foreman 1986). Neuropeptide Y (NPY), neurotransmitter found in brain and autonomic nervous system, stimulates dural mast cells to histamine release (Ottosson and Edvinsson 1997).

It is also established that somatostatin can stimulate rat peritoneal (Piotrowski and Foreman 1985, Theoharides and Douglas 1978) and human skin (Lowman et al. 1988) mast cells to histamine release, and neurotensin (NT) can elicit secretory response of rat peritoneal (Carraway et al. 1982, Kurose and Saeki 1981) and human skin (Lowman et al. 1988) mast cells. Barrocas et al. (1999) and Feldberg et al. (1998) showed that NT-induced mast cell secretion is receptor-mediated, pertussis-toxin sensitive and requires activation of phospholipase C (PKC). Mast cells release histamine also in response to challenge with vasoactive intestinal peptide (VIP) (Brzezińska-Błaszczyk et al. 1998, Lowman et al. 1988, Ottosson and Edvinsson 1997, Piotrowski and Foreman 1985) and pituitary adenylate cyclase activating polypeptide (PACAP) (Mori et al. 1994, Odum et al. 1998, Seebeck et al. 1998).

It should be stressed that the widespread distribution of neuropeptides in tissues coupled with the frequent localization of mast cells in close proximity of nerve endings suggests a neurocrine control of mast cell secretion. In turn, mast cell mediators can influence neuronal activity. These nerve-mast cells effects, together with the anatomical association between them, are assumed to be important for the promotion and regulation of many inflammatory diseases (Theoharides 1996, Theoharides and Cochranc 2004).

11.3.2.3 Cytokines and Chemokines

It is unquestionable that cytokines regulate a number of physiological and pathological processes, by influencing a lot of different cellular activities. It is becoming more and more evident that cytokines not only play a central role in mast cell development, but also significantly modulate mast cell functions. There is some data showing that some cytokines, directly or indirectly, influence mast cell degranulation and histamine release.

It was shown that SCF, one of key factors of mast cell differentiation and maturation, can directly stimulate rat (Nakajima et al. 1992) and mouse (Coleman et al. 1993) peritoneal mast cells, as well as human cutaneous (Columbo et al. 1992) and lung (Takaishi et al. 1994) mast cells to rapid degranulation. Also TNF, an important proinflammatory cytokine, activates human skin (van Overveld et al. 1991) and rat peritoneal (Brzezińska-Błaszczyk et al. 2000, Olejnik and Brzezińska-Błaszczyk 1998) mast cells to degranulation and histamine release. It was stated, that NGF induces histamine release from rat peritoneal mast cells (Pearce and Thompson 1986) and murine BMMCs (Horigome et al. 1993), as well. On the contrary, a number of cytokines, such as IL-3, IL-4, IL-5, IL-9 (Bischoff and Dahinden 1992, Takaishi et al. 1994), IL-15 (Jackson et al. 2005), IL-33 (Ho et al. 2007), and GM-CSF (Takaishi et al. 1994) do not stimulate mast cell degranulation.

From pathophysiological point of view it is of great importance that some cytokines regulate mast cell degranulation and preformed mediators, including histamine release. It is now well established that preincubation of mast cells with SCF enhances histamine release from human (Bischoff and Dahinden 1992, Columbo et al. 1992, Louis et al. 1994, 1995, Takaishi et al. 1994), and rat (Coleman et al. 1993) mast cells in response to IgE receptor crosslinking. This cytokine potentiates SP-induced degranulation (Columbo et al. 1992) and causes an increase of mast cell degranulation to the stimulation with calcium ionophore A23187 (Lin et al. 1996), as well. Hughes et al. (1995) observed an increase of histamine release from mast cells challenged with antigen, previously pretreated with TNF, and we noticed that pretreatment of mast cells with TNF significantly reduces concanavalin (Con)-A-stimulated release of histamine (Brzezińska-Błaszczyk et al. 2000, Olejnik and Brzezińska-Błaszczyk 1998). It is also documented that IFNs modulate mast cell degranulation. Bissonnette et al. (1995) documented that pretreatment of rat peritoneal mast cells with IFN-α/β or IFN-γ significantly reduces antigen-stimulated histamine release and Yanagida et al. (1996) stated that IFN-γ-pretreatment of cultured human mast cells causes an enhancement in histamine release to the challenge with anti-IgE. NGF potentiates antigen-, ConA-, and calcium ionophore A23187-induced rat peritoneal mast cell degranulation (Ferjan and Carman-Krzan 2000, Tomioka et al. 1988), IL-5 and IL-6 enhance IgE-anti-IgE-challenged degranulation of human mast cells (Yanagida et al. 1995) and GM-CSF potentiates histamine release from human lung mast cells activated through FcεRI (Louis et al. 1995). Recently, Nagasaka et al. (2008) stated that osteopontin significantly augments IgE-mediated degranulation of mast cells.

More and more data indicate that mast cell activity is controlled by some of regulatory cytokines, such as IL-10 and TGF-β1, and, to a lesser extent, by IL-4. Using murine BMMCs Gillespie et al. (2004) found that IL-10 significantly reduces FcεRI surface expression through the decrease of β chain protein level. Also TGF-β1 considerably reduces IgE receptor expression on mouse BMMCs, through regulating protein synthesis, with kinetics that is similar to IL-10 (Gomez et al. 2005). Ryan et al. (1998) stated that IL-4 exhibits a signal transducers and activator of transcription (STAT)6-dependent decrease in FcεRI expression on mouse BMMCs; however, IL-4 up-regulates expression in this receptor on human mast cells (Toru et al. 1996, Xia et al. 1997, Yamaguchi et al. 1999). Moreover, the ability of IgE to upregulate FcεRI expression is reduced by both IL-10 (Gillespie et al. 2004) and TGF-β1 (Gomez et al. 2005) stimulation. The downregulation of FcεRI expression should affect anaphylactic mast cell activation, i.e., degranulation and preformed mediator release, as well as synthesis and release of newly generated mediators that is arachidonic acid metabolites, cytokines and chemokines. Bissonnette et al. (1997) showed that antigen-induced histamine and TNF release from rat peritoneal mast cells are inhibited by TGF-β1, whereas Gomez et al. (2005) stated that this cytokine suppresses IgE-mediated degranulation as well as TNF and IL-6 production. Meade et al. (1992) documented that in vivo treatment with TGF-β1 inhibits IgE-mediated mast cell-dependent immediate hypersensitivity in mice. On the contrary, Kim and Lee (1999) reported that TGF-β1 potentiates IgE-dependent anaphylaxis. Surprisingly, IL-10 does not influence mast cell degranulation and histamine release (Gillespie et al. 2004, Marshall et al. 1996), despite reduction in IgE receptor levels. In contrast, IL-10 reduces IgE-induced TNF production and secretion (Gillespie et al. 2004). Ryan et al. (1998) noticed that the IL-4-induced decrease in FcεRI expression on mouse BMMCs is coupled with reduction both IgE-mediated degranulation and the induction of mRNA for IL-4, IL-5, IL-6, and IL-13. However, there is some data that IL-4 increases not only FcεRI expression (Toru et al. 1996, Xia et al. 1997, Yamaguchi et al. 1999) but also upregulates mast cell responsiveness. Bischoff et al. (1999) stated that IL-4 itself enhances the release of histamine, as well as LTC_4 and IL-5, in human mast cells triggered by IgE crosslinking and Yamaguchi et al. (1999) documented that this cytokine increases IgE-dependent mediator secretion. Taking into account the data mentioned above Ryan et al. (2007) suggested that TGF-β1, IL-10 and IL-4 strongly regulate mast cell homeostasis and can considerably influence mast cell mediator release, especially evoked by anaphylactic reaction.

By definition, chemokines are chemotactic cytokines orchestrating leukocyte recruitment in physiological and pathological conditions. However, binding of chemokines to their specific receptors can induce a number of different cellular activities depending on the target cell (Bonecchi et al. 2009). Besides migration, chemokines promote adhesion by regulating the expression of integrins, and stimulate release of proinflammatory mediators from leukocytes. It is now well established that mast cells express a considerable number of chemokine receptors (Juremalm and Nilsson 2005) and that some chemokines, such as CCL2, CCL5, CCL11 (eotaxin), CXCL1 (growth-related oncogene, GRO-α), CXCL4 (platelet factor 4, PF4), CXCL7 (neutrophil activating peptide, NAP-2), CXCL8, CXCL10 (interferon inducible protein, IP-10), CXCL12 (stromal cell-derived factor-1, SDF-1), and CX3CL1 (fractalcine) stimulate mast cell migration (rev. in Brzezińska-Błaszczyk and Misiak-Tłoczek (2007). However, chemokines do not seem to be an important mast cell secretagogues. It is documented that CCL2, CCL3, CCL4, CCL5, CCL7 (MCP-3), CCL8 (MCP-2), CXCL1, CXCL4, CXCL8, and CXCL10 do not induce human mast cells to histamine release (Füreder et al. 1995b, Hartmann et al. 1995, Nitschke et al. 1996, Takaishi et al. 1994). Alam et al. (1992) stated that CCL3, in a dose-dependent manner, induces the release of histamine from mouse peritoneal mast cells, and Conti et al. (1995) observed the marked, dose-dependent, CCL2-induced degranulation of rat peritoneal mast cells. It is also established that chemokines do not modulate IgE-dependent mast cell degranulation. Human lung mast cell priming with CCL2 or CCL5 (Takaishi et al. 1994) and human skin mast cell priming with CCL2, CCL3, CCL4, CCL5, CCL7, or CCL8 (Hartmann et al. 1995) does not enhance histamine release in response to anti-IgE challenge. Nitschke et al. (1996) observed that out of many chemokines, such as CCL2, CCL3, CXCL4, CCL5, and CXCL8, only CCL5 exhibits a weak, but potentially significant effect on IgE-mediated activation of human skin mast cells. Toda et al. (2004) showed that costimulation through FcεRI engagement with IgE/antigen and CCR1 engagement with CCL3 synergistically enhances degranulation in BRL-2H3 cells. Pretreatment with CCL2 does not influence anti-IgE induced histamine release from rat peritoneal mast cells (Conti et al. 1995).

11.3.2.4 Other Cell-Derived Peptides

ET-1, a 21-amino acid peptide, was initially identified as a potent vasoconstructive peptide derived from endothelial cells. Increasing evidence implicates, however, that ET-1 serves as cytokine-like agent taking part in various physiological and pathological conditions, involving inflammatory processes (Kedzierski and Yanagisawa 2001). Thus, of great importance are observations that ET-1 is one of the most potent histamine releasers in mouse (Egger et al. 1995, Yamamura et al. 1994a, b, 1995) and guinea pig (Uchida et al. 1992) mast cells. Matsushima et al. (2004b) documented that murine fetal skin-derived cultured mast cells (FSMCs) express both ET receptors at mRNA and protein levels, whereas BMMCs express lower levels of

ET_A, and little, if any, ET_B. What is more, these authors stated that ET-1 induces degranulation of FSMCs, IgE-sensitized mast cells are more susceptible to ET-1 action, and ET-1 pretreatment significantly downregulates mast cell degranulation induced by FcεRI aggregation. Matsushima et al. (2004b) also indicated that ET-1 stimulates FSMCs to TNF, IL-6 and VEGF production.

It is also established that natriuretic peptides (NPs), a family of ring-shaped powerful vasoactive hormones, can induce mast cell degranulation. An A-type natriuretic peptide (ANP) (Chai et al. 2000, Opgenorth et al. 1990, Yoshida et al. 1996) as well as B-type (BNP) and, to a lesser extend, C-type natriuretic peptide (CNP) (Yoshida et al. 1996) induce, in a concentration-dependent manner, degranulation and histamine release from rat peritoneal mast cells.

Mast cell histamine release is also observed in response to challenge with hormones such as CRH (Theoharides et al. 1998, Cao et al. 2005), CRH-related urocortin (Singh et al. 1999), and parathormone (Tsakalos et al. 1983). Rat peritoneal mast cells release histamine in response to bradykinin (Bueb et al. 1990), as well.

Mast cells and eosinophils are believed to interact during the late and chronic stages of allergic inflammation. From this point of view it seems very interesting that some of eosinophil granule-associated proteins can activate mast cells to degranulation and preformed mediator release. It is well documented that eosinophil-derived major basic protein (MPB) can induce mast cell degranulation and preformed mediator release (Furuta et al. 1998, O'Donnell et al. 1983, Patella et al. 1996, 1997, Zheutlin et al. 1984). Piliponsky et al. (2001, 2003) showed that MBP can reactivate, previously activated in IgE-dependent manner, mast cells to histamine release and this process is dependent on the membrane form of SCF. Out of other eosinophil granule-derived proteins, the ability to induce mast cell degranulation has eosinophil cationic protein (ECP), but not eosinophil-derived neurotoxin (EDN) and eosinophil peroxidase (EPO) (Patella et al. 1996, 1997, Zheutlin et al. 1984).

Tryptase, the most abundant protein product of human mast cells, belongs to preformed mediators stored in cytoplasmic granules, stimulates, in a concentration-dependent manner the release of histamine from human tonsillar (He et al. 1998) and synovial (He et al. 2001) mast cells as well as from guinea pig skin and lung mast cells (He et al. 1997). Moreover, pretreatment of mast cells with tryptase causes inhibition of their responsiveness to challenge with anti-IgE and calcium ionophore A23187 (He et al. 1998). These data suggest that tryptase might regulate mast cell activity in autocrine manner.

11.3.3 Pathogens as Mast Cell Stimulants

Mast cells are resident cells within tissues and are particularly frequent in close proximity to epithelial surfaces in skin, respiratory system, and gastrointestinal mucosa. This strategic localization of mast cells at the portals of pathogen entry ensures early contact of these cells with invading microorganisms. Thus, mast cells may represent one of the first inflammatory cells encountered by an invading pathogen. In fact nowadays there is clear evidence that mast cells play a critical protection role in the host defense against pathogens, especially against bacteria.

Mast cells have the ability to phagocytose (Arock et al. 1998, Malaviya et al. 1994b, Sher et al. 1979) and subsequently kill bacteria, via oxidative and non-oxidative systems (Malaviya et al. 1994b). Moreover, these cells are capable of processing bacterial antigens following phagocytosis for presentation through class I and II MHC molecules (Frandji et al. 1993, Malaviya et al. 1996) which leads to the development of adaptive immunity against bacteria. Recently, von Köckritz-Blickwede et al. (2008) documented that mast cells can kill bacteria independently of phagocytosis by entrapping them in extracellular structures which are composed of DNA, histones, tryptase and antimicrobial cathelicidin LL-37. The production of antimicrobial peptides by mast cells, such as β-defensin-4 and cathelicidins LL-37 and CRAMP, that act as a broad-spectrum antibiotics, is another potentially important aspect of their function in host defense against bacteria (Di Nardo et al. 2003, 2008). Moreover, mast cells can exert their bactericidal function by production of nitric oxide and superoxide radicals (Bissonnette et al. 1991, Gilchrist et al. 2004, Malaviya et al. 1994b). It seems, however, that the major function of mast cells in response to bacterial infections is to induce the development of inflammation by the action of mast cell-derived proinflammatory mediators released in response to bacteria or their products, at the place of bacteria entry.

11.3.3.1 Bacteria and Their Products as Mast Cell Activators

It is now well recognized that whole bacteria can activate mast cells to degranulation and preformed mediator release. Gram-positive bacteria, such as *Staphylococcus aureus* (Jensen et al. 1984, Norn et al. 1984) and *S. epidermidis* (Church et al. 1987) induce rat and human mast cell degranulation. Formalin-killed Gram-negative bacteria, such as *Escherichia coli*, *Enterobacter cloacae*, *Proteus vulgaris*, *Klebsiella oxytoca*, and *K. pneumoniae* stimulate human lung and tonsillar mast cells to degranulation (Church et al. 1987). Intestinal-associated bacteria, such as *Bacteroides thetaiotaomicron*, *B. fragilis*, *Bifidobacterium adolescentis* and *E. coli* activate rat peritoneal mast cells to histamine release (Brzezińska-Błaszczyk and Olejnik 1999). Mast cells are stimulated to degranulation by atypical bacteria, i.e., *Mycoplasma hominis*, *M. pneumoniae* and *Ureaplasma urealyticum*, as well (Brzezińska-Błaszczyk and Wasiela 2002, Hoek et al. 2002, Wasiela and Brzezińska-Błaszczyk 2000). It is also reported that viable bacteria, such as *Mycobacterium tuberculosis* (Muñoz et al. 2003), *Streptococcus pneumoniae* (Barbuti et al. 2006), and *Borrelia burgdorferi* (Talkington and Nickell 1999) cause degranulation of mast cells and preformed mediator release.

It is also indicated that *S. aureus* antigens activate human adenoidal and mesenteric mast cells to histamine release (Brzezińska-Błaszczyk et al. 1988a), and antigens of *S. aureus*, *S. viridans*, *Haemophilus influence*, and *Branhamella catarrhalis* induce histamine release from human pulmonary mast cells (Brzezińska-Błaszczyk et al. 1988b). Yamamoto et al. (1999) observed dose-dependent rat peritoneal mast cell degranulation in response to *Helicobacter pylori* water extract, and Montemurro et al. (2002) noticed degranulation of mast cells to challenge with neutrophil-activating protein (NAP) of this bacteria. Dalldorf et al. (1988) showed degranulation of mast cells in response to group A streptococcal polysaccharide.

Some bacterial toxins can also stimulate mast cell degranulation and preformed mediator release. Adusu et al. (1994) documented that *Pasteurella haemolytica* leukotoxin induces histamine release from bovine pulmonary mast cells. It was also proven that staphylococcal enterotoxin B (Komisar et al. 1992), as well as streptococcal exotoxin B (Watanabe et al. 2002) can induce mast cell degranulation. Mast cell degranulation and histamine release is observed in response to challenge with *E. coli*, *Serratia marcescens*, *Aeromonas hydrophila*, and *Listeria monocytogenes* hemolysins (Gross-Weege et al. 1988, Scheffer et al. 1988). The streptococcal exotoxin streptolysin O induces the release of histamine from murine BMMCs (Stassen et al. 2003), and metalloprotease secreted by *Vibro vulnificus* stimulates histamine release from rat mast cells (Miyoshi et al. 2003).

The majority of experiments with the use of purified bacterial cell wall components indicate that these constituents have no ability to induce mast cell degranulation. Lipopolysaccharides (LPS), the main bacterial cell wall components of Gram-negative bacteria do not activate neither immature (Ikeda and Funaba 2003, Mrabet-Dahbi et al. 2009, Supajatura et al. 2001, 2002, Varadaradjalou et al. 2003) nor mature (Mrabet-Dahbi et al. 2009, Wierzbicki and Brzezińska-Błaszczyk 2009) mast cells to degranulation and preformed mediator release. Lipoarabinomannan (LAM), one of the most characteristic components of mycobacterial cell wall, has no ability to induce histamine release from mature rat peritoneal mast cells (Wierzbicki and Brzezińska-Błaszczyk 2009). Lipoteichoic acids (LTA) of Gram-positive bacteria do not stimulate immature (Mrabet-Dahbi et al. 2009) or mature (Brzezińska-Błaszczyk and Rdzany 2007) mast cells to degranulation. It is also indicated that peptydoglican (PGN), main bacterial cell wall component of Gram-positive bacteria, does not induce degranulation of neither immature (Ikeda and Funaba 2003, McCurdy et al. 2003) nor mature (Wierzbicki and Brzezińska-Błaszczyk 2009) mast cells. However, Supajatura et al. (2002) observed degranulation of murine BMMCs after stimulation with PGN, and Varadaradjalou et al. (2003) noticed histamine release from PGN-activated human cord blood-derived mast cells (CBMCs).

It should be pointed out that some bacteria or bacterial cell wall components can stimulate mast cells to synthesis de novo of many different cytokines, including proinflammatory cytokines. For example murine BMMCs activated with LPS produce and release TNF, IL-1β, IL-5, IL-6, IL-10, and IL-13 (Masuda et al. 2002, Supajatura et al. 2001, 2002). PGN-stimulated murine BMMCs release TNF, IL-4, IL-5, IL-6, and IL-13 (Supajatura et al. 2002) and human CBMCs produce GM-CSF and IL-1β to PGN activation (McCurdy et al. 2003). Murine mature mast cells produce and release IL-1, IL-6, IL-10, IL-17, TNF, IFN-γ and GM-CSF, when stimulated with LTA and IL-6, IL-10, GM-CSF, and TNF in response to activation with LPS (Mrabet-Dahbi et al. 2009). LPS, but not PGN, induces human mast cells to production of IL-1β, IL-6, IL-8, and IL-12 (Kirshenbaum et al. 2008). It is also established that upon bacterial stimulation mast cells can generate arachidonic acid metabolites. For example PGN induces human CBMCs and rat mature mast cells to

LTC_4 synthesis (McCurdy et al. 2003, Wierzbicki and Brzezińska-Błaszczyk 2009), as well as murine BMMCs to LTC_4 and PGD_2 release (Kikawada et al. 2007). LTA strongly stimulates rat peritoneal mast cells to LTC_4 release (Brzezińska-Błaszczyk and Rdzany 2007) and murine peritoneal mast cells to PGD_2 generation (Mrabet-Dahbi et al. 2009). It is also reported that mature rat mast cells generate significant amounts of LTC_4 in response to LPS and LAM challenge (Wierzbicki and Brzezińska-Błaszczyk 2009).

It becomes increasingly apparent that mast cell secretory response to bacterial stimulation is highly selective. For example some bacterial cell wall components can induce arachidonic acid metabolite production without substantial degranulation (Brzezińska-Błaszczyk and Rdzany 2007, McCurdy et al. 2003, Wierzbicki and Brzezińska-Błaszczyk 2009), and microbial challenge can stimulate mast cells to production de novo of cytokines independently of degranulation (Marshall et al. 1996, McCurdy et al. 2003, Supajatura et al. 2001).

At the center of detection mechanisms for invading microorganisms lies the family of TLRs. Functional expression of TLRs has been described in human and rodent mast cells (Kikawada et al. 2007, Masuda et al. 2002, McCurdy et al. 2001, Supajatura et al. 2001, 2002, Varadaradjalou et al. 2003). What is more, it is well documented that TLR2 is involved in PGN-dependent mast cell stimulation (Supajatura et al. 2002, Varadaradjalou et al. 2003), and TLR4 is involved in LPS-induced activation of mast cells (McCurdy et al. 2001, Masuda et al. 2002, Varadaradjalou et al. 2003). It should be also stressed that secretory mast cell response to fimbriated Gram-negative bacteria depend on bacterial expression of FimH protein, a mannose-binding subunit on type I fimbriae expressed by enterobacteriaceae that directly binds to CD48 molecule (Malaviya and Abraham 2000, Malaviya et al. 1994a, 1999).

It should be stressed that some bacterial proteins can act as superantigens. Protein A, a staphylococcal surface protein, and protein L, a cell wall protein from *Peptostreptococcus magnus*, induce degranulation of human mast cells isolated from heart, skin or lung parenchyma (Genovese et al. 2000, Patella et al. 1990). The activity of protein A seems to be mediated by binding to the V_H3 region of IgE, whereas protein L interacts with the κ light chain of IgE (Genovese et al. 2000).

11.3.3.2 Viruses as Mast Cell Activators

It is now established that mast cells are able to be infected with several viruses, including HIV, dengue viruses, cytomegaloviruses, reoviruses, and adenoviruses. What is more, there is evidence that mast cells can express TLR3, TLR7, and TLR9 (Kulka et al. 2004, Matsushima et al. 2004a, Orinska et al. 2005), that interact with double-stranded (ds)RNA, single-stranded (ss)RNA, and CpG-containig DNA, respectively. Thus, it is supposed that mast cells may be activated in response to viruses; however, the studies in this area are sparse.

Burke et al. (2008) observed that human CBMC produce chemokines, such as CCL3, CXCL8, and CXCL10 in response to dsRNA virus infection, and Hosoda et al. (2002) stated that rhonovirus (RV14) infection induces mast cells to synthesis of CXCL8 and GM-CSF. It was also documented that dengue virus activates mast cells to chemokines, such as CCL3, CCL4, and CCL5 production (King et al. 2002), and mast cell stimulation with TLR3, TLR7, or TLR9 ligands induces IL-6, CCL3, CCL5, CXCL1, and TNF synthesis (Matsushima et al. 2004a). Activation of mast cells through TLR3 causes IFN-α, IFN-β, and IFN-γ production (Kulka et al. 2004, Orinska et al. 2005). Thus, it may be concluded that viral activation induces a unique profile of mediator release by mast cells, when compared to other means of stimulation, and is dominated by chemokines and proinflammatory cytokines, and by IFNs, which are important for mounting antiviral response. Virus-induced mast cell activation is not correlated with mast cell degranulation (King et al. 2002, Kulka et al. 2004, Matsushima et al. 2004a, Orinska et al. 2005). However, Hosoda et al. (2002) documented that RV14 infection may prime mast cells to enhanced histamine release in response to other stimuli.

It seems very interesting that protein Fv, an endogenous protein produced in liver and released during viral hepatitis B and C, induces human skin, lung (Patella et al. 1993) and heart (Genovese et al. 2003) mast cells to histamine release as well as to tryptase secretion and PGD_2 and LTC_4 production. It is documented that protein Fv acts as endogenous immunoglobulin superantigen by interacting with the V_H3 domain of IgE.

11.4 Histamine and Mast Cells

Histamine is one of the most important mediators involved in various physiological and pathological conditions, including neurotransmission and numerous brain functions, secretion of pituitary hormones, and regulation of gastrointestinal and circulating functions (Repka-Ramirez and Baraniuk 2002). What is more, it is now well established that histamine is a key player in inflammatory reactions; it stimulates the secretion of proinflammatory cytokines as well as some chemokines in several cell types, enhances adhesion molecule expression, and regulates granulocyte accumulation in tissues (MacGlashan 2003, Repka-Ramirez and Baraniuk 2002). Increasing evidence suggest that this amine strongly modulates mechanisms of immunological reactions by the regulation of monocytes, dendritic cells and granulocytes activities (Jutel et al. 2002, 2006, Schneider et al. 2002) and by the influence of Th1/Th2 balance (Jutel et al. 2001a, b). Taking into account that mast cells are involved in the course of inflammatory processes and take part in different immune responses, it seems extremely important to get to examine and describe the influence of histamine on mast cell activity.

11.4.1 Mast Cell Histamine Receptors

It is know well established that histamine exerts its effects by activating specific histamine receptors (HRs) of which 4 subtypes (HR1, HR2, HR3, and HR4)

Table 11.2 Expression and functional characteristics of HRs on mast cells

HR type	Expression	Effect on mast cells
H1	+ rat peritoneal mast cells, RBL-2H3 cells, HMC-1 line	modulation of cytokine production? cAMP increase
H2	+ rat peritoneal mast cells, HMC-1 line, human skin mast cells	modulation of cytokine production? cAMP increase modulation of histamine secretion?
H3	–	
H4	+ mouse BMMCs, HMC-1 line, human skin mast cells	intracellular Ca^{2+} mobilization chemotaxis enhancement of CXCLI2-induced chemotaxis modulation of H4 expression?

are recognized. All of these receptors belong to G protein-coupled receptor family, comprising 7 transmembrane domains, NH_2-terminal glycosylation sites, and phosphorylation sites for protein kinases (Table 11.2).

Data regarding the type of histamine receptor expressed by mast cells in different organs and species are variable and in part even contradictory. Wescott et al. (1982) stated that rat mast cells have H1 receptor, which is probably involved in histamine-induced cAMP increase and Alm et al. (1984) documented that histamine receptors present on rat peritoneal mast cells are mainly of H1-type. Pharmacological studies with the use of specific histamine receptor antagonists indicated that both RBL-2H3 cells (Hide et al. 1997) and HMC-1line (Lippert et al. 1995, 2000, Zhao et al. 2005) express H1 receptors. Lippert et al. (2004) stated that, despite description of mRNA, H1 receptor protein is only moderately expressed in HMC-1 cells and is virtually absent in human skin mast cells. The expression of this type of histamine receptor was shown using both RT-PCR and Western blotting in human fully mature mast cells as well as HMC-1 cell line (Godot et al. 2007).

The data prove the presence of H2 receptors on mature rat peritoneal mast cells (Antohe et al. 1988, Bissonnette 1996, Masini et al. 1982) as well as on immature HMC-1 cells (Lippert et al. 2000). Recently, Lippert et al. (2004) stated that both HMC-1 cells and mast cells isolated from normal human skin express H2 receptor at mRNA and protein levels, and that radiolabelled histamine binding is strongly inhibited by ranitidine, H2 receptor specific antagonist. Godot et al. (2007) documented the presence of H2 receptors in mature human mast cells and in HMC-1 line by the use both RT-PCR and Western blotting.

H3 receptors were initially found on rat peritoneal mast cells (Bissonnette 1996, Kohno et al. 1993, 1994), rat cutaneous mast cells (Ohkubo et al. 1994), as well as on human adenoidal mast cells (Bent et al. 1991). Rożniecki et al. (1999) suggested the presence of this type of histamine receptor on rat brain mast cells. It should be pointed out, however, that in all studies mentioned above thioperamide was used as a specific H3 receptor antagonist, and it is now well established that both mouse and human H4 receptor can bind thioperamide, as well (Liu et al. 2001). According to more recent data it seems that H3 receptor is not expressed on mast cells. Hofstra et al. (2003) documented that H3 receptor is undetectable by Northern blot analysis and RT-PCR on murine BMMCs. Gantner et al. (2002), using mRNA expression studies, stated that H3 receptor mRNA is completely absent in HMC-1 cells. Lippert et al. (2004) documented that H3 receptor mRNA and receptor protein are undetectable both on HMC-1 and human skin mast cells, and immunohistochemistry of cutaneous tissue showed absence of H3 receptor in these cells.

The expression of the H4 receptor on mast cells was suggested by Zhu et al. (2001). Gantner et al. (2002) indicated that HMC-1 cells do express this type of histamine receptor. Later on, Lippert et al. (2004) unambiguously documented the presence of H4 receptors on HMC-1 line and human skin mast cells, both at mRNA and protein levels. Furthermore, these authors indicated that H4 receptors are detectable by Western blot analysis of HMC-1 cells and that radiolabelled histamine binding is strongly inhibited by H3/H4 (FUB-108) specific antagonist. The expression of H4 receptor on immature and mature human mast cells was also observed by Godot et al. (2007) and Hofstra et al. (2003). There is also evidence that H4 receptor is present in mouse BMMCs (Hofstra et al. 2003, Takeshita et al. 2003, Thurmond et al. 2004).

11.4.2 Histamine Influences Mast Cell Activity

Basing on the given data it can be stated that mast cells express H1, H2, and H4 receptors, but not H3 receptors. Therefore histamine, acting through these specific receptors, might modulate different aspects of mast cell activity. However, currently there is only limited data on the influence of histamine on mast cells.

Some data indicate that histamine, through H1 and/or H2 receptors, might modulate cytokine secretion from mast cells. Bissonnette (1996) stated that pretreatment of rat peritoneal mast cells with histamine results in inhibition of TNF-dependent cytotoxicity. The blockage of H2 receptors with specific antagonists, such as ranitidine and clemastine, abrogates the inhibitory effect of histamine on mast cell TNF-dependent cytotoxicity. What is more, blockage of H2 receptors with ranitidine increases the release of TNF from rat mast cells stimulated with antigen, suggesting that histamine released by mast cells in response to antigen stimulation downregulates the subsequent release of TNF. Considering these observations the authors suggested that histamine may act as an autocrine regulator of cytokine release by mast cells. Hide et al. (1997) documented that azelastine, H1 receptor antagonist, inhibits both TNF release and TNF mRNA expression and TNF protein synthesis by antigen- and ionomycin-stimulated mast cells. Also Lippert et al. (1995, 2000) observed that H1- and H2-receptor antagonists cause dose-dependent inhibition of TNF, and, to a lesser extent, CXCL8, IL-6 and IL-3 release from HMC-1 cell line after stimulation with phorbol myristate acetate (PMA) and calcium ionophore A23187.

It was also suggested that histamine, through H2 receptors, can regulate its own secretion by induction of cAMP increase in mast cells. Histamine causes a concentration-dependent increase in cAMP level in HMC-1, and famotidine, H2 receptor antagonist, almost completely abrogates this effect (Lippert et al. 2004). Ranitidine inhibits histamine-induced cAMP increase in murine BMMCs (Hofstra et al. 2003). Also Masini et al. (1982) hinted the existence of H2-mediated inhibitory feedback regulation of histamine release. There is also some data indicating that histamine probably modulates its own release through H3 receptors. Kohno et al. (1994) documented, with the use of thioperamide, that this amine can block anaphylactic histamine release through H3 receptors and Ohkubo et al. (1994), applying the same histamine receptor antagonist, indicated that histamine, through H3 receptors, influences its own secretion in neurogenic inflammation. However, it is important to keep in mind that H3 and H4 receptors exhibit 40% homology, are functionally related, and H3 receptor inhibitors, for example thioperamide, also bind to H4 receptors (Liu et al. 2001). In view of the lack of H3 receptor on mast cells and the cross-reactivity of H3 receptor antagonists with H4 receptors it might be speculated that histamine can modulate its own secretion not only through H2 receptors, but through H4 receptors, as well.

Regarding the information available it seems to be well documented that histamine, through H4 receptors, mediates mast cell migration. Hofstra et al. (2003) indicated that histamine, in a concentration-dependent manner, induces murine BMMCs chemotaxis and thioperamide completely inhibits mast cells chemotaxis in response to histamine. Also Venable et al. (2005) stated that H4 receptor antagonists demonstrate efficacy in in vitro mast cell chemotaxis assay. Thurmond et al. (2004) observed histamine-induced migration of mast cells in vivo. Upon administration of histamine, there is an increase in the number of mast cells per tracheal section and apparent migration of mast cells toward tracheal epithelium. This effect is blocked by s.c. administration of JNJ7777120 and thioperamide, but is not affected by H1-, H2-, or H3 selective antagonists. Extremely interesting data was presented by Godot et al. (2007). The authors established that histamine enhances CXCL12 chemotactic activity on immature mast cells. The synergy between histamine and CXCL12 is not observed with mature mast cells. The authors also stated that histamine does not modulate chemotactic activity of SCF and LTB_4 on immature mast cells and does not change the level of CXCR4 expression on mast cells. The effect of histamine on CXCL12-induced mast cell migration is mediated through H4 receptor; pretreatment of mast cells with H1 or H2 receptor antagonists has no effect on the synergistic effects of histamine on both HMC-1 cells and immature mast cells, and after incubation of cells with thioperamide or JNJ7777120 the synergy between histamine and CXCL12 is substantially inhibited in the first case and totally abrogated in the second case. When H4 receptor is blocked by selective antagonists during migration assay, the effect of histamine disappeared. What is more, Godot et al. (2007) established that when H1 receptor is blocked during migration of immature mast cells, synergistic effect of histamine on CXCL12-induced migration is markedly enhanced. This finding implies that H1 receptor can exert a negative control in immature mast cell migration and recruitment.

It is also established that histamine, in a concentration-dependent manner, induces calcium mobilization in mast cells (Hofstra et al. 2003, Thurmond et al. 2004), and neither H1 receptor antagonists nor H2 receptor blockers alter histamine-induced calcium mobilization, and thioperamide inhibits this effect of histamine. What is more, histamine stimulation of BMMCs generated from $H4R^{-/-}$ mice does not result in calcium mobilization (Hofstra et al. 2003). Thus, it can be concluded that histamine induces calcium mobilization in mast cells through H4 receptor. Histamine mediates the release of calcium from intracellular calcium stores in mast cells (Hofstra et al. 2003). H4 receptor and histamine do not seem to be involved in antigen-induced degranulation nor in de novo production of LTB_4 and PGs (Hofstra et al. 2003).

A commonly used model of acute inflammation is the mouse model of zymosan-induced peritonitis in mice (Doherty et al. 1985, Kołaczkowska et al. 2001a) that culminates in peritoneal neutrophil influx. What is more, mast cells and histamine have been shown to be critical for zymosan-induced inflammation in rodents (Kołaczkowska 2002, Kołaczkowska et al. 2001a, b). Takeshita et al. (2003) stated that mice pretreated with H1 receptor antagonist, pyrilamine, or with H2 receptor antagonist, cimetidine, prior to zymosan injection into the pleural cavity, show no change in the neutrophil influx. In contrast, pretreatment of mice with thioperamide, H3/H4 antagonist, significantly reduces the inflammatory response in a dose-dependent manner. Moreover, mice deficient in mast cells, major cellular source of histamine, also show an 80% reduction in neutrophilia upon zymosan challenge, and maximum efficacy is similar to that observed in thioperamide-treated mice. The authors also investigated the potential link between mast cell- and H4 receptor-mediated neutrophil recruitment after zymosan stimulation and looked for potential chemoattractant mediators being released into the pleural cavity of zymosan-challenged mice. Increasing amounts of a variety of both mast cell- and monocyte-derived factors, such as TNF, IL-1β, IL-6, IL-10, IL-12, and LTB_4, in the pleural fluid within 1.5 h after challenge are observed, i.e., before significant neutrophilia. A significant reduction in LTB_4 level, one of the most potent known chemoattractants for neutrophils, is noted in H4 receptor antagonist-treated animals, and LTB_4 levels are similarly reduced in mast cell-deficient mice. The authors also documented that in mice lacking MyD88, a pivotal signaling molecule linked to TLRs, including mast cell-expressed zymosan receptor, TLR2, neutrophilia is dramatically reduced in zymosan-challenged mice. A similar reduction of neutrophilia is observed upon pretreatment of mice with antibody direct against TLR2. Collectively, these carefully planed and accomplished conducted experiments led the authors to the conclusion that histamine released from mast cells after TLR2-triggered MyD88 activation by zymosan acts in an autocrine fashion on mast cell-expressed H4 receptor, thereby leading to the release of chemoattractants for neutrophils, including LTB_4. Also Thurmond et al. (2004) documented that if mice are injected intraperitoneally with zymosan, there is a dramatic extravasation of polymorphonuclear cells, but when these mice are pretreated s.c. with JNJ7777120 or thioperamide prior to injection of zymosan, there is a significant reduction in neutrophil accumulation. Recently, Strakhova et al. (2009) established that there is an expression of H4 receptor mRNA in cells derived from peritoneal lavage of naïve mice, and this level of expression is significantly lower in cells derived from mice that are devoid of mast cells. These authors also stated that intraperitoneal challenge with zymosan results in an increase of both histamine and PGD_2 levels in peritoneal lavage fluid. Pharmacological studies showed that H1 receptor antagonists loratidine and terfenadine, H2 receptor antagonist cimetidine, and H3 receptor antagonist ABT-239 had no effect on neutrophil influx. Only H4 receptor antagonist JNJ7777120 significantly reverse neutrophil influx to levels comparable to those obtained with dexamethasone. A-940894, the novel H4 receptor antagonist, given s.c., prior to injection of zymosan, results in almost complete inhibition of neutrophil myeloperoxidase (MPO) activity in lavages, as well. A-940894 and JNJ7777120 dose-dependently reduce PGD_2 and PGE_2 levels, but not LTB_4 and CXCL1 levels, in peritoneal lavage fluid.

11.5 Concluding Remarks

Mast cells, widely distributed within the body, are main and very potent cellular source of histamine. It should be stressed that mast cell degranulation and histamine release can be induced not only by IgE-antigen-FcεRI signaling, but also by diverse endogenous stimuli, such as IgG, C3a and C5a peptides, superantigens, defensins and cathelicidins, neuropeptides, as well as by some cytokines and chemokines, hormones and different other cell-derived peptides. Moreover, mast cells release histamine in response to bacteria and bacterial products (Fig. 11.1). Therefore, mast cell-derived histamine, together with other humoral factors, is involved in complex

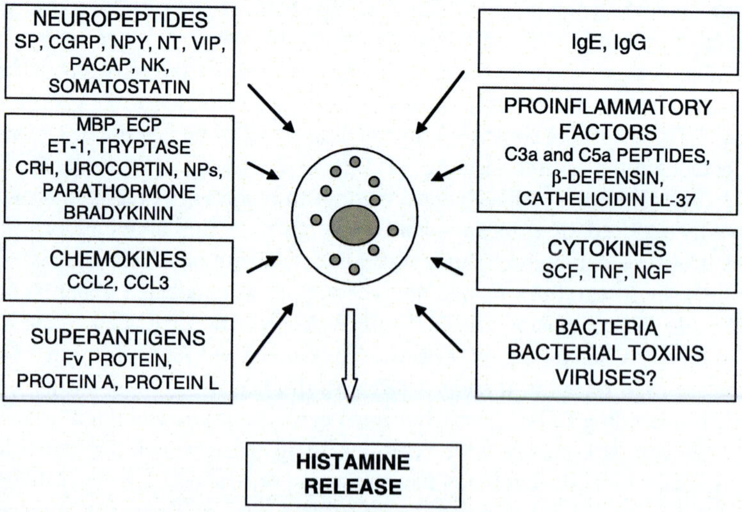

Fig. 11.1 Triggers of mast cell histamine release

network regulating homeostasis, physiological processes, immune reactions, as well as diverse pathological processes, including inflammation.

Within the last few years there has been enormous progress in the understanding of mast cell biology and function. Apart from histamine, mast cells can produce and release a lot of powerful mediators, cytokines and chemokines exerting diversity of effects on surrounding cells and tissues. Thereby, it is not surprising that mast cells are involved in physiological processes and maintenance of homeostasis, and take part in many diseases characterized by inflammation and tissue remodeling. What is more, mast cells play a critical role in host defense. That is why recognition of factors influencing mast cell homeostasis and activity is crucial. From this point of view, of special interest are findings proving that mast cells express specific histamine receptors H1, H2, and H4 (Table 11.2). Thus, it can be presumed that histamine, together with other humoral factors such as IL-10, TGF-β, IL-4 and SCF, might affect tissue mast cells homeostasis and reactivity, and might regulate its own secretion, as well.

Acknowledgements The author wishes to thank Łukasz Konopka, MD, PhD and Waciej Wierzbicki, PhD for their involvement in the creation of references for this chapter.

References

Adusu TE, Conlon PD, Shewen PE et al (1994) *Pasteurella haemolytica* leukotoxin induces histamine release from bovine pulmonary mast cells. Can J Vet Res 58: 1–5

Alam R, Forsythe PA, Stafford S et al (1992) Macrophage inflammatory protein-1α activates basophils and mast cells. J Exp Med 176:781–786

Ali H, Leung KB, Pearce FL et al (1986) Comparison of the histamine-releasing action of substance P on mast cells and basophils from different species and tissues. Int Arch Allergy Appl Immunol 79:413–418

Alm E, Bloom GD, Fredriksson BA (1984) Surface histamine receptors in rat peritoneal mast cells. Separation of receptor-bearing cells *via* binding to a histamine-protein conjugate, Cell-ect. Agents Actions 14:370–372

Antohe F, Dobrila LN, Heltianu C (1988) Histamine receptor on mast cells. Microcirc Endothelium Lymphatics 4:469–488

Arock M, Ross E, Lai-Kuen R et al (1998) Phagocytic and tumor necrosis factor alpha response of human mast cells following exposure to gram-negative and gram-positive bacteria. Infect Immun 66:6030–6034

Arrang JM, Garbarg M, Schwartz JC (1983) Auto-inhibition of brain histamine release mediated by a novel class (H_3) of histamine receptor. Nature 302:832–837

Asai K, Kitaura J, Kawakami Y et al (2001) Regulation of mast cell survival by IgE. Immunity 14:791–800

Barbuti G, Moschioni M, Censini S et al (2006) *Streptococcus pneumoniae* induces mast cell degranulation. Int J Med Microbiol 296:325–329

Barrocas AM, Cochrane DE, Carraway RE et al (1999) Neurotensin stimulation of mast cell secretion is receptor-mediated, pertussis-toxin sensitive and requires activation of phospholipase C. Immunopharmacology 41:131–137

Bauer O, Razin E (2000) Mast cell-nerve interactions. News Physiol Sci 15:213–218

Befus AD, Mowat C, Gilchrist M et al (1999) Neutrophil defensins induce histamine secretion from mast cells: mechanisms of action. J Immunol 163:947–953

Bent S, Fehling U, Braam U et al (1991) The influence of H1-, H2- and H3-receptors on the spontaneous and ConA induced histamine release from human adenoidal mast cells. Agents Actions 33:67–70

Bischoff SC, Dahinden CA (1992) *c-kit* ligand: a unique potentiator of mediator release by human lung mast cells. J Exp Med 175:237–244

Bischoff SC, Sellge G, Lorentz A et al (1999) IL-4 enhances proliferation and mediator release in mature human mast cells. Proc Natl Acad Sci USA 96:8080–8085

Bissonnette EY (1996) Histamine inhibits tumor necrosis factor α release by mast cells through H_2 and H_3 receptors. Am J Respir Cell Mol Biol 14:620–626

Bissonnette EY, Chin B, Befus AD (1995) Interferons differentially regulate histamine and TNF-alpha (TNF-α) in rat intestinal mucosal mast cells. Immunology 86:12–17

Bissonnette EY, Enciso JA, Befus AD (1997) TGF-β1 inhibits the release of histamine and tumor necrosis factor-α from mast cells through an autocrine pathway. Am J Respir Cell Mol Biol 16:275–282

Bissonnette EY, Hogaboam CM, Wallace JL et al (1991) Potentiation of tumor necrosis factor-α-mediated cytotoxicity of mast cells by their production of nitric oxide. J Immunol 147: 3060–3065

Bonecchi R, Galliera E, Borroni EM et al (2009) Chemokines and chemokine receptors: an overview. Front Biosci 14:540–551

Borkowski TA, Jouvin MH, Lin SY et al (2001) Minimal requirements for IgE-mediated regulation of surface FcεRI. J Immunol 167:1290–1296

Bradding P, Okayama Y, Howarth PH et al (1995) Heterogeneity of human mast cells based on cytokine content. J Immunol 155:297–307

Brzezińska-Błaszczyk E, Misiak-Tłoczek A (2007) The regulation of mast cell migration. Part 2: mast cell chemoattractants. Postepy Hig Med Dosw 61:493–499

Brzezińska-Błaszczyk E, Olejnik AK (1999) Intestinal mucosa-associated bacteria modulate rat mast cell reactivity. Int J Immunopathol Pharmacol 12:31–36

Brzezińska-Błaszczyk E, Rdzany RS (2007) Lipoteichoic acids selectively stimulate rat mast cells to cysteinyl leukotriene generation and affect mast cell migration after tumor necrosis factor (TNF)-priming. Immunol Lett 109:138–144

Brzezińska-Błaszczyk E, Wasiela M (2002) Vaginal bacterial flora activates rat peritoneal mast cells. Int J Immunopathol Pharmacol 15:233–238

Brzezińska-Błaszczyk E, Zalewska A (1998) In vitro reactivity of mast cells in urticaria pigmentosa skin. Arch Dermatol Res 290:14–17

Brzezińska-Błaszczyk E, Czuwaj M, Wyczółkowska J (1988a) Histamine release from human adenoidal and mesenteric mast cells induced by bacterial antigens. Agents Actions 23:230–232

Brzezińska-Błaszczyk E, Gaik A, Czuwaj M et al (1988b) Histamine release from human pulmonary mast cells induced by bacterial antigens. Allergol Immunopathol 16:375–378

Brzezińska-Błaszczyk E, Forczmański M, Pietrzak A (2000) The action of tumor necrosis factor-α on rat mast cells. J Interferon Cytokine Res 20:377–382

Brzezińska-Błaszczyk E, Wasowska-Królikowska K, Dynowski J et al (1998) Intestinal mast cell response to neuropeptide stimulation. Int J Immunopathol Pharmacol 11:23–28

Bueb JL, Mousli M, Landry Y et al (1990) A pertussis toxin-sensitive G protein is required to induce histamine release from rat peritoneal mast cells by bradykinin. Agents Actions 30: 98–101

Burke SM, Issekutz TB, Mohan K et al (2008) Human mast cell activation with virus-associated stimuli leads to the selective chemotaxis of natural killer cells by a CXCL8-dependent mechanism. Blood 111:5467–5476

Cao J, Papadopoulou N, Kempuraj D et al (2005) Human mast cells express corticotropin-releasing hormone (CRH) receptors and CRH leads to selective secretion of vascular endothelial growth factor. J Immunol 174:7665–7675

Carraway R, Cochrane DE, Lansman JB et al (1982) Neurotensin stimulates exocytotic histamine secretion from rat mast cells and elevates plasma histamine levels. J Physiol 323:403–414

Chai OH, Lee YH, Han EH et al (2000) Atrial natriuretic peptide induces rat peritoneal mast cell activation by cGMP-independent and calcium uptake-dependent mechanism. Exp Mol Med 32:179–186

Chong HJ, Andrew Bouton L, Bailey DP et al (2003) IL-4 selectively enhances FcγRIII expression and signaling on mouse mast cells. Cell Immunol 224:65–73

Church MK, Norn S, Pao GJ et al (1987) Non-IgE-dependent bacteria-induced histamine release from human lung and tonsillar mast cells. Clin Allergy 17:341–353

Cocchiara R, Albeggiani G, Lampiasi N et al (1999) Histamine and tumor necrosis factor production from purified rat brain mast cells mediated by substance P. Neuroreport 10:575–578

Coleman JW, Holliday MR, Kimber I et al (1993) Regulation of mouse peritoneal mast cell secretory function by stem cell factor, IL-3 or IL-4. J Immunol 150:556–562

Columbo M, Horowitz EM, Botana LM et al (1992) The human recombinant *c-kit* receptor ligand, rhSCF, induces mediator release from human cutaneous mast cells and enhances IgE-dependent mediator release from both skin mast cells and peripheral blood basophils. J Immunol 149: 599–608

Columbo M, Horowitz EM, Kagey-Sobotka A et al (1996) Substance P activates the release of histamine from human skin mast cells through a pertussis toxin-sensitive and protein kinase C-dependent mechanism. Clin Immunol Immunopathol 81:68–73

Conti P, Boucher W, Letourneau R et al (1995) Monocyte chemotactic protein-1 provokes mast cell aggregation and [^{3}H]5HT release. Immunology 86:434–440

Cruse G, Cockerill S, Bradding P (2008) IgE alone promotes human lung mast cell survival through the autocrine production of IL-6. BMC Immunol. doi:10.1186/1417-2172-9-2

Cruse G, Kaur D, Yang W et al (2005) Activation of human lung mast cells by monomeric immunoglobulin E. Eur Respir J 25:858–863

Daëron M, Bonnerot C, Latour S et al (1992) Murine recombinant FcγRIII, but not FcγRII, trigger serotonin release in rat basophilic leukemia cells. J Immunol 149:1365–1373

Daëron M, Malbec O, Latour S et al (1995) Regulation of high-affinity IgE receptor-mediated mast cell activation by murine low-affinity IgG receptors. J Clin Invest 95:577–585

Dalldorf FG, Anderle SK, Brown RR et al (1988) Mast cell activation by group A streptococcal polysaccharide in the rat and its role in experimental arthritis. 132:258–264

Dastych J, Hardison MC, Metcalfe DD (1997) Aggregation of low affinity IgG receptors induces mast cell adherence to fibronectin: requirement for the common FcR γ-chain. J Immunol 158:1803–1809

Di Nardo A, Vitiello A, Gallo RL (2003) Cutting edge: mast cell antimicrobial activity is mediated by expression of cathelicidin antimicrobial peptide. J Immunol 170:2274–2278

Di Nardo A, Yamasaki K, Dorschner RA et al (2008) Mast cell cathelicidin antimicrobial peptide prevents invasive group A Streptococcus infection of the skin. J Immunol 180:7565–7573

Doherty NS, Poubelle P, Borgeat P et al (1985) Intraperitoneal injection of zymosan in mice induces pain, inflammation and the synthesis of peptidoleukotrienes and prostaglandin E_2. Prostaglandins 30:769–789

Dy M, Lebel B (1983) Skin allografts generate an enhanced production of histamine and histamine-producing cell-stimulating factor (HCSF) by spleen cells in response to T cell mitogens. J Immunol 130:2343–2347

Dy M, Lebel B, Kamoun P et al (1981) Histamine production during the anti-allograft response. Demonstration of a new lymphokine enhancing histamine synthesis. J Exp Med 153: 293–309

Egger D, Geuenich S, Denzlinger C et al (1995) IL-4 renders mast cells functionally responsive to endothelin-1. J Immunol 154:1830–1837

el-Lati SG, Dahinden CA, Church MK (1994) Complement peptides C3a- and C5a-induced mediator release from dissociated human skin mast cells. J Invest Dermatol 102:803–806

Erdei A, Pecht I (1996) Complement peptides and mast cell triggering. Immunol Lett 54:109–112

Erdei A, Kerekes K, Pecht I (1997) Role of C3a and C5a in the activation of mast cells. Exp Clin Immunogenet 14:16–18

Falus A, Hegyesi H, Lázár-Molnár E et al (2001) Paracrine and autocrine interactions in melanoma: histamine is a relevant player in local regulation. Trends Immunol 22:648–652

Feldberg RS, Cochrane DE, Carraway RE et al (1998) Evidence for a neurotensin receptor in rat serosal mast cells. Inflamm Res 47:245–250

Ferjan HI, Carman-Krzan M (2000) Differential effect of interleukin-3, stem cell factor and nerve growth factor on histamine and serotonin release from rat mast cells. Inflamm Res 49:S15–S16

Fewtrell CM, Foreman JC, Jordan CC et al (1982) The effects of substance P on histamine and 5-hydroxytryptamine release in the rat. J Physiol 330:393–411

Fong DC, Malbec O, Arock M et al (1996) Selective in vivo recruitment of the phosphatidylinositol phosphatase SHIP by phosphorylated FcγRIIB during negative regulation of IgE-dependent mouse mast cell activation. Immunol Lett 54:83–91

Frandji P, Oskéritzian C, Cacaraci F et al (1993) Antigen-dependent stimulation by bone marrow-derived mast cells of MHC class II-restricted T cell hybridoma. J Immunol 151:6318–6328

Furuichi K, Rivera J, Isersky C (1985) The receptor for immunoglobulin E on rat basophilic leukemia cells: effect of ligand binding on receptor expression. Proc Natl Acad Sci USA 82:1522–1525

Furuno T, Ito A, Koma Y et al (2005) The spermatogenic Ig superfamily/synaptic cell adhesion molecule mast-cell adhesion molecule promotes interaction with nerves. J Immunol 174: 6934–6942

Furuta GT, Ackerman SJ, Lu L et al (1998) Stem cell factor influences mast cell mediator release in response to eosinophil-derived granule major basic protein. Blood 92:1055–1061

Füreder W, Agis H, Willheim M et al (1995a) Differential expression of complement receptors on human basophils and mast cells. Evidence for mast cell heterogeneity and CD88/C5aR expression on skin mast cells. J Immunol 155:3152–3160

Füreder W, Agis H, Semper H et al (1995b) Differential response of human basophils and mast cells to recombinant chemokines. Ann Hematol 70:251–258

Galli SJ, Tsai M (2008) Mast cells: versatile regulators of inflammation, tissue remodeling, host defense and homeostasis. J Dermatol Sci 49:7–19

Gantner F, Sakai K, Tusche MW et al (2002) Histamine H_4 and H_2 receptors control histamine-induced interleukin-16 release from human $CD8^+$ T cells. J Pharmacol Exp Ther 303:300–307

Genovese A, Borgia G, Bouvet JP et al (2003) Protein Fv produced during viral hepatitis is an endogenous immunoglobulin superantigen activating human heart mast cells. Int Arch Allergy Immunol 132:336–345

Genovese A, Bouvet JP, Florio G et al (2000) Bacterial immunoglobulin superantigen proteins A and L activate human heart mast cells by interacting with immunoglobulin E. Infect Immun 68:5517–5524

Gilchrist M, McCauley SD, Befus AD (2004) Expression, localization, and regulation of NOS in human mast cell lines: effects on leukotriene production. Blood 104:462–469

Gilfillan AM, Tkaczyk C (2006) Integrated signalling pathways for mast-cell activation. Nat Rev Immunol 6:218–230

Gillespie SR, DeMartino RR, Zhu J et al (2004) IL-10 inhibits FcεRI expression in mouse mast cells. J Immunol 172:3181–3188

Godot V, Arock M, Garcia G et al (2007) H_4 histamine receptor mediates optimal migration of mast cell precursors to CXCL12. J Allergy Clin Immunol 120:827–834

Gomez G, Ramirez CD, Rivera J et al (2005) TGF-β1 inhibits mast cell FcεRI expression. J Immunol 174:5987–5993

Gross Weege W, König W, Scheffer J et al (1988) Induction of histamine release from rat mast cells and human basophilic granulocytes by clinical *Escherichia coli* isolates and relation to hemolysin production and adhesin expression. J Clin Microbiol 26:1831–1837

Haas HL, Sergeeva OA, Selbach O (2008) Histamine in the nervous system. Physiol Rev 88: 1183–1241

Hallgren J, Gurish MF (2007) Pathways of murine mast cell development and trafficking: tracking the roots and routes of the mast cell. Immunol Rev 217:8–18

Hartmann K, Beiglböck F, Czarnetzki BM et al (1995) Effect of CC chemokines on mediator release from human skin mast cells and basophils. Int Arch Allergy Immunol 108:224–230

He S, Walls AF (1997) Human mast cell tryptase: a stimulus of microvascular leakage and mast cell activation. Eur J Pharmacol 328:89–97

He S, Gaça MD, Walls AF (1998) A role for tryptase in the activation of human mast cells: modulation of histamine release by tryptase and inhibitors of tryptase. J Pharmacol Exp Ther 286:289–297

He S, Gaça MD, Walls AF (2001) The activation of synovial mast cells: modulation of histamine release by tryptase and chymase and their inhibitors. Eur J Pharmacol 412: 223–229

Hide I, Toriu N, Nuibe T et al (1997) Suppression of TNF-α secretion by azelastine in a rat mast (RBL-2H3) cell line: evidence for differential regulation of TNF-alpha release, transcription, and degranulation. J Immunol 159:2932–2940

Ho LH, Ohno T, Oboki K et al (2007) IL-33 induces IL-13 production by mouse mast cells independently of IgE-FcεRI signals. J Leukoc Biol 82:1481–1490

Hoek KL, Cassell GH, Duffy LB et al (2002) *Mycoplasma pneumoniae*-induced activation and cytokine production in rodent mast cells. J Allergy Clin Immunol 109:470–476

Hofstra CL, Desai PJ, Thurmond RL et al (2003) Histamine H_4 receptor mediates chemotaxis and calcium mobilization of mast cells. J Pharmacol Exp Ther 305:1212–1221

Horigome K, Pryor JC, Bullock ED et al (1993) Mediator release from mast cells by nerve growth factor. Neurotrophin specificity and receptor mediation. J Biol Chem 268:14881–14887

Hosoda M, Yamaya M, Suzuki T et al (2002) Effects of rhinovirus infection on histamine and cytokine production by cell lines from human mast cells and basophils. J Immunol 169: 1482–1491

Hsu C, MacGlashan D Jr (1996) IgE antibody up-regulates high affinity IgE binding on murine bone marrow-derived mast cells. Immunol Lett 52:129–134

Hughes JM, Stringer RS, Black JL et al (1995) The effects of tumour necrosis factor α on mediator release from human lung. Pulm Pharmacol 8:31–36

Ikeda T, Funaba M (2003) Altered function of murine mast cells in response to lipopolysaccharide and peptidoglycan. Immunol Lett 88:21–26

Irani AA, Schechter NM, Craig SS et al (1986) Two types of human mast cells that have distinct neutral protease compositions. Proc Natl Acad Sci USA 83:4464–4468

Ito A, Hagiyama M, Oonuma J (2008) Nerve-mast cell and smooth muscle-mast cell interaction mediated by cell adhesion molecule-1, CADM1. J Smooth Muscle Res 44:83–93

Jackson NE, Wang HW, Tedla N et al (2005) IL-15 induces mast cell migration *via* a pertussis toxin-sensitive receptor. Eur J Immunol 35:2376–2385

Jensen C, Norn S, Stahl Skov P et al (1984) Bacterial histamine release by immunological and non-immunological lectin-mediated reactions. Allergy 39:371–377

Juremalm M, Nilsson G (2005) Chemokine receptor expression by mast cells. Chem Immunol Allergy 87:130–144

Jutel M, Blaser K, Akdis CA (2006) The role of histamine in regulation of immune responses. Chem Immunol Allergy 91:174–187

Jutel M, Klunker S, Akdis M et al (2001a) Histamine upregulates Th1 and downregulates Th2 responses due to different patterns of surface histamine 1 and 2 receptor expression. Int Arch Allergy Immunol 124:190–192

Jutel M, Watanabe T, Akdis M et al (2002) Immune regulation by histamine. Curr Opin Immunol 14:735–740

Jutel M, Watanabe T, Klunker S et al (2001b) Histamine regulates T-cell and antibody responses by differential expression of H1 and H2 receptors. Nature 413:420–425

Kalesnikoff J, Galli SJ (2008) New developments in mast cell biology. Nat Immunol 9:1215–1223

Kase K, Hua J, Yokoi H et al (2009) Inhibitory action of roxithromycin on histamine release and prostaglandin D2 production from β-defensin 2-stimulated mast cells. Int J Mol Med 23: 337–340

Katz HR, Lobell RB (1995) Expression and function of FcγR in mouse mast cells. Int Arch Allergy Immunol 107:76–78

Katz HR, Arm JP, Benson AC et al (1990) Maturation-related changes in the expression of FcγRII and FcγRIII on mouse mast cells derived in vitro and in vivo. J Immunol 145:3412–3417

Katz HR, Raizman MB, Gartner CS et al (1992) Secretory granule mediator release and generation of oxidative metabolites of arachidonic acid via Fc-IgG receptor bridging in mouse mast cells. J Immunol 148:868–871

Kawaguchi-Nagata K, Okamura H, Tamura T et al (1985) Induction of histidine decarboxylase activity in the spleen of mice treated with staphylococcal enterotoxin A and demonstration of its non-mast cell origin. Biochem Biophys Res Commun 129:187–192

Kawakami T, Galli SJ (2002) Regulation of mast-cell and basophil function and survival by IgE. Nat Rev Immunol 2:773–786

Kedzierski RM, Yanagisawa M (2001) Endothelin system: the double-edged sword in health and disease. Annu Rev Pharmacol Toxicol 41:851–876

Kempuraj D, Papadopoulou NG, Lytinas M et al (2003) Corticotropin-releasing hormone and its structurally related urocortin are synthesized and secreted by human mast cells. Endocrinology 145:43–48

Kepley CL, Taghavi S, Mackay G et al (2004) Co-aggregation of FcγRII with FcεRI on human mast cells inhibits antigen-induced secretion and involves SHIP-Grb2-Dok complexes. J Biol Chem 279:35139–35149

Kiener HP, Baghestanian M, Dominkus M et al (1998) Expression of the C5a receptor (CD88) on synovial mast cells in patients with rheumatoid arthritis. Arthritis Rheum 41:233–245

Kikawada E, Bonventre JV, Arm JP (2007) Group V secretory PLA_2 regulates TLR2-dependent eicosanoid generation in mouse mast cells through amplification of ERK and $cPLA_2\alpha$ activation. Blood 110:561–567

Kim HM, Lee YM (1999) Role of TGF-β 1 on the IgE-dependent anaphylaxis reaction. J Immunol 162:4960–4965

Kinet JP (1999) The high-affinity receptor (FcεRI): from physiology to pathology. Annu Rev Immunol 17:931–972.

King CA, Anderson R, Marshall JS (2002) Dengue virus selectively induces human mast cell chemokine production. J Virol 76:8408–8419

Kirshenbaum AS, Kessler SW, Goff JP et al (1991) Demonstration of the origin of human mast cells from $CD34^+$ bone marrow progenitor cells. J Immunol 146:1410–1415

Kirshenbaum AS, Goff JP, Semere T et al (1999) Demonstration that human mast cells arise from a progenitor cell population that is $CD34^+$, c-kit^+, and expresses aminopeptidase N (CD13). Blood 94:2333–2342

Kirshenbaum AS, Swindle E, Kulka M et al (2008) Effect of lipopolysaccharide (LPS) and peptidoglycan (PGN) on human mast cell numbers, cytokine production, and protease composition. BMC Immunol 9:45. doi: 10.1186/1471–2172–9-45

Kitamura Y (1989) Heterogeneity of mast cells and phenotypic change between subpopulations Annu Rev Immunol 7:59–76

Kitaura J, Eto K, Kinoshita T et al (2005) Regulation of highly cytokinergic IgE-induced mast cell adhesion by Src, Syk, Tec, and protein kinase C family kinases. J Immunol 174: 4495–4504

Kitaura J, Xiao W, Maeda-Yamamoto M et al (2004) Early divergence of Fcε receptor I signals for receptor up-regulation and internalization from degranulation, cytokine production, and survival. J Immunol 173:4317–4323

Kohno S, Nakao S, Ogawa K et al (1994) Possible participation of histamine H_3-receptors in the regulation of anaphylactic histamine release from isolated rat peritoneal mast cells. Jpn J Pharmacol 66:173–180

Kohno S, Ogawa K, Nabe T et al (1993) Dimaprit, a histamine H_2-agonist, inhibits anaphylactic histamine release from mast cells and the decreased release is restored by thioperamide (H_3-antagonist), but not by cimetidine (H_2-antagonist). Jpn J Pharmacol 62:75–79

Kohno M, Yamasaki S, Tybulewicz VL et al (2005) Rapid and large amount of autocrine IL-3 production is responsible for mast cell survival by IgE in the absence of antigen. Blood 105:2059–2065

Kołaczkowska E (2002) Shedding light on vascular permeability during peritonitis: role of mast cell histamine versus macrophage cysteinyl leukotrienes. Inflamm Res 51:519–521

Kołaczkowska E, Seljelid R, Płytycz B (2001a) Role of mast cells in zymosan-induced peritoneal inflammation in Balb/c and mast cell-deficient WBB6F1 mice. J Leukoc Biol 69:33–42

Kołaczkowska E, Seljelid R, Płytycz B (2001b) Critical role of mast cells in morphine-mediated impairment of zymosan-induced peritonitis in mice. Inflamm Res 50:415–421

Komisar J, Rivera J, Vega A et al (1992) Effects of staphylococcal enterotoxin B on rodent mast cells. Infect Immun 60:2969–2975

Krishnaswamy G, Kelley J, Johnson D et al (2001) The human mast cell: functions in physiology and disease. Front Biosci 6:D1109–D1127

Kubo Y, Nakano K (1999) Regulation of histamine synthesis in mouse $CD4^+$ and $CD8^+$ T lymphocytes. Inflamm Res 48:149–153

Kubo S, Matsuoka K, Taya C et al (2001) Drastic up-regulation of FcεRI on mast cells is induced by IgE binding through stabilization and accumulation of FcεRI on the cell surface. J Immunol 167:3427–3434

Kubota Y (1992) The effect of human anaphylatoxins and neutrophils on histamine release from isolated human skin mast cells. J Dermatol 19:19–26

Kulka M, Alexopoulou L, Flavell RA et al (2004) Activation of mast cells by double-stranded RNA: evidence for activation through Toll-like receptor 3. J Allergy Clin Immunol 114: 174–182

Kurose M, Saeki K (1981) Histamine release induced by neurotensin from rat peritoneal mast cells. Eur J Pharmacol 76:129–136

Lam V, Kalesnikoff J, Lee CW et al (2003) IgE alone stimulates mast cell adhesion to fibronectin via pathways similar to those used by IgE + antigen but distinct from those used by Steel factor. Blood 102:1405–1413

László V, Rothe G, Hegyesi H et al (2001) Increased histidine decarboxylase expression during in vitro monocyte maturation; a possible role of endogenously synthesised histamine in monocyte/macrophage differentiation. Inflamm Res 50:428–434

Lau AH, Chow SS, Ng YS (2001) Immunologically induced histamine release from rat peritoneal mast cells is enhanced by low levels of substance P. Eur J Pharmacol 414:295–303

Legler DF, Loetscher M, Jones SA et al (1996) Expression of high- and low-affinity receptors for C3a on the human mast cell line, HMC-1. Eur J Immunol 26:753–758

Lin TJ, Bissonnette EY, Hirsh A et al (1996) Stem cell factor potentiates histamine secretion by multiple mechanisms, but does not affect tumour necrosis factor-α release from rat mast cells. Immunology 89:301–307

Lippert U, Artuc M, Grützkau A et al (2004) Human skin mast cells express H2 and H4, but not H3 receptors. J Invest Dermatol 123:116–123

Lippert U, Krüger-Krasagakes S, Möller A et al (1995) Pharmacological modulation of IL-6 and IL-8 secretion by the H_1-antagonist decarboethoxy-loratadine and dexamethasone by human mast and basophilic cell lines. Exp Dermatol 4:272–276

Lippert U, Möller A, Welker P et al (2000) Inhibition of cytokine secretion from human leukemic mast cells and basophils by H_1- and H_2-receptor antagonists. Exp Dermatol 9:118–124

Liu C, Ma X, Jiang X et al (2001) Cloning and pharmacological characterization of a fourth histamine receptor H_4 expressed in bone marrow. Mol Pharmacol 59:420–426

Liu Y, Yamada H, Ochi J (1998) Immunocytochemical studies on endothelin in mast cells and macrophages in the rat gastrointestinal tract. Histochem Cell Biol 109:301–307

Louis R, Dowlati A, Weber T et al (1994) Modulation of immunological histamine release from human lung fragments by stem cell factor, IL-3, IL-5 and GM-CSF: comparison with human leukocytes. Int Arch Allergy Immunol 105:18–25

Louis R, Tilkin P, Poncelet M et al (1995) Regulation of histamine release from human bronchoalveolar lavage mast cells by stem cell factor in several respiratory diseases. Allergy 50:340–348

Lowman MA, Benyon RC, Church MK (1988) Characterization of neuropeptide-induced histamine release from human dispersed skin mast cells. Br J Pharmacol 95:121–130

Lukacs NW, Hogaboam CM, Kunkel SL et al (1998) Mast cells produce ENA-78, which can function as a potent neutrophil chemoattractant during allergic airway inflammation. J Leukoc Biol 63:746–751

MacGlashan D Jr (2003) Histamine: a mediator of inflammation. J Allergy Clin Immunol 112: S53–S59

Malaviya R, Abraham SN (2000) Role of mast cell leukotrienes in neutrophil recruitment and bacterial clearance in infectious peritonitis. J Leukoc Biol 67:841–846

Malaviya R, Gao Z, Thankavel K et al (1999) The mast cell tumor necrosis factor alpha response to FimH-expressing *Escherichia coli* is mediated by the glycosylphosphatidylinositol-anchored molecule CD48. Proc Natl Acad Sci USA 96:8110–8115

Malaviya R, Ross E, Jakschik BA et al (1994a) Mast cell degranulation induced by type 1 fimbriated *Escherichia coli* in mice. J Clin Invest 93:1645–1653

Malaviya R, Ross EA, MacGregor JI et al (1994b) Mast cell phagocytosis of FimH-expressing enterobacteria. J Immunol 152:1907–1914

Malaviya R, Twesten NJ, Ross EA et al (1996) Mast cells process bacterial Ags through a phagocytic route for class I MHC presentation to T cells. J Immunol 156:1490–1496

Mao SY, Alber G, Rivera J et al (1992) Interaction of aggregated native and mutant IgE receptors with the cellular skeleton. Proc Natl Acad Sci USA 89:222–226

Marshall JS, Leal-Berumen I, Nielsen L et al (1996) Interleukin (IL)-10 inhibits long-term IL-6 production but not preformed mediator release from rat peritoneal mast cells. J Clin Invest 97:1122–1128

Masini E, Blandina P, Brunelleschi S et al (1982) Evidence for H2-receptor-mediated inhibition of histamine release from isolated rat mast cells. Agents Actions 12:85–88

Masuda A, Yoshikai Y, Aiba K et al (2002) Th2 cytokine production from mast cells is directly induced by lipopolysaccharide and distinctly regulated by c-Jun N-terminal kinase and p38 pathways. J Immunol 169:3801–3810

Maślińska D, Gujski M, Laure-Kamionowska M et al (2004) Subcellular localization of histamine in articular cartilage chondrocytes of rheumatoid arthritis patients. Inflamm Res 53: S35–S36

Matsuda K, Piliponsky AM, Iikura M et al (2005) Monomeric IgE enhances human mast cell chemokine production: IL-4 augments and dexamethasone suppresses the response. J Allergy Clin Immunol 116:1357–1363

Matsushima H, Yamada N, Matsue H et al (2004a) TLR3-, TLR7-, and TLR9-mediated production of proinflammatory cytokines and chemokines from murine connective tissue type skin-derived mast cells but not from bone marrow-derived mast cells. J Immunol 173:531–541

Matsushima H, Yamada N, Matsue H et al (2004b) The effects of endothelin-1 on degranulation, cytokine, and growth factor production by skin-derived mast cells. Eur J Immunol 34: 1910–1919

Maurer M, Theoharides T, Granstein RD et al (2003) What is the physiological function of mast cells? Exp Dermatol 12:886–910

McCurdy JD, Lin TJ, Marshall JS (2001) Toll-like receptor 4-mediated activation of murine mast cells. J Leukoc Biol 70:977–984

McCurdy JD, Olynych TJ, Maher LH et al (2003) Cutting edge: distinct Toll-like receptor 2 activators selectively induce different classes of mediator production from human mast cells. J Immunol 170:1625–1629

Meade R, Askenase PW, Geba GP et al (1992) Transforming growth factor-β1 inhibits murine immediate and delayed type hypersensitivity. J Immunol 149:521–528

Metcalfe DD, Baram D, Mekori YA (1997) Mast cells. Physiol Rev 77:1033–1079

Metz M, Maurer M (2007) Mast cells – key effector cells in immune responses. Trends Immunol 28:234–241

Metz M, Grimbaldeston MA, Nakae S et al (2007) Mast cells in the promotion and limitation of chronic inflammation. Immunol Rev 217:304–328

Miyoshi S, Kawata K, Hosokawa M et al (2003) Histamine-releasing reaction induced by the N-terminal domain of *Vibrio vulnificus* metalloprotease. Life Sci 72:2235–2242

Montemurro P, Nishioka H, Dundon WG et al (2002) The neutrophil-activating protein (HP-NAP) of *Helicobacter pylori* is a potent stimulant of mast cells. Eur J Immunol 32:671–676

Mori T, Kawashima T, Beppu Y et al (1994) Histamine release induced by pituitary adenylate cyclase activating polypeptide from rat peritoneal mast cells. Arzneimittelforschung 44:1044–1046

Mousli M, Bronner C, Bueb JL et al (1989) Activation of rat peritoneal mast cells by substance P and mastoparan. J Pharmacol Exp Ther 250:329–335

Mousli M, Hugli TE, Landry Y et al (1992) A mechanism of action for anaphylatoxin C3a stimulation of mast cells. J Immunol 148:2456–2461

Mrabet-Dahbi S, Metz M, Dudeck A et al (2009) Murine mast cells secrete a unique profile of cytokines and prostaglandins in response to distinct TLR2 ligands. Exp Dermatol 18:437–444

Muñoz S, Hernández-Pando R, Abraham SN et al (2003) Mast cell activation by *Mycobacterium tuberculosis*: mediator release and role of CD48. J Immunol 170:5590–5596

Nagasaka A, Matsue H, Matsushima H et al (2008) Osteopontin is produced by mast cells and affects IgE-mediated degranulation and migration of mast cells. Eur J Immunol 38:489–499

Nakajima K, Hirai K, Yamaguchi M et al (1992) Stem cell factor has histamine releasing activity in rat connective tissue-type mast cells. Biochem Biophys Res Commun 183:1076–1083

Nilsson G, Johnell M, Hammer CH et al (1996) C3a and C5a are chemotaxins for human mast cells and act through distinct receptors via a pertussis toxin-sensitive signal transduction pathway. J Immunol 157:1693–1698

Nitschke M, Sohn K, Dieckmann D et al (1996) Effects of basophil-priming and stimulating cytokines on histamine release from isolated human skin mast cells. Arch Dermatol Res 288:463–468

Niyonsaba F, Someya A, Hirata M et al (2001) Evaluation of the effects of peptide antibiotics human beta-defensins-1/-2 and LL-37 on histamine release and prostaglandin D_2 production from mast cells. Eur J Immunol 31:1066–1075

Norn S, Stahl Skov P, Jensen C et al (1984) Lectin-mediated reactions in histamine release caused by bacteria. Agents Actions 14:481–483

O'Donnell MC, Ackerman SJ, Gleich GJ et al (1983) Activation of basophil and mast cell histamine release by eosinophil granule major basic protein. J Exp Med 157:1981–1991

Odum L, Petersen LJ, Skov PS et al (1998) Pituitary adenylate cyclase activating polypeptide (PACAP) is localized in human dermal neurons and causes histamine release from skin mast cells. Inflamm Res 47:488–492

Ogawa K, Nabe T, Yamamura H et al (1999) Nanomolar concentrations of neuropeptides induce histamine release from peritoneal mast cells of a substrain of Wistar rats. Eur J Pharmacol 374:285–291

Ohkubo T, Shibata M, Inoue M et al (1994) Autoregulation of histamine release via the histamine H3 receptor on mast cells in the rat skin. Arch Int Pharmacodyn Ther 328:307–314

Oka T, Hori M, Tanaka A et al (2004) IgE alone-induced actin assembly modifies calcium signaling and degranulation in RBL-2H3 mast cells. Am J Physiol Cell Physiol 286:C256–C263

Okayama Y, Kawakami T (2006) Development, migration, and survival of mast cells. Immunol Res 34:97–115

Okayama Y, Hagaman DD, Metcalfe DD (2001a) A comparison of mediators released or generated by IFN-gamma-treated human mast cells following aggregation of FcγRI or FcεRI. J Immunol 166:4705–4712

Okayama Y, Hagaman DD, Woolhiser M et al (2001b) Further characterization of FcγRII and FcγRIII expression by cultured human mast cells. Int Arch Allergy Immunol 124:155–157

Okayama Y, Kirshenbaum AS, Metcalfe DD (2000) Expression of a functional high-affinity IgG receptor, FcγRI, on human mast cells: up-regulation by IFN-γ. J Immunol 164:4332–4339
Okayama Y, Tkaczyk C, Metcalfe DD et al (2003) Comparison of FcεRI and FcγRI-mediated degranulation and TNF-alpha synthesis in human mast cells: selective utilization of phosphatidylinositol-3-kinase for FcγRI-induced degranulation. Eur J Immunol 33: 1450–1459
Okumura S, Sagara H, Fukuda T et al (2005) FcεRI-mediated amphiregulin production by human mast cells increases mucin gene expression in epithelial cells. J Allergy Clin Immunol 115: 272–279
Olejnik AK, Brzezińska-Błaszczyk E (1998) Tumor necrosis factor alpha (TNF-α) modulates rat mast cell reactivity. Immunol Lett 64:167–171
Opgenorth TJ, Budzik GP, Mollison KW et al (1990) Atrial peptides induce mast cell histamine release. Peptides 11:1003–1007
Orinska Z, Bulanova E, Budagian V et al (2005) TLR3-induced activation of mast cells modulates $CD8^+$ T-cell recruitment. Blood 106:978–987
Oskeritzian CA, Zhao W, Min HK et al (2005) Surface CD88 functionally distinguishes the MCTC from the MCT type of human lung mast cell. J Allergy Clin Immunol 115:1162–1168
Ottosson A, Edvinsson L (1997) Release of histamine from dural mast cells by substance P and calcitonin gene-related peptide. Cephalalgia 17:166–174
Pandey V, Mihara S, Fensome-Green A et al (2004) Monomeric IgE stimulates NFAT translocation into the nucleus, a rise in cytosol Ca^{2+}, degranulation, and membrane ruffling in the cultured rat basophilic leukemia-2H3 mast cell line. J Immunol 172:4048–4058
Pardo J, Wallich R, Ebnet K et al (2007) Granzyme B is expressed in mouse mast cells in vivo and in vitro and causes delayed cell death independent of perforin. Cell Death Differ 14:1768–1779
Patella V, Bouvet JP, Marone G (1993) Protein Fv produced during vital hepatitis is a novel activator of human basophils and mast cells. J Immunol 151:5685–5698
Patella V, Casolaro V, Björck L et al (1990) Protein L. A bacterial Ig-binding protein that activates human basophils and mast cells. J Immunol 145:3054–3061
Patella V, de Crescenzo G, Marinò I et al (1996) Eosinophil granule proteins activate human heart mast cells. J Immunol 157:1219–1225
Patella V, de Crescenzo G, Marinò I et al (1997) Eosinophil granule proteins are selective activators of human heart mast cells. Int Arch Allergy Immunol 113:200–2002
Pearce FL, Thompson HL (1986) Some characteristics of histamine secretion from rat peritoneal mast cells stimulated with nerve growth factor. J Physiol 372:379–393
Piliponsky AM, Gleich GJ, Nagler A et al (2003) Non-IgE-dependent activation of human lung- and cord blood-derived mast cells is induced by eosinophil major basic protein and modulated by the membrane form of stem cell factor. Blood 101:1898–1904
Piliponsky AM, Pickholtz D, Gleich GJ et al (2001) Human eosinophils induce histamine release from antigen-activated rat peritoneal mast cells: a possible role for mast cells in late-phase allergic reactions. J Allergy Clin Immunol 107:993–1000
Piotrowski W, Foreman JC (1985) On the actions of substance P, somatostatin, and vasoactive intestinal polypeptide on rat peritoneal mast cells and in human skin. Naunyn Schmiedebergs Arch Pharmacol 331:364–368
Piotrowski W, Foreman JC (1986) Some effects of calcitonin gene-related peptide in human skin and on histamine release. Br J Dermatol 114:37–46
Piquet-Pellorce C, Dy M (1991) Effect of lipopolysaccharides on histamine synthesis by hematopoietic cells. Cell Immunol 135:360–371
Prinz C, Zanner R, Gratzl M (2003) Physiology of gastric enterochromaffin-like cells. Annu Rev Physiol 65:371–382
Rao KN, Brown MA (2008) Mast cells: multifaceted immune cells with diverse roles in health and disease. Ann NY Acad Sci 1143:83–104
Repka-Ramirez MS, Baraniuk JN (2002) Histamine in health and disease. Clin Allergy Immunol 17:1–25

Rivera J, Gilfillan AM (2006) Molecular regulation of mast cell activation. J Allergy Clin Immunol 117:1214–1225

Robertson D, Holowka D, Baird B (1986) Cross-linking of immunoglobulin E-receptor complexes induces their interaction with the cytoskeleton of rat basophilic leukemia cells. J Immunol 136:4565–4572

Rodewald HR, Dessing M, Dvorak AM et al (1996) Identification of a committed precursor for the mast cell lineage. Science 271:818–822

Rożniecki JJ, Letourneau R, Sugiultzoglu M et al (1999) Differential effect of histamine 3 receptor-active agents on brain, but not peritoneal, mast cell activation. J Pharmacol Exp Ther 290: 1427–1435

Ryan JJ, DeSimone S, Klisch G et al (1998) IL-4 inhibits mouse mast cell FcεRI expression through a STAT6-dependent mechanism. J Immunol 161:6915–6923

Ryan JJ, Kashyap M, Bailey D et al (2007) Mast cell homeostasis: a fundamental aspect of allergic disease. Crit Rev Immunol 27:15–32

Scheffer J, König W, Braun V et al (1988) Comparison of four hemolysin-producing organisms (*Escherichia coli*, *Serratia marcescens*, *Aeromonas hydrophila*, and *Listeria monocytogenes*) for release of inflammatory mediators from various cells. J Clin Microbiol 26:544–551

Schneider E, Pollard H, Lepault F et al (1987) Histamine-producing cell-stimulating activity. Interleukin 3 and granulocyte-macrophage colony-stimulating factor induce de novo synthesis of histidine decarboxylase in hemopoietic progenitor cells. J Immunol 139:3710–3717

Schneider E, Rolli-Derkinderen M, Arock M et al (2002) Trends in histamine research: new functions during immune responses and hematopoiesis. Trends Immunol 23:255–263

Schulman ES, Post TJ, Henson PM et al (1988) Differential effects of the complement peptides, C5a and C5a des Arg on human basophil and lung mast cell histamine release. J Clin Invest 81:918–923

Seebeck J, Kruse ML, Schmidt-Choudhury A et al (1998) Pituitary adenylate cyclase activating polypeptide induces degranulation of rat peritoneal mast cells via high-affinity PACAP receptor-independent activation of G proteins. Ann NY Acad Sci 865:141–146

Sher A, Hein A, Moser G et al (1979) Complement receptors promote the phagocytosis of bacteria by rat peritoneal mast cells. Lab Invest 41:490–499

Shiraishi M, Hirasawa N, Oikawa S et al (2000) Analysis of histamine-producing cells at the late phase of allergic inflammation in rats. Immunology 99:600–606

Singh LK, Boucher W, Pang X et al (1999) Potent mast cell degranulation and vascular permeability triggered by urocortin through activation of corticotropin-releasing hormone receptors. J Pharmacol Exp Ther 288:1349–1356

Sonobe Y, Nakane H, Watanabe T et al (2004) Regulation of Con A-dependent cytokine production from $CD4^+$ and $CD8^+$ T lymphocytes by autosecretion of histamine. Inflamm Res 53: 87–92

Soruri A, Grigat J, Kiafard Z et al (2008) Mast cell activation is characterized by upregulation of a functional anaphylatoxin C5a receptor. BMC Immunol 9:29 doi:10.1186/1471-2172-9-29

Stassen M, Müller C, Richter C et al (2003) The streptococcal exotoxin streptolysin O activates mast cells to produce tumor necrosis factor alpha by p38 mitogen-activated protein kinase- and protein kinase C-dependent pathways. Infect Immun 71:6171–6177

Stead RH, Dixon MF, Bramwell NH et al (1989) Mast cells are closely apposed to nerves in the human gastrointestinal mucosa. Gastroenterology 97:575–585

Stead RH, Tomioka M, Quinonez G et al (1987) Intestinal mucosal mast cells in normal and nematode-infected rat intestines are in intimate contact with peptidergic nerves. Proc Natl Acad Sci USA 84:2975–2979

Strakhova MI, Cuff CA, Manelli AM et al (2009) In vitro and in vivo characterization of A-940894: a potent histamine H_4 receptor antagonist with anti-inflammatory properties. Br J Pharmacol 157:44–54

Supajatura V, Ushio H, Nakao A et al (2001) Protective roles of mast cells against enterobacterial infection are mediated by Toll-like receptor 4. J Immunol 167:2250–2256

Supajatura V, Ushio H, Nakao A et al (2002) Differential responses of mast cell Toll-like receptors 2 and 4 in allergy and innate immunity. J Clin Invest 109:1351–1359

Suzuki R, Furuno T, Teshima R et al (2001) Bi-directional relationship of in vitro mast cell-nerve communication observed by confocal laser scanning microscopy. Biol Pharm Bull 24:291–294

Suzuki A, Suzuki R, Furuno T et al (2004) N-cadherin plays a role in the synapse-like structures between mast cells and neurites. Biol Pharm Bull 27:1891–1894

Szeberényi JB, László V, Pállinger E et al (2001a) Intracellular histamine content increases during in vitro dendritic cell differentiation. Inflamm Res 50:S112–S113

Szeberényi JB, Pállinger E, Zsinkó M et al (2001b) Inhibition of effects of endogenously synthesized histamine disturbs in vitro human dendritic cell differentiation. Immunol Lett 76:175–182

Takaishi T, Morita Y, Hirai K et al (1994) Effect of cytokines on mediator release from human dispersed lung mast cells. Allergy 49:837–842

Takamatsu S, Nakashima I, Nakano K (1996) Modulation of endotoxin-induced histamine synthesis by cytokines in mouse bone marrow-derived macrophages. J Immunol 156:778–785

Takeshita K, Sakai K, Bacon KB et al (2003) Critical role of histamine H_4 receptor in leukotriene B_4 production and mast cell-dependent neutrophil recruitment induced by zymosan *in vivo*. J Pharmacol Exp Ther 307:1072–1078

Talkington J, Nickell SP (1999) *Borrelia burgdorferi* spirochetes induce mast cell activation and cytokine release. Infect Immun 67:1107–1115

Tam SW, Demissie S, Thomas D et al (2004) A bispecific antibody against human IgE and human FcγRII that inhibits antigen-induced histamine release by human mast cells and basophils. Allergy 59:772–780

Tanaka S, Takasu Y, Mikura S et al (2002) Antigen-independent induction of histamine synthesis by immunoglobulin E in mouse bone marrow-derived mast cells. J Exp Med 196:229–235

Theoharides TC (1996) The mast cell: a neuroimmunoendocrine master player. Int J Tissue React 18:1–21

Theoharides TC, Cochrane DE (2004) Critical role of mast cells in inflammatory diseases and the effect of acute stress. J Neuroimmunol 146:1–12

Theoharides TC, Douglas WW (1978) Somatostatin induces histamine secretion from rat peritoneal mast cells. Endocrinology 102:1637–1640

Theoharides TC, Kalogeromitros D (2006) The critical role of mast cells in allergy and inflammation. Ann NY Acad Sci 1088:78–99

Theoharides TC, Singh LK, Boucher W et al (1998) Corticotropin-releasing hormone induces skin mast cell degranulation and increased vascular permeability, a possible explanation for its proinflammatory effects. Endocrinology 139:403–413

Thurmond RL, Desai PJ, Dunford PJ et al (2004) A potent and selective histamine H_4 receptor antagonist with anti-inflammatory properties. J Pharmacol Exp Ther 309:404–413

Tkaczyk C, Okayama Y, Metcalfe DD et al (2004) Fcγ receptors on mast cells: activatory and inhibitory regulation of mediator release. Int Arch Allergy Immunol 133:305–315

Toda M, Dawson M, Nakamura T et al (2004) Impact of engagement of FcεRI and CC chemokine receptor 1 on mast cell activation and motility. J Biol Chem 279:48443–48448

Tomioka M, Stead RH, Nielsen L et al (1988) Nerve growth factor enhances antigen and other secretagogue-induced histamine release from rat peritoneal mast cells in the absence of phosphatidylserine. J Allergy Clin Immunol 82:599–607

Toru H, Ra C, Nonoyama S et al (1996) Induction of the high-affinity IgE receptor (FcεRI) on human mast cells by IL-4. Int Immunol 8:1367–1373

Tsakalos ND, Theoharides TC, Kops SK et al (1983) Induction of mast cell secretion by parathormone. Biochem Pharmacol 32:355–360

Uchida Y, Ninomiya H, Sakamoto T et al (1992) ET-1 released histamine from guinea pig pulmonary but not peritoneal mast cells. Biochem Biophys Res Commun 189:1196–1201

Váczi A, László V, Pállinger E et al (2001) Detection of histamine and histidine decarboxylase in human platelets by flow cytometry. Inflamm Res 50:S91–S92

Valent P, Schernthaner GH, Sperr WR et al (2001) Variable expression of activation-linked surface antigens on human mast cells in health and disease. Immunol Rev 179:74–81

van der Kleij HP, Ma D, Redegeld FA et al (2003) Functional expression of neurokinin 1 receptors on mast cells induced by IL-4 and stem cell factor. J Immunol 171:2074–2079

van Overveld FJ, Jorens PG, Rampart M et al (1991) Tumour necrosis factor stimulates human skin mast cells to release histamine and tryptase. Clin Exp Allergy 21:711–714

Van Nassauw L, Adriaensen D, Timmermans JP (2007) The bidirectional communication between neurons and mast cells within the gastrointestinal tract. Auton Neurosci 133:91–103

Varadaradjalou S, Féger F, Thieblemont N et al (2003) Toll-like receptor 2 (TLR2) and TLR4 differentially activate human mast cells. Eur J Immunol 33:899–906

Venable JD, Cai H, Chai W et al (2005) Preparation and biological evaluation of indole, benzimidazole, and thienopyrrole piperazine carboxamides: potent human histamine H_4 antagonists. J Med Chem 48: 8289–8298

von Köckritz-Blickwede M, Goldmann O, Thulin P et al (2008) Phagocytosis-independent antimicrobial activity of mast cells by means of extracellular trap formation. Blood 111:3070–3080

Wang SW, Oh CK, Cho SH et al (2005) Amphiregulin expression in human mast cells and its effect on the primary human lung fibroblasts. J Allergy Clin Immunol 115:287–294

Wasiela M, Brzezińska-Błaszczyk E (2000) The influence of anaerobic bacteria and mycoplasma isolated from the genital tract on mast cell activation. Med Dosw Mikrobiol 52:389–396

Watabe K, Ito A, Koma Y et al (2004) Distinct roles for the SgIGSF adhesion molecule and c-kit receptor tyrosine kinase in the interaction between mast cells and the mesentery. Biochem Biophys Res Commun 324:782–788

Watanabe Y, Todome Y, Ohkuni H et al (2002) Cysteine protease activity and histamine release from the human mast cell line HMC-1 stimulated by recombinant streptococcal pyrogenic exotoxin B/streptococcal cysteine protease. Infect Immun 70:3944–3947

Welle M (2005) Development, significance, and heterogeneity of mast cells with particular regard to the mast cell-specific proteases chymase and tryptase. J Leukoc Biol 61:233–245

Wescott SL, Hunt WA, Kaliner M (1982) Histamine H_1 receptors on rat peritoneal mast cells. Life Sci 31:1911–1919

Wierzbicki M, Brzezińska-Błaszczyk E (2009) Diverse effect of bacterial cell wall component on mast cell degranulation, cysteinyl leukotriene generation and migration. Micriobiol Immunol 53:694–703

Wojtecka-Łukasik E, Maśliński S (1992) Fibronectin and fibrinogen degradation products stimulate PMN-leukocyte and mast cell degranulation. J Physiol Pharmacol 43:173–181

Woolhiser MR, Okayama Y, Gilfillan AM et al (2001) IgG-dependent activation of human mast cells following up-regulation of FcγRI by IFN-γ. Eur J Immunol 31:3298–3307

Woolhiser MR, Brockow K, Metcalfe DD (2004) Activation of human mast cells by aggregated IgG through FcγRI: additive effects of C3a. Clin Immunol 110:172–180

Xia HZ, Du Z, Craig S et al (1997) Effect of recombinant human IL-4 on tryptase, chymase, and Fcε receptor type I expression in recombinant human stem cell factor-dependent fetal liver-derived human mast cells. J Immunol 159:2911–2921

Yamaguchi M, Lantz CS, Oettgen HC et al (1997) IgE enhances mouse mast cell FcεRI expression In Vitro and In Vivo: evidence for a novel amplification mechanism in IgE-dependent reactions. J Exp Med 185:663–672

Yamaguchi K, Motegi K, Endo Y (2000a) Induction of histidine decarboxylase, the histamine-forming enzyme, in mice by interleukin-12. Toxicology 156:57–65

Yamaguchi K, Motegi K, Kurimoto M et al (2000b) Induction of the activity of the histamine-forming enzyme, histidine decarboxylase, in mice by IL-18 and by IL-18 plus IL-12. Inflamm Res 49:513–519

Yamaguchi M, Sayama K, Yano K et al (1999) IgE enhances Fcε receptor I expression and IgE-dependent release of histamine and lipid mediators from human umbilical cord blood-derived mast cells: synergistic effect of IL-4 and IgE on human mast cell Fc epsilon receptor I expression and mediator release. J Immunol 162:5455–5465

Yamamoto J, Watanabe S, Hirose M et al (1999) Role of mast cells as a trigger of inflammation in *Helicobacter pylori* infection. J Physiol Pharmacol 50:17–23

Yamamura H, Nabe T, Kohno S et al (1994a) Endothelin-1 induces release of histamine and leukotriene C4 from mouse bone marrow-derived mast cells. Eur J Pharmacol 257:235–242

Yamamura H, Nabe T, Kohno S et al (1994b) Endothelin-1, one of the most potent histamine releasers in mouse peritoneal mast cells. Eur J Pharmacol 265:9–15

Yamamura H, Nabe T, Kohno S et al (1995) Mechanism of histamine release by endothelin-1 distinct from that by antigen in mouse bone marrow-derived mast cells. Eur J Pharmacol 288:269–275

Yanagida M, Fukamachi H, Ohgami K et al (1995) Effects of T-helper 2-type cytokines, interleukin-3 (IL-3), IL-4, IL-5, and IL-6 on the survival of cultured human mast cells. Blood 86:3705–3714

Yanagida M, Fukamachi H, Takei M et al (1996) Interferon-gamma promotes the survival and FcεRI-mediated histamine release in cultured human mast cells. Immunology 89:547–552

Yoshida H, Inagaki Y, Yamaki K et al (1996) Histamine release induced by human natriuretic peptide from rat peritoneal mast cells. Regul Pept 61:45–49

Yoshimoto T, Tsutsui H, Tominaga K et al (1999) IL-18, although antiallergic when administered with IL-12, stimulates IL-4 and histamine release by basophils. Proc Natl Acad Sci USA 96:13962–13966

Zalewska A, Brzezińska-Błaszczyk E, Omulecki A et al (1997) Functional studies of skin mast cells in lichen planus. Arch Dermatol Res 289:261–264

Zhao W, Kepley CL, Morel PA et al (2006) FcγRIIa, not FcγRIIb, is constitutively and functionally expressed on skin-derived human mast cells. J Immunol 177:694–701

Zhao Y, van Hasselt CA, Woo KS et al (2005) Effects of budesonide, desloratadine and dexamethasone on interleukine-4 release and expression from human mast cell line. Zhonghua Er Bi Yan Hou Tou Jing Wai Ke Za Zhi 40:124–127

Zheutlin LM, Ackerman SJ, Gleich GJ et al (1984) Stimulation of basophil and rat mast cell histamine release by eosinophil granule-derived cationic proteins. J Immunol 133:2180–2185

Zhu Y, Michalovich D, Wu H et al (2001) Cloning, expression, and pharmacological characterization of a novel human histamine receptor. Mol Pharmacol 59:434–441

Zwadlo-Klarwasser G, Vogts M, Hamann W et al (1998) Generation and subcellular distribution of histamine in human blood monocytes and monocyte subsets. Inflamm Res 47:434–439

Chapter 12
Histamine H1 Receptor Gene Expression Mechanism as a Novel Therapeutic Target of Allergy

Hiroyuki Fukui and Hiroyuki Mizuguchi

Abstract The histamine H1 receptor is a unique G-protein coupled receptor because the stimulation of the receptor induced the receptor up-regulation through increase in gene expression. Histamine-induced up-regulation of H1 receptor was mediated by protein kinase C-δ signaling. This increase was induced in the nasal mucosa by the provocation of the nasal hypersensitivity model rats. Therapeutics for allergy such as dexamethasone, antihistamines, suplatast tosillate, Sho-seiryu-to and Kujin (*Sophorae flavescensis*) extract suppressed histamine H1 receptor gene expression by different degrees. Short-term treatment of antihistamines showed partial suppression of H1 receptor gene expression. Long-term treatment showed almost complete suppression with improvement of symptom. Correlation between symptom and histamine H1 receptor mRNA level was observed, and the data strongly suggest that histamine H1 receptor gene is an allergic disease-sensitive gene. Drugs for allergy also showed strong suppression of IL-4 and IL-5 gene expression besides H1 receptor gene expression. Histamine H1 receptor signaling is regulated by allergic network and novel strategy of therapy for allergy is highly expected using synergistic suppression by different drugs with different mechanisms of gene expression.

Keywords Histamine receptor · Gene expression · Allergy

Abbreviations

GPCR	G-protein coupled receptor
PKC	protein kinase C
PMA	phorbol 12-myristate, 13-acetate
TDI	toluene 2, 4-diisocyanate
IL	interleukin

H. Fukui (✉)
Department of Molecular Pharmacology, Institute of Health Biosciences, The University of Tokushima Graduate School, 1-78-1 Shomachi, Tokushima 770-8505, Japan
e-mail: hfukui@ph.tokushima-u.ac.jp

M. Shahid et al. (eds.), *Biomedical Aspects of Histamine*,
DOI 10.1007/978-90-481-9349-3_12,

Contents

12.1 Introduction

Population of allergic diseases is increasing, and the prevalence of allergic rhinitis was reported over 10–20% (Okuda 2003). Histamine is a major mediator of allergy. Symptoms of allergy are mainly mediate by the histamine H1 receptor. Antihistamines (histamine H1 receptor antagonists) have been used for the therapy of allergic diseases. Expression level of the histamine H1 receptor plays a key role in the regulation of receptor-mediated signaling. Most G-protein coupled receptors (GPCRs) are down-regulated by repetitive stimulation with their agonist as a step of receptor desensitization. The histamine H1 receptor is a unique GPCR because the receptor was up-regulated through the activation of its gene expression (Das et al. 2007).

Allergic diseases are multi-factorial, and involved with abnormal expression of disease-related genes. Therapeutics targeting the expression mechanism of the disease-sensitive gene is highly expected. The gene expression of the histamine H1 receptor was elevated in allergy model rats (Kitamura et al. 2004). The histamine H1 receptor gene is thought a strong candidate of allergic disease-sensitive gene by additional data (Mizuguchi et al. 2008). The mechanisms of the histamine H1 receptor gene expression, evidences of the histamine H1 receptor gene as an allergic disease-sensitive gene and novel strategy for the therapy of allergy are described in this chapter.

12.2 Desensitization of the Histamine H1 Receptor

Most GPCRs are desensitized after repetitive stimulation of receptors with agonist. It is well-known that the histamine H1 receptor is desensitized. Involvement of receptor down-regulation is reported as a step of desensitization, and the histamine H1 receptor was also down-regulated by the receptor stimulation (Horio et al. 2004a). Five residues of serine and threonine seem to be the key phosphorylation sites for the receptor down-regulation because the mutant histamine H1 receptor lacking these five residues showed no down-regulation (Fig. 12.1) (Horio

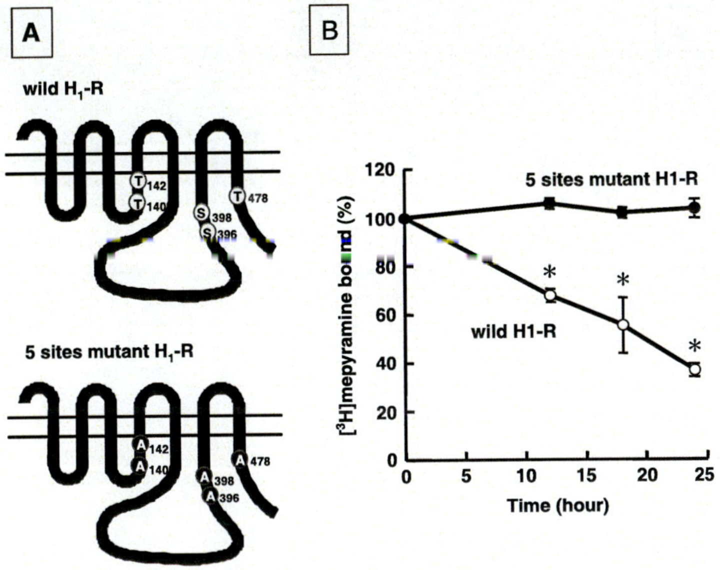

Fig. 12.1 Histamine-induced down-regulation of the histamine H1 receptor. (**a**) Illustration of wild (*upper*) and mutant (*lower*) histamine H1 receptors. Putative phosphorylation sites (S: serine and T: threonine) in wild H1 receptor (wild H1-R) are displaced by As: alanines in the mutant H1 receptor (5 sites mutant H1-R). (**b**) Time course of histamine H1 receptor expression level by the stimulation of wild (●) and mutant (○) H1 receptors. *p<0.001 vs. 5 sites mutant H1-R (n=6)

et al. 2004b). The histamine H1 receptor was phosphorylated by various kinases including protein kinase C (PKC), Ca^{2+}/calmodulin-dependent protein kinase II, protein kinase G and protein kinase A (Kawakami et al. 2003). Heterologous down-regulation of the histamine H1 receptor was induced by the stimulation of M_3 muscarinic and β_2-adrenergic receptors (Kawakami et al. 2004, Miyoshi et al., 2004a, b).

12.3 Up-Regulation of the Histamine H1 Receptor at the Cellular Level

Stimulation of the histamine H1 receptor induced H1 receptor up-regulation in HeLa cells naturally bearing histamine H1 receptors was observed (Fig. 12.2) (Das et al. 2007). Increases in histamine H1 receptor mRNA expression and H1 receptor gene promoter activity were involved. Simultaneously, histamine H1 receptor-mediated H1 receptor down-regulation is supposed to be induced (Horio et al. 2004a). However, up-regulation is dominant in HeLa cells (Fig. 12.3). Up-regulation of the histamine H1 receptor was also induced by the stimulation of PKC-activating phorbol ester, phorbol 12-myristate, 13-acetate (PMA) (Fig. 12.4). Histamine-induced

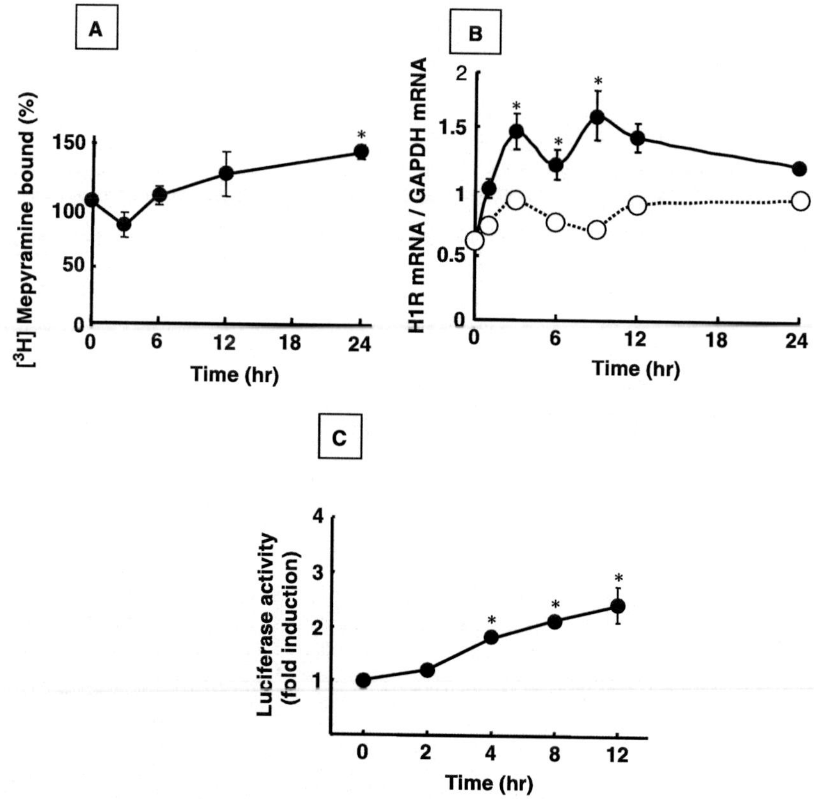

Fig. 12.2 Histamine-induced up-regulation of the histamine H1 receptor. Time course of the H1 receptor expression (**a**), H1 receptor mRNA (**b**) and H1 receptor prompter activity (**c**) was determined. HeLa cells were starved with serum free medium for 24 h at 37°C before the treatment of 10 μM histamine. (**a**) The amount of H1R is shown as a percentage of the control [^{3}H]mepyramine binding activity (130 fmol/mg protein) in the untreated cell membrane. *p<0.05 vs. control (n = 4). (**b**) The histamine H1 receptor mRNA was determined by quantitative real-time RT-PCR. The data were normalized by GAPDH mRNA levels. Histamine (●), control (○). *p<0.05 vs. control (n = 4). (**c**) HeLa cells were co-transfected with pH1R and pRL-MPK vector. The histamine H1 receptor promoter activity was measured as luciferase activity by the dual-luciferase assay system. The data are expressed as fold of the control luminescence. *p<0.05 vs. control (n=4)

elevation of H1 receptor mRNA was suppressed by an inhibitor of PKC, Ro31-8220. When the histamine H1 receptor was up-regulated, histamine-induced inositol phosphate accumulation was increased in proportion to the expression level of the histamine H1 receptor.

Heterologous up-regulation and down-regulation of H1 receptor by M_3 muscarinic and β_2 adrenergic receptors, respectively, were observed (Miyoshi et al.

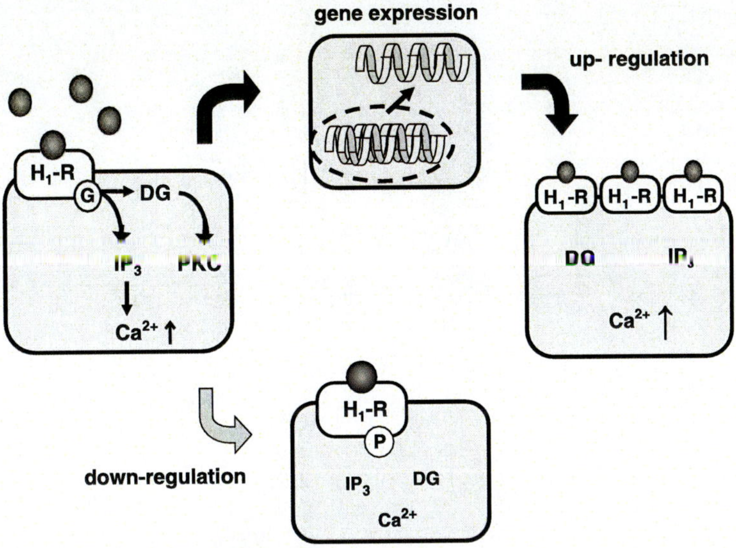

Fig. 12.3 Two regulatory mechanisms of histamine H1 receptor expression level by up-regulation through the elevation of gene expression and down-regulation

2007, 2008). The data suggest the autonomic regulation of histamine H1 receptor gene expression. Down-regulation of H1 receptor by β_2 adrenergic receptor agonists is induced not only by the suppression of H1 receptor gene expression but also by the receptor phosphorylation, a desensitization mechanism, beneficial for the therapy of asthma, and is seems to have aided affect for the therapy of asthma.

12.4 Up-Regulation of the Histamine H1 Receptor in Allergy Model Rats

Various allergy model animals have been developed. In the present study, a convenient and reproducible method of nasal hypersensitivity model rats was developed (Kitamura et al. 2004). Six weeks old male Brown Norway rats weighing about 200–250 g were used. Sensitization was performed by the application of 10 μl of 10% solution of toluene 2, 4-diisocyanate (TDI) in ethyl acetate bilaterally on the nasal vestibule of each rat once a day for five consecutive days (Fig. 12.5). This sensitization procedure was then repeated after 2-days interval. Nine days after the second sensitization, 10 μl of 10% TDI solution was again applied to the nasal vestibule to provoke nasal allergy-like symptoms.

The histamine H1 receptor mRNA level was elevated several-fold in nasal mucosa of nasal hypersensitivity model rats after the provocation by TDI (Fig. 12.6).

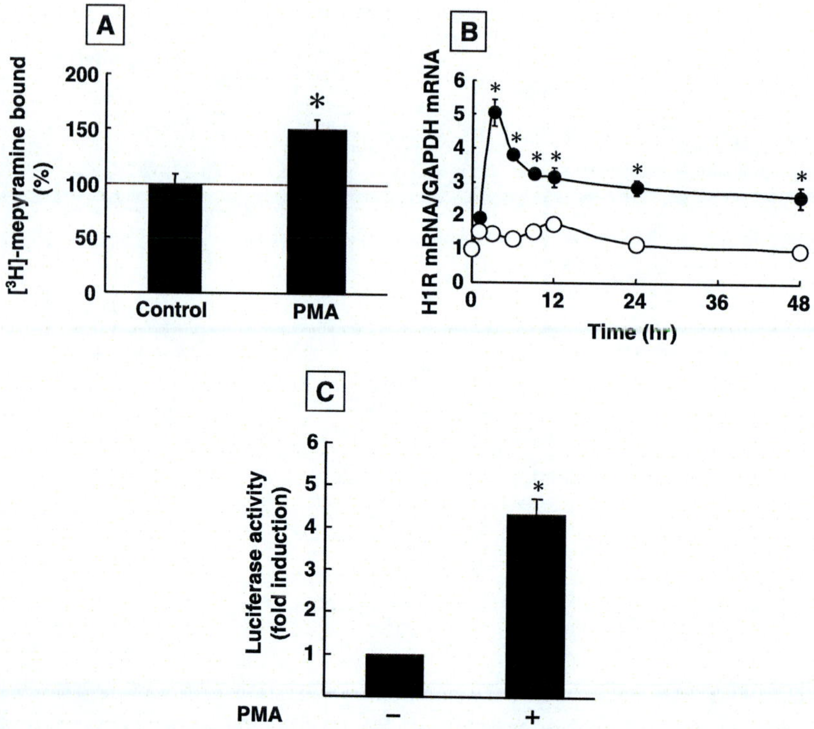

Fig. 12.4 Effect of protein kinase C activator on the histamine H1 receptor expression level (**a**), histamine H1 receptor mRNA (**b**), and histamine H1 receptor promoter activity (**c**). A. HeLa cells were treated with 1 μM of PMA for 24 h. The histamine H1 receptor expression level was determined by [^{3}H]mepyramine binding. The activity is shown as percentage of [^{3}H]mepyramine binding activity in untreated cell membrane (30 fmol/mg protein). *p<0.05 vs. control (n=4). B: HeLa cells were treated with 1 μM of PMA, and the histamine H1 receptor mRNA was determined by quantitative real-time RT-PCR. Histamine H1 receptor mRNA levels were normalized by GAPDH mRNA levels. (●) PMA; (○) control. *p<0.05 vs. respective control (n=4). (**c**) HeLa cells were co-transfected with pH1R and pRL-MPK vector and treated with 1 μM of PMA for 4 h. The luciferase activity was measured by the dual-luciferase assay system. Data are expressed as fold of the control luminescence. *p<0.05 vs. control (n=4)

The expression reached to its peak level in-between 3 and 5 h after the provocation, and the level was declined thereafter. Up-regulation of histamine H1 receptor was observed 24 h after the provocation.

Dexamethasone showed almost complete suppression of the mRNA elevation and up-regulation of the H1 receptor (Kitamura et al. 2004). Antihistamines also suppressed the mRNA elevation (Mizuguchi et al. 2008). The degree of suppression by antihistamines, however, was smaller than that of dexamethasone.

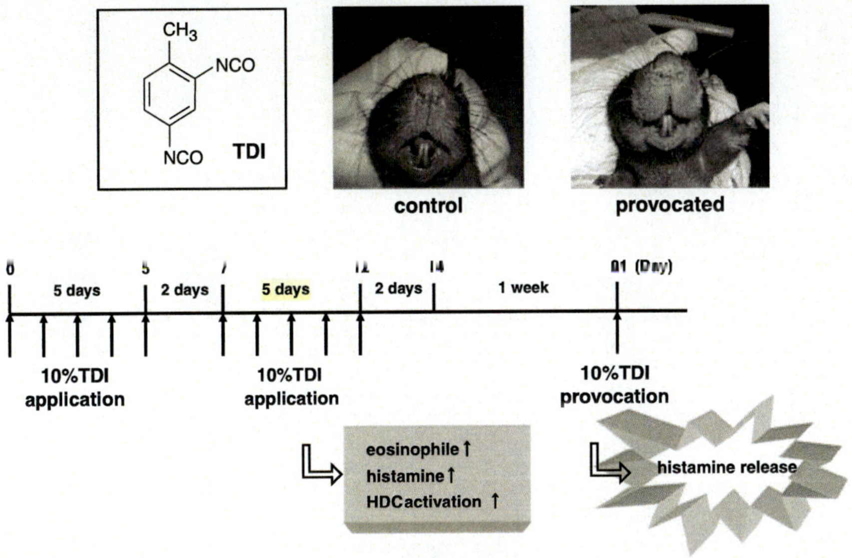

Fig. 12.5 Toluene 2,4-diisocyanate (TDI)-sensitizaed nasal hypersensitivity model rat. Chemical structure of TDI is shown in the rectangle. Two pictures show the control rat (*left picture*) and the model rat provocated with TDI (*right picture*). Lower panel shows the schedule for the preparation of TDI-sensitized nasal hypersensitivity model rat

12.5 Prophylactic Treatment with Antihistamines

Prophylactic treatment with antihistamines, anti-releasers, anti-leukotrienes or Th2 cytokine suppresser (suplatast tosilate) is recommended by starting it about 2 weeks before pollen season in Japan (Baba et al. 2008). The mechanism of this treatment remains to be elucidated. Studies of prophylactic treatment with an antihistamine were performed using TDI-sensitized nasal hypersensitivity model rats (Mizuguchi et al. 2008). Treatments were started 3 days, 1 week, 3 weeks and 5 weeks before the provocation, and effect on symptoms (number of sneezing) and the level of histamine H1 receptor mRNA elevation were examined (Fig. 12.7). Treatment with an antihistamine just before 3 days of the provocation showed partial suppression of symptoms and H1 receptor mRNA elevation. Treatment more than 1 week before the provocation showed stronger suppression of the symptoms and histamine H1 receptor mRNA elevation (Fig. 12.8). Simultaneously, prophylactic treatment showed similar suppression profile to IL-4 mRNA elevation. These data suggest that nasal hypersensitivity symptoms are linked to gene expression of histamine H1 receptor and IL-4. Allergic signal circuit between histamine H1 receptor and IL-4 is postulated, and considered to worsen the allergy symptom. Application of IL-4 bilaterally in the nasal cavity of rats induced histamine H1 receptor mRNA elevation in 6 h (Shahriar et al. 2009). While, histamine could induce IL-4 mRNA

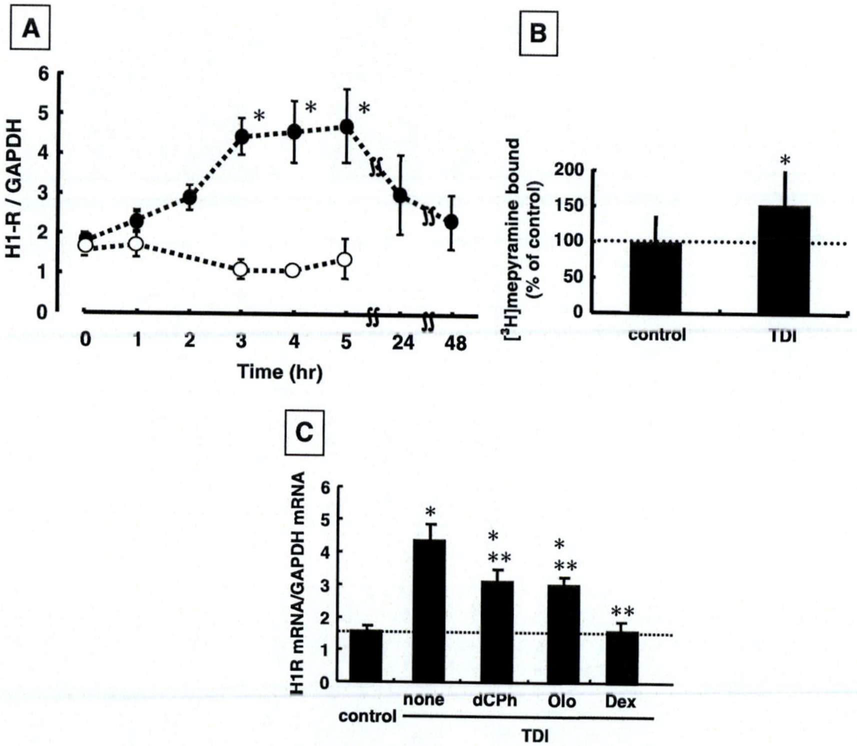

Fig. 12.6 Up-regulation of histamine H1 receptor and suppression by therapeutics for allergy. (**a**) Time course of the histamine H1 receptor mRNA elevation in the nasal mucosa of hypersensitivity rats after the provocation of TDI. Nasal hypersensitivity rats (●), control rats (○). $^*p<0.01$ vs. control ($n=4$). (**b**) Up-regulation of histamine H1 receptor expression by TDI. $^*p<0.01$ vs. control ($n=4$). (**c**) Suppression by d-chlorpheniramine (dCPh), olopatadine (Olo) and dexamethasone (Dex). $^*p<0.01$ vs. control ($n=4$), $^{**}p<0.01$ vs. TDI-none ($n=4$)

elevation by daily treatment for 1 week (Shahriar et al. 2009). The mechanism of histamine-induced IL-4 seems important for the elucidation of allergy symptom.

12.6 Various Drugs Targeting Histamine H1 Receptor Gene Expression Mechanism

Suplatast tosilate is reported as a suppressor of IL-4 and IL-5 production, IgE production and eosionophil function (Mimura et al. 2005). Suplatast suppressed histamine H1 receptor up-regulation and gene expression of H1 receptor besides that of IL-4 and IL-5 in TDI-sensitized nasal hypersensitivity rats (Fig. 12.9) (Shahriar et al. 2009). Both Sho-seiryu-to, a Kampo medicine used for the therapy of respiratory disorders, and Kujin (a Chinese natural medicine, *Sophorae flavescensis*) also

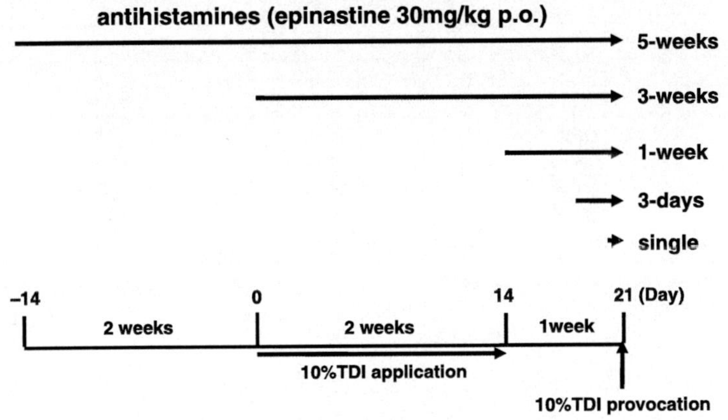

Fig. 12.7 Protocol for TDI sensitization and schedule for anti-histamine pre-treatment. Rats were sensitized with 10 μl of 10% TDI in ethyl acetate for 2 weeks. One week later, they were treated with 10% TDI in ethyl acetate. Control rats were treated similarly with ethyl acetate only. Antihistamines were administered orally 1 hr before provocation or once a day for 3 days, 1 week, 3 weeks, or 5 weeks before provocation with TDI

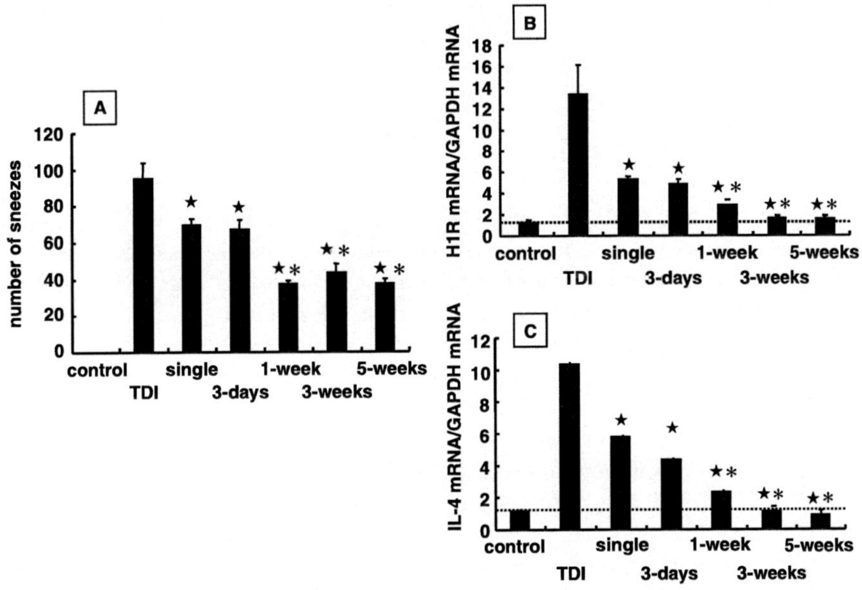

Fig. 12.8 Effect of repeated pre-treatment with epinastine before provocation on TDI-induced sneezing (**a**), up-regulations of histamine H1 receptor mRNA (**b**) and IL-4 mRNA (**c**) in TDI-sensitized rats. (**a**) The numbers of sneezes were counted for 10 min just after TDI-provocation. Epinastine (30 mg/kg/day) was administered orally. ★$p<0.05$ vs. TDI and *$p<0.05$ vs. single treatment ($n=3$). (**b**) Nasal mucosa was collected 4 h after provocation. Total RNA was extracted and the mRNA levels of histamine H1 receptor (**b**) and IL-4 (**c**) were determined by real-time quantitative RT-PCR. ★$p<0.05$ vs. TDI and *$p<0.05$ vs. single treatment ($n=4$)

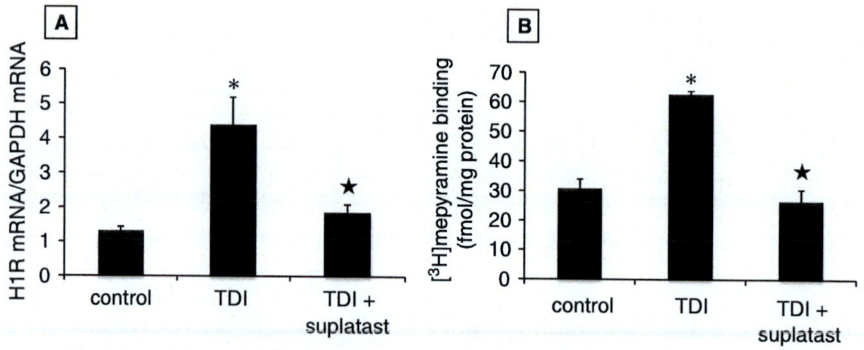

Fig. 12.9 Suppression by suplatast tosilate of histamine H1 receptor up-regulation. Suplatast blocks TDI-induced up-regulations of histamine H1 receptor mRNA (**a**) and H1 receptor expression (**b**) in nasal mucosa of TDI-sensitized nasal hypersensitivity rats. (**a**) Rats were sacrificed 4 h after TDI provocation and the H1 receptor mRNA was determined. (**b**) Rats were sacrificed 24 h after provocation and [^{3}H]mepyramine binding activity was determined. *$p<0.01$ vs. control, ★$p<0.01$ vs. TDI

showed strong suppression to histamine H1 receptor up-regulation and gene expression of H1 receptor, IL-4 and IL-5 (Das et al. 2009, Dev et al. 2009). These drugs also potently improved the symptoms of TDI-sensitized nasal hypersensitivity rats.

12.7 Concluding Remarks

It is quite obvious that the histamine H1 receptor signaling is very important in allergic diseases. Allergic diseases are multi-factorial disease, and development of new therapeutics targeting disease-sensitive gene is highly expected. The data in this chapter strongly suggest that histamine H1 receptor gene is an allergy-sensitive gene. Histamine H1 receptor signaling is increased when H1 receptor is up-regulated, and increase in histamine H1 receptor signaling is suggested to worsen the allergy symptoms. Current therapeutics for allergic diseases revealed to have potent suppressive effect on gene expression. These drugs suppressed IL-4 and IL-5 gene expression in addition to the suppression of H1 receptor. Cross-talk between histamine H1 receptor signaling and IL-4 signaling was strongly suggested. It is suggested that histamine H1 receptor signaling is regulated by allergy network. Target molecules of antihistamine, suplatast tosilate, Sho-seiryu-to and Kujin are considered quite different, although these drugs suppress similar gene expression pattern. Novel strategy of the therapy for allergic diseases is highly expected through synergistic suppression of gene expression by the combination use.

Acknowledgements This work was financially supported by a Grant-in Aid for Scientific Research from Japan Society for the Promotion of Science (18390167 to H.F.) and by grants from the Osaka Medical Research Foundation for Incurable Diseases. We highly appreciate collaborators.

References

Baba K, Konno A, Takenaka H (eds) (2008) Committee of guideline for the therapy of nasal allergy 2009. In: Guideline for the therapy of nasal allergy 2009 – perennial rhinitis and pollinosis (Japanese), Life Science (publisher)

Das AK, Mizuguchi H, Kodama M et al (2009) Sho-seiryu-to suppresses histamine signaling at the trascription level in TDI-sentitized nasal allergy model rats. Allergol Int 58:81–88

Das AK, Yoshimura S, Mishima R et al (2007) Stimulation of histamine H_1 receptor up-regulates histamine H_1 receptor itself through activation of receptor gene transcription. J Pharmacol Sci 103:374–382

Dev S, Mizuguchi H, Das AK et al (2009) Kujin suppresses histamine signaling at transcriptional level in toluene 2,4-diisocyanate-sensitized rats. J Pharmacil Sci 109:606–617

Horio S, Kato T, Ogawa M et al (2004b) Two threonine residues and two serine residues in the second and third loops are both involved in histamine H_1 receptor downregulation. FEBS Lett 573:226–230

Horio S, Ogawa M, Kawakami N et al (2004a) Identification of amino acid residues responsible for agonist-induced down-regulation of histamine H_1 receptors. J Pharmacol Sci 94:410–419

Kawakami N, Miyoshi K, Horio S et al (2003) Direct phosphorylation of histamine H_1 receptor by various protein kinases in vitro. Methods Findings Exp Clin Pharmacol 25:685–693

Kawakami N, Miyoshi K, Horio S et al (2004) β_2-Adrenergic receptor-mediated histamine H_1 receptor down-regulation: another possible advantage of β_2 agonists in asthmatic therapy. J Pharmacol Sci 94:449–458

Kitamura Y, Miyoshi A, Murata Y et al (2004) Effect of glucocorticoid on upregulation of histamine H_1 receptor mRNA in nasal mucosa of rats sensitized by exposure to toluene diisocyanate. Acta Otolaryngol 124:1053–1058

Mimura T, Shinozaki Y, Kawasaki H et al (2005) JTP-27536 [(+)-1,3-dihydroxy-2-hydroxymethylpropyl-2-ammonium 2-[(R)-3-cyclo-hexyl-1-phenylpropyl]-1,3-dioxo-2,3-di-hydro-1H-isoindole-5-carboxylate monohydrate], a novel inhibitor of immunoglobulins and interleukin-5 with anti-inflammatory properties in mouse allergic dermatitis model. J Pharmacol Exp Ther 314:293–301

Miyoshi K, Kawakami N, Das AK et al (2007) Heterologous up-regulation of the histamine H_1 receptor by M_3 muscarinic receptor – mediated activation of H_1 receptor gene transcription. J Pharm Pharmacol 59:843–848

Miyoshi K, Kawakami N, Horio S et al (2004b) Homologous and heterologous phosphorylation of human histamine H_1 receptor in intact cells. J Pharmacol Sci 96:474–482

Miyoshi K, Kawakami N, Wakayama Y et al (2004a) Histamine H_1 receptor down-regulation mediated by M_3 muscarinic acetylcholine receptor subtype. J Pharmacol Sci 95:426–434

Miyoshi K, Kawakami N, Umehara H et al (2008) Down-regulation of histamine H_1 receptor by β_2-adrenoceptor-mediated inhibition of H_1 receptor gene transcription. J Pharm Pharmacol 60:747–752

Mizuguchi H, Hatano M, Matsushita C et al (2008) Repeated pre-treatment with antihistamines suppresses transcriptional up-regulations of histamine H_1 receptor and interleukin-4 genes in toluene-2,4-diisocyanate–sensitized rats. J Pharmacol Sci 108:480–486

Okuda M (2003) Epidemiology – prevalence of allergic rhinitis in Japan and the world. In: Konno A (ed) Chapter 1. Outline and epidemiology of allergic rhinitis, (Japanese), Saishin-igaku Bessatsu: ABC of new diagnosis and therapy 12/immunology 2, Saishin-igakusha (Publisher), pp 18–26

Shahriar M, Mizuguchi H, Maeyama K et al (2009) Suplatast tosilate inhibits histamine signaling by direct and indirect down-regulation of histamine H_1 receptor gene expression through suppression of histidine decarboxylase and interleukin-4 gene transcriptions. J Immunol 183:2133–2141

Part VIII
Histamine in the Nervous System

Chapter 13
The Neuronal Histamine and it's Receptors as New Therapeutic Targets for Food Intake and Obesity

Takayuki Masaki

Abstract Histamine neurons and histamine receptors have distributed in the brain and addressed in their implications of regulatory energy homeostasis. Several studies using agonist/antagonist of neuronal histamine and it's receptors demonstrated that they have been shown to be involved in food intake and obesity. In addition, adipocytokine leptin regulates food intake and obesity partially via neuronal histamine and it's receptors. Furthermore, recent studies have provided evidence that regulation of the diurnal rhythm of food intake through neuronal histamine is a crucial factor in the development of obesity. Thus, we focused on these roles of the neuronal histamine and it's receptors in regulating the food intake and obesity.

Keywords Neuronal histamine · Histamine receptors · Food intake · Obesity

Abbreviations

TMN	tuberomammillary nucleus
HDC	histidine decarboxylase
IP3	inositol-1,4,5-triphosphate
DAG	1,2-diacylglycerol
cAMP	cyclic adenosine monophosphate
α-FMH	alpha-fluoromethylhistidine
PVN	paraventricullar nucleus
UCPs	uncoupling proteins
IAs	inverse agonists
VLPO	ventrolateral preoptic nucleus
REM	rapid eye movement
WT	wild-type

T. Masaki (✉)
Department of Internal Medicine, Oita University, 1-1 Idaigaoka, Yufu-Hasama, Oita, 879-5593 Japan
e-mail: masaki@med.oita-u.ac.jp

M. Shahid et al. (eds.), *Biomedical Aspects of Histamine*,
DOI 10.1007/978-90-481-9349-3_13,

ARC arcuate nucleus
VMH ventromedial nucleus

Contents

13.1 Introduction

Histamine neurons exist in tuberomammillary nucleus (TMN) of hypothalamus and project to whole brain including thalamus, hippocampus, basal ganglia and cortex (Brown et al. 2001, Haas and Panula 2003, Schwartz et al. 1991). Histamine is synthesized in the brain from l-histidine by the enzyme histidine decarboxylase (HDC). The termination of histamine's action in the brain may require its catabolism to telemethylhistamine by the enzyme histamine N-methyltransferase. Four types of histamine receptors, H1-receptor, H2-receptor, H3-receptor and H4-receptor (H1-R, H2-R, H3-R and H4-R), have been cloned and identified (Arrang et al. 1983, Birdsall 1991, de Esch et al. 2005, Nguyen et al. 2001, Timmerman 1992). Neuronal histamine is involved in a variety of hypothalamic functions such as locomoter activity, circadian rhythm, memory, drinking and food intake through H1-R, H2-R and H3-R (Inoue et al. 1996, Masaki and Yoshimatsu 2006, 2007a, b, Parmentier et al. 2002).

Histamine H1-R are present in areas involved in thalamus, cortex, cholinergic cell groups in the mesopontine tegmentum and in the basal forebrain as well as the locus coeruleus and raphe nuclei. In addition, high densities of H1-Rs are present in the limbic system, including many nuclei of the hypothalamus, most septal nuclei, medial amygdala and several hippocampal areas (Brown et al. 2001, Haas and Panula 2003, Schwartz et al. 1991, Terao et al. 2004). Histamine H2-Rs are located postsynaptically and high densities H2-Rs are found in hippocampus, and basal ganglia (Brown et al. 2001, Haas and Panula 2003, Schwartz et al. 1991, Terao et al. 2004). Histamine H3-Rs are located on the somata and axon terminals of histamine neurons where they serve as autoreceptors to modulate histamine synthesis and release, and are also located pre- and post-synaptically in other brain regions (Arrang et al. 1983).

Based on these accumulated data from anatomical studies, a role for histamine receptors have been suggested to be involved in many physiological functions throughout the brain.

13.2 The Signaling of Histamine Receptors

The gene for the H1-R encodes a member of 7-transmembrane spanning, G-protein-associated receptor family (Brown et al. 2001). Intracellularly, stimulation of H1-R leads to the hydrolysis of phosphatidyl 4,5-biphosphate and the formation of inositol-1,4,5-triphosphate (IP3) and 1,2-diacylglycerol (DAG). DAG potentiates the activity of protein kinase C, whilst IP3 binds to the IP3 receptor located on the endoplasmic reticulum. IP3 mobilizes intracellular calcium, and DAG activates protein kinase C. In this way, histamine induces the production of inositol phosphates and, activation of H1-R has been shown to increase intracellular calcium. In addition, histamine H1-R activation can lead to the formation of AA, most likely through the action of phospholipase A2 and to the formation of cGMP. The increase in intracellular calcium explains the pharmacological effects of H1-R stimulation. It has been suggested that H1-R stimulation–dependent elevation in intracellular calcium leads to increased cyclic adenosine monophosphate (cAMP) levels (Brown et al. 2001, Haas and Panula 2003, Schwartz et al. 1991). The gene for the H2-R also encodes a 7-transmembrane domain, G-protein coupled receptor (Brown et al. 2001, Haas and Panula 2003, Schwartz et al. 1991). The Gs G-protein is associated with the receptor, activation of which leads to stimulation of adenylyl cylase and enhanced production of the second messenger molecule cAMP. One prominent target of cAMP is the cAMP-dependent PKA which can phosphorylate target proteins in the cytosol, in the cell membrane or translocate to the nucleus and activate the transcription factor CREB. The H3-R was described as a G-protein coupled receptor which is pertussis-toxin sensitive, similar to many other presynaptic inhibitory receptors. Interestingly, the H3-R gene shows a low overall homology to all other biogenic amine receptors. In various cell lines, H3-R activation led to an inhibition of forskolin-stimulated cAMP formation.

13.3 Neuronal Histamine and H1-R on Food Intake and Obesity

Physiological and pharmacological experiments have demonstrated that the neuronal histamine system plays a critical role in the regulation of obesity and diabetes (Fulop et al. 2003, Jorgensen et al. 2006, Lecklin et al. 1998, Masaki et al. 2001a, b, 2004, Mollet et al. 2001, Takahashi et al. 2002). Central injection of histamine suppress food intake in rodents (Lecklin et al. 1998, Masaki et al. 2001b). The peripheral injection of histidine, a precursor of histamine, also had the same effect on food intake in rodents (Kasaoka et al. 2004, Yoshimatsu et al. 2002). It is suggested that histidine can penetrate the blood brain barrier and it is converted into histamine in the brain by HDC (Yoshimatsu et al. 2002). Thus, the histidine-induced suppression of food intake results from an elevation of the histamine level in brain. In contrast, application of alpha-fluoromethylhistidine (α-FMH), HDC suicide inhibitor, increase short-term food intake (Tuomisto et al. 1994).

Experiments using histamine H1-R-agonists and antagonists also showed that H1-Rs also control food intake in rodents (Sakata et al. 1988). Histamine H1-R-agonist 2-(3-trifluoromethylphenyl) histamine (betahistine) injected centrally decreased food intake and activated the c-*fos* like immunoreactivity in paraventricullar nucleus (PVN) (Masaki et al. 2004). Contrary, central administration of the H1-R-antagonists chlorpheniramine or pyrilamine elicit food intake in rats (Sakata et al. 1988). From these observations, neuronal histamine and histamine H1-Rs may be involved in neural regulation of food intake.

13.4 Effects of Neuronal Histamine on Sympathetic Nerve Activity and the Expression Uncoupling Proteins (UCPs)

Obesity is also regulated by energy expenditure in addition to food intake. Uncoupling proteins especially in brown adipose tissue are crucial roles in energy expenditure both in rodent (Feldmann et al. 2009, Masaki et al. 1999, 2000a, b) and human (Cypess et al. 2009, van Marken Lichtenbelt et al. 2009, Virtanen et al. 2009). Expression of the molecule is regulated by neuronal and humoral factors. The sympathetic nervous activity also has been well documented to regulate of energy expenditure. Central administration of histamine affected the activity of sympathetic nerves innervating BAT (Yasuda et al. 2004b). Histamine H1-R agonist also increased the expression of UCP1 mRNA in BAT (Masaki et al. 2004). It is indicated that neuronal histamine and H1-Rs are involved in the central regulation of energy homeostasis (Table 13.1).

A central injection of histamine increased glycerol concentration in the perfusate from the adipose tissue in rat (Tsuda et al. 2002). Central infusion of thioperamide activates histamine neurons to increase synthesis and release of neuronal histamine, mimicked histamine action in the augmented lipolysis. Similarly, intraperitoneal administration of histidine activated the BAT sympathetic nerve activity (Yasuda et al. 2004a). Furthermore, sustained central infusion of histamine reduced body adiposity independently food intake (Masaki et al. 2001b, 2003). Collectively, hypothalamic histamine neurons and/or histamine H1-R agonist regulate peripheral lipid and energy metabolism through the accelerating of sympathetic nerve activity and UCP in adipose tissues (Masaki et al. 2001a).

Table 13.1 Neuronal histamine, histamine H1 receptor and obesity

	Effect or phenotype	References
Neuronal Histamine	Decreased food intake and body weight	Masaki et al. (2001b, 2003)
Histidine	Decreased food intake and body weight	Yoshimatsu et al. (2002), Kasaoka et al. (2004)
Inhibitor of histidine decarboxylase	Increased food intake	Tuomisto et al. (1994)
Agonist of histamine H1 receptor in rodents	Decreased food intake and body weight	Lecklin et al. (1998)
Agonist of histamine H1 receptor in human	Decreased body weight in women	Barak et al. (2008)
Antagonist of histamine H1 receptor	Increased food intake	Sakata et al. (1988)
Histidine decarboxylase deficient mice	Increased food intake and obesity	Fulop et al. (2003), Jorgensen et al. (2006)
Histamine H1 receptor deficient mice	Increased food intake and obesity	Mollet et al. (2001), Masaki et al. (2004)

13.5 Neuronal Histamine and H3-R on Food Intake and Obesity

H3-Rs are pharmacologically identified and predominantly expressed in the brain, where they negatively regulate histamine release (Arrang et al. 1983). Therefore, H3-R antagonists/inverse agonists (IAs) have therapeutic potential for treating obesity (Table 13.2). Investigations into the role of histamine as a neurotransmitter have shown that histamine inhibits its own neuronal synthesis and release from depolarized slices of the rat cortex via presynaptic feedback mechanisms (Arrang et al. 1983, Leurs et al. 2005). H3-R IAs are believed to suppress appetite by activating H1-Rs in post-synaptic areas, because H3-Rs negatively regulate the release of HA in the brain (Arrang et al. 1983, Leurs et al. 2005). To address the therapeutic potential of H3-R ligands as anti-obesity agents, several studies have reported the pharmacological profiles of H3-R IAs in animal studies.

Thioperamide, an imidazole-containing H3-R IAs, suppressed food intake in spontaneous, fast-induced, schedule-induced, and NPY-induced feeding in rodents (Itoh et al. 1999). In addition, thioperamide, clobenpropit and ciproxifan, imidazole-based compounds, both decreased short-term or long-term food intake (Attoub et al. 2001, Hancock and Brune 2005, Morimoto et al. 2001). Contrary, administration of imetit, H3-R agonist, to hamsters in the lean state increased food intake (Jethwa et al. 2009). Although these reports have suggested the therapeutic potential of H3-R IAs, their anti-obesity effects remain controversial. Administration of thioperamide enhanced HA release in the brain, but the treatment did not decrease

Table 13.2 Histamine H3 receptor and obesity

	Effect or phenotype	References
Antagonist of histamine H3 receptor		
Thioperamide	Decreased food intake	Itoh et al. (1999), Attoub et al. (2001), Jethwa et al. (2009)
	Increased food intake	Yoshimoto et al. (2006)
A-331440	Decreased food intake and body weight	Hancock et al. (2004)
NNC 0038-1049	Decreased food intake and body weight	Malmlof et al. (2005)
NNC 0038-1202	Decreased food intake and body weight	Malmlof et al. (2006)
Histamine H3 receptor deficient mice	Increased food intake and obesity	Takahashi et al. (2002)
Agonist of histamine H3 receptor		
Imetit	Increased food intake	Jethwa et al. (2002)
	Decreased food intake and body weight	Yoshimoto et al. (2006)

food intake (Yoshimoto et al. 2006). In addition, the H3-R agonist imetit reduces adiposity in DIO mice by inhibiting food intake and increasing energy expenditure (Yoshimoto et al. 2006). The anti-obese effects of the H3-R agonist were also confirmed using an H3-R agonist, *R*-methylhistamine. Moreover, both intraperitoneal and oral administration of thioperamide enhanced HA release in the brain, while only IP administration caused significant reductions in food intake (Sindelar et al. 2004). Further studies are needed to clarify the involvement of H3-Rs in food intake and obesity.

13.6 The Studies Using Histamine Receptors or HDC Deficient Mice

Although drugs exert their primary actions by interacting with the specific target molecules, they also have other actions. No drug causes only a single specific effect. At higher concentrations, most drugs can interact with a wide variety of biological molecules, often resulting in functional alterations. For investigators that utilize mammals as experimental systems, the technical development of production of animals with specific genetic alteration has promised an unprecedented opportunity for a wide variety of investigation in animals to be done in a much more sophisticated manner.

The cloning of the gene for the H1-R has enabled the production of mice lacking this gene (Inoue et al. 1996). The use of H1-R deficient mice makes it possible to clarify the possible physiological roles of H1-R more clearly than classical pharmacological studies, which affect other neurotransmitter systems as described above. These mice appeared to develop normally but had deficits in the normal circadian rhythm of locomotor activity and reduced exploratory behaviour in a novel environment (Inoue et al. 1996). H1-R deficient mice showed no significantly change in daily food intake, growth curve, body weight, or adiposity in younger age (Masaki et al. 2004). However, H1-R deficient mice develop aging-related obesity accompanied with hyperphagia (Masaki et al. 2004, Mollet et al. 2001). Loading of high-fat diet to H1-R deficient mice increased fat deposition more than that in wild mice (Masaki et al. 2004). These results provide insights into control of energy homeostasis that H1-R deficient mice are models of diet-induced and aging-related obesity and H1-R is a key receptor that contributes to regulation of food intake and obesity.

Gene expressions of UCP1 in brown adipose tissues, respectively, were up-regulated more in diet-induced and *db/db* obese mice with the central histamine infusion than those in the pair-fed controls (Masaki et al. 2001b). Chronic central treatment with histamine thus makes it possible to restore the distorted food intake and expenditure. Actions of histamine neuron systems and H1-R systems in the brain may be useful in the development of therapeutic approaches to obesity.

Similar with reports of H1-R deficient mice, mutations of pre-synaptic histamine H3-R and HDC have also been reported to induce abdominal obesity (Fulop et al. 2003, Jorgensen et al. 2006, Takahashi et al. 2002). The study of histamime H3-R deficient mice demonstrated that H3-R inactivation in mice alters the regulation of food intake, and energy expenditure and leads to an obese hyperphagic mise. In addition, the regulation of UCP expression in BAT was attenuated in histamine H3-R deficient mice (Takahashi et al. 2002). However, several lines of histamine H3-R deficient mice did not display abdominal obesity (Toyota et al. 2002). HDC deficient mice display a metabolic phenotype characterized by abdominal obesity and increased white and brown fat depots, supporting the important role that histamine plays in regulation of food intake and energy expenditure. Cold-exposure regulation of body temperature and up-regulation of UCP expression was attenuated in HDC deficient mice (Fulop et al. 2003).

From these observations, it has been accepted that HDC, histamine H3-R and histamine H1-R all contribute to the regulation of food intake and energy expenditure.

13.7 Relationship Between Neuronal Histamine and Adipocytokine Leptin in Controlling Food Intake and Obesity

Obesity is an increasingly health problem since it clusters with type-2 diabetes, hypertension and hyperlipidemia in the metabolic syndrome. The molecular mechanisms underlying obesity have not been fully clarified, and effective therapeutic approaches are currently of general interest. The development of obesity in general is regulated by genetic and environmental factors (Ahima 2005, Balthasar et al. 2004, Bouret and Simerly 2004, Flier 2004, Friedman 2004, Takahashi and Cone 2005, Unger 2004). A number of studies have revealed that the hypothalamic functions that regulate energy balance play a central role in the development of obesity. Several orexigenic and anorexigenic neuropeptides in the hypothalamus are involved in feeding and obesity, although the contribution of each peptide to the development of obesity is different (Ahima 2005, Balthasar et al. 2004, Bouret and Simerly 2004, Flier 2004, Friedman 2004, Takahashi and Cone 2005, Unger 2004).

From the discovery of leptin and its receptors, obesity research has been sparked all over the world (Ahima 2005, Bouret and Simerly 2004, Flier 2004, Friedman 2004, Unger 2004). Leptin was discovered through the identification of the mutation responsible for producing obesity in the *ob/ob* mouse (Ahima 2005, Bouret and Simerly 2004, Flier 2004, Friedman 2004, Unger 2004). Leptin binding sites, which correspond to various classes of leptin receptor, have been identified in the hypothalamus, predominantly the ventromedial nucleus and arcuate nucleus. There is increasing evidence that the effects of leptin are governed by a number of hypothalamic mediators including orexigenic substances such as neuropeptide Y, and agouti-related protein, in addition to anorexigenic substances, such as, proopiomelanocortin and melanocortin-4 receptor and neuronal histamine (Balthasar et al. 2004, Takahashi et al. 2005, Yoshimatsu et al. 1999).

Leptin and histamine are both satiety factors, and we postulated that leptin expresses the anorectic effect through the histaminergic system. Concentrations of hypothalamic histamine and *t*-MH were lowered in *db/db* obese mice, since the mice are known to be deficient in leptin receptors (Yoshimatsu et al. 1999). Akin to *db/db* obese mice, leptin-deficient *ob/ob* obese mice also showed lower histamine turnover as well, albeit the insufficient turnover was recovered by leptin injection (Morimoto et al. 2000).

A central injection of leptin elevated turnover rate of neuronal histamine in the hypothalamus (Morimoto et al. 2000, Yoshimatsu et al. 1999). The administration of FMH prior to the injection of leptin attenuated leptin-induced suppression of food intake in rodent (Morimoto et al. 1999, 2000, Toftegaard et al. 2003), suggesting the involvement of the central histaminergic system as a target for leptin in its control of food intake. In addition, in wild type mice, leptin reduced food intake and obesity, whereas in H1-R deficient mice, the effect of leptin attenuated (Masaki et al. 2001a). Taken together, leptin may affect the food intake through activation of the central histaminergic system via H1-R.

13.8 Neuronal Histamine H1-R as a Potential Regulator of Sleep-Wakeful Cycle

It is well known that activation of the histaminergic system promotes wake-sleep rhythm through activation of histamine H1-R. The histaminergic neurons are located in the TMN and histamine promotes cortical wakefulness through direct cortical projections or by tonic control over the sleep-generating mechanisms in the preoptic/anterior hypothalamus (Sherin et al. 1998). Sleep-wakeful neurons in the ventrolateral preoptic nucleus (VLPO) as sleep center, projection of GABA or glutamate containing neurons, provide a major input to the TMN (Sherin et al. 1998). VLPO axons could be also traced into the brainstem, where they provided terminals in the serotoninergic dorsal and median raphe nuclei, and the core of the noradrenergic locus coeruleus. Furthermore, the descending projection from the VLPO selectively targets the cell bodies and proximal dendrites of the histaminergic TMN. Thus, these monoaminergic populations are known to fire during slow wave sleep and to cease firing during rapid eye movement (REM) sleep. The VLPO is an attractive candidate for simultaneously hyperpolarizing neurons in these monoaminergic neurons that regulates sleep-wakeful cycle (McGinty and Szymusiak 2000, Mignot et al. 2002).

The histaminergic neuron and H1-R are also involved in orexin-induced sleep-wakeful cycle (Huang et al. 2001). Orexin A and B were isolated and identified from rat hypothalamic extracts, and implicated in feeding, energy homeostasis, and sleep-awake cycle (Mieda and Sakurai 2009). Immunohistochemical studies have shown that orexin neurons project widely throughout the entire neuroaxis. Orexin containing neuron in the LHA, one of important modulator for arousal system, also project to histamine neurons in the TMN, in which orexin-2 receptors are involved (Yamanaka et al. 2002). Perfusion of orexin A into the TMN of rats through a microdialysis probe promptly increased wakefulness, concomitant with a reduction in rapid eye movement (REM) and non-REM sleep. Microdialysis studies showed that application of orexin A to the TMN increased histamine release from both the medial preoptic area and the frontal cortex. Orexin A also increased arousal in wild-type mice, but not in H1-R deficient mice. It is indicate that the arousal effect of orexin A depends on the activation of histaminergic neurotransmission mediated by histamine H1-R (Huang et al. 2001). Finally, neuronal histamine regulates sleep-wakeful cycle through its projection to the SCN (Michelsen et al. 2005), center of biological clock. Thus, this input-output organization indicates the importance of neuronal histamine in regulation of biological rhythm.

13.9 Diurnal Rhythm of Food Intake by Hypothalamic Histamine and Histamine H1-R

Similar to the sleep-awake cycle, food intake is also regulated by circadian rhythm (Kalra and Kalra 2004, Xu et al. 2008). Previous studies have demonstrated that the circadian rhythm of food intake is a crucial factor in the development of obesity, and abnormalities in the rhythm of feeding are associated with obesity (Masaki et al. 2004, Masaki and Yoshimatsu 2006, Mistlberger et al. 1998). In addition, correcting disturbances in circadian feeding rhythms can partially reverse obesity and related metabolic disorders (Mistlberger et al. 1998, Masaki et al. 2004). Several neuronal factors such as NPY have been shown to crossly regulate by circadian rhythm (Kalra and Kalra 2004).

As for neuronal histamine, since the concentrations of neuronal histamine across the sleep-wake cycle in H1-R deficient mice are significantly altered, it is possible that an altered circadian rhythm in H1-R deficient mice affects their feeding behavior and consequently contributes to the development of obesity. Indeed, histamine H1-R deficient mice had abnormal circadian rhythms of food intake relative to wild-type (WT) controls (Masaki and Yoshimatsu 2006, Masaki et al. 2004). The feeding behavior of H1-R deficient mice differed from that of WT mice. Daily food consumption was the same for WT and H1-R deficient mice between 1 and 32 weeks of age, but was slightly greater in H1-R deficient mice at 48 weeks of age. At 12 weeks of age, the total amount of food that was consumed per day was the same in WT and H1-R deficient mice. However, the ratio of food consumption in the light versus dark phase was smaller in 12-week-old H1-R deficient mice, as compared to WT mice of the same age; this difference was even greater at 48 weeks of age. In addition, the total amount of food consumed per day was greater for 48-week-old H1-R deficient mice (Masaki et al. 2004).

Scheduled feeding had no effect on the increase in body mass of WT mice when compared to control animals that were fed ad libitum. However, the scheduled feeding attenuated the increase in body mass in comparison to H1-R deficient controls that were fed ad libitum, although the cumulative food consumption of each group was the almost same. Serum concentrations of glucose and insulin and *ob* mRNA expression in WAT were the same in WT mice that were fed either according to a schedule or ad libitum. By contrast, serum concentrations of insulin and expression of *ob* mRNA in WAT were both significantly lower in schedule-fed H1-R deficient mice, as compared to H1-R deficient controls that were fed ad libitum. It is indicated that the disruption of feeding rhythm in H1-R deficient mice contributed to the obesity. In addition, central administration of histamine caused a significant increase in SCN c-fos-like immunoreactivity in WT mice. The effect of histamine on c-fos-like immunoreactivity in the SCN was attenuated in H1-R deficient mice (Masaki et al. 2004).

Zucker obese rats also exhibited hyperphagia, disruption of feeding rhythm and severe obesity (Mistlberger et al. 1998). Ad libitum fed Zucker obese rats gained more weight compared with scheduled feeding groups, although food intake did not differ significantly between groups. It is suggesting that disruption of feeding rhythm may contribute to body weight regulation in Zucher obese rats. Abnormalities in Zucker obese rats including disruptions of circadian feeding patterns and adaptive behaviors mimicked those in the H1-R deficient mice. In fact, studies in Zucker obese rats revealed deficiency in both histamine concentration and HDC activity in the hypothalamus (Machidori et al. 1992). So, the abnormalities in the rhythm of feeding in Zucker obese rats are due to the disturbance of neuronal histamine.

Recently, the CLOCK and BMAL-1 both can regulate circadian nutrient homeostasis (Ando et al. 2005, Shimba et al. 2005, Turek et al. 2005). The neuronal circadian clock located within the hypothalamic SCN regulates the cycles in the physiological rhythm including feeding behavior. CLOCK mutant mice have an attenuated diurnal feeding rhythm, are hyperphagic and obese, and develop a metabolic syndrome of hyperleptinemia, hyperlipidemia and hyperglycemia (Turek et al. 2005). These results suggest that the circadian CLOCK gene network play an important role in feeding behavior, glucose and lipid metabolism.

Taken together, the diurnal rhythm of food intake can be an independently and crucial factor for regulation of obesity.

13.10 Neuronal Histamine and Psychotropic Drug-Related Weight Gain

The use of anti-psychotic drug is associated with metabolic side effects including weight gain and diabetes mellitus (Gentile 2009, Tardieu et al. 2003). It has been shown that several anti-psychotic drugs had side effects of appetite stimulation and weight gain. These drugs were proved to involve in histamine H1-R receptor, conversely the increased feeding and obesity appeared to result from blockade of H1-R. Atypical anti-psychotics such as clozapine and olanzapine also had side effects of appetite stimulation and weight gain via histamine H1-R signaling. Atypical anti-psychotics clozapine and olanzapine both caused the hyperphagia and body weight gain and it is suggested that the relative receptor affinities of the atypical anti-psychotics for histamine H1-R appear to be the most robust correlate of the obesity (Han et al. 2008, Wirshing et al. 1999). Atypical anti-psychotic olanzapine caused the hyperphagia and body weight gain and it is suggested that the relative receptor affinities of the atypical anti-psychotics for histamine H1-R appear to be the most robust correlate of the obesity. Orexigenic atypical antipsychotic drugs activate hypothalamic AMP-kinase, an action abolished in mice with deletion of H1-R (Kim et al. 2007). The study demonstrated that the effects of antipsychotic drug treatment on weight gain and H1-R expression in the brain (Kim et al. 2007). There were negative correlations between the levels of histamine H1-R mRNA expression, and body weight gain and energy efficiency in the arcuate nucleus (ARC) and ventromedial nucleus (VMH) after antipsychotic treatments. In addition, H1-R mRNA expression in the ARC showed a negative correlation with food intake and fat mass. Furthermore, there were negative correlations between H1-R binding density in the VMH and total fat mass and body weight gain after antipsychotic treatment. The finding suggested that downregulated VMH and ARC H1-R expression might be a key factor contributing to antipsychotic drug-induced obesity. Thus, the involvement of histamine and H1-R in antipsychotics-induced hyperphagia and obesity might be tightly related.

13.11 Clinical Studies of Brain Histamine and H1-R in Feeding and Obesity

Betahistine is a centrally acting H1-R agonist with partial H3-R antagonistic activity and no H2-R-binding effects. Betahistine has been studied mainly as a vasodilator for conditions such as cluster headaches, vascular dementia and Meniere's disease, for which it is still used. The unique pharmacologic properties of betahistine point to its potential use as an antiobesity agent (Barak 2008). Recent study showed that betahistine induced significant weight loss with minimal adverse events in women (Barak et al. 2008).

Several pharmaceutical companies have developed non-imidazole H3-R IAs (Celanire et al. 2005, Esbenshade et al. 2006, Hancock and Brune 2005). As observed in A-331440, A-349821, A-417022 and A-423579, specific isoforms interacting in different intensities with similar ligands, may have a distinct influence on efficacy in different models (Celanire et al. 2005, Esbenshade et al. 2006, Hancock and Brune 2005). Among these, A-331440 suppresses food intake and body weight gain in diet-induced obese mice (Hancock et al. 2004). Other imidazole-based H3 antagonists, including GT-2394, reduce cumulative food intake in obese rodents (Celanire et al. 2005). In addition, NNC-0038-1049 and NNC-0038-1202, structurally distinct H3-R antagonists, reduced food intake and body weight (Malmlof et al. 2005, 2006). Contrary, ABT-239 and JNJ-5207852 showed no anti-obesity effects. Although, these observations may explain why some classes of H3-R IA exert anti-obesity activity, potentially unknown off-target activity of specific compounds might contribute to their anorectic effects and thus further investigation is required. Following this substantial differences of the outcome, further investigations have to prove the so far unclear concept of H3-R antagonists in the treatment of obesity and weight gain. Further studies are needed to examine the relationship human obesity and neuronal histamine.

13.12 Concluding Remarks

The activation of histamine neurons suppressed food intake and body weight through histamine H1-R in the brain. The histamine neuron and H1-R accelerated lipolysis in the visceral adipose tissue and up-regulated gene expression of UCP1 in BAT. The signals of histamine neurons and H1-R to regulate food intake and UCP1 were observed as down stream of adipocytokine leptin. It is indicated that energy homeostasis is tightly maintained through the formation of a loop bridged between histamine neuron and adipocytokine leptin. The diurnal rhythm of food intake by histamine neuron and receptors are also crucial factor for regulation of obesity. Taken together, histamine neuron and receptors regulation implicate possible maintenance of food intake, feeding rhythm and obesity in rodents. In the future, therapeutic application of activating of histamine neuron and receptors might be effective and promising therapy to reduce visceral adiposity in obese humans.

References

Ahima RS (2005) Central actions of adipocyte hormones. Trends Endocrinol Metab 16:307–313

Ando H, Yanagihara H, Hayashi Y et al (2005) Rhythmic messenger ribonucleic acid expression of clock genes and adipocytokines in mouse visceral adipose tissue. Endocrinology 146: 5631–5636

Arrang JM, Garbarg M, Schwartz JC (1983) Auto-inhibition of brain histamine release mediated by a novel class (H3) of histamine receptor. Nature 302:832–837

Attoub S, Moizo L, Sobhani I et al (2001) The H3 receptor is involved in cholecystokinin inhibition of food intake in rats. Life Sci 69:469–478

Balthasar N, Coppari R, McMinn J et al (2004) Leptin receptor signaling in POMC neurons is required for normal body weight homeostasis. Neuron 42:983–991

Barak N (2008) Betahistine: what's new on the agenda? Expert Opin Investig Drugs 17:795–804

Barak N, Greenway FL, Fujioka K et al (2008) Effect of histaminergic manipulation on weight in obese adults: a randomized placebo controlled trial. Int J Obes (Lond) 32:1559–1565

Birdsall NJ (1991) Cloning and structure function of the H2 histamine receptor. Trends Pharmacol Sci 12:9–10

Bouret SG, Simerly RB (2004) Minireview: leptin and development of hypothalamic feeding circuits. Endocrinology 145:2621–2626

Brown RE, Stevens DR, Haas HL (2001) The physiology of brain histamine. Prog Neurobiol 63:637–672

Celanire S, Wijtmans M, Talaga P (2005) Histamine H3 receptor antagonists reach out for the clinic. Drug Discov Today 10:1613–1627

Cypess AM, Lehman S, Williams G et al (2009) Identification and importance of brown adipose tissue in adult humans. N Engl J Med 360:1509–1517

de Esch IJ, Thurmond RL, Jongejan A et al (2005) The histamine H4 receptor as a new therapeutic target for inflammation. Trends Pharmacol Sci 26:462–469

Esbenshade TA, Fox GB, Cowart MD (2006) Histamine H3 receptor antagonists: preclinical promise for treating obesity and cognitive disorders. Mol Interv 6:77–88

Feldmann HM, Golozoubova V, Cannon B et al (2009) UCP1 ablation induces obesity and abolishes diet-induced thermogenesis in mice exempt from thermal stress by living at thermoneutrality. Cell Metab 9:203–209

Flier JS (2004) Obesity wars: molecular progress confronts an expanding epidemic. Cell 116: 337–350

Friedman JM (2004) Modern science versus the stigma of obesity. Nat Med 10:563–569

Fulop AK, Foldes A, Buzas E et al (2003) Hyperleptinemia, visceral adiposity, and decreased glucose tolerance in mice with a targeted disruption of the histidine decarboxylase gene. Endocrinology 144:4306–4314

Gentile S (2009) Contributing factors to weight gain during long-term treatment with second-generation antipsychotics. A systematic appraisal and clinical implications. Obes Rev 10: 527–542

Haas H, Panula P (2003) The role of histamine and the tuberomamillary nucleus in the nervous system. Nat Rev Neurosci 4:121–130

Han M, Deng C, Burne TH et al (2008) Short- and long-term effects of antipsychotic drug treatment on weight gain and H1 receptor expression. Psychoneuroendocrinology 33:569–580

Hancock AA, Bennani YL, Bush EN et al (2004) Antiobesity effects of A-331440, a novel non-imidazole histamine H3 receptor antagonist. Eur J Pharmacol 487:183–197

Hancock AA, Brune ME (2005) Assessment of pharmacology and potential antiobesity properties of H3 receptor antagonists/inverse agonists. Expert Opin Investig Drugs 14:223–241

Huang ZL, Qu WM, Li WD et al (2001) Arousal effect of orexin A depends on activation of the histaminergic system. Proc Natl Acad Sci USA 98:9965–9970

Inoue I, Yanai K, Kitamura D et al (1996) Impaired locomotor activity and exploratory behavior in mice lacking histamine H1 receptors. Proc Natl Acad Sci USA 93:13316–13320

Itoh E, Fujimiya M, Inui A (1999) Thioperamide, a histamine H3 receptor antagonist, powerfully suppresses peptide YY-induced food intake in rats. Biol Psychiatry 45:475–481

Jethwa PH, Barrett P, Turnbull Y et al (2009) The role of histamine 3 receptors in the control of food intake in a seasonal model of obesity: the Siberian hamster. Behav Pharmacol 20:155–165

Jorgensen EA, Vogelsang TW, Knigge U et al (2006) Increased susceptibility to diet-induced obesity in histamine-deficient mice. Neuroendocrinology 83:289–294

Kalra SP, Kalra PS (2004) NPY and cohorts in regulating appetite, obesity and metabolic syndrome: beneficial effects of gene therapy. Neuropeptides 38:201–211

Kasaoka S, Tsuboyama-Kasaoka N, Kawahara Y et al (2004) Histidine supplementation suppresses food intake and fat accumulation in rats. Nutrition 20:991–996.

Kim SF, Huang AS, Snowman AM et al (2007) Antipsychotic drug-induced weight gain mediated by histamine H1 receptor-linked activation of hypothalamic AMP-kinase. Proc Natl Acad Sci USA 104:3456–3459

Lecklin A, Etu-Seppala P, Stark H (1998) Effects of intracerebroventricularly infused histamine and selective H1, H2 and H3 agonists on food and water intake and urine flow in Wistar rats. Brain Res 793:279–288

Leurs R, Bakker RA, Timmerman H et al (2005) The histamine H3 receptor from gene cloning to H3 receptor drugs. Nat Rev Drug Discov 4:107–120

Machidori H, Sakata T, Yoshimatsu H et al (1992) Zucker obese rats: defect in brain histamine control of feeding. Brain Res 590:180–186

Malmlof K, Golozoubova V, Peschke B et al (2006) Increase of neuronal histamine in obese rats is associated with decreases in body weight and plasma triglycerides. Obesity (Silver Spring) 14:2154–2162

Malmlof K, Zaragoza F, Golozoubova V et al (2005) Influence of a selective histamine H3 receptor antagonist on hypothalamic neural activity, food intake and body weight. Int J Obes (Lond) 29:1402–1412

Masaki T, Chiba S, Yasuda T et al (2004) Involvement of hypothalamic histamine H_1-receptor in the regulation of feeding rhythm and obesity. Diabetes 53:2250–2260

Masaki T, Chiba S, Yoshimichi G et al (2003) Neuronal histamine regulates food intake, adiposity, and uncoupling protein expression in agouti yellow (A(y)/a) obesemice. Endocrinology 144:2741–2748

Masaki T, Yoshimatsu H (2006) The hypothalamic H1 receptor: a novel therapeutic target for disrupting diurnal feeding rhythm and obesity. Trends Pharmacol Sci 27:279–284

Masaki T, Yoshimatsu H (2007a) Neuronal histamine and its receptors in food intake and obesity. Mini Rev Med Chem 7:821–825

Masaki T, Yoshimatsu H (2007b) Neuronal histamine and its receptors in obesity and diabetes. Current Diabetes Rev 3:212–221

Masaki T, Yoshimatsu H, Chiba S et al (2000b) Impaired response of UCP family to cold exposure in diabetic (db/db) mice. Am J Physiol Regul Integr Comp Physiol 279:R1305-R1309

Masaki T, Yoshimatsu H, Chiba S et al (2001a) Targeted disruption of histamine H1-receptor attenuates regulatory effects of leptin on feeding, adiposity, and UCP family in mice. Diabetes 50:385–391

Masaki T, Yoshimatsu H, Chiba S et al (2001b) Central infusion of histamine reduces fat accumulation and up-regulates UCP family in leptin resistant obese mice. Diabetes 50:376–384

Masaki T, Yoshimatsu H, Kakuma T et al (1999) Induction of rat uncoupling protein-2 gene treated with tumour necrosis factor alpha *in vivo*. Eur J Clin Invest 29:76–82

Masaki T, Yoshimatsu H, Sakata T (2000a) Expression of rat uncoupling protein family mRNA levels by chronic treatment with thyroid hormone. Int J Obes Relat Metab Disord 24: S162-S164

McGinty D, Szymusiak R (2000) The sleep-wake switch: a neuronal alarm clock. Nat Med 6: 510–511

Michelsen KA, Lozada A, Kaslin J et al (2005) Histamine-immunoreactive neurons in the mouse and rat suprachiasmatic nucleus. Eur J Neurosci 22:1997–2004

Mieda M, Sakurai T (2009) Integrative physiology of orexins and orexin receptors. CNS Neurol Disord Drug Targets 8:281–295

Mignot E, Taheri S, Nishino S (2002) Sleeping with the hypothalamus: emerging therapeutic targets for sleep disorders. Nat Neurosci 5:1071–1075

Mistlberger RE, Lukman H, Nadeau BG (1998) Circadian rhythms in the Zucker obese rat: assessment and intervention. Appetite 30:255–267

Mollet A, Lutz TA, Meier S et al (2001) Histamine H1 receptors mediate the anorectic action of the pancreatic hormone amylin. Am J Physiol Regul Integr Comp Physiol 281:R1442–R1448
Morimoto T, Yamamoto Y, Mobarakeh JI et al (1999) Involvement of the histaminergic system in leptin-induced suppression of food intake. Physiol Behav 67:679–683
Morimoto T, Yamamoto Y, Yamatodani A (2000) Leptin facilitates histamine release from the hypothalamus in rats. Brain Res 868:367–369
Morimoto T, Yamamoto Y, Yamatodani A (2001) Brain histamine and feeding behavior. Behav Brain Res 124:145–150
Nguyen T, Shapiro DA, George SR et al (2001) Discovery of a novel member of the histamine receptor family. Mol Pharmacol 59:427–433
Parmentier R, Ohtsu H, Djebbara-Hannas Z et al (2002) Anatomical, physiological, and pharmacological characteristics of histidine decarboxylase knock-out mice: evidence for the role of brain histamine in behavioral and sleep-wake control. J Neurosci 22:7695–7711
Sakata T, Ookuma K, Fukagawa K et al (1988) Blockade of the histamine H1-receptor in the rat ventromedial hypothalamus and feeding elicitation. Brain Res 441:403–407
Schwartz JC, Arrang JM, Garbarg M et al (1991) Histaminergic transmission in the mammalian brain. Physiol Rev 71:1–51
Sherin JE, Elmquist JK, Torrealba F et al (1998) Innervation of histaminergic tuberomammillary neurons by GABAergic and galaninergic neurons in the ventrolateral preoptic nucleus of the rat. J Neurosci 18:4705–4721
Shimba S, Ishii N, Ohta Y et al (2005) Brain and muscle Arnt-like protein-1 (BMAL1), a component of the molecular clock, regulates adipogenesis. Proc Natl Acad Sci USA 102: 12071–12076
Sindelar DK, Shepperd ML, Pickard RT et al (2004) Central H3R activation by thioperamide does not affect energy balance. Pharmacol Biochem Behav 78:275–283
Takahashi KA, Cone RD (2005) Fasting induces a large, leptin-dependent increase in the intrinsic action potential frequency of orexigenic arcuate nucleus NPY/AgRP neurons. Endocrinology 146:1043–1047
Takahashi K, Suwa H, Ishikawa T et al (2002) Targeted disruption of H3 receptors results in changes in brain histamine tone leading to an obese phenotype. J Clin Invest 110:1791–1799
Tardieu S, Micallef J, Gentile S et al (2003) Weight gain profiles of new anti-psychotics: public health consequences. Obes Rev 4:129–38
Terao A, Steininger TL, Morairty SR et al (2004) Age-related changes in histamine receptor mRNA levels in the mouse brain. Neurosci Lett 355:81–84
Timmerman H (1992) Cloning of the H1 histamine receptor. Trends Pharmacol Sci 13:6–7
Toftegaard CL, Knigge U, Kjaer A et al (2003) The role of hypothalamic histamine in leptin-induced suppression of short-term food intake in fasted rats. Regul Pept 111:83–90
Toyota H, Dugovic C, Koehl M et al (2002) Behavioral characterization of mice lacking histamine H_3 receptors. Mol Pharmacol 62:389–397
Tsuda K, Yoshimatsu H, Niijima A et al (2002) Hypothalamic histamine neurons activate lipolysis in rat adipose tissue. Exp Biol Med (Maywood) 227:208–213
Tuomisto L, Yamatodani A, Jolkkonen J et al (1994) Inhibition of brain histamine synthesis increases food intake and attenuates vasopressin response to salt loading in rats. Methods Find Exp Clin Pharmacol 16:355–359
Turek FW, Joshu C, Kohsaka A et al (2005) Obesity and metabolic syndrome in circadian Clock mutant mice. Science 308:1043–1045
Unger RH (2004) The hyperleptinemia of obesity-regulator of caloric surpluses. Cell 117:145–146
van Marken Lichtenbelt WD, Vanhommerig JW, Smulders NM et al (2009) Cold-activated brown adipose tissue in healthy men. N Engl J Med 360:1500–1508
Virtanen KA, Lidell ME, Orava J et al (2009) Functional brown adipose tissue in healthy adults. N Engl J Med 360:1518–1525
Wirshing DA, Wirshing WC, Kysar L et al (1999) Novel antipsychotics: comparison of weight gain liabilities. J Clin Psychiatry 60:358–363

Xu K, Zheng X, Sehgal A et al (2008) Regulation of feeding and metabolism by neuronal and peripheral clocks in Drosophila. Cell Metab 8:289–300

Yamanaka A, Tsujino N, Funahashi H et al (2002) Orexins activate histaminergic neurons via the orexin 2 receptor. Biochem Biophys Res Commun 290:1237–1245

Yasuda T, Masaki T, Chiba S et al (2004a) L-histidine stimulates sympathetic nerve activity to brown adipose tissue in rats. Neurosci Lett 362:71–74

Yasuda T, Masaki T, Sakata T et al (2004b) Hypothalamic neuronal histamine regulates sympathetic nerve activity and expression of uncoupling protein 1 mRNA in brown adipose tissue in rats. Neuroscience 125:535–540

Yoshimatsu H, Chiba S, Tajima D et al (2002) Histidine suppresses food intake through its conversion into neuronal histamine. Exp Biol Med (Maywood) 227:63–68

Yoshimatsu H, Itateyama E, Kondou S et al (1999) Hypothalamic neuronal histamine as a target of leptin in feeding behavior. Diabetes 48:2286–2291

Yoshimoto R, Miyamoto Y, Shimamura K et al (2006) Therapeutic potential of histamine H3 receptor agonist for the treatment of obesity and diabetes mellitus. Proc Natl Acad Sci USA 103:13866–13671

Chapter 14
Implications of Histaminergic System in Brain Histamine Dysfunction

Aijaz Ahmed Khan, Trivendra Tripathi, Mohammed Shahid, Haris M. Khan, and Rahat Ali Khan

Abstract Histamine a signaling molecule synthesized in a variety of cells and is involved in a broad spectrum of functions both in health and disease. It is a hydrophobic molecule composed of an imidazole ring and an amino group connected by two methylene groups. It is synthesized in a wide variety of cells including mast cells, basophils, platelets, enterochromaffin-like cells, endothelial cells and neurons from L-histidine by the enzyme L-histidine decarboxylase. Histamine is believed to stimulate nociceptive afferent fibers in a variety of tissues such as dura mater, heart, joints, jejunum and skin. It activates itch receptors in the skin to produce scratching. Histamine is present in the central nervous system (CNS) of invertebrates, lower vertebrates and mammals and is stored in at least two classes of cells including neurons and mast cells. In the CNS, histamine acts as a key neurotransmitter and involved in the regulation of most of the brain activities in the physiological and pathological states. The cell bodies of the histaminergic neuronal system are concentrated in the tuberomamillary nucleus (TMN) of hypothalamus from which axons reach to innervate almost all regions of the central nervous system from cortex to the spinal cord. Histamine neurons are involved in many functions of central nervous system such as spontaneous locomotion, arousal in wake-sleep cycle, appetite control, seizures, learning and memory, aggressive behavior, emotion, thermoregulation, respiratory and cardiovascular control, neuroendocrine responses, drug sensitization, ischemic lesions, stress, and pain. In this chapter we review the reported actions of histamine in different pathophysiological states of brain.

Keywords Histamine · Histamine receptors · Histaminergic system · Pathophysiology of brain

---

A.A. Khan (✉)
Department of Anatomy, Jawaharlal Nehru Medical College and Hospital, Aligarh Muslim University, Aligarh 202002, UP, India
e-mail: aijazahmedkhan7@live.com

M. Shahid et al. (eds.), *Biomedical Aspects of Histamine*,
DOI 10.1007/978-90-481-9349-3_14,

Abbreviations

CNS	central nervous system
TMN	tuberomamillary nucleus
HDC	histidine decarboxylation
GABA	gamma-aminobutyric acid
KO	knock out
α-FMH	α-fluoromethyl-histidine
HMT	histamine N-methyl transferase
CVA	cerebrovascular accidents
BBB	blood-brain barrier
EEG	electroencephalogram
PET	positron emission tomography
REM	rapid eye movement
VLPO	ventrolateral preoptic nucleus
CRH	corticotropin-releasing hormone
VTA	ventral tegmental area
PD	Parkinson's disease
6-OHDA	6-hydroxydopamine
AMPK	AMP-activated protein kinase

Contents

14.1 Introduction

Histamine affects various central nervous system (CNS) functions not only through its specific receptors but also through its interaction with other neurotransmitter which is very subtle but complex. Histamine is an evolutionary signaling molecule, is the product of histidine decarboxylation (HDC) and has been studied for nearly a century. It plays an important role in gastric acid secretion, immunomodulation, bronchoconstriction, vasodilation and neurotransmission, and occurs in cells of neuroepithelial and hematopoietic origin (Shahid et al. 2009). These actions have important implications for gastrointestinal, immune, cardiovascular, and reproductive functions (Haas et al. 2008). Histamine is stored in the mast cells of peripheral tissues, and it has been implicated in the pathogenesis of various inflammatory reactions (Takahashi et al. 2002). Histamine is an aminergic neurotransmitter that is localized in the CNS and the peripheral nervous system. In the CNS, the only neurons to synthesize histamine are found in the tuberomamillary nucleus of the posterior hypothalamus (the only location where HDC activity has been detected), from which projection reach towards the rest of the brain. Thus, histamine has become just another neurotransmitter. The morphological characteristics of the histaminergic system are similar to those of other biogenic amine systems e.g., norepinephrine, serotonin. It also possesses a compact neuronal nucleus from which many fibers emerge in all directions. There are four histamine receptors that have been identified: H1R, H2R, H3R and H4R (Shahid et al. 2009). Histamine interacts within the CNS with specific H1Rs, H2Rs, H3Rs and H4Rs to induce wide range activities. In contrast to H1Rs, H2Rs and H4Rs, histamine H3Rs are predominantly expressed in the CNS (Lovenberg et al. 1999, Oda et al. 2000), act as autoreceptors in presynaptic neurons, and control histamine turnover. In addition H3Rs have also been shown to act as heteroreceptors in dopamine-, serotonin-, noradrenaline-, gamma-aminobutyric acid (GABA), and acetylcholine-containing neurons (Schlicker et al. 1994). Since H3Rs are located predominantly in the CNS, it has been suggested that H3Rs mediate various CNS functions by modulating brain histaminergic tone and possibly by also collaborating with H1- and H2-receptors. Histamine has been implicated in the regulation of arousal state, locomotor activity, cardiovascular control, water intake, food intake, and memory formation (Blandina et al. 1996, Clapham and Kilpatrick 1994, Imamura et al. 1996, Lecklin et al. 1998, Leurs et al. 1998, Lin et al. 1990). In fact, H1Rs knockout (KO) mice have been shown to have disturbed circadian rhythms, locomotor activities and exploratory behavior. This suggests that H1Rs are important in some functions of histamine (Inoue et al. 1996, Takahashi et al. 2002). Like other aminergic cells, the histamine neurons through H3Rs act on their own somata, dendrites, and axon varicosities. Haas et al. (2008) described the role of histamine in almost all parts of central nervous system including spinal cord, brainstem, cerebellum, thalamus, hypothalamus, basal ganglia, amygdala, hippocampus and also in some parts peripheral nervous system in addition to its role in synaptic plasticity and blood-brain barrier.

Animals with a loss of histamine receptors exhibit subtle abnormalities in their basic physiology or behavior and require additional factors to come into picture to reveal the function of histamine dysfunction in such diseases. Several studies have showed that histidine decarboxylase (HDC)-(KO) and histamine receptor-KO mice exhibit defects in the adaptation of brain functions when exposed to various challenges (Ma et al. 2002, Masaki and Yoshimatsu 2006, Parmentier et al. 2002). Thus, histamine dysfunction may be one of the important factors for brain that demonstrates several defects in brain functions such as: (i) homeostatic brain functions including behavioral state, biological rhythms, thermoregulation in hibernation, feeding rhythms and energy metabolism, fluid intake and balance, stress, thyroid axis, somatotrope axis, bone physiology and calcium homeostasis, and reproduction; and (ii) higher brain functions including sensory and motor systems, mood and cognition (such as anxiety and aversion, pleasure and reward), and learning and memory (Haas et al. 2008).

Thus, many studies suggest that the interactions of the histaminergic system are very numerous and complex, and that the system exerts its different effects by activating different receptor subtypes in different brain regions.

14.2 Role of Histamine in Pathophysiology of Brain

14.2.1 Role of Histamine in Pain

The role of H3R in nociception, analgesia, hyperalgesia and pruritus is quite subtle and complex but recent studies have tried to identify these receptors as potential targets for pain management in future. Histamine is found to mediate itch and modulates pain in the CNS and in the periphery (Ikoma et al. 2006, McMahon and Koltzenburg 1992). Histamine activates and sensitizes itch-specific nociceptive C fibers in the periphery (Schmelz et al. 1997). Histamine and opioid, both can generate itch, whereas scratch induced pain and antidepressants with antihistaminic properties can eliminate itch (Sawynok et al. 2001). The CNS also plays an important role in antinociception and stress-induced analgesia, in contrast to actions of histamine on nociceptive fibers (Cannon et al. 2007, Hough et al. 2000). Histamine modulated central sites of itch and pain comprise first-order itch-specific lamina I neurons in the dorsal horn of the spinal cord and spinothalamic itch sensitive pathways up to higher order cortical and subcortical circuitries (Andrew and Craig 2001, Drzezga et al. 2001, Mochizuki et al. 2003).

Histamine has analgesic effect into the cerebral ventricles or periaquaeductal grey (Glick and Crane 1978, Malmberg-Aiello et al. 1994, Thoburn et al. 1994). H2R mediated analgesic effects and H1R mediated hyperalgesic effects are in keeping with altered pain sensitivity in H1R- and H2R-deficient mice (Malmberg-Aiello et al. 1994, 1998, Mobarakeh et al. 2005). Histaminergic transmission modifies analgesic or nociceptive effects of several neuropeptides (Haas et al. 2008). Morphine can enhance the release and metabolism of histamine in brain when applied systemically or locally in the periaquaductal grey and slightly depolarizes TMN neurons, while the opioid peptide (nociceptin) causes a hyperpolarization that may contribute to the antagonism of opioid-induced analgesia (Barke and Hough 1994, Darland et al. 1998, Eriksson et al. 2000). Histamine release has been demonstrated to be under the control of facilitatory presynaptic μ-opioid receptors and inhibitory κ-opioid receptors (Gulat-Marnay et al. 1990, Itoh et al. 1988). κ-opioid receptors are also gating GABAergic inputs on TMN neurons by orexins/hypocretins (Eriksson et al. 2004). Reductions of histamine levels in brain by administration of H3R-agonists or α-fluoromethyl-histidine (α-FMH) promote nociception (Malmberg-Aiello et al. 1994, 1998). Increases of histamine in brain produced by loading with L-histidine or histamine *N*-methyl transferase (HMT) inhibitors or H3R-antagonists have analgesic effects (Malmberg-Aiello et al. 1994, 1998). Thus, H3R represent a potential target in pain therapy (Cannon et al. 2007).

14.2.2 Effects of Histamine in Neuroinflammation

Various experimental studies in mince involving KOs for HDC, H1R, H2R and H3R have revealed that autoimmunity and allergy are no more antipodal and particularly H3R as potential target for neuroinflammatory and neurodegenerative diseases. Histamine and HRs cooperate on multiple arms of autoimmune and allergic responses (Haas et al. 2008). HDC-KO mice have increased levels of proinflammatory cytokines, and develop a severe experimental allergic encephalomyelitis (EAE) and multiple sclerosis (MS) (Musio et al. 2006). HDC in various tissues is downregulated by glucocorticoids (a gold standard in the therapy of inflammatory CNS diseases), known to protect the brain during innate immune responses. A lack of histamine synthesis and downregulation of H1R and H2R mRNA levels by dexamethasone was found in cerebral endothelial cells (Haas et al. 2008). In sympathetic ganglia, an antigen-induced release of histamine from mast cells or endocrine cells can modulate vegetative nervous transmission (Weinreich et al. 1995). The gene locus encoding the H1R is identical to that for autoimmune disease locus *Bordetella* pertussis toxin-sensitization (Bphs), and controls both histamine-mediated autoimmune T-cell and vascular responses after pertussis toxin sensitization (Ma et al. 2002). H1R- and H2R-KO mice have a lower susceptibility to develop EAE (Ma et al. 2002, Teuscher et al. 2004, 2007). H1Rs and H2Rs are reciprocally up and down regulated on Th1 cells, which is reactive to myelin proteolipid protein. This challenge demonstrates the pathogenetic concepts of autoimmunity, which previously thought to be antipodal to allergy (Pedotti et al. 2003). H1R are raised 4.6-fold in chronic silent cases of MS (Lock et al. 2002). H1R-antagonists have been approved for treatment of allergy, urticaria and vestibular dysfunction; may be useful in diagnosis of MS (Alonso et al. 2006). EAE is attenuated in mast cell-KO mice and it has been noticed that augmented mast cell-proteases are found in both EAE and MS. This advocates a major contribution of mast cells in inflammatory CNS diseases (Haas et al. 2008). However recent study highlights the role of the central histamine systems and H3R in inflammatory CNS diseases (Haas et al. 2008). In H3R-KO mice, neuroinflammation is worsened, and disease severity and progression are increased (Teuscher et al. 2007), which not only control brain histaminergic tone but also act as gatekeepers for the immigration of immune cells into the immunoprivileged CNS (Haas et al. 2008, Teuscher et al. 2007). Aggravation of inflammatory brain disorders by acute stress (CRH excess) or nutritional-metabolic loads (leptin surges) are in keeping with the sensitivity and function of the brain histamine system in these contexts (Musio et al. 2006, Theoharides and Konstantinidou 2007). Thus, the brain histamine system and particularly H3R are candidate targets for the development of drugs treating neuroinflammatory and neurodegenerative conditions related with blood-brain barrier (BBB) and/or transmigration of blood cells into the brain (Haas et al. 2008).

14.2.3 Role of Histamine in Brain Injury

Histamine has been linked with a wide range of clinical conditions involving dilatation of blood vessels and opening of blood-brain barrier (BBB) as Cerebrovascular accidents (CVA), trauma, neoplasm, and vascular headache but histamine antagonists do not show expected beneficial effects in such conditions suggesting its indirect role and hence, interestingly enough, HRs-agonist are under trial for some of these conditions as vascular headache. Histamine contributes to the pathophysiology of brain injury related with hypoxia, ischemia, stroke and trauma or neoplasms (Dux et al. 1984, Hiraga et al. 2007, Lefranc et al. 2006, Lozada et al. 2005a, b, Mohanty et al. 1989). In all of these condition, histamine-arbitrated recruitment of immune cells into damaged tissue and functions of HRs have been observed to be altered (Hiraga et al. 2007, Lozada et al. 2005a). H1Rs and H2Rs on endothelial cells directly participate in acute hyperemic response to physiological and pathological stimuli, which require BBB opening, however without affecting cerebrovascular protein permeability (Haas et al. 2008). Vascular H1Rs and H2Rs is downregulated by dexamethasone (a glucocorticoids) which is used to treat brain edema (Karlstedt et al. 1999). Cimetidine (H2Rs-antagonist) exhibits unexpected properties as an antitumor agent with potential for the treatment of glioblastoma likely by inhibiting growth-promoting and immunomodulatory effects of histamine. Furthermore, histamine interferes with neurovascular and BBB functions implicated in aseptic neurogenic inflammations underlying vascular headaches (Haas et al. 2008). Histamine operates on both peripheral and central components of the trigeminovascular system that includes trigeminal nuclei, ganglia and nerve terminals, blood vessel endothelial and mast cells (Haas et al. 2008). Histamine released from vascular endothelia induces nitric oxide and prostaglandin E2 (PGE2) synthesis and its release from mast cells sensitizes a subset of mechanoinsensitive nociceptive afferents of meninges, along with blood vessel dilatation (Akerman et al. 2002, Dux et al. 2002, Lassen et al. 2003, Schwenger et al. 2007, Theoharides et al. 2005). Intravenous injection of histamine causes cluster headache, migraine and neuralgias (Lassen et al. 1996, Mayor 1965, Neubauer et al. 1997). Cluster headache is called histaminic cephalalgia (Horton's headache) and is linked with a hypothalamic dysfunction, disturbed biological rhythms and sleep (Fanciullacci 2006, Montagna 2006, Vetrugno et al. 2007). Nitric oxide and alcohol, both of which have been implicated with histaminergic functions precipitates histaminic cephalalgia. Conversely, antihistamines do not appear to be an effective treatment of acute primary headaches (Haas et al. 2008). On the contrary, triptans (5-HT1B/D agonists) grant a pharmacological treatment of migraine and other vascular headaches (Levy et al. 2004). Thus, histamine may interfere with primary headaches indirectly, by the actions on serotonergic transmission or other migraine susceptibility gene products (Jost and Selbach 2002). Migraine is a failure of normal sensory processing, is compatible with the role of the central histamine system in sensory gating, itch, and antinociception (Goadsby 2007, Hough et al. 2005, Mobarakeh et al. 2005). Several clinical trials evaluating H3R-agonists in neurogenic edema and migraine prophylaxis are under way (Haas et al. 2008).

14.2.4 Role of Histamine in Encephalopathy

Histamine levels in the brain are determined by the availability of histidine. It is augmented several fold in patients with liver cirrhosis and in animal models of that disease with a portacaval shunt which is believe to be due to highly elevated histamine levels in the hypothalamus along with modest changes in tele-methylhistamine and histamine-*N*-methyltransferase (HMT) activity (Fogel et al. 1991, 2002, Haas et al. 2008). H1R upregulation is responsible for changes in hepatic encephalopathy [such as disorders of circadian rhythms and sleep electroencephalogram (EEG)] (Lozeva et al. 1999). Thus, H1R-antagonists have been proposed for prevention and treatment of circadian rhythm and sleep abnormalities caused by histaminergic hyperactivity, which may contribute to disorder of thalamocortical processing and clinical symptoms of human hepatic encephalopathy (Lozeva et al. 2001). Similarly, portacaval shunted rats exhibited behavioral abnormalities prototypic for hepatic encephalopathy along with a striking impairment in H3R-mediated corticostriatal synaptic long-term depression (Sergeeva et al. 2005a). The release of histamine from nerve terminals and other vasoactive substances from granulocytes may be responsible for thiamine deficiency induced vascular breakdown and perivascular edema within the thalamus of rats (Langlais et al. 2002). This suggests an important role of histamine in the pathogenesis of thalamic lesions in Wernicke's encephalopathy that is related with shrinkage of hypothalamic mamillary bodies in humans. Mamillary abnormalities have also been observed in schizophrenia. Moreover, thiamine deficiency promotes muricidal behavior in rats (Haas et al. 2008). Thus, brain histamine plays a role in the pathophysiology of several brain disorders ranging from disturbed circadian rhythms to behavioral disorders.

14.2.5 Role of Histamine in Mood Disorders

14.2.5.1 Histamine in Schizophrenia

Several studies have suggested a role of brain histamine in schizophrenia. Schizophrenics have elevated levels of *N*-tele-methylhistamine, the major histamine metabolite in the cerebrospinal fluid in line with enhanced histamine turnover in most genetic, pharmacological and lesion-based animal models of schizophrenia (Haas et al. 2008, Prell et al. 1995, 1996a). In post mortem brain samples, H1R binding sites are diminished in the frontal and cingulate cortex or PET studies along with abnormalities in hypothalamic paraventricular and mamillary body morphology, and implies augmented histamine release and turnover in schizophrenia (Goldstein et al. 2007, Iwabuchi et al. 2005, Nakai et al. 1991, Yanai and Tashiro 2007). Moreover, H2R antagonist (Famotidine) decreased negative symptoms in schizophrenics, irrespective of drug interactions with antipsychotic medication (Karnushina et al. 1980, Martinez 1999, Prell et al. 1996b). None of the polymorphisms in H2R or HMT has been consistently linked to psychotic symptoms in schizophrenia (Haas et al. 2008). The idea that antipsychotics act on dopamine D2R have supported the proposition of dopaminergic supersensitivity as a major factor in disease susceptibility and pathogenesis and of novel pharmaceutical targets interfering with both brain dopamine and histamine systems (Korotkova et al. 2007, Seeman et al. 2006, Sergeeva et al. 2007a). Additionally, *N*-methyl-D-aspartate receptor antagonists increase histamine neuron activity in rodent brain and demonstrated that histamine in brain contributes to glutamatergic dysfunction in schizophrenia (Faucard et al. 2006). Thioperamide (a H3R-antagonist/partial H4R-agonist) has antipsychotic-like properties in mice (Akhtar et al. 2006). Ciproxifan (a H3R antagonist) has been demonstrated to potentiate neurochemical and behavioral effects of haloperidol in the rat and modulates the effects of methamphetamine on neuropeptide mRNA expression in the rat striatum (Pillot et al. 2002a, 2003). Sedative antipsychotics bind to H1R, whereas atypical antipsychotics have H3R antagonistic properties thus increasing histamine outflow and its turnover. Moreover, activation of hypothalamic H1R and AMPK pathways are believed to be responsible for weight gain induced by atypical neuroleptics (Haas et al. 2008).

14.2.5.2 Histamine in Depression

Pharmacological or genetic loss of histamine or HRs has demonstrated their role in depression (Dai et al. 2007, Ito et al. 1999, Nath et al. 1988, Song et al. 1996). Histaminergic neurons in the TMN are sensitive to many, if not all, neuroendocrine signals mixed up with depression including biogenic amines, peptides and steroid hormones as well as antidepressant medication (Haas et al. 2008). Histamine neurons are stimulated by 5-HT2C (a serotonin receptor) that undergoes posttranscriptional editing that correlates with suicide (Schmauss 2003, Sergeeva et al. 2007b). Positron emission tomography (PET) studies using [11C]doxepin (an antidepressant with high affinity to H1R) revealed decreased H1R binding in frontal and prefrontal cortices and the cingulate gyrus correlating with the severity of clinical depression (Haas et al. 2008). Abnormalities in histamine metabolism may account for endogenous depression in humans, and the connection of depression and atopy is in line with convergent functions of histamine in immune and stress responses (Gagne et al. 1982, Steinman 2004, Theoharides and Konstantinidou 2007, Timonen et al. 2003). Several antidepressants have H1R and H2R antihistaminic properties that do not account for their therapeutic efficacy but in fact a number of serious adverse effects such as sedation, weight gain and cardiovascular dysfunctions (Haas et al. 2008). Dose-dependent H1R-antagonists properties of antidepressants may be useful to treat insomnia (Singh and Becker 2007). Endogenous histamine and H1R-agonists have antidepressant-like properties (Lamberti et al. 1998). Some of the first-generation antihistamines and H3R-antagonists act as serotonin reuptake inhibitors in animals and humans (Barbier et al. 2007, Kanof and Greengard 1978, Perez-Garcia et al. 1999). Currently available antidepressant pharmacological interventions have a rather slow onset (2–3 weeks). In contrast, sleep deprivation exerts well-known rapid but transient antidepressive effects, which may rely on a histamine mechanism in arousal control. Thus, modulation of histaminergic transmission may prove to be useful in the treatment of depression and related mood disorders (Haas et al. 2008).

14.2.6 Effect of Histamine in Sleep Disorders

Since histaminergic system has been linked to various sleep disorders, in future various HRs agonists and antagonists are expected to be the potential targets for treatment of sleep disorders ranging from insomnia to hypersomnia. In the central nervous system (CNS), histamine is known as wake-promoting neurotransmitter and an important regulator of behavioral state. Thus, histamine is considered to be responsible for the pathogenesis of sleep disorders. However, several studies in animals and humans, such as in von Economo's encephalitis lethargica, in early hypersomnia or insomnia after brain region-specific lesions in the posterior or anterior hypothalamus suggested a central role of the hypothalamus and histamine in sleep control (Bayer et al. 2007, Mignot et al. 2002). 24-h sleep and wake under undisturbed conditions but a striking inability to stay awake in novel environments, along with slowing of EEG activity and wake fragmentation. Increased rapid eye movement (REM) sleep has been observed in H1R-deficient or HDC-deficient mice (Huang et al. 2001, Parmentier et al. 2002), similar to that of hypocretin-deficient animals (a model of human narcolepsy) (Haas et al. 2008). It has been documented that components of a hypothalamic sleep switch comprising GABAergic inputs from sleep-active ventrolateral preoptic nucleus (VLPO) neurons to the histamine neurons in TMN is an important key targets for the sedative effects of general anesthetics (Lin 2000, Lin et al. 1988, Nelson et al. 2002, Saper et al. 2005, Szymusiak et al. 2007). In histaminergic TMN neurons, hypnotics targeting VLPO projection sites with specific GABAA receptor subtypes deserve for a specific treatment of insomnia, lacking some side effects of currently used benzodiazepines (Sergeeva et al. 2005b). H1R-agonists and H3R-antagonists for hypersomnia and H1R-antagonists and H3R-agonists for insomnia are promising treatment targets in future (Barbier and Bradbury 2007, Mignot et al. 2002). Since clinically used antihistamines were not designed to treat insomnia, antihistamines find limited use in sleep medicine due to their long half-lives and peripheral side effects (Barbier and Bradbury 2007, Mignot et al. 2002). Several effective H1R-antagonists acting on dopamine and serotonin receptors play a role in the treatment of psychoses (Haas et al. 2008). Drugs such as (amphetamines and modafinil) which enhance dopaminergic effects mainly treat hypersomnia; can promote wakefulness by activating TMN histamine neurons (Scammell et al. 2000). H3Rs have been identified to control histaminergic activity and outflow, and showed their most promising roles to treat hypersomnia (Leurs et al. 2005). H3Rs deficients demonstrate excessive muscle activity reminiscent of REM behavior disorder. It has been suggested that there is a specific contribution of H3Rs in the control of REM sleep phenomena and related disorders, such as narcolepsy (Haas et al. 2008, Tuomisto and Mannisto 1985).

14.2.7 Role of Histamine in Addiction and Compulsion

Addiction and compulsion primary result from an almost complete takeover of biological machinery controlling learning and memory and their reinforcement by pleasure and aversion. Histaminergic modulation of either function may precipitate drug dependence, addiction and compulsion. Moreover, it is noteworthy that histamine-dependent modulation of pain and memory functions through novelty-induced arousal may be important for the vicious cycle of relapse and withdrawal that includes hyper arousal, pain and psychosis (delirium) (Haas et al. 2008). Several of the drugs such as benzodiazepines, alcohol, morphine, cannabinoids and cocaine interfering with behavioral and metabolic state are addictive and interfere with TMN histamine neuron activity (Nath and Gupta 2001). Though the detailed mechanisms of how the brain histamine system is concerned in addiction and compulsion are poorly understood but likely depend on histamine effects in decisive brain targets such as hypothalamic hypocretin and corticotropin-releasing hormone (CRH) neurons, ventral tegmental area (VTA), accumbens and hippocampus (see Haas et al. 2008). Histamine H3-receptors cooperate with dopamine D2 receptors in the regulation of striatal gene expression (Pillot et al. 2002b). Related interactions of histamine with dopamine, other amines, glutamate and GABA may be significant for learning and memory as well as addiction and compulsion (Selbach et al. 1997, 2007). In a study, rats selected for ethanol preference show highly increased brain histamine levels and turnover, and demonstrate augmented density of histamine-immunoreactive nerve fibers, lower H1R expression and lower H1R and H3R binding in some brain areas (Lintunen et al. 2001). In addition, thioperamide and clobenpropit decrease and *R*-α-methylhistamine enhances ethanol intake in these rats and thereby suggesting that H3Rs control operant responding to ethanol. However, H3R antagonist-stimulated dopamine release was not further augmented by ethanol. In contrast, rats bred selectively for sensitivity to ethanol-induced motor impairment display notably lower brain histamine levels than the ethanol-tolerant rat line and demonstrate higher receptor expression and G protein signaling of H1R and H3R. Lowering the brain histamine levels notably enhances ethanol sensitivity of tolerant rats. Thus, these data provide evidence that a HMT polymorphism has been linked to alcoholism in humans (Haas et al. 2008, Lintunen et al. 2002, Reuter et al. 2007).

14.2.8 Role of Histamine in Dementia

In Alzheimer's disease, numerous subcortical ascending projections including histaminergic neurons display degeneration and tangle formation. In the hypothalamus, neurofibrillary tangles occur exclusively in the TMN accompanied by decreased numbers of large neurons (Airaksinen et al. 1991a, b, Nakamura et al. 1993, Swaab et al. 1998). Decreasing histamine levels and/or HDC activity has been seen in Alzheimer's disease and Down's syndrome (Ishunina et al. 2003, Seidl et al. 1997). Functional imaging studies demonstrate decreased brain H1R occupancy in Alzheimer's disease compared with age-matched healthy controls in keeping with cognitive impairments induced by chlorpheniramine (H1R-antagonist) (Okamura et al. 2000). In contrast to other amines, histamine and its metabolite levels in the spinal fluid augment with increasing age (Prell et al. 1988). Long-term treatment with H2R antagonists did not demonstrate consistent protection in Alzheimer's disease (Haas et al. 2008, Zandi et al. 2002). Thus, loss or degeneration of histaminergic neurons and H1R antagonists have shown clinical features of dementia very akin to Alzheimer.

14.2.9 Role of Histamine in Movement Disorders

Movement disorders like Parkinson's disease have interesting association with brain levels of histamine and specific HRs. The level of histamine in Parkinson patients is raised in the putamen, substantia nigra and external globus pallidus, but tele-methylhistamine levels are unchanged in the substantia nigra suggesting limited histamine transport capacity (Haas et al. 2008, Rinne et al. 2002). The TMN neuron morphology and HDC activity were found normal in patients suffering from Parkinson's disease, however morphology and density of histaminergic fibers in the substantia nigra showed occurrence of histamine-containing terminal fibers around the degenerating nigral neurons (Anichtchik et al. 2000a, Garbarg et al. 1983, Nakamura et al. 1996). H3R expression is strong in the putamen, moderate in the globus pallidus and low in the substantia nigra of the human basal ganglia (Anichtchik et al. 2001). Moreover, H3Rs binding is abnormally high in the substantia nigra of Parkinson's disease (PD), and this phenomenon is seen in rats after depletion of nigrostriatal dopamine stores using 6-hydroxydopamine (6-OHDA) (Anichtchik et al. 2000b, Ryu et al. 1994). H3R activation affects GABA and serotoninergic outflow of both direct and indirect basal ganglia pathways and the signaling of H3Rs are suggestive of their being promising drug targets for the therapy of basal ganglia disorders and many other neurodegenerative diseases. In Huntington's disease, there is a specific loss of H2R particularly in the putamen and globus pallidus in keeping with animal data on neurotoxin-lesioned striatal neurons (Haas et al. 2008).

14.2.10 Role of Histamine in Epilepsy

Histamine protects against convulsions in animal epilepsy models (Chen et al. 2002, 2003, Yokoyama 2001). Treatments that increase histamine levels in brain ameliorate a form of hereditary temporal lobe epilepsy, which can be elicited by weekly vestibular stimulation, whereas intraperitoneal injection of the H1R-antagonist (diphenhydramine) aggravates seizures (Yawata et al. 2004). Lesion of the TMN E2 region attenuates postictal seizure protection, whereas blockade of H1R promotes convulsions in animal models and humans (Haas et al. 2008, Jin et al. 2007). Proconvulsant effects of H1R-anatagonists have been detected in children and seizures may be promoted by treatment with H2R-antihistamine (famotidine) (Simons 2004, Starke et al. 2005, Von Einsiedel et al. 2002). H3R-antagonists that facilitate histamine release are anticonvulsant (Kukko-Lukjanov et al. 2006, Yawata et al. 2004). The antiepileptic network effects of histaminergic transmission is believe to rely on H1R-mediated excitation of interneurons and inhibition of hippocampal principal neurons, which outbalance excitatory histamine effects on cortical excitability, potentiation of NMDA receptors and the

H2R-mediated potentiation of excitability (Haas et al. 2008). Furthermore, H1R activation in line with their antiepileptic properties is neuroprotective in vitro and restrains excitotoxic glutamatergic actions (Haas et al. 2008). In contrast, histamine can promote excitotoxicity by its excitation potentiating actions on the NMDA receptor (Saybasili et al. 1995, Skaper et al. 2001, Yanovsky et al. 1995). Thus the antiepileptic actions of histamine and HRs-agonists, and epileptogenic action of HRs-antagonists are multipronged.

14.2.11 Role of Histamine in Eating Disorders and Metabolic Syndrome

Histamine and some of the HRs play subtle but important role in a complex manner to regulate feeding behaviour, body weight and associated metabolic syndromes both in experimental and clinical settings. Histamine in brain controls appetite, feeding rhythms and energy metabolism (Haas et al. 2008). Thus, its role has been documented in eating disorders and metabolic syndromes (Jorgensen et al. 2007, Masaki and Yoshimatsu 2006, Sakata et al. 1997). Haas et al. (2008) demonstrated the compulsive eating in bulimia and binge-eating disorders relate to histamine outcomes on brain reward systems. Several H3Rs-ligands are clinically tested for application in eating disorders (Leurs et al. 2005, Steffen et al. 2006). Histamine and HRs-knock out (KO) animals have shown hyperphagia and disruption of feeding circadian rhythm. These animals develop fundamental features of metabolic syndromes such as obesity, diabetes mellitus, hyperlipidemia, hyperinsulinemia, and disturbance of thermoregulation and cardiovascular functions (Fulop et al. 2003, Jorgensen et al. 2006, Masaki and Yoshimatsu 2006, Tanimoto et al. 2006, Yoshimoto et al. 2006). Depletion of neuronal histamine from the hypothalamus mimics behavioral and metabolic abnormalities in obese Zucker rats (Sakata et al. 2003). Food intake, adiposity, and uncoupling protein expression are regulated by neuronal histamine in agouti yellow obese mice (Masaki et al. 2003). It has been observed that mice with a targeted disruption of the HDC gene illustrate hyperleptinemia, visceral adiposity, decreased glucose tolerance, and augmented susceptibility to high-fat diet-induced obesity (Fulop et al. 2003, Jorgensen et al. 2006). Disturbed H1R-dependent diurnal feeding rhythms and sleep precipitated autonomic dysfunction and late onset obesity has been reported to implicate alterations in humoral arousal and satiety factors (Haas et al. 2008). Brain histamine is partially responsible for the adipocytokine leptin that regulates feeding and obesity. Disturbed H1R function attenuates leptin outcomes on feeding, adiposity and uncoupling protein expression (Masaki et al. 2001). AMP-activated protein kinase (AMPK) activation and hypothalamic H1R are mainly responsible for antipsychotic-induced weight gain (Masaki and Yoshimatsu 2006). H3R-deficient has been demonstrated to display hyperphagia and late-onset obesity associated with hyperinsulinemia and leptinemia (Yoshimoto et al. 2006). Thus, H3R-antagonists have been developed to counter weight gain (Leurs et al. 2005, Yoshimoto et al. 2006).

Moreover, it has been well documented that cardiovascular dysfunction and hypertension linked to metabolic syndromes are related with a wide variety of functional changes in the hypothalamus, probably reflecting an integrated compensatory natriuretic response to the kidney's impaired ability to excrete sodium (De Wardener 2001).

14.3.13 Role of Histamine in Vestibular Disorders

Histamine antagonists are effective treatments of motion sickness and emesis by blocking histaminergic signals from vestibular nuclei to the vomiting center in the medulla (Simons 2004, Takeda et al. 1986, 1993, 2001). The effect of histamine in brain is in agreement with the autonomic responses, vestibular nucleus-induced hypothalamic neuronal activity in the guinea pig is modulated by H1R and H2R-antagonists (Inokuchi et al. 1999). Furthermore, histamine plays significant role in the central plasticity encompassing vestibular compensation, and responsible for long term changes in expression of HDC in the TMN and H3R binding in vestibular nuclei (Pan et al. 1998, O'Neill et al. 1999, Tighilet et al. 2006). Betahistine (a partial agonist for H1R and antagonist for H3R) upregulates histamine turnover and its release. It reduces histaminergic excitation of medial vestibular neurons and therefore, it is frequently prescribed for treatment of motion sickness and vertigo (Kingma et al. 1997, Tighilet et al. 2002).

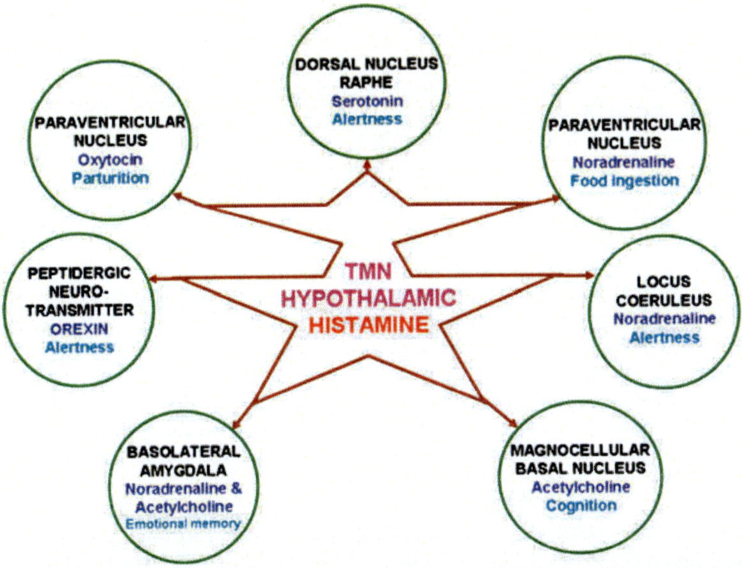

Fig. 14.1 Interactions of brain histamine system with other neurotransmitter systems in brain

14.3 Conclusion

In brief, important actions of histamine interaction may be summarized as: (i) Modulation of release of acetylcholine, (ii) Modulation of emotional memory acquisition, (iii) Modulation of alertness, (iv) Regulation of food intake, (v) Stimulation of food intake, (vi) Control of oxytocin (Fig. 14.1). In conclusion, it may be stated that the interactions of the histaminergic system are very complex, which exerts its various effects by not only stimulating different histamine receptors (H1R, H2R, H3R and H4R) in different brain regions but also indirectly by its interaction with other neurotransmitters.

References

Airaksinen MS, Paetau A, Paljarvi L et al (1991a) Histamine neurons in human hypothalamus: anatomy in normal and Alzheimer diseased brains. Neuroscience 44:465–481

Airaksinen MS, Reinikainen K, Riekkinen P et al (1991b) Neurofibrillary tangles and histamine-containing neurons in Alzheimer hypothalamus. Agents Actions 33:104–107

Akerman S, Williamson DJ, Kaube H et al (2002) The role of histamine in dural vessel dilation. Brain Res 956:96–102

Akhtar M, Uma DP, Ali A et al (2006) Antipsychoticlike profile of thioperamide, a selective H3-receptor antagonist in mice. Fundam Clin Pharmacol 20:373–378

Alonso A, Jick SS, Hernan MA (2006) Allergy, histamine 1 receptor blockers, the risk of multiple sclerosis. Neurology 66:572–575

Andrew D, Craig AD (2001) Spinothalamic lamina I neurons selectively sensitive to histamine: a central neural pathway for itch. Nat Neurosci 4:72–77

Anichtchik OV, Huotari M, Peitsaro N et al (2000b) Modulation of histamine H3 receptors in the brain of 6-hydroxydopamine-lesioned rats. Eur J Neurosci 12:3823–3832

Anichtchik OV, Peitsaro N, Rinne JO et al (2001) Distribution and modulation of histamine H(3) receptors in basal ganglia and frontal cortex of healthy controls and patients with Parkinson's disease. Neurobiol Dis 8:707–716

Anichtchik OV, Rinne JO, Kalimo H et al (2000a) An altered histaminergic innervation of the substantia nigra in Parkinson's disease. Exp Neurol 163:20–30

Barbier AJ, Aluisio L, Lord B et al (2007) Pharmacological characterization of JNJ-28583867, a histamine H(3) receptor antagonist and serotonin reuptake inhibitor. Eur J Pharmacol 576: 43–54

Barbier AJ, Bradbury MJ (2007) Histaminergic control of sleep-wake cycles: recent therapeutic advances for sleep and wake disorders. CNS Neurol Disord Drug Targets 6:31–43

Barke KE, Hough LB (1994) Characterization of basal and morphine induced histamine release in the rat periaqueductal gray. J Neurochem 63:238–244

Bayer L, Serafin M, Muhlethaler M (2007) Histamine excite melanin concentrating hormone neurons and has no effect on hypocretin/orexin neurons. Soc Neurosci Abstr 633.5

Blandina P, Giorgetti M, Bartolini L et al (1996) Inhibition of cortical acetylcholine release and cognitive performance by histamine H3 receptor activation in rats. Br J Pharmacol 119. 1656–1664

Cannon KE, Leurs R, Hough LB (2007) Activation of peripheral and spinal histamine H(3) receptors inhibits formalin-induced inflammation and nociception, respectively. Pharmacol Biochem Behav 88:122–129

Chen Z, Li WD, Zhu LJ et al (2002) Effects of histidine, a precursor of histamine, on pentylenetetrazole-induced seizures in rats. Acta Pharmacol Sin 23:361–366

Chen Z, Li Z, Sakurai E et al (2003) Chemical kindling induced by pentylenetetrazol in histamine H(1) receptor gene knockout mice [H(1)KO], histidine decarboxylase-deficient mice [HDC (–/–)] and mast cell-deficient W/W(v) mice. Brain Res 968:162–166

Clapham J, Kilpatrick GJ (1994) Thioperamide, the selective histamine H3 receptor antagonist, attenuates stimulant-induced locomotor activity in the mouse. Eur J Phamacol 259:107–114

Dai H, Kaneko K, Kato H et al (2007) Selective cognitive dysfunction in mice lacking histamine H1 and H2 receptors. Neurosci Res 57:306–313

Darland T, Heinricher MM, Grandy DK (1998) Orphanin FQ/nociceptin: a role in pain and analgesia, but so much more. Trends Neurosci 21:215–221

De Wardener HE (2001) The hypothalamus and hypertension. Physiol Rev 81:1599–1630

Drzezga A, Darsow U, Treede RD et al (2001) Central activation by histamine-induced itch: analogies to pain processing: a correlational analysis of O-15 H_2O positron emission tomography studies. Pain 92:295–305

Dux M, Schwenger N, Messlinger K (2002) Possible role of histamine (H1- and H2-) receptors in the regulation of meningeal blood flow. Br J Pharmacol 137:874–880

Dux E, Temesvari P, Joo F et al (1984) The blood-brain barrier in hypoxia: ultrastructural aspects and adenylate cyclase activity of brain capillaries. Neuroscience 12:951–958

Eriksson KS, Sergeeva OA, Selbach O et al (2004) Orexin (hypocretin)/dynorphin neurons control GABAergic inputs to tuberomammillary neurons. Eur J Neurosci 19:1278–1284

Eriksson KS, Stevens DR, Haas HL (2000) Opposite modulation of histaminergic neurons by nociceptin and morphine. Neuropharmacology 39:2492–2498

Fanciullacci M (2006) When cluster headache was called histaminic cephalalgia (Horton's headache). J Headache Pain 7:231–234

Faucard R, Armand V, Heron A et al (2006) N-methyl-D-aspartate receptor antagonists enhance histamine neuron activity in rodent brain. J Neurochem 98:1487–1496

Fogel WA, Andrzejewski W, Maslinski C (1991) Brain histamine in rats with hepatic encephalopathy. J Neurochem 56:38–43

Fogel WA, Michelsen KA, Granerus G et al (2002) Neuronal storage of histamine in the brain and tele-methylimidazoleacetic acid excretion in portocaval shunted rats. J Neurochem 80:375–382

Fulop AK, Foldes A, Buzas E et al (2003) Hyperleptinemia, visceral adiposity, decreased glucose tolerance in mice with a targeted disruption of the histidine decarboxylase gene. Endocrinology 144:4306–4314

Gagne MA, Wollin A, Navert H et al (1982) Anomaly of histamine methylation in endogenous depression. Prog Neuropsychopharmacol Biol Psychiatry 6:483–486

Garbarg M, Javoy-Agid F, Schwartz JC et al (1983) Brain histidine decarboxylase activity in Parkinson's disease. Lancet 1:74–75

Glick SD, Crane LA (1978) Opiate-like and abstinence-like effects of intracerebral histamine administration in rats. Nature 273:547–549

Goadsby PJ (2007) Recent advances in understanding migraine mechanisms, molecules and therapeutics. Trends Mol Med 13:39–44

Goldstein JM, Seidman LJ, Makris N et al (2007) Hypothalamic abnormalities in schizophrenia: sex effects and genetic vulnerability. Biol Psychiatry 61:935–945

Gulat-Marnay C, Lafitte A, Arrang JM et al (1990) Modulation of histamine release in the rat brain by kappa-opioid receptors. J Neurochem 55:47–53

Haas HL, Sergeeva OA, Selbach O (2008) Histamine in the nervous system. Physiol Rev 88: 1183–1241

Hiraga N, Adachi N, Liu K et al (2007) Suppression of inflammatory cell recruitment by histamine receptor stimulation in ischemic rat brains. Eur J Pharmacol 557:236–244

Hough LB, Nalwalk JW, Barnes WG (2000) A third life for burimamide. Discovery and characterization of a novel class of non-opioid analgesics derived from histamine antagonists. Ann NY Acad Sci 909:25–40

Hough LB, Nalwalk JW, Lu Q et al (2005) Antinociceptive, brain-penetrating derivatives related to improgan, a non-opioid analgesic. Eur J Pharmacol 522:38–46

Huang ZL, Qu WM, Li WD et al (2001) Arousal effect of orexin A depends on activation of the histaminergic system. Proc Natl Acad Sci USA 98:9965–9970

Ikoma A, Steinhoff M, Stander S et al (2006) The neurobiology of itch. Nat Rev Neurosci 7: 535–547

Imamura M, Smith NC, Garbarg M et al (1996) Histamine H3-receptor-mediated inhibition of calcitonin gene-related peptide release from cardiac C fibers. A regulatory negative-feedback loop. Circ Res 78:863–869

Inokuchi A, Liu F, Yokomitsu S et al (1999) Effects of the antihistaminergic drugs diphenhydramine and zolantidine on vestibular-induced hypothalamic neuronal activity in the guinea pig. Eur Arch Otorhinolaryngol 256(Suppl 1):S22–S26

Inoue I, Yanai K, Kitamura D et al (1996) Impaired locomotor activity and exploratory behavior in mice lacking histamine H1 receptors. Proc Natl Acad Sci USA 93:13316–13320

Ishunina TA, van Heerikhuize JJ, Ravid R et al (2003) Estrogen receptors and metabolic activity in the human tuberomamillary nucleus: changes in relation to sex, aging and Alzheimer's disease. Brain Res 988:84–96

Ito C, Shen H, Toyota H et al (1999) Effects of the acute and chronic restraint stresses on the central histaminergic neuron system of Fischer rat. Neurosci Lett 262:143–145

Itoh Y, Oishi R, Nishibori M et al (1988) Involvement of Mu receptors in the opioid-induced increase in the turnover of mouse brain histamine. J Pharmacol Exp Ther 244:1021–1026

Iwabuchi K, Ito C, Tashiro M et al (2005) Histamine H1 receptors in schizophrenic patients measured by positron emission tomography. Eur Neuropsychopharmacol 15:185–191

Jin CL, Zhuge ZB, Wu DC et al (2007) Lesion of the tuberomammillary nucleus E2-region attenuates postictal seizure protection in rats. Epilepsy Res 73:250–258

Jorgensen EA, Knigge U, Warberg J et al (2007) Histamine and the regulation of body weight. Neuroendocrinology 86:210–214

Jorgensen EA, Vogelsang TW, Knigge U et al (2006) Increased susceptibility to diet-induced obesity in histamine-deficient mice. Neuroendocrinology 83:289–294

Jost WH, Selbach O (2002) Therapy of migraine. UNI-MED, Bremen

Kanof PD, Greengard P (1978) Brain histamine receptors as targets for antidepressant drugs. Nature 272:329–333

Karlstedt K, Sallmen T, Eriksson KS et al (1999) Lack of histamine synthesis and downregulation of H1 and H2 receptor mRNA levels by dexamethasone in cerebral endothelial cells. J Cereb Blood Flow Metab 19:321–330

Karnushina IL, Palacios JM, Barbin G et al (1980) Studies on a capillary-rich fraction isolated from brain: histaminic components and characterization of the histamine receptors linked to adenylate cyclase. J Neurochem 34:1201–1208

Kingma H, Bonink M, Meulenbroeks A et al (1997) Dose dependent effect of betahistine on the vestibulo-ocular reflex: a double-blind, placebo controlled study in patients with paroxysmal vertigo. Acta Otolaryngol 117:641–646

Korotkova TM, Klyuch BP, Ponomarenko AA et al (2007) Modafinil inhibits rat midbrain dopaminergic neurons through D2-like receptors. Neuropharmacology 52:626–633

Kukko-Lukjanov TK, Soini S, Taira T et al (2006) Histaminergic neurons protect the developing hippocampus from kainic acid-induced neuronal damage in an organotypic coculture system. J Neurosci 26:1088–1097

Lamberti C, Ipponi A, Bartolini A et al (1998) Antidepressant-like effects of endogenous histamine and of two histamine H1 receptor agonists in the mouse forced swim test. Br J Pharmacol 123:1331–1336

Langlais PJ, McRee RC, Nalwalk JA et al (2002) Depletion of brain histamine produces regionally selective protection against thiamine deficiency-induced lesions in the rat. Metab Brain Dis 17:199–210

Lassen LH, Christiansen I, Iversen HK et al (2003) The effect of nitric oxide synthase inhibition on histamine induced headache and arterial dilatation in migraineurs. Cephalalgia 23: 877–886

Lassen LH, Heinig JH, Oestergaard S et al (1996) Histamine inhalation is a specific but insensitive laboratory test for migraine. Cephalalgia 16:550–553

Lecklin A, Etu-Seppala P, Stark H et al (1998) Effects of intracerebroventricularly infused histamine and selective H1, H2, and H3 agonists on food and water intake and urine flow in Wistar rats. Brain Res 793:279–288

Lefranc F, Yeaton P, Brotchi J et al (2006) Cimetidine, an unexpected anti-tumor agent, its potential for the treatment of glioblastoma (review). Int J Oncol 28:1021–1030

Leurs R, Bakker RA, Timmerman H et al (2005) The histamine H3 receptor: from gene cloning to H3 receptor drugs. Nat Rev Drug Discov 4:107–120

Leurs R, Blandina P, Tedford C et al (1998) Therapeutic potential of histamine H3 receptor agonists and antagonists. Trends Pharmacol Sci 19:177–184

Levy D, Jakubowski M, Burstein R (2004) Disruption of communication between peripheral and central trigeminovascular neurons mediates the antimigraine action of 5HT 1B/1D receptor agonists. Proc Natl Acad Sci USA 101:4274–4279

Lin JS (2000) Brain structures and mechanisms involved in the control of cortical activation and wakefulness, with emphasis on the posterior hypothalamus and histaminergic neurons. Sleep Med Rev 4:471–503

Lin JS, Sakai K, Jouvet M (1988) Evidence for histaminergic arousal mechanisms in the hypothalamus of cat. Neuropharmacology 27:111–122

Lin JS, Sakai K, Vanni-Mercier G et al (1990) Involvement of histaminergic neurons in arousal mechanisms demonstrated with H3-receptor ligands in the cat. Brain Res 523:325–330

Lintunen M, Hyytia P, Sallmen T et al (2001) Increased brain histamine in an alcohol-preferring rat line and modulation of ethanol consumption by H(3) receptor mechanisms. FASEB J 15: 1074–1076

Lintunen M, Raatesalmi K, Sallmen T et al (2002) Low brain histamine content affects ethanol-induced motor impairment. Neurobiol Dis 9:94–105

Lock C, Hermans G, Pedotti R et al (2002) Gene-microarray analysis of multiple sclerosis lesions yields new targets validated in autoimmune encephalomyelitis. Nat Med 8:500–508

Lovenberg TW, Roland BL, Wilson SJ et al (1999) Cloning and functional expression of the human histamine H3 receptor. Mol Pharmacol 55:1101–1107

Lozada A, Maegele M, Stark H et al (2005a) Traumatic brain injury results in mast cell increase and changes in regulation of central histamine receptors. Neuropathol Appl Neurobiol 31: 150–162

Lozada A, Munyao N, Sallmen T et al (2005b) Postischemic regulation of central histamine receptors. Neuroscience 136:371–379

Lozeva V, Tuomisto L, Sola D et al (2001) Increased density of brain histamine H(1) receptors in rats with portacaval anastomosis and in cirrhotic patients with chronic hepatic encephalopathy. Hepatology 33:1370–1376

Lozeva V, Valjakka A, Anttila E et al (1999) Brain histamine levels and neocortical slow-wave activity in rats with portacaval anastomosis. Hepatology 29:340–346

Ma RZ, Gao J, Meeker ND et al (2002) Identification of Bphs, an autoimmune disease locus, as histamine receptor H1. Science 297:620–623

Malmberg-Aiello P, Lamberti C, Ghelardini C et al (1994) Role of histamine in rodent antinociception. Br J Pharmacol 111:1269–1279

Malmberg-Aiello P, Lamberti C, Ipponi A et al (1998) Evidence for hypernociception induction following histamine H1 receptor activation in rodents. Life Sci 63:463–476

Martinez MC (1999) Famotidine in the management of schizophrenia. Ann Pharmacother 33: 742–747

Masaki T, Chiba S, Yoshimichi G et al (2003) Neuronal histamine regulates food intake, adiposity, uncoupling protein expression in agouti yellow [A(y)/a] obese mice. Endocrinology 144: 2741–2748

Masaki T, Yoshimatsu H (2006) The hypothalamic H1 receptor: a novel therapeutic target for disrupting diurnal feeding rhythm and obesity. Trends Pharmacol Sci 27:279–284

Masaki T, Yoshimatsu H, Chiba S et al (2001) Targeted disruption of histamine H1-receptor attenuates regulatory effects of leptin on feeding, adiposity, UCP family in mice. Diabetes 50:385–391
Mayor O (1965) The use of intravenous histamine in typical neuralgias of the face. Ann Otol Rhinol Laryngol 74:1085–1090
McMahon SB, Koltzenburg M (1992) Itching for an explanation. Trends Neurosci 15:497–501
Mignot E, Taheri S, Nishino S (2002) Sleeping with the hypothalamus: emerging therapeutic targets for sleep disorders. Nat Neurosci 5:1071–1075
Mobarakeh JI, Takahashi K, Sakurada S et al (2005) Enhanced antinociception by intracerebroventricularly administered orexin A in histamine H1 or H2 receptor gene knockout mice. Pain 118:254–262
Mochizuki H, Tashiro M, Kano M et al (2003) Imaging of central itch modulation in the human brain using positron emission tomography. Pain 105:339–346
Mohanty S, Dey PK, Sharma HS et al (1989) Role of histamine in traumatic brain edema. An experimental study in the rat. J Neurol Sci 90:87–97
Montagna P (2006) Hypothalamus, sleep and headaches. Neurol Sci 27:S138–S143
Musio S, Gallo B, Scabeni S et al (2006) A key regulatory role for histamine in experimental autoimmune encephalomyelitis: disease exacerbation in histidine decarboxylase-deficient mice. J Immunol 176:17–26
Nakai T, Kitamura N, Hashimoto T et al (1991) Decreased histamine H1 receptors in the frontal cortex of brains from patients with chronic schizophrenia. Biol Psychiatry 30:349–356
Nakamura S, Ohnishi K, Nishimura M et al (1996) Large neurons in the tuberomammillary nucleus in patients with Parkinson's disease and multiple system atrophy. Neurology 46: 1693–1696
Nakamura S, Takemura M, Ohnishi K et al (1993) Loss of large neurons and occurrence of neurofibrillary tangles in the tuberomammillary nucleus of patients with Alzheimer's disease. Neurosci Lett 151:196–199
Nath C, Gulati A, Dhawan KN et al (1988) Role of central histaminergic mechanism in behavioural depression (swimming despair) in mice. Life Sci 42:2413–2417
Nath C, Gupta MB (2001) Role of central histaminergic system in lorazepam withdrawal syndrome in rats. Pharmacol Biochem Behav 68:777–782
Nelson LE, Guo TZ, Lu J et al (2002) The sedative component of anesthesia is mediated by GABA(A) receptors in an endogenous sleep pathway. Nat Neurosci 5:979–984
Neubauer D, Kuhar M, Ravnik IM (1997) Antihistamine responsive cluster headache in a teenaged girl. Headache 37:296–298
Oda T, Morikawa N, Saito Y et al (2000) Molecular cloning and characterization of a novel type of histamine receptor preferentially expressed in leukocytes. J Biol Chem 275:36781–36786
Okamura N, Yanai K, Higuchi M et al (2000) Functional neuroimaging of cognition impaired by a classical antihistamine, D-chlorpheniramine. Br J Pharmacol 129:115–123
O'Neill AB, Pan JB, Sullivan JP et al (1999) Pharmacological evaluation of an in vivo model of vestibular dysfunction in the rat. Methods Find Exp Clin Pharmacol 21:285–289
Pan JB, O'Neill AB, Hancock AA et al (1998) Histaminergic ligands attenuate barrel rotation in rats following unilateral labyrinthectomy. Methods Find Exp Clin Pharmacol 20: 771–777
Parmentier R, Ohtsu H, Djebbara-Hannas Z et al (2002) Anatomical, physiological, pharmacological characteristics of histidine decarboxylase knock-out mice: evidence for the role of brain histamine in behavioral and sleep-wake control. J Neurosci 22:7695–7711
Pedotti R, De Voss JJ, Steinman L et al (2003) Involvement of both "allergic" and "autoimmune" mechanisms in EAE, MS and other autoimmune diseases. Trends Immunol 24:479–484
Perez-Garcia C, Morales L, Cano MV et al (1999) Effects of histamine H3 receptor ligands in experimental models of anxiety and depression. Psychopharmacology 142:215–220
Pillot C, Heron A, Cochois V et al (2002b) A detailed mapping of the histamine H(3) receptor and its gene transcripts in rat brain. Neuroscience 114:173–193

Pillot C, Heron A, Schwartz JC et al (2003) Ciproxifan, a histamine H3-receptor antagonist/inverse agonist, modulates the effects of methamphetamine on neuropeptide mRNA expression in rat striatum. Eur J Neurosci 17:307–314

Pillot C, Ortiz J, Heron A et al (2002a) Ciproxifan, a histamine H3-receptor antagonist/inverse agonist, potentiates neurochemical and behavioral effects of haloperidol in the rat. J Neurosci 22:7272–7280

Prell GD, Green JP, Elkashef AM et al (1996a) The relationship between urine excretion and biogenic amines and their metabolites in cerebrospinal fluid of schizophrenic patients. Schizophr Res 19:171–176

Prell GD, Green JP, Kaufmann CA et al (1995) Histamine metabolites in cerebrospinal fluid of patients with chronic schizophrenia: their relationships to levels of other aminergic transmitters and ratings of symptoms. Schizophr Res 14:93–104

Prell GD, Khandelwal JK, Burns RS et al (1988) Histamine metabolites in cerebrospinal fluid of the rhesus monkey (Macaca mulatta): cisternal-lumbar concentration gradients. J Neurochem 50:1194–1199

Prell GD, Rosse RB, Deutsch SI (1996b) Apparent absence of famotidine-antipsychotic drug interactions in patients with chronic schizophrenia. J Psychiatry Neurosci 21:61–62

Reuter M, Jeste N, Klein T et al (2007) Association of THR105Ile, a functional polymorphism of histamine N-methyltransferase (HNMT), with alcoholism in German Caucasians. Drug Alcohol Depend 87:69–75

Rinne JO, Anichtchik OV, Eriksson KS et al (2002) Increased brain histamine levels in Parkinson's disease but not in multiple system atrophy. J Neurochem 81:954–960

Ryu JH, Yanai K, Watanabe T (1994) Marked increase in histamine H3 receptors in the striatum and substantia nigra after 6-hydroxydopamine-induced denervation of dopaminergic neurons: an autoradiographic study. Neurosci Lett 178:19–22

Sakata T, Yoshimatsu H, Kurokawa M (1997) Hypothalamic neuronal histamine: implications of its homeostatic control of energy metabolism. Nutrition 13:403–411

Sakata T, Yoshimatsu H, Masaki T et al (2003) Anti-obesity actions of mastication driven by histamine neurons in rats. Exp Biol Med 228:1106–1110

Saper CB, Scammell TE, Lu J (2005) Hypothalamic regulation of sleep and circadian rhythms. Nature 437:1257–1263

Sawynok J, Esser MJ, Reid AR (2001) Antidepressants as analgesics: an overview of central and peripheral mechanisms of action. J Psychiatry Neurosci 26:21–29

Saybasili H, Stevens DR, Haas HL (1995) pH-dependent modulation of N-methyl-D-aspartate receptor-mediated synaptic currents by histamine in rat hippocampus in vitro. Neurosci Lett 199:225–227

Scammell TE, Estabrooke IV, McCarthy MT et al (2000) Hypothalamic arousal regions are activated during modafinil-induced wakefulness. J Neurosci 20:8620–8628

Schlicker E, Malinowska B, Kathmann M et al (1994) Modulation of neurotransmitter release via histamine H3 heteroreceptors. Fundam Clin Pharmacol 8:128–137

Schmauss C (2003) Serotonin 2C receptors: suicide, serotonin, runaway RNA editing. Neuroscientist 9:237–242

Schmelz M, Schmidt R, Bickel A et al (1997) Specific C-receptors for itch in human skin. J Neurosci 17:8003–8008

Schwenger N, Dux M, de Col R et al (2007) Interaction of calcitonin gene-related peptide, nitric oxide and histamine release in neurogenic blood flow and afferent activation in the rat cranial dura mater. Cephalalgia 27:481–491

Seeman P, Schwarz J, Chen JF et al (2006) Psychosis pathways converge via D2 high dopamine receptors. Synapse 60:319–346

Seidl R, Hauser E, Bernert G et al (1997) Auditory evoked potentials in young patients with Down syndrome. Event-related potentials (P3) and histaminergic system. Cogn Brain Res 5:301–309

Selbach O, Brown RE, Haas HL (1997) Long-term increase of hippocampal excitability by histamine and cyclic AMP. Neuropharmacology 36:1539–1548

Selbach O, Stehle J, Haas HL (2007) Hippocampal long-term synaptic plasticity is controlled by histamine, hypocretins (orexins) and clock genes. Soc Neurosci Abstr 928.13

Sergeeva OA, Amberger BT, Haas HL (2007b) Editing of AMPA and serotonin 2C receptors in individual central neurons, controlling wakefulness. Cell Mol Neurobiol 27:669–680

Sergeeva OA, Andreeva N, Garret M et al (2005b) Pharmacological properties of GABAA receptors in rat hypothalamic neurons expressing the epsilon-subunit. J Neurosci 25: 88–95

Sergeeva OA, Klyuch BP, Vandael D et al (2007a) Dopaminergic excitation of histaminergic tuberomamillary neurons. Acta Physiol 189:S653

Sergeeva OA, Schulz D, Doreulee N et al (2005a) Deficits in cortico-striatal synaptic plasticity and behavioral habituation in rats with portacaval anastomosis. Neuroscience 134:1091–1098

Shahid M, Tripathi T, Sobia F et al (2009) Histamine, histamine receptors and their role in immunomodulation: an updated systematic review. The Open Immunol J 2:9–41

Simons FE (2004) Advances in H1-antihistamines. N Engl J Med 351:2203–2217

Singh H, Becker PM (2007) Novel therapeutic usage of low-dose doxepin hydrochloride. Expert Opin Investig Drugs 16:1295–1305

Skaper SD, Facci L, Kee WJ et al (2001) Potentiation by histamine of synaptically mediated excitotoxicity in cultured hippocampal neurones: a possible role for mast cells. J Neurochem 76:47–55

Song C, Earley B, Leonard BE (1996) Behavioural and immunological effects of the antihistamine terfenadine in olfactory bulbectomized rats. Eur Neuropsychopharmacol 6:157–162

Starke PR, Weaver J, Chowdhury BA (2005) Boxed warning added to promethazine labeling for pediatric use. N Engl J Med 352:2653

Steffen KJ, Roerig JL, Mitchell JE et al (2006) Emerging drugs for eating disorder treatment. Expert Opin Emerg Drugs 11:315–336

Steinman L (2004) Elaborate interactions between the immune and nervous systems. Nat Immunol 5:575–581

Swaab DF, Lucassen PJ, Salehi A et al (1998) Reduced neuronal activity and reactivation in Alzheimer's disease. Prog Brain Res 117:343–377

Szymusiak R, Gvilia I, McGinty D (2007) Hypothalamic control of sleep. Sleep Med 8:291–301

Takahashi K, Suwa H, Ishikawa T et al (2002) Targeted disruption of H3 receptors results in changes in brain histamine tone leading to an obese phenotype J Clin Invest 110:1791–1799

Takeda N, Morita M, Hasegawa S et al (1993) Neuropharmacology of motion sickness and emesis. A review. Acta Otolaryngol Suppl 501:10–15

Takeda N, Morita M, Horii A et al (2001) Neural mechanisms of motion sickness. J Med Invest 48:44–59

Takeda N, Morita M, Kubo T et al (1986) Histaminergic mechanism of motion sickness. Neurochemical and neuropharmacological studies in rats. Acta Otolaryngol 101:416–421

Tanimoto A, Sasaguri Y, Ohtsu H (2006) Histamine network in atherosclerosis. Trends Cardiovasc Med 16:280–284

Teuscher C, Poynter ME, Offner H et al (2004) Attenuation of Th1 effector cell responses and susceptibility to experimental allergic encephalomyelitis in histamine H2 receptor knockout mice is due to dysregulation of cytokine production by antigen-presenting cells. Am J Pathol 164:883–892

Teuscher C, Subramanian M, Noubade R et al (2007) Central histamine H3 receptor signaling negatively regulates susceptibility to autoimmune inflammatory disease of the CNS. Proc Natl Acad Sci USA 104:10146–10151

Theoharides TC, Donelan J, Kandere-Grzybowska K et al (2005) The role of mast cells in migraine pathophysiology. Brain Res 49:65–76

Theoharides TC, Konstantinidou AD (2007) Corticotropin-releasing hormone and the blood-brain-barrier. Front Biosci 12:1615–1628

Thoburn KK, Hough LB, Nalwalk JW et al (1994) Histamine induced modulation of nociceptive responses. Pain 58:29–37

Tighilet B, Trottier S, Mourre C et al (2002) Betahistine dihydrochloride interaction with the histaminergic system in the cat: neurochemical and molecular mechanisms. Eur J Pharmacol 446:63–73

Tighilet B, Trottier S, Mourre C et al (2006) Changes in the histaminergic system during vestibular compensation in the cat. J Physiol 573:723–739

Timonen M, Jokelainen J, Hakko H et al (2003) Atopy and depression: results from the Northern Finland 1966 Birth Cohort Study. Mol Psychiatry 8:738–744

Tuomisto J, Mannisto P (1985) Neurotransmitter regulation of anterior pituitary hormones. Pharmacol Rev 37:249–332

Vetrugno R, Pierangeli G, Leone M et al (2007) Effect on sleep of posterior hypothalamus stimulation in cluster headache. Headache 47:1085–1090

Von Einsiedel RW, Roesch-Ely D, Diebold K et al (2002) H(2)-histamine antagonist (famotidine) induced adverse CNS reactions with long-standing secondary mania and epileptic seizures. Pharmacopsychiatry 35:152–154

Weinreich D, Undem BJ, Taylor G et al (1995) Antigen-induced long-term potentiation of nicotinic synaptic transmission in the superior cervical ganglion of the guinea pig. J Neurophysiol 73:2004–2016

Yanai K, Tashiro M (2007) The physiological and pathophysiological roles of neuronal histamine: an insight from human positron emission tomography studies. Pharmacol Ther 113:1–15

Yanovsky Y, Reymann K, Haas HL (1995) pH-dependent facilitation of synaptic transmission by histamine in the CA1 region of mouse hippocampus. Eur J Neurosci 7:2017–2020

Yawata I, Tanaka K, Nakagawa Y et al (2004) Role of histaminergic neurons in development of epileptic seizures in EL mice. Brain Res 132:13–17

Yokoyama H (2001) The role of central histaminergic neuron system as an anticonvulsive mechanism in developing brain. Brain Dev 23:542–547

Yoshimoto R, Miyamoto Y, Shimamura K et al (2006) Therapeutic potential of histamine H3 receptor agonist for the treatment of obesity and diabetes mellitus. Proc Natl Acad Sci USA 103:13866–13871

Zandi PP, Anthony JC, Hayden KM et al (2002) Reduced incidence of AD with NSAID but not H2 receptor antagonists: the Cache County study. Neurology 59:880–886

Part IX
Histamine H3 Receptor: A Target for Momentous Brain Research

Chapter 15
Pre-Synaptic Control by Histamine H3 Receptors of Neurotransmitter Release

Angélica Osorio-Espinoza, Judith Ramos-Jiménez, and José-Antonio Arias-Montaño

Abstract Histamine regulates pre- and post-synaptically several brain functions, through the interaction with G protein-coupled receptors. Four such receptors (H1–H4) have been cloned, and three of them (H1, H2, and H3) are widely distributed in the mammalian nervous system. The histamine H3 receptor (H3R) was first identified in 1983 by Arrang and colleagues as an auto-receptor controlling histamine synthesis and release. Although H3Rs can be found in the periphery, mainly on axons of sympathetic and parasympathetic neurons, the central nervous system contains the great majority of such receptors, and the comparison with mRNA levels indicates that in most areas H3Rs are expressed on nerve terminals. Several lines of evidence have shown that in addition to its function as auto-receptor, the H3R regulates as a hetero-receptor the release of a number of neuroactive substances, namely acetylcholine, 5-hydroxytryptamine (5-HT, serotonin), noradrenaline, dopamine, glutamate, γ-aminobutyric acid (GABA) and substance P. In this work we review the reported actions of H3R activation on neurotransmitter release.

Keywords Histamine · H3 receptors · neurotransmitter release · brain · glutamate · GABA

Abbreviations

Acn	acetylcholine
CNS	central nervous system
EC_{50}	half maximal effective concentration
EPSCs	excitatory post-synaptic currents
EPSPs	excitatory post-synaptic potentials
IPSCs	inhibitory post-synaptic currents
IPSPs	inhibitory post-synaptic potentials

J.-A. Arias-Montaño (✉)
Departamento de Fisiología, Biofísica y Neurociencias, Cinvestav-IPN, México, D.F. 07000, México
e-mail: jaarias@fisio.cinvestav.mx

M. Shahid et al. (eds.), *Biomedical Aspects of Histamine*,
DOI 10.1007/978-90-481-9349-3_15, © Springer Science+Business Media B.V. 2010

GABA	γ-aminobutyric acid
GPCRs	G protein-coupled receptors
5-HT	5-hydroxytryptamine (serotonin)
H3R	histamine H3 receptor
hH3R	human histamine H3 receptor
rH3R	rat histamine H3 receptor
HPLC	high-performance liquid chromatography
IC_{50}	half maximal inhibitory concentration
K_d	dissociation constant
K_i	inhibition constant
K_B	antagonist dissociation constant
MAPKs	mitogen-activated protein kinases
NAMH	N^{α}-methylhistamine
NEM	*N*-ethylmaleimide
pA_2	$-\log_{10} K_B$ (estimated from a Schild plot)
pD_2	$-\log_{10}$ EC_{50} or IC_{50}
pK_i	$-\log_{10}$ of the inhibition constant
PTX	*pertussis* toxin
RAMH	(*R*)-α-methylhistamine
SNr	*substantia nigra pars reticulata*
TTX	tetrotoxin

Contents

15.1 Introduction

In the mammalian central nervous system (CNS) histamine-releasing neurons are located exclusively in the tuberomamillary nucleus of the hypothalamus and project to all major areas of the brain where participate in functions such as the regulation of sleep/wakefulness, locomotor activity, autonomic and vestibular functions, feeding and drinking, analgesia and memory. The typical morphology of chemical synapses is rarely seen for histaminergic fibers, and most axon endings do not make close contact with post-synaptic sites, in a pattern similar to that reported for other biogenic amines. Histamine actions in the mammalian brain are mostly mediated by metabotropic receptors. Four such receptors (H1–H4) have been cloned to date, and three of them (H1, H2 and H3) are widely distributed in the CNS (Haas and Panula 2003, Leurs et al. 2005).

The CNS contains the great majority of histamine H3 receptors (H3Rs), although these receptors can also be found in the periphery, mainly on axons of sympathetic and parasympathetic neurons (Leurs et al. 2005, Poli et al. 1991, Silver et al. 2002). High densities of H3Rs are found in the neocortex, basal ganglia (striatum, globus pallidus and *substantia nigra pars reticulata*, SNr), entorhinal cortex, nucleus accumbens, thalamic association nuclei and the amiygdaloid complex (Pillot et al. 2002). The comparison with mRNA levels indicates that in most areas H3Rs are expressed on nerve terminals, but in striatum, cerebral cortex and hippocampus H3Rs appear to be also located on neuronal bodies and dendrites.

In this work we first describe the main characteristics of H3Rs to then review the evidence for H3R-mediated modulation of synaptic transmission by regulating at the pre-synaptic level the release of several transmitters, namely histamine itself, acetylcholine, noradrenaline, 5-hydrotryptamine (5-HT, serotonin), dopamine, glutamate, γ-aminobutyric acid (GABA) and substance P.

15.2 General Characteristics of the Histamine H3 Receptor

The H3R was identified pharmacologically by Arrang et al. (1983) as an autoreceptor modulating histamine release from depolarized rat cerebro-cortical slices. Further work showed that H3Rs also modulated histamine synthesis in rat cerebrocortical slices and synaptosomes, and in slices from the posterior hypothalamus (Arrang et al. 1987).

15.2.1 Molecular Structure

In 1999 Lovenberg et al. cloned the human H3R (hH3R) cDNA, which encoded a 445 amino acid protein with all the hallmarks of the family A, rhodopsin-like G protein-coupled receptors, GPCRs (Fig. 15.1). The hH3R gene is located on

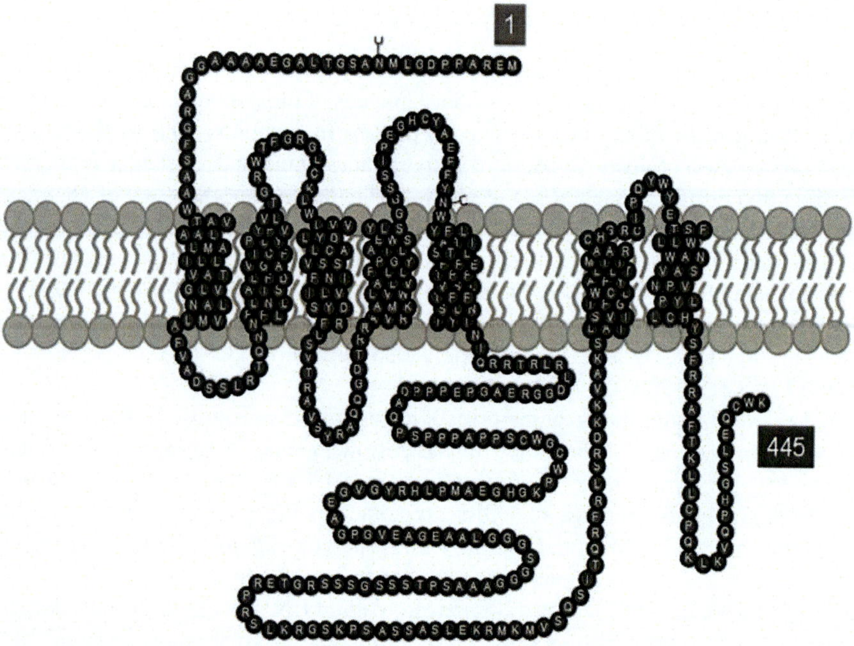

Fig. 15.1 Molecular structure of the human histamine H3 receptor ($hH3R_{445}$)

chromosome 20 at location 20q13.33 (HRH3 GeneID: 11255) and the coding region has been suggested to consist of three exons and two introns (GenBank accession number *AL078633*). In the coding region for the hH3R exon 1 codes for transmembrane domain (TM) 1 and half of TM2, exon 2 codes for the second half of TM2 and the entire TM3, and exon 3 codes for TM domains 4–7 (Bongers et al. 2007a).

Alternative splicing at exon-intron junctions generates at least 20 H3R isoforms in rodent and human brain, although some of these isoforms lack those regions necessary for agonist binding and receptor activation (reviewed by Bakker 2004 and Bongers et al. 2007a). Functional H3R isoforms reported for different species are the following (number of aminoacids between parentheses); human: $hH_{3(445)}$, $hH_{3(453)}$, $hH_{3(373)}$ and $hH_{3(365)}$ (Bongers et al. 2007b, Coge et al. 2001, Tardivel-Lacombe et al. 2001, Wellendorph et al. 2002); rat: $rH_{3A(445)}$, $rH_{3B(413)}$ and $rH_{3C(397)}$ (Drutel et al. 2001, Morisset et al. 2001); guinea pig: $H_{3L(445)}$ and $H_{3S(415)}$ (Tardivel-Lacombe et al. 2000); 3) mouse: $mH_{3(445)}$, $mH_{3(413)}$ and $mH_{3(397)}$ (Rouleau et al. 2004); monkey: $H_{3(445)}$, $H_{3(335)}$, $H_{3(413)}$ and $H_{3(410)}$ (Strakhova et al. 2008). For a significant number of H3R isoforms neither binding nor signaling capability has yet been determined. In addition, some splice variants which are abundantly expressed in rodent brain do not bind histamine but reduce the cell surface expression levels of functional H3Rs (Bakker et al. 2006).

15.2.2 Constitutive Activity

GPCRs appear to exist in equilibrium between active and non-active conformations. Active conformations are promoted and stabilized by agonists, but also exist in the absence of agonists, leading to constitutive or spontaneous activity. H3Rs exhibit constitutive activity when expressed in different cell lines, a property that has also been reported for native receptors. This issue has been comprehensively reviewed by Arrang et al. (2007), and only a few aspects are therefore referred to herein. H3R constitutive activity appears to rely on a consensus motive (Arg-Leu-Ser-Arg-Asp-Arg/Lys-Lys-Val-Ala-Lys-Ser-Leu) on the carboxyl terminus of the third intracellular loop, which is highly conserved among species (Sander et al. 2008). A number of classical H3R antagonists such as thioperamide, clobenpropit and ciproxyfan reverse constitutive receptor activity and are thus H3R inverse agonists (Bongers et al. 2007b, Leurs et al. 2005). In the CNS, constitutive activity of H3 auto-receptors exert a tonic inhibitory control on histamine synthesis and release (Morisset et al. 2000) and appears to account for the thioperamide-induced increase in firing rate of histaminergic neurons (Haas and Panula 2003).

15.2.3 Signaling

Upon activation the H3R triggers several signal transduction pathways through actions at diverse signaling proteins such as adenylyl cyclases, voltage-operated Ca^{2+} channels, Akt kinase, mitogen-activated protein kinases (MAPKs) and the Na^+/H^+ exchanger (Fig. 15.2).

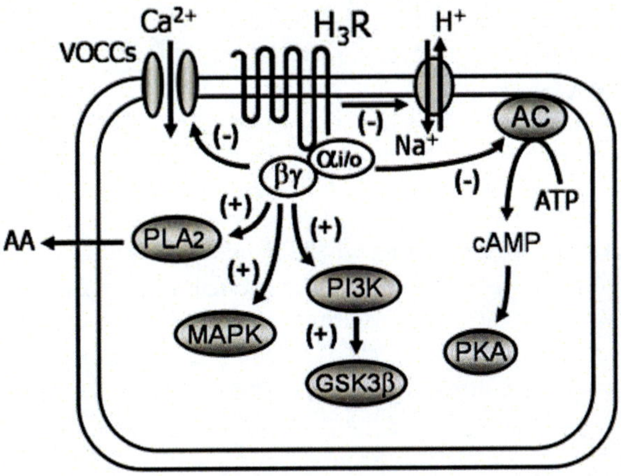

Fig. 15.2 Signaling pathways of the histamine H3 receptor (H3R). (+), Stimulation; (–), inhibition; AA, araquidonic acid; AC, adenylyl cyclase; cAMP, cyclic AMP; MAPK, mitogen-activated kinases; PI3K, phosphatidyl-inositol 3-kinase; GSK3β, glycogen synthase 3β-kinase; PKA, protein kinase A; PLA_2, phospholipase A_2; VOCCs, voltage-operated Ca^{2+} channels

15.2.3.1 Inhibition of Adenylyl Cyclase Activity

Several lines of evidence have shown that H3Rs couple to $G\alpha_{i/o}$ proteins and thus to the inhibition of cAMP formation in a *pertussis* toxin (PTX)-sensitive manner, leading to a subsequent reduction in the activity of protein kinase A (PKA), which participates in a variety of biological responses including gene expression, cell growth and proliferation, and synaptic plasticity (Bongers et al. 2007a).

15.2.3.2 Modulation of Voltage-Operated Ca^{2+} Channels

H3Rs have been shown to reduce depolarization-induced Ca^{2+} influx through voltage-operated channels in hypothalamic histaminergic neurons (Takeshita et al. 1998), human neuroblastoma SH-SY5Y cells (Silver et al. 2001) and rat striatal synaptosomes (Molina-Hernández et al. 2001). Likewise other $G\alpha_{i/o}$ protein-coupled receptors this effect most likely involves a direct action of $G_{\beta\gamma}$ dimers on the pore-forming α_1 subunit of N- and P/Q-type voltage-operated Ca^{2+} channels (Tedford and Zamponi 2006).

15.2.3.3 Inhibition of Na^+/H^+ Exchange

The Na^+/H^+ exchanger (NHX) regulates physiological intracellular pH by equimolarly exchanging intracellular H^+ ions for extracellular Na^+ ions and preventing thereby acidification. H3R activation inhibits neuronal NHX activity and this pathway may reduce the excessive release of noradrenaline during prolonged myocardial ischemia (Silver et al. 2001). The mechanism responsible for H3R-mediated inhibition of NHX activity remains to be fully elucidated although a direct interaction with $G\alpha_{i/o}$ proteins has been suggested.

15.2.3.4 MAPK Activation

Activation of $G\alpha_{i/o}$ proteins leads to the release of $G_{\beta\gamma}$ subunits which in turn may stimulate MAPKs (Marinissen and Gutkind 2001), known to have effects on cellular growth, differentiation and survival, as well as on neuronal plasticity and memory processes. Activation of H3Rs induces MAPK phosphorylation in cells transfected with the rat H3R, cardiac sympathetic nerve terminals and cultured rat cortical neurons (Bongers et al. 2007c, Levi et al. 2007, Mariottini et al. 2009). Whether this action is solely due to $G_{\beta\gamma}$ dimers, crosstalk with growth factor receptors or the use of scaffold proteins like β-arrestins, remains to be elucidated (Bongers et al. 2007a).

15.2.3.5 Activation of the Akt/GSK-3β Axis

H3R activation has been reported to modulate the activities of Akt kinase and glycogen synthase kinase 3β (GSK-3β) in a neuroblastoma cell line, primary cultures of cortical neurons and rat striatal slices through phospho-inositol-3-kinase (PI3K) and

MAPK stimulation via activated $G\alpha_{i/o}$ proteins (Bongers et al. 2007c, Mariottini et al. 2009).

15.2.3.6 Modulation of K^+ Channels

G protein-gated inwardly rectifying K^+ channels (GIRKs) are activated by $G_{\beta\gamma}$ dimers released in response to the stimulation of $G\alpha_{i/o}$ protein-coupled receptors, and there exits a report showing that H3Rs activate channels formed by the GIRK1 (Kir3.1) and GIRK4 (Kir3.4) subunits expressed in *Xenopus* oocytes (Sahlholm et al. 2007).

15.2.4 Pharmacology

H3Rs bind the endogenous ligand histamine with high affinity ($pK_i = 8.0$), similar to that reported for the H4 receptor ($pK_i = 7.8$), but in marked contrast with the affinity of either H1- or H2-receptors ($pK_i = 5.9$ and $pK_i = 5.7$, respectively; Gillard et al. 2002, Leurs et al. 1994). In addition, a relatively large number of compounds acting at the H3R have been synthesized.

15.2.4.1 H3R Agonists

All H3R agonists closely resemble histamine and contain a 4(5)-substituted imidazole moiety (Fig. 15.3). Typical agonists include N^{α}-methylhistamine (NAMH, $pK_i = 9.8$ at hH3R), (*R*)-α-methylhistamine (RAMH, $pK_i = 8.4$ at hH3R), imetit ($pK_i = 9.2$) and immepip ($pK_i = 9.3$) (Leurs et al. 2005, Lovenberg et al. 2000).

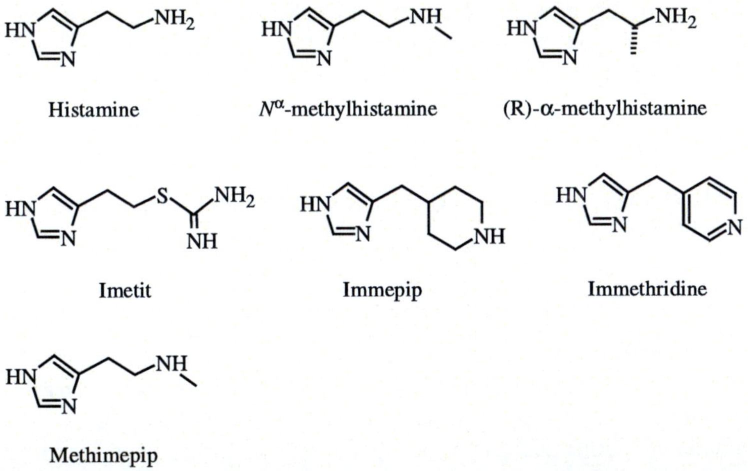

Fig. 15.3 Histamine H3 receptor agonists

However, with the recent discovery of the H4 receptor, it also became clear that these drugs show limited selectivity (27–55-fold) for the H3R over the related H4-receptor (Leurs et al. 2005). Agonists with improved selectivity are immethridine ($pK_i = 9.1$, 300-fold selectivity) and methimepip ($pK_i = 9.0$, 2,000-fold selectivity).

15.2.4.2 H3R Antagonists

Imidazole-Containing H3R Antagonists

The first potent H3R antagonist to be described that lacked H1- and H2-receptor activity was thioperamide (Fig. 15.4). As mentioned before, thioperamide and several other compounds initially identified as H3R antagonists have been re-classified as H3R antagonists/inverse agonists (Leurs et al. 2005). Thioperamide shows high affinity for the rH3R ($pK_i = 8.4$), but proved to be less active at the hH3R ($pK_i = 7.2$) and binds with similar potency at the human H4 receptor ($pK_i = 7.3$). Another imidazole-containing antagonist that has been extensively used for H3R characterization is clobenpropit ($pK_i = 9.4$, hH3R). Proxyfan was initially identified as a neutral H3R antagonist ($pK_i = 8.0$, rH3R), but also behaves as H3R antagonist and inverse agonist, depending on the signaling assay tested, and is therefore considered to be a protean ligand. The structurally related compound ciproxifan is a potent inverse agonist at the rH3R ($pK_i = 9.2$), but shows moderate affinity for the hH3R ($pK_i = 7.2$). Other imidazole-containing antagonists are cipralisant (GT-2331, $pK_i = 9.9$, rH3R; $pK_i = 8.4$, hH3R) and SCH-79687 ($pK_i = 8.7$, rH3R).

Non-Imidazole H3R Antagonists

Most of the imidazole-containing antagonists interact with cytochrome P450, an undesirable effect in drug development which has led to the synthesis of non-imidazole H3R antagonists. Examples of these drugs are the following (Leurs et al. 2005): UCL-1972 ($pK_i = 7.4$, rH3R), VU-F5391 ($pK_i = 8.2$, rH3R), FUB-649 ($pK_i = 7.8$, rH3R), A-317920 ($pK_i = 9.2$, rH3R; $pK_i = 7.0$, hH3R), A-331440 (inverse agonist; $pK_i = 7.8$, rH3R; $pK_i = 8.6$, hH3R), ABT-239 (potent inverse agonist; $pK_i = 8.9$, rH3R; $pK_i = 9.3$, hH3R), JNJ-5207852 ($pK_i = 9.5$, hH3R), JNJ-10181457 ($pK_i = 9.1$, hH3R), and NNC-0038-0000-1202 (inverse agonist; $pK_i = 8.3$, hH3R).

15.2.4.3 Species-Related Pharmacological Differences

As illustrated by data shown above, the comparison of affinities for different ligands points out to the existence of receptor heterogeneity among species, particularly between human and rat receptors, the latter the prototype for drug characterization. Mutational studies and molecular modeling approaches have identified two aminoacids located in the third transmembrane domain of rat (Ala^{119} and Val^{122}) and human (Thr^{119} and Ala^{122}) receptors that appear responsible for the observed pharmacological differences (Leurs et al. 2005, Sander et al. 2008).

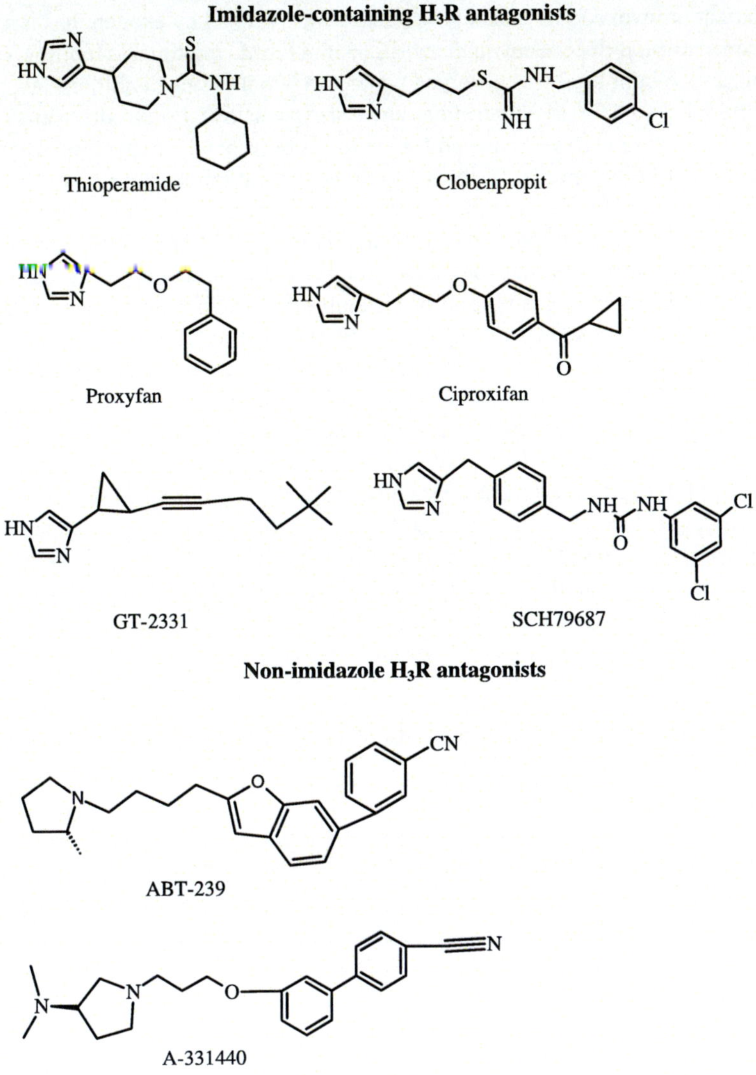

Fig. 15.4 Histamine H3 receptor antagonists

15.3 Modulation by Histamine H3 Receptors of Neurotransmitter Release

15.3.1 Modulation of Histamine Release

As mentioned before, the first experimental evidence for the existence of a third histamine receptor was provided in 1983 by Arrang et al. who showed that in rat cerebro-cortical slices labeled with [^{3}H]-histidine, Ca^{2+}-dependent, depolarization-evoked [^{3}H]-histamine release was reduced by exogenous histamine in a concentration-dependent manner (IC_{50} = 41 nM, maximal inhibition 61%). The histamine inhibition was observed under two depolarizing conditions, exposure to 30 mM K^+ or 10 μM veratridine, and was insensitive to tetrodotoxin (TTX), which by blocking voltage-activated Na^+ currents prevents the generation and propagation of action potentials. In the same work, the inhibitory action of histamine was mimicked by NAMH, and the concentration-response curve for histamine was shifted to the right by impromidine and burimamide, with potencies significantly different from those reported for blockade of H2-receptors. Based on these data, it was proposed that auto-inhibition of histamine release in rat brain was mediated by a novel class of histamine receptor named H3 (Arrang et al. 1983). This study was extended to show an inverse relationship between the magnitude of inhibition and the concentration of K^+ and Ca^{2+} ions in the incubation medium (Arrang et al. 1985), suggesting that the histamine effect was related to Ca^{2+} entry into the histaminergic axon terminals (see Table 15.1). In the latter study, auto-inhibition of K^+-evoked [^{3}H]-histamine release was also demonstrated for slices of rat striatum (–49%), hippocampus (–47%) and hypothalamus (–64%), and in isolated nerve terminals (synaptosomes) from cerebral cortex (–30%), in which the IC_{50} estimate was similar to that obtained in cerebro-cortical slices (200 ± 50 and 130 ± 20 nM, respectively). Following these studies, auto-inhibition of [^{3}H]-histamine release evoked by electrical stimulation of brain slices was also reported (Van der Werf et al. 1987).

Table 15.1 Summary of the effect of histamine H3 receptors on neurotransmitter release in the nervous system

Neurotransmitter	Species and tissue	References
1. Histamine	In vitro studies	
	Rat	
	cerebral cortex slices (↓)	1, 2, 3, 5
	cerebral cortex synaptosomes (↓)	2, 4
	striatum slices (↓)	2
	hippocampus slices (↓)	2
	hypothalamus slices (↓)	2
	Mouse	
	cerebral cortex synaptosomes (↓)	4
	In vivo studies	
	Rat	
	hypothalamus (↓)	6
	cerebral cortex (↓)	7, 8
	tuberomammillary nucleus (↓)	7
	nucleus basalis magnocellularis (↓)	7
2. Acetylcholine	In vitro studies	
	Guinea-pig	
	ileum (↓)	9, 10, 11
	smooth muscle-myenteric plexus (↓)	12
	sub-mucous neurons (↓)	13

Table 15.1 (continued)

Neurotransmitter	Species and tissue	References
	Rat	
	cerebral cortex slices (↓)	2, 14
	cerebral cortex synaptosomes (no effect)	2
	hippocampus slices (no effect)	15
	In vivo studies	
	Rat	
	cerebral cortex (↓)	16
	hippocampus (↓)	17, 18
	ventral striatum (↑)	19
3. Noradrenaline	In vitro studies	
	Guinea-pig	
	mesenteric artery (↓)	20
	heart (↓)	21
	cardiac synaptosomes (↓)	22, 23
	retina discs (↓)	24
	cerebral cortex slices (↓)	25
	cerebellum slices (↓)	25
	hippocampus slices (↓)	25
	hypothalamus slices (↓)	25
	Dog heart (↓)	26
	Human	
	cardiac synaptosomes (↓)	27
	cerebral cortex slices (↓)	28
	Rat	
	cerebral cortex slices (↓)	24, 29
	spinal cord slices (↓)	30
	Mouse cerebral cortex slices (↓)	31
	In vivo studies	
	Rat	
	hippocampus (↓)	32
	cerebral cortex (↓)	33
4. 5-HT	In vitro studies	
	Rat	
	cerebral cortex slices (↓)	34, 35
	sustantia nigra, midbrain slices (↓)	36
5. Dopamine	In vitro studies	
	Mouse striatum slices (↓)	37
	Rat	
	sustantia nigra slices (↓)	38
	striatum slices (no effect)	37
	Rabbit striatum slices (no effect)	39
	In vivo studies	
	Rat	
	nucleus accumbens (↑ by H3R antagonists)	40
	cerebral cortex (↑ by H3R antagonists)	41, 42, 33
6. Glutamate	In vitro studies	
	Rat	
	hippocampus slices (↓)	43, 44

Table 15.1 (continued)

Neurotransmitter	Species and tissue	References
	striatum slices (↓)	45
	striatum synaptosomes (↓)	46
	amygdala slices (↓)	47
	thalamus slices and synaptosomes (↓)	48
	Mouse striatum slices (↓)	49
7. GABA	In vitro studies	
	Rat	
	sustantia nigra slices (↓)*	50
	striatum slices (↓)*	51, 52
	medial vestibular nucleus slices (↓)	53
	hypothalamus, dissociated neurons (↓)	54
	cultured cerebro-cortical neurons (↓)	55
	thalamus slices and synaptosomes (no effect)	56
	globus pallidus slices and synaptosomes (no effect)	57
8. Substance P	In vitro studies	
	Guinea-pig ileum (↓)	58
	Rabbit lung (↓)	59
	In vivo studies	
	Guinea-pig respiratory system (↓)	60
	Rat hindpaw (↓)	61, 62

↓, inhibition; ↑, facilitation

* Inhibition of the facilitatory action of dopamine D_1-like receptors

[1]Arrang et al. (1983), [2]Arrang et al. (1985), [3]Moreno-Delgado et al. (2009), [4]Morisset et al. (2000), [5]Van der Werf et al. (1987), [6]Jansen et al. (1998), [7]Giannoni et al. (2009), [8]Leineweber et al. (2007), [9]Hew et al. (1990), [10]Leurs et al. (1991), [11]Trzeciakowski (1987), [12]Poli et al. (1991), [13]Frieling et al. (1994), [14]Clapham and Kilpatrick (1992), [15]Alves-Rodrigues et al. (1998), [16]Blandina et al. (1996), [17]Bacciottini et al. (2002), [18]Mochizuki et al. (1994), [19]Prast et al. (1999), [20]Ishikawa and Sperelakis (1987), [21]Endou et al. (1994), [22]Seyedi et al. (2005), [23]Silver et al. (2002), [24]Schlicker et al. (1990), [25]Timm et al. (1998), [26]Mazenot et al. (1999), [27]Imamura et al. (1995), [28]Schlicker et al. (1999), [29]Schlicker et al. (1994), [30]Celuch (1995), [31]Schlicker et al. (1989), [32]Di et al. (2000), [33]Medhurst et al. (2007), [34]Fink et al. (1990), [35]Schlicker et al. (1988), [36]Threlfell et al. (2004), [37]Schlicker et al. (1993), [38]García et al. (1997), [39]Smits and Mulder (1991), [40]Munzar et al. (2004), [41]Fox et al. (2005), [42]Ligneau et al. (2007), [43]Brown and Haas (1999), [44]Brown and Reymann (1996), [45]Doreulee et al. (2001), [46]Molina-Hernández et al. (2001), [47]Jiang et al. (2005), [48]Garduño-Torres et al. (2007), [49]Doreulee et al. (2001), [50]García et al. (1997), [51]Arias-Montaño et al. (2001), [52]Arias-Montaño et al. (2007), [53]Bergquist et al. (2006), [54]Jang et al. (2001), [55]Dai et al. (2007), [56]Garduño-Torres et al. (2007), [57]Osorio-Espinoza et al. (2009), [58]Taylor and Kilpatrick (1992), [59]Nemmara et al. (1999), [60]Ichinose and Barnes (1998), [61]Ohkubo et al. (1995a), [62]Ohkubo and Shibata (1995)

Recently, Moreno-Delgado et al. (2009) showed that depolarization-evoked $[^3H]$-histamine release from rat cerebro-cortical slices involves Ca^{2+} entry and the activation of CamKII, a serine/threonine protein kinase primarily regulated by the Ca^{2+}/calmodulin complex. In this work, blockade of N- and P/Q-type voltage operated Ca^{2+} channels reduced $[^3H]$-histamine release by 30 and 60% respectively, indicating the participation of these channels in H3R-mediated auto-inhibition of histamine release.

From the initials reports by Arrang et al. (1983, 1985), auto-inhibition of [^{3}H]-histamine release from brain slices or synaptosomes labeled with either [^{3}H]-histidine or [^{3}H]-histamine has become a standard assay to test the pharmacological properties of drugs acting at H3Rs.

Auto-inhibition of histamine release has also been addressed by in vivo studies based on microdialysis and the measurement of histamine content in the perfusates by high-performance liquid chromatography (HPLC). As mentioned in the introductory section, all histaminergic neurons are located in the hypothalamus and perfusion of the H3R agonist immepip into the anterior hypothalamic area reduced basal histamine release in a concentration-dependent manner with suppression at 100 nM. Conversely, the H3R antagonist clobenpropit increased histamine levels to ~200% at 100 nM (Jansen et al. 1998). As the anterior hypothalamic area is enriched with histaminergic fibers, the effect of the H3R agonist is likely to be caused by their action at pre-synaptic H3Rs. In line with this, the antagonist effect may be explained by blockade of tonic auto-inhibition of release by endogenous histamine or by an action as inverse agonist at constitutively active H3Rs shown to control [^{3}H]-histamine release from rat and mouse cerebro-cortical synaptosomes submitted to a strong depolarizing (40–55 mM K^+) stimulus (Morisset et al. 2000).

H3 auto-receptors also appear to control histamine release in the cerebral cortex in vivo. Microdialysis in free-moving rats shows that the systemic administration of the H3R agonist immepip (5 or 10 mg/kg, i.p.) induces a significant decrease in cortical histamine efflux with a peak inhibition of 27–37% from the baseline (Lamberty et al. 2003). Gently handling resulted in increased histamine levels in prefrontal cortex dialysates and this effect was reduced (–80%) by the infusion of 1 μM TTX (Westerink et al. 2002). Handling-induced increase in extracellular histamine was markedly reduced by infusion of the H3R agonist RAMH (10 μM), and enhanced by the antagonist thioperamide (10 μM), indicating that H3 auto-receptors modulate histamine release during natural stimulatory conditions.

A recent microdialysis study used either a single-probe implanted in a number of rat brain areas (hypothalamic tuberomamillary nucleus, nucleus basalis magnocellularis, nucleus accumbens, striatum and cerebral cortex) to monitor local changes in histamine release induced by drug-perfusion, or a dual-probe system that allowed for drug administration into the tuberomamillary nucleus and monitoring histamine release in nuclei receiving histaminergic innervation (Giannoni et al. 2009). In the dual-probe experiments, perfusion with the H3R antagonist/inverse agonist thioperamide of the tuberomamillary nucleus increased histamine release in this nucleus and in nucleus basalis magnocellularis and cerebral cortex, but not in nucleus accumbens and striatum. This pattern was confirmed by single-probe determinations, leading to the rather interesting conclusion that histaminergic neurons are organized into functionally distinct circuits that influence different brain regions, and display selective control mechanisms.

15.3.2 Modulation of Acetylcholine (ACh) Release

Modulation by H3Rs of cholinergic transmission was first demonstrated in the peripheral nervous system. In 1987, Trzeciakowski reported that the electrically-induced contraction of guinea-pig ileum segments in which the contractile action of H1-receptors had been prevented by mepyramine, was inhibited by both histamine and NMHA with EC_{50} values of 64 and 1.7 nM, respectively. NMHA did not alter contractions produced by exogenous ACh, and its inhibitory action on contraction was blocked by impromidine in a competitive manner with a K_B estimate of 26 nM, similar to that reported previously for H3 auto-receptors in rat cerebral cortex (Arrang et al. 1983, 1985). In the longitudinal smooth muscle-myenteric plexus preparation the H3R agonist RAMH produced a marked inhibition of the twitch contractions elicited by electrical transmural stimulation of segments of guinea-pig ileum ($EC_{50} = 6.7$ nM, maximal inhibition ~90%). The RAMH inhibition was antagonized by thioperamide ($K_B = 1.1$ nM) but not by H1- or H2-receptor antagonists. In line with the study by Trzeciakowski (1987), RAMH had no effect on the contractile responses to carbachol, supporting that H3Rs inhibited the release of ACh from pre-synaptic myenteric nerve terminals (Hew et al. 1990). In a similar study using muscle strips of guinea-pig large and small intestine RAMH inhibited by 57–69% the electrically-evoked contraction in duodenum, ileum, jejunum and colon with pD_2 values in the range 8.09–8.27, and the agonist effect was antagonized by thioperamide with pA_2 values in the range 8.09–8.36 (Leurs et al. 1991).

More direct evidence for H3R-mediated modulation of ACh release in the intestine was provided by two reports. The first one used the longitudinal smooth muscle-myenteric plexus preparation pre-loaded with $[^3H]$-choline. In the presence of H1- and H2-receptors antagonists, electrically-stimulated $[^3H]$-ACh release was inhibited in a concentration-dependent manner by histamine and RAMH, and the effect of histamine was blocked by the H3R antagonists thioperamide and impromidine (Poli et al. 1991). In the second report, the electrical stimulation of inter-ganglionic fiber tracts resulted in excitatory post-synaptic potentials (EPSPs) in sub-mucous neurons that were abolished by histamine, an effect mimicked by NMHA and blocked by burimamide, indicating that H3R activation inhibited pre-synaptically ACh release in nicotinic synapses (Frieling et al. 1993).

Early in vitro evidence for H3R-mediated regulation of cholinergic transmission in the CNS was provided by experiments examining K^+-stimulated $[^3H]$-ACh release from rat entorhinal cortex slices pre-loaded with $[^3H]$-choline. Whereas the H3R agonist RAMH inhibited release (maximal inhibition ~40%), the H3R antagonist thioperamide competitively antagonized the RAMH action ($pK_B = 8.4$) and on its own (1 μM) augmented the depolarization-stimulated release by 23% (Clapham and Kilpatrick 1992). These findings were confirmed by Arrang et al. using entorhinal cortex slices in which RAMH reduced K^+-evoked $[^3H]$-ACh release with maximal inhibition of 39% and IC_{50} of 25 nM, and thioperamide antagonized this effect with K_i of 22 nM. However, in synaptosomes from the same region, K^+-stimulated $[^3H]$-ACh release remained unaltered in the presence of the H3R agonists imetit and RAMH, questioning the presence of H3Rs on cholinergic nerve terminals (Arrang et al. 1995). Further, H3R-mediated modulation of ACh release depends on the brain region studies, because in rat hippocampus, where the presence of H3Rs was detected by radioligand binding, RAMH failed to modify K^+-stimulated [^{3}H]-ACh release from slices pre-loaded with [^{3}H]-choline, but significantly inhibited depolarization-evoked [^{3}H]-noradrenaline release (Alves-Rodrigues et al. 1998).

The first evidence for a regulatory role of H3Rs on brain ACh release in vivo was reported in 1996. Microdialysis from the fronto-parietal cortex of freely moving rats showed that histamine did not affect spontaneous but inhibited K^+ (100 mM)-stimulated ACh release in a concentration-dependent manner with maximal inhibition of ∼50%. The H3R agonists RAMH, imetit and immepip mimicked the histamine effect, which was blocked by the H3R antagonist clobenpropit but not by H1- or H2-receptor antagonists (Blandina et al. 1996). Other studies have shown that H3R activation also regulates ACh in a number of brain regions, namely hippocampus (Bacciottini et al. 2002, Mochizuki et al. 1994), ventral striatum (Prast et al. 1999) and basolateral amygdala (Passani et al. 2001). In contrast to the inhibitory action of H3Rs on ACh release reported for rat cerebral cortex and hippocampus, in the ventral striatum histamine and H3R agonists and antagonists increase the release of ACh, presumably by an indirect effect (Prast et al. 1999, see below).

Likewise studies in brain slices or synaptosomes, in vivo studies indicate that H3R-mediated modulation of brain ACh release involves trans-synaptic effects rather than a direct action at receptors located on cholinergic neurons. In the study by Blandina et al. (1996) TTX perfusion had no significant effect on 100 mM K^+-evoked ACh release, but prevented the H3R-mediated inhibition, suggesting that receptors modulating ACh release are not located on cholinergic nerve terminals, in accord with the failure of H3R agonists to alter K^+-evoked release of [^{3}H]-ACh from rat entorhinal cortex synaptosomes (Arrang et al. 1995). In addition to H3R-mediated inhibition of ACh release in rat cerebral cortex being both TTX-sensitive and prevented by $GABA_A$ receptor blockade by bicuculline, the H3R agonist immepip increased K^+-evoked GABA release in vivo (Giorgetti et al. 1997). These authors have therefore proposed that post-synaptic H3Rs facilitate the release of GABA which, in turn, inhibits ACh release. In the ventral striatum histamine increased ACh release and this effect was mimicked by both H3R agonists (immepip and imetit) and antagonists (thioperamide and clobenpropit), and prevented by the $GABA_A$ receptor antagonist bicuculline. The effect of H3R agonists was suppressed by blocking dopamine D_1- and D_2-like receptors and by inhibiting histamine synthesis with α-fluoromethylhistidine (FMH), while the effect of H3R antagonists was also prevented by D_1- and D_2-like receptor blockade but proved resistant to FMH (Prast et al. 1999). These results can be explained by a dual action of histamine at H3 auto- and hetero-receptors, with the latter reducing GABAergic transmission by either a direct effect on GABAergic nerve terminals (García et al. 1997) or by acting at dopaminergic axon terminals where they would inhibit dopamine release (Schlicker et al. 1993) which in turn would decrease GABA release (Arias-Montaño et al. 2001, 2007), finally resulting in enhanced ACh release.

As mentioned above, H3R activation decreases the cholinergic tone in the frontal cortex and the hippocampus and this action may be important in learning and memory. In that respect, the use of H3R antagonists may represent a potential therapy to correct the deficits resulting from cholinergic hypofunction, and H3Rs antagonists have been shown to exert procognitive effects in several behavioral assays. For example, the selective H3Rs antagonists ABT-239, BF2.649, GSK189254 and JNJ-10181457 increased ACh release from rodent frontal cortex and/or dorsal hippocampus, associated with procognitive efficacy in behavioral animal models. These results provide support to the hypothesis that H3Rs antagonists may have clinical use in cognitive-related disorders, especially those in which cholinergic neurotransmission is compromised (reviewed by Esbenshade et al. 2008).

15.3.3 Modulation of Noradrenaline Release

There is substantial evidence for H3R regulating noradrenaline release in both peripheral and central nervous systems. The first of such reports was carried out in the guinea-pig mesenteric artery to show that histamine depressed electrically-stimulated transmitter release from perivascular sympathetic nerve terminals, without modifying the passive membrane properties of the post-synaptic smooth muscle cells (Ishikawa and Sperelakis 1987). The histamine effect was mimicked by the agonist NAMH and was antagonized by impromidine with a pA_2 value similar to that obtained for antagonism of histamine-induced inhibition of $[^3H]$-histamine release from depolarized rat cerebro-cortical slices (Arrang et al. 1983).

Functional H3Rs have been identified on the adrenergic nerve endings in the heart of the guinea-pig (Endou et al. 1994), dog (Mazenot et al. 1999) and humans (Imamura et al. 1995). In the isolated guinea-pig atria, the H3R agonist RAMH attenuates the chronotropic and inotropic response to transmural stimulation of adrenergic nerve endings, effects prevented by the antagonist thioperamide, reduced by pre-treatment with PTX and potentiated by ω-conotoxin, a blocker of N-type voltage-operated Ca^{2+} channels. Further, transmural sympathetic nerve stimulation elicited Ca^{2+}-dependent noradrenaline release which was significantly reduced by the H3R agonist NAMH with the agonist action being prevented by the antagonist thioperamide and decreased by PTX pre-treatment (Endou et al. 1994). Taken together, these findings indicate that pre-junctional H3Rs modulate depolarization-dependent noradrenaline release from myocardial sympathetic nerve endings, through a mechanism dependent on $G\alpha_{i/o}$ protein activation and reduction of voltage-activated Ca^{2+} currents.

In the anaesthetized dog Mazenot et al. (1999) found that the increase in noradrenaline content in coronary sinus blood after electrical stimulation of the right cardiac sympathetic nerves was decreased by intravenously administered RAMH (0.2 and 2 μmol/kg, 75–80% inhibition) and this effect was partially prevented by the H3R antagonist SC-359 (1 mg/kg, i.v.). In sympathetic nerve endings (cardiac synaptosomes) isolated from surgical specimens of human right atria, depolarization-evoked noradrenaline release was prevented by blockade of N-type Ca^{2+} channels and markedly reduced (–65%) by the H3R agonist RAMH. The effect of the latter drug was mimicked by immepip and the action of both agonists was prevented by the H3R antagonist thioperamide (Imamura et al. 1995).

Depolarization-induced noradrenaline release from guinea-pig cardiac synaptosomes is sensitive to blockade of N-type Ca^{2+} channels and reduced by H3R activation, the latter effect being prevented by PTX pre-treatment (Seyedi et al. 2005, Silver et al. 2002). In the cardiac synaptosome preparation activation of the cAMP/PKA pathway elicits noradrenaline release which is also reduced by H3R stimulation in a PTX-sensitive manner (Seyedi et al. 2005). These data indicate that in sympathetic cardiac nerves H3R control neurotransmitter release by inhibiting the increase in intracellular Ca^{2+} levels through $G\alpha_{i/o}$ protein-mediated actions at both voltage-operated Ca^{2+} channels and adenylyl cyclases. The effects on either pathway are most likely due to the $G\alpha_{\beta\gamma}$ complexes and $G\alpha_{i/o}$ subunits, respectively (Morrey et al. 2008, Seyedi et al. 2005).

As stated before, H3R stimulation induces MAPK activation through the $G\alpha_{\beta\gamma}$ complexes released upon $G\alpha_{i/o}$ protein activation. For cardiac sympathetic nerve terminals R. Levi and colleagues have shown that in addition to their actions at voltage-operated Ca^{2+} channels and adenylyl cyclases, H3Rs modulate noradrenaline release through trans-activation of the prostanoid receptor EP_3R, also coupled to $G\alpha_{i/o}$ proteins. The proposed pathway involves MAPK-mediated phosphorylation of cytosolic phospholiphase A_2 ($cPLA_2$) which is then translocated to the cellular membrane, with the consequent formation of arachidonic acid from membrane phospholipids, and the subsequent production of PGE_2 via cyclooxygenase. In turn, PGE_2 activates membranal EP_3Rs and the $G\alpha_{\beta\gamma}$ complexes released on $G\alpha_{i/o}$ protein activation contribute to the inhibition of Ca^{2+} entry, thus attenuating noradrenaline exocytosis (Levi et al. 2007).

Activation of H3Rs also inhibits noradrenaline release in animal models of acute and protracted myocardial ischemia, in which sympathetic over-activity with excessive noradrenaline release is a prominent cause of cardiac dysfunction and arrhythmias. In acute ischemia the H3R antagonist thioperamide enhances Ca^{2+}-dependent noradrenaline release at reperfusion with no effect of the agonist RAMH, indicating that H3Rs become fully activated during the ischemic period. In the protracted ischemia model, noradrenaline release is Ca^{2+}-independent and carrier-mediated (Imamura et al. 1994, 1996, Levi and Smith 2000). Under this condition, ATP depletion promotes Na^+ accumulation in sympathetic nerve endings and prevents the vesicular storage of noradrenaline, leading to reversal of the noradrenaline transporter (NET) from an inward to an outward direction and massive carrier-mediated noradrenaline release (Du and Dart 1993, Schömig 1990). H3R-induced attenuation of transporter-mediated noradrenaline release probably involves the inhibition of the Na^+/H^+ exchanger, reducing thus intraterminal Na^+ accumulation and noradrenaline efflux (Imamura et al. 1996, Leineweber et al. 2007). However, the mechanism involved remains unclear, and in addition to the inhibition of the Na^+/H^+ exchanger, modulation of voltage-dependent Na^+ channels may participate in the H3R action (Hatta et al. 1997). In summary, pre-synaptic H3Rs are likely to serve a modulatory role in cardiac adrenergic function in normal conditions as well as in pathophysiological scenarios such as myocardial ischemia and arrhythmic dysfunction, and for the latter conditions H3R-mediated attenuation of noradrenaline release appears to play a protective role.

An inhibitory action of H3R activation on electrically-induced [^{3}H]-noradrenaline release has also been reported for pig retina discs (Schlicker et al. 1990). The evoked-release of [^{3}H]-noradrenaline was most likely originated in the vascular postganglionic sympathetic nerve fibers and required the blockade of α_2-adrenoceptors.

As to the CNS, histamine decreased [^{3}H]-noradrenaline release from rat cerebro-cortical slices induced by electrical or chemical (20 mM K^+) stimulation. The evoked [^{3}H]-noradrenaline overflow was mimicked by the H3R agonist RAMH, and the concentration-response curves of both agonists were shifted to the right by thioperamide, impromidine and burimamide with apparent pA_2 values of 8.37, 6.86 and 7.05, respectively (Schlicker et al. 1989). Inhibition by H3R activation of electrically-evoked [^{3}H]-noradrenaline release from pre-labeled slices has also been reported for mouse cerebral cortex (Schlicker et al. 1992), rat spinal cord (Celuch 1995), guinea-pig cerebral cortex, cerebellum, hippocampus and hypothalamus (Timm et al. 1998), and human cerebral cortex (Schlicker et al. 1999).

In rat cerebro-cortical slices H3R-mediated inhibition of electrically-evoked [^{3}H]-noradrenaline release shows an inverse relationship with both the stimulation frequency (0.1–3 Hz) and the Ca^{2+} concentration (0.8–2.6 mM) in the perfusion buffer. Further, tissue pre-incubation with *N*-ethylmaleimide (NEM), which by alkylation of SH groups inactivates a series of G proteins, significantly reduced the inhibitory effect of H3R activation (Schlicker et al. 1994). These pieces of evidence are compatible with H3Rs inhibiting neurotransmitter release by reducing Ca^{2+} availability in the axon terminals through a mechanism that involves the action of $G\alpha_{i/o}$ proteins.

H3R-mediated modulation of noradrenaline release has also been demonstrated in vivo. In rat hippocampus the perfusion of the H3R agonist RAMH (1 and 100 μM) resulted in short-lasting and dose-dependent reduction in extracellular NA levels (peak inhibition 31 and 45%, respectively), assessed in freely moving rats by microdialysis and HPLC. The effect of RAMH was reversed by the addition of thioperamide to the perfusion solution as well as by the systemic administration of the H3R antagonist (Di Carlo et al. 2000). In another brain microdialysis study, oral administration of GSK-189254 (1 and 3 mg/kg), a H3R antagonist with good CNS penetration, induces significant (~180% of baseline) and sustained increases in noradrenaline efflux in the anterior cingulate subregion of the rat prefrontal cortex (Medhurst et al. 2007).

H3R-mediated inhibition of noradrenaline release from central and peripheral neurons is enhanced by blockade of α_2-autoreceptors (reviewed by Schlicker and Göthert 1998). This effect is most likely explained by convergence at a common site of action since both H3Rs and α_2-adrenoceptors couple to $G\alpha_{i/o}$ proteins. However, other interactions, such as receptor hetero-dimerization can not be ruled out.

15.3.4 Modulation of 5-Hydroxytryptamine (5-HT) Release

Reports on H3R-mediated modulation of 5-HT release have been primarily limited to in vitro studies. The first of such reports showed that electrically-evoked, TTX-sensitive and Ca^{2+}-dependent release of [^{3}H]-5-HT from perfused rat cerebro-cortical slices was decreased by histamine in a concentration-dependent manner and that this effect was antagonized by impromidine (H3R antagonist/H2R partial agonist) and burimamide (H3R antagonist/H2R antagonist), but not by selective antagonists at H1- or H2-receptors (Schlicker et al. 1988). Two years later, Fink et al. reported that the inhibitory action of histamine on electrically-evoked [^{3}H]-5-HT release from rat cerebro-cortical slices was mimicked by two selective H3R agonists (NAMH and RAMH) and was antagonized by thioperamide. Further, in both cerebro-cortical slices and synaptomes Ca^{2+}-dependent, K^+-induced [^{3}H]-5-HT release was inhibited by histamine and this effect was blocked by thioperamide.

By monitoring 5-HT release with fast-scan cyclic voltammetry at carbon-fiber microelectrodes in rat midbrain slices, it was shown that in *substantia nigra pars reticulata* (SNr) the electrically-evoked release of 5-HT was potently reduced by the H3R agonists RAMH (–49%, $IC_{50} = 23$ nM) and immepip (–39%, $IC_{50} = 43$ nM). The agonist attenuation of 5-HT release was concentration-dependent, prevented by thioperamide and not affected by GABA- or glutamate-receptor antagonists, indicating that the effect was due to a direct action on serotonergic terminals (Threlfell et al. 2004).

Treatments for depression include inhibitors of 5-HT reuptake (Savitz et al. 2009), and the evidence for a role of H3Rs in controlling neuronal 5-HT release has therefore led to substantial interest for drugs that by combining H3R antagonism with 5-HT uptake inhibition increase brain 5-HT levels as an antidepressant therapy (Esbenshade et al. 2008). In this regard the drug JNJ-28583867, a selective and potent H3R antagonist and inhibitor of 5-HT transport, showed antidepressant-like activity in mice (Barbier et al. 2007).

Enterochromaffin cells of the digestive tract are responsible for the production and storage of the largest pool of 5-HT in the body, and when the transmitter is released by exocytosis can act on the intrinsic nerves and vagal endings (Bertrand and Bertrand 2010). Histamine has been shown to regulate 5-HT release through H3Rs, that appear to be located on the enterochromaffin cells (reviewed by Racke et al. 1996).

15.3.5 Modulation of Dopamine Release

In superfused mouse striatal slices, electrically evoked [^{3}H]-dopamine release was reduced (–18 $\pm$ 3%) by histamine, and the extent of inhibition was increased to 38 $\pm$ 4% when the D_2-like receptor antagonist haloperidol was included in the perfusion medium (Schlicker et al. 1993). The histamine effect was mimicked by NAMH and attenuated by thioperamide but not by H1- or H2-receptor antagonists, indicating the participation of H3Rs. Inhibition by H3R activation (–30%) was also observed when [^{3}H]-dopamine release was induced by adding Ca^{2+} ions to continuously depolarized mouse striatal slices.

H3R-mRNA has been detected in rat *substantia nigra* (Pillot et al. 2002) supporting the expression of H3R receptor by nigro-striatal dopaminergic neurons, and we showed that in *substantia nigra pars reticulata* slices K^+-evoked [^{3}H]-dopamine release was significantly reduced (–38%) by the H3R agonist immepip suggesting that some H3Rs are located on the dendrites of the dopaminergic neurons (García et al. 1997). In contrast, H3R activation failed to inhibit depolarization-evoked [^{3}H]-dopamine release from rat or rabbit striatal slices or synaptosomes (Schlicker et al. 1993, Smits and Mulder 1991, and unpublished results of our own). Taken together, these data point out to inter-species and inter-region differences in H3R expression.

Modulation of dopamine release by H3Rs has also been approached by in vivo microdialysis studies. Systemic administration of the H3R antagonists thioperamide or clobenprobit had no effect on basal extracellular dopamine, but potentiated methamphetamine-induced dopamine release in the nucleus accumbens shell as did the local perfusion of thioperamide. However, the effect of intra-accumbal perfusion of thioperamide was smaller than those elicited by its systemic administration (Munzar et al. 2004), indicating that the observed potentiation may also include actions at the level of other neurotransmitter systems. On the other hand, H3R-mRNA is not expressed in the ventral tegmental area (Pillot et al. 2002), the main source of dopaminergic innervation to nucleus accumbens (Wise 2004), questioning a direct action of histamine at pre-synaptic H3Rs located on accumbal dopaminergic nerve terminals. Further, the systemic administration of the H3R agonist immepip significantly attenuated the behavioral-stimulant effects of methamphetamine in mice but not in monkeys (Banks et al. 2009), re-inforcing the hypothesis of species-related differences in the action of H3R ligands.

Microdialysis studies have also demonstrated enhanced dopamine release in rat prefrontal cortex after the administration of the H3R antagonists ABT-239 (Fox et al. 2005), BF2.649 (Ligneau et al. 2007) and GSK-189254 (Medhurst et al. 2007). Dopamine release was not affected by the H3R antagonist ABT-239 in the striatum of anaesthetized rats (Fox et al. 2005).

A study of our own showed that H3R activation also exerted an inhibitory influence on depolarization-evoked dopamine synthesis in rat striatal slices (Molina-Hernández et al. 2000). In line with this observation, the H3R agonist imetit reduces L-DOPA-induced increase in dopamine content in microdialysis samples from rat striatum (Nowak et al. 2008). While these results support a direct action of pre-synaptic H3Rs located on dopaminergic nigro-striatal terminals, the lack of effect of H3R-receptor activation on dopamine release from rat striatal slices discussed before leads to considering alternative mechanisms such as trans-synaptic effects of H3R agonists or modulation of dopamine synthesis occurring in non-dopaminergic neurons, such as 5-HT-releasing neurons (Tanaka et al. 1999).

15.3.6 Modulation of Glutamate Release

The first evidence for H3R-mediated modulation of glutamate release was provided by Brown and Reymann (1996), who showed that histamine reduced by 24% the slope of both field excitatory postsynaptic potentials (fEPSPs) and excitatory postsynaptic currents (EPSCs) in the molecular layer of the rat hippocampal dentate gyrus. Depression of fEPSPs was mimicked by RAMH and blocked by thioperamide, but not by H1- or H2-receptor antagonists. Histamine increased the EPSC coefficient of variation, had no effect on EPSCs evoked by activating glutamate AMPA receptors and enhanced paired-pulse facilitation of both fEPSPs and EPSCs, all these actions being consistent with a pre-synaptic effect.

This study was extended to show that histamine-induced depression of fEPSPs was inversely related to the extracellular Ca^{2+} concentration, and insensitive to ω-conotoxin GVIA or ω-agatoxin. The K^+-channel blocker 4-aminopyridine (4-AP) increased the size of fEPSPs but had not effect on the histamine depression indicating that this effect did not involve H3R-mediated activation of pre-synaptic K^+ channels. Histamine inhibition was occluded by activating adenosine A_1 receptors supporting a pre-synaptic locus of action (Brown and Haas 1999). Further, miniature excitatory postsynaptic currents (mEPSCs) recorded from the somata of granule cells using the whole-cell configuration of the patch clamp technique were slightly reduced in frequency by histamine without effect on mEPSC amplitude.

Electrophysiological evidence for histamine modulation of glutamatergic transmission has also been provided for rat striatum, basolateral amygdala and thalamus. In rat striatum histamine decreased extracellular field potentials (FPs) by 30% ($IC_{50} = 1.6\ \mu M$), an effect mimicked by RAMH and prevented by thioperamide. In intracellular recordings from GABAergic striatal projection neurons with a paired-pulse protocol, histamine and RAMH reduced the slope of the first EPSP but increased paired-pulse facilitation (Doreulee et al. 2001). Histamine also depressed FPs in mouse striatum but to a lesser extent (–10%), indicating species-related differences.

In slices of the rat amygdala, histamine reduced by ~30% the amplitude of the EPSPs induced by stimulation in the external capsula ($EC_{50} = 0.47\ \mu M$), and this action was mimicked by RAMH and blocked by thioperamide. In addition, histamine increased paired-pulse facilitation of the slope of EPSPs, attenuated both the NMDA- and the AMPA/kainate-receptor component of EPSPs, and the latter effect was also abolished by thioperamide (Jiang et al. 2005). In rat thalamus, glutamatergic field potentials evoked by stimulation of the internal capsula showed inhibition of the second response in the paired-pulse protocol. The selective H3R agonist immepip reduced the first response and significantly increased the FP2/FP1 ratio, suggesting a pre-synaptic action prevented by the H3R antagonist clobenpropit (Garduño-Torres et al. 2007).

In rat striatal synaptosomes the Ca^{2+}-dependent release of endogenous glutamate evoked by 4-aminopyridine (4-AP), which by blockade of K^+ channels produces TTX-sensitive repetitive firing and neurotransmitter release (Tibbs et al. 1989), was inhibited by immepip (–60%, $IC_{50} = 68$ nM) and this effect was blocked by the antagonist thioperamide with $K_i = 4$ nM (Molina-Hernández et al. 2001). H3R-mediated inhibition of endogenous glutamate release was also shown in rat thalamus synaptosomes (Garduño-Torres et al. 2007).

The synaptosomal preparation allows for the measurement of changes in the levels of intraterminal Ca^{2+} ($[Ca^{2+}]_i$), and in fura 2-loaded striatal synaptosomes depolarization with 4-AP resulted in a significant increase in $[Ca^{2+}]_i$ ($\Delta[Ca^{2+}]_i = 88 \pm 15$ nM), which was reduced (~30%) by immepip, with this effect being prevented by thioperamide (Molina-Hernández et al. 2001).

15.3.7 Modulation of GABA Release

The first evidence for the participation of H3Rs in regulating GABA release (García et al. 1997) was obtained in the *substantia nigra pars reticulata* (SNr), a neuronal nucleus intimately involved in the control of motor behavior and that expresses one of the highest levels of H3Rs in mammalian brain.

In rat SNr slices [^{3}H]-GABA release induced by depolarization with 15 mM K^+ was inhibited (–70%) by the dopamine D_1-like receptor antagonist SCH-23390, consistent with a large component of release dependent on the activation of these receptors by endogenous dopamine. Both histamine and the H3R selective agonist immepip inhibited K^+-evoked [^{3}H]-GABA release by ~80%, and the effect was prevented by the H3R antagonist thioperamide, while in the presence of SCH-23390 depolarization-induced [^{3}H]-GABA release was not affected by H3R activation. Further, in rats depleted of dopamine by pretreatment with reserpine, immepip no longer inhibited depolarization-induced [^{3}H]-GABA release, but in the presence of the D_1-like receptor agonist SKF-38393, which produced a 7-fold stimulation of release, immepip reduced the release to control levels (García et al. 1997). Striato-nigral neurons posses collaterals that remain in the striatum, and Ca^{2+}-dependent, K^+-evoked release of [^{3}H]-GABA from striatal slices from reserpinized rats was also greatly increased by D_1-like receptor activation. This action was markedly inhibited by histamine (–78%; $IC_{50} = 1.3$ μM) and immepip (–81%; $IC_{50} = 16$ nM), and the effect of the latter was reversed by the H3R antagonists thioperamide and clobenpropit (Arias-Montaño et al. 2001). Taken together these pieces of evidence indicate that in the nerve terminals of striato-nigral neurons, previously shown to express both D_1-like and H3-receptors (Ryu et al. 1994), H3R activation inhibits the same component of [^{3}H]-GABA release enhanced by D_1-like receptor stimulation.

In slices of rat medial vestibular nucleus Bergquist et al. (2006) showed that the increase in endogenous GABA release evoked by perfusion with high (60 mM) K^+ was also significantly reduced (~50%) by immepip ($IC_{50} = 0.2$ nM) and histamine, with the immepip effect being blocked by an equimolar concentration of the H3R antagonist clobenpropit.

Supporting a role for H3Rs in modulating GABA release, this action has also been shown in dissociated or cultured neurons. In mechanically dissociated neurons from the ventromedial nucleus of the rat hypothalamus the application of histamine

(IC_{50} = 440 nM) or the H3R agonist imetit (IC_{50} = 4.7 nM) reduced by 25% the frequency of GABAergic spontaneous inhibitory postsynaptic currents (sIPSCs) without affecting the mean current amplitude. The imetit effect was completely abolished by the H3R antagonists clobenpropit and thioperamide (Jang et al. 2001). In primary cultures of rat cerebro-cortical neurons (Dai et al. 2007), clobenpropit (100 nM) enhanced the release of endogenous GABA to 268% of controls, with the action being reversed by the H3R agonist RAMH (100 μM). The clobenpropit-induced enhancement of neurotransmitter release could be explained by either the blockade of tonic activation of H3Rs by endogenous histamine or by the expression of constitutively active H3Rs.

Finally, Welty and Shoblock (2009) report that in the rat prefrontal cortex perfusion with 100 mM K^+ increases the content of GABA in microdialysis perfusates with systemically administered thioperamide attenuating this effect. The action of the antagonist/inverse agonist thioperamide is opposite to that expected from previous reports and, as pointed out by the authors, it may involve an action at post-synaptic H3Rs located on GABA interneurons or trans-synaptic processes that may even rely on neuronal loops between the prefrontal cortex and histaminergic neurons located in the tuberomamillary nucleus.

In contrast with these pieces of information, two studies of our own failed to shown any significant action of H3R activation on Ca^{2+}-dependent, K^+-evoked [^{3}H]-GABA release from slices and synaptosomes of rat thalamus and globus pallidus (Garduño-Torres et al. 2007, Osorio-Espinoza et al. 2009). These results suggest that H3R-mediated regulation of GABA release depends on the brain region studied and that not all GABAergic neurons express H3Rs.

Several lines of evidence indicate that when present H3R-mediated modulation of GABA release involves an action of $G\alpha_{i/o}$ proteins at P/Q-type voltage-operated Ca^{2+}channels. In dissociated neurons from the hypothalamic ventromedial nucleus the GTP-binding protein inhibitor *N*-ethylmaleimide (NEM) prevented the histaminergic inhibition of GABAergic sIPSCs, while elimination of external Ca^{2+} reduced sIPSC frequency, but no the distribution of current amplitudes, and abolished the inhibitory effect of imetit on sIPSC frequency (Jang et al. 2001). Further, the H3R-mediated reduction in GABAergic sIPSC frequency was occluded by the P/Q-type Ca^{2+} channel blocker ω-agatoxin IVA, but not by the N-type Ca^{2+} channel blocker ω-conotoxin GVIA or the L-type Ca^{2+} channel blocker nicardipine. As discussed before, depolarization-induced [^{3}H]-GABA release from striatal slices is facilitated by dopamine D_1-like receptor activation, and this effect was mimicked by 8-bromo-cyclic AMP (Br-cAMP) and inhibited by the protein kinase A (PKA) inhibitor H-89 (Arias-Montaño et al. 2007). [^{3}H]-GABA release stimulated by D_1-receptor activation was markedly reduced by ω-agatoxin TK, a P/Q-type channel blocker, while neither ω-conotoxin MVIIA (N-type channel Ca^{2+} channel blocker) nor nimodipine (L-type Ca^{2+} channel blocker) had significant effects. The stimulatory effects of D_1-like receptor activation and Br-cAMP on [^{3}H]-GABA release were practically abolished by H3R receptor activation. These observations indicate that D_1-like receptor-mediated facilitation and H3R receptor-mediated inhibition of GABA release from striatal terminals converge at P/Q-type Ca^{2+} channels.

15.3.8 Modulation of Substance P Release

Non-adrenergic, non-cholinergic broncho-constriction in guinea-pig induced in vivo by vagal stimulation was reduced by the systemic administration of either histamine or the selective H3R agonist RMHA (maximal inhibition 46% at 10 mg/kg i.v.), with the effect of the latter being blocked by the H3R antagonist thioperamide. RAMH did not affect bronchoconstriction induced by exogenous substance P (Ichinose and Barnes 1989). Likewise, non-adrenergic non-cholinergic contraction elicited by electric field stimulation of the guinea-pig isolated ileum longitudinal muscle-myenteric plexus preparation was blocked by neurokinin NK_1 receptor antagonists as well as by histamine and the H3R agonists RAMH and NAMH. H3R antagonists caused parallel concentration-related rightward shifts in the agonist concentration-response curve (Taylor and Kilpatrick 1992). These studies suggested that H3R activation inhibited the release of neuropeptides (SP and neurokinins) from sensory nerve endings.

Support for a role for H3R in controlling neuropeptide release was provided by two studies in which the levels of substance P were determined by radioimmunoassay. Antidromic electrical stimulation of the sciatic nerve resulted in an increase in substance P content in subcutaneous perfusates in the rat hindpaw and the systemic administration of the H3R agonist RAMH inhibited this action in a dose-related manner while thioperamide antagonized this effect (Ohkubo et al. 1995). Likewise, in perfused rabbit lungs the capsaicin-induced increase in substance P release was prevented by imetit (Nemmara et al. 1999). These results indicate that via presynaptic H3Rs histamine regulates substance P release from peripheral endings of sensory nerves.

In a second study by Ohkubo and Shibata (1995) the H3R-mediated inhibition of substance P release in the rat hindpaw was significantly antagonized by the ATP-sensitive K^+ channel blocker glibenclamide and by tetraethylammonium, a general K^+ channel blocker, leading the authors to postulate that the control by H3Rs of substance P release from sensory nerve endings was achieved by activating ATP-sensitive K^+ channels. However, the only report in the literature for H3R-mediated modulation of K^+ channels refers to a different type of channels, the G protein-gated inwardly rectifying channels (GIRKs; Sahlholm et al. 2007).

15.4 Final Remarks

Evidence is accumulating for a significant role for histamine in modulating nervous system function through H3Rs whose activation controls the release of several important neurotransmitters. The increasing knowledge of the role played by H3Rs both in normal and pathophysiological conditions have targeted drug discovery efforts to the receptor and several pharmaceutical companies are currently active in this field.

H3R agonists might have therapeutic use in sleep disorders, pain relief, prevention and treatment of myocardial ischaemic arrhythmias, and neurogenic inflammatory processes involved in migraine, while antagonists are being tested for the treatment of obesity and sleep and cognitive disorders (Leurs et al. 2005). In particular, the potential therapeutic use for cognitive disorders is based on the ability of H3R antagonists to enhance the release of neurotransmitters such as histamine, ACh, noradrenaline and dopamine that play critical roles in cognitive processes, and bears special interest for the treatment of attention deficit hyperactivity disorder, Alzheimer's disease and schizophrenia. The integration of drugs acting at H3Rs into effective treatment of neurological disorders requires of continued research efforts that further our insight into the H3R function.

References

Alves-Rodrigues A, Timmerman H, Willems E et al (1998) Pharmacological characterization of the histamine H_3 receptor in the rat hippocampus. Brain Res 788:179–186

Arias-Montaño J-A, Florán B, Florán L et al (2007) Dopamine D_1 receptor facilitation of depolarisation-induced release of γ-aminobutyric acid (GABA) in rat striatum is mediated predominantly via P/Q-type calcium channels. Synapse 61:310–319

Arias-Montaño J-A, Florán B, García M et al (2001) Histamine H_3 receptor-mediated inhibition of depolarisation-induced, dopamine D_1 receptor-dependent release of [^{3}H]-γ-aminobutyric acid in rat striatum. Br J Pharmacol 133:165–171

Arrang J-M, Drutel G, Schwartz J-C (1995) Characterization of histamine H_3 receptors regulating acetylcholine release in rat entorhinal cortex. Br J Pharmacol 114:1518–1522

Arrang J-M, Garbarg M, Schwartz J-C (1983) Auto-inhibition of brain histamine release mediated by a novel class (H_3) of histamine receptor. Nature 302:832–837

Arrang JM, Garbarg M, Schwartz J-C (1985) Autoregulation of histamine release in brain by presynaptic H_3-receptors. Neuroscience 15:553–562

Arrang J-M, Garbarg M, Schwartz J-C (1987) Autoinhibition of histamine synthesis mediated by presynaptic H_3-receptors. Neuroscience 23:149–157

Arrang J-M, Morisset S, Gbahou S (2007) Constitutive activity of the histamine H_3 receptor. Trends Pharmacol Sci 28:350–357

Bacciottini L, Passani MB, Giovannelli L et al (2002) Endogenous histamine in the medial septum-diagonal band complex increases the release of acetylcholine from the hippocampus: a dual-probe microdialysis study in the freely moving rat. Eur J Neurosci 15:1669–1680

Bakker RA (2004) Histamine H_3-receptor isoforms. Inflamm Res 53:509–516

Bakker RA, Flores-Lozada A, van Marle A et al (2006) Discovery of naturally occurring splice variants of the rat histamine H_3 receptor that act as dominant-negative isoforms. Mol Pharmacol 69:1194–1206

Banks ML, Manvich DF, Bauzo RM et al (2009) Effects of histamine H_3 receptor activation on the behavioral-stimulant effects of methamphetamine and cocaine in mice and squirrel monkeys. Pharmacology 83:164–169

Barbier AJ, Aluisio L, Lord B et al (2007) Pharmacological characterization of JNJ-28583867, a histamine H_3 receptor antagonist and serotonin reuptake inhibitor. Eur J Pharmacol 576: 43–54

Bergquist F, Ruthven A, Ludwig M et al (2006) Histaminergic and glycinergic modulation of GABA release in the vestibular nuclei of normal and labyrinthectomised rats. J Physiol 577:857–868

Bertrand PP, Bertrand RL (2010) Serotonin release and uptake in the gastrointestinal tract. Auton Neurosci 153:47–57

Blandina P, Giorgetti M, Bartolini L et al (1996) Inhibition of cortical acetylcholine release and cognitive performance by histamine H_3 receptor activation in rats. Br J Pharmacol 8:1656–1664

Bongers G, Bakker RA, Leurs R (2007a) Molecular aspects of the histamine H_3 receptor. Biochem Pharmacol 73:1195–1204

Bongers G, Krueger KM, Miller TR et al (2007b) A 80 amino acid deletion in the third intracellular loop of a naturally occurring human histamine H_3 isoform confers pharmacological differences and constitutive activity. J Pharmacol Exp Ther 323:888–898

Bongers G, Sallmen T, Passani MB et al (2007c) The Akt/GSK-3β axis as a new signaling pathway of the histamine H_3 receptor. J Neurochem 103:248–258

Brown RE, Haas HL (1999) On the mechanism of histaminergic inhibition of glutamate release in the rat dentate gyrus. J Physiol 515:777–786

Brown RE, Reymann KG (1996) Histamine H_3 receptor-mediated depression of synaptic transmission in the dentate gyrus of the rat *in vitro*. J Physiol 496:175–184

Celuch SM (1995) Possible participation of histamine H_3 receptors in the modulation of noradrenaline release from rat spinal cord slices. Eur J Pharmacol 287:127–133

Clapham J, Kilpatrick GJ (1992) Histamine H_3 receptors modulate the release of [^{3}H]-acetylcholine from slices of rat entorhinal cortex: evidence for the possible existence of H_3 receptor subtypes. Br J Pharmacol 107:919–923

Coge F, Guenin SP, Audinot V et al (2001) Genomic organization and characterization of splice variants of the human histamine H_3 receptor. Biochem J 355:279–288

Dai H, Fu Q, Shen Y et al (2007) The histamine H_3 receptor antagonist clobenpropit enhances GABA release to protect against NMDA-induced excitotoxicity through the cAMP/protein kinase A pathway in cultured cortical neurons. Eur J Pharmacol 563:117–123

Di Carlo G, Ghi P, Orsetti M (2000) Effect of R-(-)-α-methylhistamine and thioperamide on *in vivo* release of norepinephrine in the rat hippocampus. Prog Neuropsychopharmacol Biol Psychiatry 24:275–284

Doreulee N, Yanovsky Y, Flagmeyer I et al (2001) Histamine H_3 receptors depress synaptic transmission in the corticostriatal pathway. Neuropharmacology 40:106–113

Drutel G, Peitsaro N, Karlstedt K et al (2001) Identification of rat H_3 receptor isoforms with different brain expression and signaling properties. Mol Pharmacol 59:1–8

Du XJ, Dart AM (1993) Mechanisms of noradrenaline release in the anoxic heart of the rat. Cardiovasc Res 27:2011–2015

Endou M, Poli E, Levi R (1994) Histamine H_3-receptor signaling in the heart: possible involvement of G_i/G_o proteins and N-type Ca^{++} channels. J Pharmacol Exp Ther 269:221–229

Esbenshade TA, Browman KE, Bitner RS et al (2008) The histamine H_3 receptor: an attractive target for the treatment of cognitive disorders. Br J Pharmacol 154: 1166–1181

Fink K, Schlicker E, Neise A et al (1990) Involvement of presynaptic H_3 receptors in the inhibitory effect of histamine on serotonin release in the rat brain cortex. Naunyn Schmiedeberg's Arch Pharmacol 342:513–519

Fox GB, Esbenshade TA, Pan JB et al (2005) Pharmacological properties of ABT-239 [4-(2-{2-[(2R)-2-Methylpyrrolidinyl]ethyl}-benzofuran-5-yl)benzonitrile]:II. Neurophysiological characterization and broad preclinical efficacy in cognition and schizophrenia of a potent and selective histamine H_3 receptor antagonist. J Pharmacol Exp Ther 313: 176–190

Frieling T, Cooke HJ, Wood JD (1993) Histamine receptors on submucous neurons in guinea pig colon. Am J Physiol 264:G74–80

García M, Florán B, Arias-Montaño J-A et al (1997) Histamine H_3 receptor activation selectively inhibits dopamine D_1 receptor-dependent [^{3}H]GABA release from depolarisation-stimulated slices of rat substantia nigra pars reticulata. Neuroscience 80:241–249

Garduño-Torres B, Treviño M, Gutiérrez R et al (2007) Presynaptic histamine H_3 receptors regulate glutamate, but not GABA release in rat thalamus. Neuropharmacology 52: 527–535

Giannoni P, Passani MB, Nosi D et al (2009) Heterogeneity of histaminergic neurons in the tuberomammillary nucleus of the rat. Eur J Neurosci 29:2363–2374

Gillard M, Van Der Perren C, Moguilevsky N et al (2002) Binding characteristics of cetirizine and levocetirizine to human H_1 histamine receptors: contribution of Lys^{191} and Thr^{194}. Mol Pharmacol 61:391–399

Giorgetti M, Bacciottini L, Bianchi L et al (1997) GABAergic mechanism in histamine H_3 receptor inhibition of K^+-evoked release of acetylcholine from rat cortex *in vivo*. Inflamm Res 46(Suppl 1):S33–S34

Haas H, Panula P (2003) The role of histamine and the tuberomamillary nucleus in the nervous system. Nature Rev Neurosci 4:121–130

Hatta E, Yasuda K, Levi R (1997) Activation of histamine H_3 receptors inhibits carrier-mediated norepinephrine release in a human model of protracted myocardial ischemia. J Pharmacol Exp Ther 283:494–500

Hew RWS, Hodgkinson CR, Hill SJ (1990) Characterization of histamine H_3-receptors in guinea-pig ileum with H_3-selective ligands. Br J Pharmacol 101:621–624

Ichinose M, Barnes PJ (1989) Histamine H_3-receptors modulate nonadrenergic non-cholinergic neural bronchoconstriction in guinea-pig *in vivo*. Eur J Pharmacol 174: 49–55

Imamura M, Lander HM, Levi R (1996) Activation of histamine H_3-receptors inhibits carrier-mediated norepinephrine release during protracted myocardial ischemia. Comparison with adenosine A_1-receptors and α_2-adrenoceptors. Circ Res 78:475–481

Imamura M, Poli E, Omoniyi AT et al (1994) Unmasking of activated histamine H_3-receptors in myocardial ischemia: their role as regulators of exocytotic norepinephrine release. J Pharmacol Exp Ther 271:1259–1266

Imamura M, Seyedi N, Lander HM et al (1995) Functional identification of histamine H_3-receptors in the human heart. Circ Res 77:206–210

Ishikawa S, Sperelakis N (1987) A novel class (H_3) of histamine receptors on perivascular nerve terminals. Nature 327:158–160

Jang I, Rhee J-S, Watanabe T et al (2001) Histaminergic modulation of GABAergic transmission in rat ventromedial hypothalamic neurons. J Physiol 534:791–803

Jansen FP, Mochizuki T, Yamamoto Y et al (1998) *In vivo* modulation of rat hypothalamic histamine release by the histamine H_3 receptor ligands, immepip and clobenpropit. Effects of intrahypothalamic and peripheral application. Eur J Pharmacol 362:149–155

Jiang X, Chen A, Li H (2005) Histaminergic modulation of excitatory synaptic transmission in the rat basolateral amygdale. Neuroscience 131:691–703

Lamberty Y, Margineanu DG, Dassesse D et al (2003) H3 agonist immepip markedly reduces cortical histamine release, but only weakly promotes sleep in the rat. Pharmacol Res 48: 193–198

Leineweber K, Heusch G, Schulz R (2007) Regulation and role of the presynaptic and myocardial Na^+/H^+ exchanger NHE1: effects on the sympathetic nervous system in heart failure. Cardiovasc Drug Rev 25:123–131

Leurs R, Bakker RA, Timmeman H et al (2005) The histamine H_3 receptor: from gene cloning to H_3 receptor drugs. Nature Rev Drug Discov 4:107–121

Leurs R, Brozius MM, Smit MJ et al (1991) Effects of histamine H_1-, H_2- and H_3-receptor selective drugs on the mechanical activity of guinea-pig small and large intestine. Br J Pharmacol 102:179–185

Leurs R, Smit MJ, Menge WM et al (1994) Pharmacological characterization of the human histamine H_2 receptor stably expressed in Chinese hamster ovary cells. Br J Pharmacol 112:847–854

Levi R, Seyedi N, Schaefer U et al (2007) Histamine H_3-receptor signaling in cardiac sympathetic nerves: identification of a novel MAPK-PLA_2-COX-PGE_2-EP_3R pathway. Biochem Pharmacol 73:1146–1156

Levi R, Smith NC (2000) Histamine H_3-receptors: a new frontier in myocardial ischemia. J Pharmacol Exp Ther 292:825–830

Ligneau X, Perrin D, Landais L et al (2007) BF2.649 [1-{3-[3-(4-Chlorophenyl)propoxy]propyl}piperidine, hydrochloride], a nonimidazole inverse agonist/antagonist at the human histamine H_3 receptor: preclinical pharmacology. J Pharmacol Exp Ther 320:365–375

Lovenberg TW, Roland BL, Wilson SJ et al (1999) Cloning and functional expression of the human histamine H_3 receptor. Mol Pharmacol 55:1101–1107

Lovenberg TW, Pyati J, Chang H, Wilson SJ, Erlander MG (2000) Cloning of rat histamine H3 receptor reveals distinct species pharmacological profiles. J Pharmacol Exp Ther 293:771–778

Marinissen MJ, Gutkind JS (2001) G-protein-coupled receptors and signaling networks: emerging paradigms. Trends Pharmacol Sci 22:368–376

Mariottini C, Scartabelli T, Bongers G et al (2009) Activation of the histaminergic H_3 receptor induces phosphorylation of the Akt/GSK-3β pathway in cultured cortical neurons and protects against neurotoxic insults. J Neurochem 110:1469–1478

Mazenot C, Ribuot C, Durand A et al (1999) *In vivo* demonstration of H_3-histaminergic inhibition of cardiac sympathetic stimulation by R-α-methyl-histamine and its prodrug BP 2.94 in the dog. Br J Pharmacol 126:264–268

Medhurst AD, Atkins AR, Beresford IJ et al (2007) GSK189254, a novel H_3 receptor antagonist that binds to histamine H_3 receptors in Alzheimer's disease brain and improves cognitive performance in preclinical models. J Pharmacol Exp Ther 321:1032–1045

Mochizuki T, Okakura-Mochizuki K, Horii A et al (1994) Histaminergic modulation of hippocampal acetylcholine release *in vivo*. J Neurochem 62:2275–2282

Molina-Hernández A, Nuñez A, Arias-Montaño J-A (2000) Histamine H_3-receptor activation inhibits dopamine synthesis in rat striatum. Neuroreport 17163–17166

Molina-Hernández A, Nuñez A, Sierra JJ et al (2001) Histamine H_3 receptor activation inhibits glutamate release from rat striatal synaptosomes. Neuropharmacology 41: 928–934

Moreno-Delgado D, Gómez-Ramírez J, Torrent-Moreno A et al (2009) Different role of cAMP dependent protein kinase and CaMKII in H_3 receptor regulation of histamine synthesis and release. Neuroscience 164:1244–1251

Morisset S, Rouleau A, Ligneau X et al (2000) High constitutive activity of native H_3 receptors regulates histamine neurons in brain. Nature 408: 860–864

Morisset S, Sasse A, Gbahou F et al (2001) The rat H_3 receptor: gene organization and multiple isoforms. Biochem Biophys Res Commun 280:75–80

Morrey C, Estephan R, Abbott GW et al (2008) Cardioprotective effect of histamine H_3-receptor activation: pivotal role of Gβγ-dependent inhibition of voltage-operated Ca^{2+} channels. Pharmacol Exp Ther 326:871–878

Munzar P, Tanda G, Justinova Z et al (2004) Histamine H_3 receptor antagonists potentiate methamphetamine self-administration and methamphetamine-induced accumbal dopamine release. Neuropsychopharmacology 29:705–717

Nemmara A, Delaunois A, Beckers JF et al (1999) Modulatory effect of imetit, a histamine H_3 receptor agonist, on C-fibers, cholinergic fibers and mast cells in rabbit lungs *in vitro*. Eur J Pharmacol 371: 23–30

Nowak P, Bortel A, Dabrowska J et al (2008) Histamine H_3 receptor ligands modulate L-dopa-evoked behavioral responses and L-dopa derived extracellular dopamine in dopamine-denervated rat striatum. Neurotox Res 13:231–240

Ohkubo T, Shibata M (1995) ATP-sensitive K^+ channels mediate regulation of substance P release via the prejunctional histamine H_3 receptor. Eur J Pharmacol 277:45–49

Ohkubo T, Shibata M, Inoue M et al (1995) Regulation of substance P release mediated via prejunctional histamine H_3 receptors. Eur J Pharmacol 273:83–88

Osorio-Espinoza A, Garcia-Ramirez M, Ramos-Jimenez J et al (2009) Modulation by presynaptic histamine H_3 receptors of glutamatergic transmission in rat globus pallidus. In: Abstracts of the British pharmacological society summer meeting 2009, Edinburgh, UK. http://www.pa2online.org/abstracts/Vol7Issue2abst004P.pdf. Retrieved November 18, 2009

Passani MB, Cangioli I, Baldi E et al (2001) Histamine H_3 receptor-mediated impairment of contextual fear conditioning and *in-vivo* inhibition of cholinergic transmission in the rat basolateral amygdala. Eur J Neurosci 14:1522–1532

Pillot C, Héron A, Cochois V et al (2002) A detailed mapping of the histamine H_3 receptor and its gene transcripts in rat brain. Neuroscience 114:173–193

Poli E, Coruzzi G, Bertaccini G (1991) Histamine H_3 receptors regulate acetylcholine release from the guinea pig ileum myenteric plexus. Life Sci 48:PL63–PL68

Prast H, Tran MH, Fischer H et al (1999) Histaminergic neurons modulate acetylcholine release in the ventral striatum: role of H_3 histamine receptors. Naunyn Schmiedeberg's Arch Pharmacol 360:558–564

Racke K, Reimann A, Schworer H et al (1996) Regulation of 5-HT release from enterochromaffin cells. Behav Brain Res 73:83–87

Rouleau A, Heron A, Cochois V et al (2004) Cloning and expression of the mouse histamine H_3 receptor: evidence for multiple isoforms. J Neurochem 90:1331–1338

Ryu JH, Yanai K, Iwata R et al (1994) Heterogenous distribution of histamine H_3, dopamine D_1 and D_2 receptors in rat brain. Neuroreport 5:621–624

Sahlholm K, Nilsson J, Marcellino D et al (2007) The human histamine H_3 receptor couples to GIRK channels in *Xenopus* oocytes. Eur J Pharmacol 567:206–210

Sander K, Kottke T, Stark H (2008) Histamine H_3 receptor antagonists go to clinics. Biol Pharm Bull 31:2163–2181

Savitz J, Lucki I, Drevets WC (2009) 5-HT_{1A} receptor function in major depressive disorders. Prog Neurobiol 88:17–31

Schlicker E, Behling A, Lümmen G et al (1992) Histamine H_{3A} receptor-mediated inhibition of noradrenaline release in the mouse brain cortex. Naunyn-Schmiedeberg's Arch Pharmacol 345:489–493

Schlicker E, Betz R, Göthert M (1988) Histamine H_3-receptor-mediated inhibition of serotonin release in the rat brain cortex. Naunyn-Schmiedeberg's Arch Pharmacol 337:588–590

Schlicker E, Fink K, Detzner M et al (1993) Histamine inhibits dopamine release in the mouse striatum via presynaptic H_3 receptors. J Neural Transm Gen Sect 93:1–10

Schlicker E, Fink K, Hinterhaner M et al (1989) Inhibition of noradrenaline release in the rat brain cortex via presynaptic H_3 receptors. Naunyn-Schmiedeberg's Arch Pharmacol 340:633–638

Schlicker E, Göthert M (1998) Interactions between the presynaptic α_2-autoreceptor and presynaptic inhibitory heteroreceptors on noradrenergic neurons. Brain Res Bull 47:129–132

Schlicker E, Kathmann M, Detzner M et al (1994) H_3 receptor-mediated inhibition of noradrenaline release: an investigation into the involvement of Ca^{2+} and K^+ ions, G protein and adenylate cyclase. Naunyn Schmiedebergs Arch Pharmacol 350:34–41

Schlicker E, Schunack W, Göthert M (1990) Histamine H_3 receptor-mediated inhibition of noradrenaline release in pig retina discs. Naunyn-Schmiedeberg's Arch Pharmacol 342:497–501

Schlicker E, Werthwein S, Zentner J (1999) Histamine H_3 receptor-mediated inhibition of noradrenaline release in the human brain. Fundam Clin Pharmacol 13:120–122

Schömig A (1990) Catecholamines in myocardial ischemia. Systemic and cardiac release. Circulation 82(Suppl II):13–22

Seyedi N, Mackins CJ, Machida T et al (2005) Histamine H_3-receptor-induced attenuation of norepinephrine exocytosis: a decreased protein kinase A activity mediates a reduction in intracellular calcium. J Pharmacol Exp Ther 312:272–280

Silver RB, Mackins CJ, Smith NC et al (2001) Coupling of histamine H_3 receptors to neuronal Na^+/H^+ exchange: a novel protective mechanism in myocardial ischemia. Proc Natl Acad Sci USA 98:2855–2859

Silver RB, Poonwasi KS, Seyedi N et al (2002) Decreased intracellular calcium mediates the histamine H_3-receptor-induced attenuation of norepinephrine exocytosis from cardiac sympathetic nerve endings. Proc Natl Acad Sci USA 99:501–506

Smits RPJM, Mulder AH (1991) Inhibitory effects of histamine on the release of serotonin and noradrenaline from rat brain slices. Neurochem Int 18:215–220

Strakhova MI, Fox GB, Carr TL et al (2008) Cloning and characterization of the monkey histamine H_3 receptor isoforms. Eur J Pharmacol 601:8–15

Takeshita Y, Watanabe T, Sakata T et al (1998) Histamine modulates high-voltage-activated calcium channels in neurons dissociated from the rat tuberomammillary nucleus. Neuroscience 87:797–805

Tanaka H, Kannari K, Maeda T et al (1999) Role of serotonergic neurons in L-DOPA-derived extracellular dopamine in the striatum of 6-OHDA-lesioned rats. Neuroreport 10:631–634
Tardivel-Lacombe J, Morisset S, Gbahou F et al (2001) Chromosomal mapping and organization of the human histamine H_3 receptor gene. Neuroreport 12:321–324
Tardivel-Lacombe J, Rouleau A, Heron A et al (2000) Cloning and cerebral expression of the guinea pig histamine H_3 receptor: evidence for two isoforms. Neuroreport 11:755–759
Taylor SJ, Kilpatrick GJ (1992) Characterization of histamine-H_3 receptors controlling non-adrenergic non-cholinergic contractions of the guinea-pig isolated ileum. Br J Pharmacol 105:667–674
Tedford HW, Zamponi GW (2006) Direct G protein modulation of Ca_v2 calcium channels. Pharmacol Rev 58:837–862
Threlfell S, Cragg SJ, Kallo I et al (2004) Histamine H_3 receptors inhibit serotonin release in substantia nigra pars reticulata. J Neurosci 24:8704 871
Tibbs GR, Barrie AP, Van Mieghem FJ et al (1989) Repetitive action potentials in isolated nerve terminals in the presence of 4-aminopyridine: effects on cytosolic free Ca^{2+} and glutamate release. J Neurochem 53:1693–1699
Timm J, Marr I, Werthwein S et al (1998) H_2 receptor-mediated facilitation and H_3 receptor-mediated inhibition of noradrenaline release in the guinea-pig brain. Naunyn-Schmiedeberg's Arch Pharmacol 357:232–239
Trzeciakowski JP (1987) Inhibition of guinea pig ileum contractions mediated by a class of histamine receptor resembling the H_3 subtype. J Pharmacol Exp Ther 243:874–880
Van der Werf JF, Bast A, Bijloo GJ et al (1987) HA autoreceptor assay with superfused slices of rat brain cortex and electrical stimulation. Eur J Pharmacol 138:199–206
Wellendorph P, Goodman MW, Burstein ES et al (2002) Molecular cloning and pharmacology of functionally distinct isoforms of the human histamine H_3 receptor. Neuropharmacology 42:929–940
Welty N, Shoblock J (2009) The effects of thioperamide on extracellular levels of glutamate and GABA in the rat prefrontal cortex. Psychopharmacology 208:265–277
Westerink BH, Cremers TI, De Vries JB et al (2002) Evidence for activation of histamine H_3 autoreceptors during handling stress in the prefrontal cortex of the rat. Synapse 43:238–243
Wise RA (2004) Dopamine, learning and motivation. Nature Rev Neurosci 5:483–494

Part X
Histamine H4 Receptor: A Noble Target for Inflammatory and Immune Research

Chapter 16
Expression of Histamine H4 Receptor in Human Synovial Cells and Dermal Tissues

Yoshiko Matsuda, Katsunori Yamaura, Masahiko Suzuki, Takao Namiki, and Koichi Ueno

Abstract The last of the four histamine receptors, H4 receptor (H4R), was identified in the year 2000. Since that time, H4R has been implicated in cellular mechanisms related to immune systems, inflammatory processes, and allergic reactions. We reported the expression of H4R in rheumatoid arthritis (RA) synovial cell cultures and human dermal tissues. In the synovial cell cultures, two specific types of cell populations, fibroblast-like and macrophage-like cells, both showed expression of H4R. We also demonstrated H4R expression in human dermal fibroblast and epidermal tissue. When investigating the effect of histamine H4R antagonists on pruritus using a mouse model, JNJ7777120, a H4R antagonist, was found to significantly reduce histamine- and substance P-induced scratching. These results suggest that H4R may be useful for treatment rheumatoid arthritis or pruritus.

Keywords Histamine H4 receptors · Rheumatoid arthritis · H4R-antagonists

Abbreviations

RA	rheumatoid arthritis
H4R	histamine H4 receptor
GPCR	G-protein coupled receptor
HSCC	human synovial cell culture

Contents

K. Ueno (✉)
Department of Geriatric Pharmacology and Therapeutics, Graduate School of Pharmaceutical Sciences, Chiba University, 1-8-1 Inohana, Chuo-ku, Chiba 260-8675, Japan
e-mail: kueno@p.chiba-u.ac.jp

M. Shahid et al. (eds.), *Biomedical Aspects of Histamine*,
DOI 10.1007/978-90-481-9349-3_16, © Springer Science+Business Media B.V. 2010

16.1 Introduction

The histamine H4 receptor (H4R) is the newest of the four histamine receptors to be identified; it belongs to the same G-protein coupled receptor (GPCR) family as other histamine receptors. It's the total H4R amino acid sequence shares approximately 37% homology with that of H3R, and 58% homology in the transmembrane regions (Oda and Matsumoto 2001). Furthermore, H4R couples to $G_{i/o}$ proteins and shows ligand affinities similar to that of H3R.

Several organs express H4R, and immune tissues such as the spleen, thymus, bone marrow and leukocytes have a wide range of expressions (Oda et al. 2000). It was reported that chemotaxis of mast cells and eosinophils is stimulated by histamine via H4R; the receptor is therefore attractive as a new target of research into allergic diseases (de Esch et al. 2005).

16.2 Expression of H4R in Rheumatoid Arthritis Synovial Cell Culture

Histamine has been implicated in rheumatoid arthritis (RA). RA consists mainly of synovial tissue inflammation that may be dispersed throughout the body, but its molecular etiology remains unclear. Macrophage infiltration and excessive formation of fibroblasts cause a variety of cytokines to be secreted from synovial membranes in RA patients, and this in turn stimulates osteolytic activity (Sweeney and Firestein 2004). There is documented evidence of significant increase in histamine concentration in synovial samples from RA patients (Frewin et al. 1986). These observations indicated potentially significant roles of H4R in the cause, progression and treatment of RA.

The presence of H1R and H2R in human synovial cell culture (HSCC) has been clearly shown by ligand binding experiments (Nagata 1991). However, there has been no definitive evidence or conclusive reports of the similar presence of H3R and H4R. Therefore, utilizing our expertise in RT-PCR techniques, we examined the H4R specific mRNA expression in HSCC obtained from 11 RA patients who underwent artificial knee replacement surgery (Ikawa et al. 2005).

After excising the synovial membrane specimen under aseptic conditions, the sample was treated with collagenase and trypsin solution to separate it into single cells. The cells were cultured in an FBS-containing medium for 2 weeks. When the culture converged, the cells were harvested and all RNA extracted. The expression of histamine receptor-specific mRNA was analyzed by the RT-PCR method. Analysis

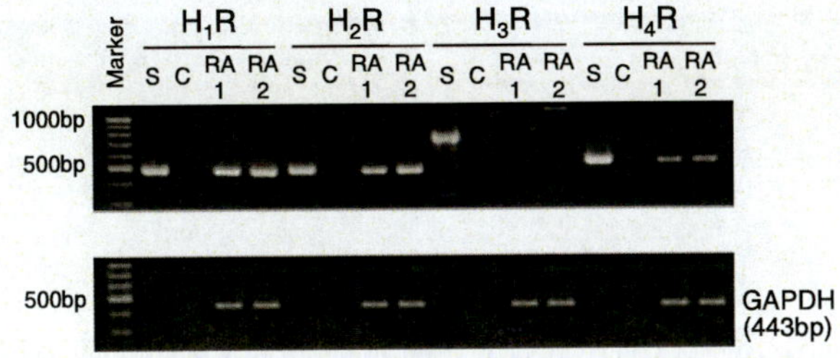

Fig. 16.1 Expression of mRNAs specific to 4 subtypes of histamine receptor (H1R, H2R, H3R and H4R) in human synovial cell cultures from 2 RA patients. The gel was loaded with 5 μL of amplified products. 100 bp DNA Ladder indicates molecular weight marker. S: standard; C: control; samples from 2 RA patients, RA1 and RA2. Figure reprinted with permission from the Pharmaceutical Society of Japan

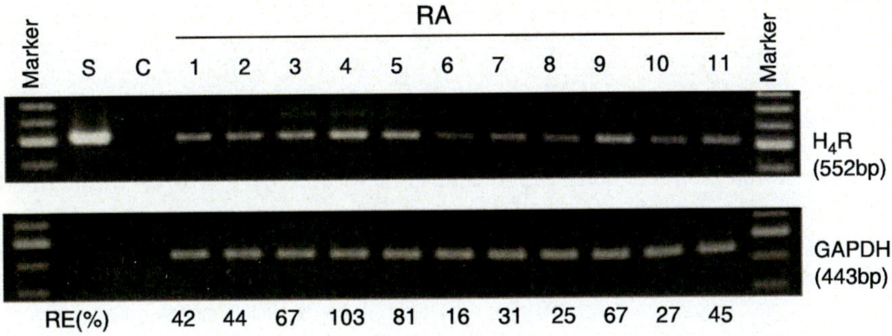

Fig. 16.2 Expression of H4R-specific mRNA in human synovial cell cultures from 11 RA patients. The gel was loaded with 5 μL of amplified products. 100 bp DNA Ladder indicates molecular weight marker. S: standard; C: control; sample from 11 different RA patients, RA1 to RA11 RE (relative expression): Relative expression of mRNA was calculated by normalizing the separated sample intensity value, taking that of the corresponding internal control (GAPDH) as 100%. Intensity values were measured using an image analyzer (IX81, OLYMPUS). Figure reprinted with permission from the Pharmaceutical Society of Japan

of expression of the 4 subtypes in 2 individual RA patients (RA1 and RA2) showed that, under the experimental conditions, H1R-, H2R- and H4R-specific mRNAs were expressed, but H3R-specific mRNA was absent (Fig. 16.1). Expression of H4R-specific mRNA was confirmed in all 11 samples, RA1–RA11 (Fig. 16.2). Notably, intensity of the separated H4R-specific mRNA bands varied considerably from one sample to another, suggesting differences in cellular concentrations of H4R between the RA patients.

Inflamed synoviocytes consist of three cell types: (1) macrophage-like cells (type A); (2) fibroblast-like cells (type B); and (3) dendritic cells (type D) (Tanaka 2005). High levels of lymphocyte infiltration have been observed in RA compared to other types of arthritis (Fonseca et al. 2005). A variety of cell types such as

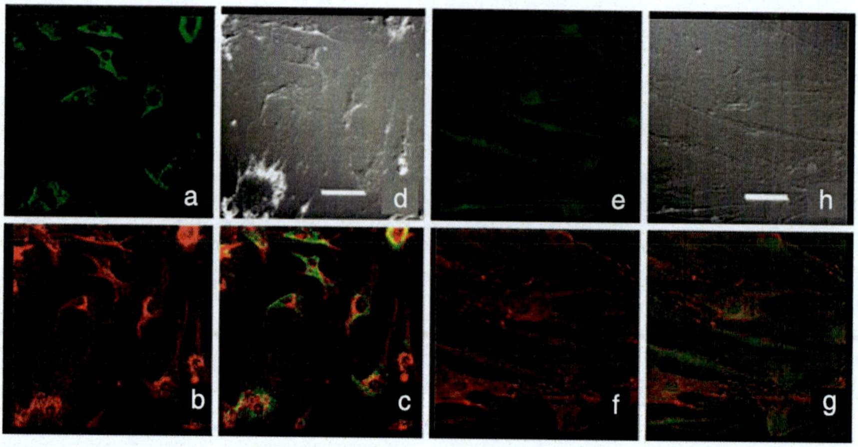

Fig. 16.3 Co-expression of H4R Protein with fibroblast-specific marker proteins. (**a**) mouse anti-PH then Cy2 anti-mouse (*green*); (**b**) rabbit anti-H4R then Cy3 anti-rabbit (*red*); (**c**) superposition of a on b; (**d**) NPCMI; (**e**) rabbit anti-H4R then Cy2 anti-rabbit (*green*); (**f**) mouse anti-CD55 (*red*); (**g**) superposition of e on f; (**h**) NPCMI. Bar: 50 μm. Figure reproduced with permission from the Pharmaceutical Society of Japan

macrophage-like cells, dendritic cells and granulocytes have also been identified in the human RA synovium. Since H4R has been reported to be present in immune cells, expression of H4R mRNA seems most likely to occur in cells derived from the hematopoietic system, i.e. macrophage-like or dendritic cells, etc. from synovial

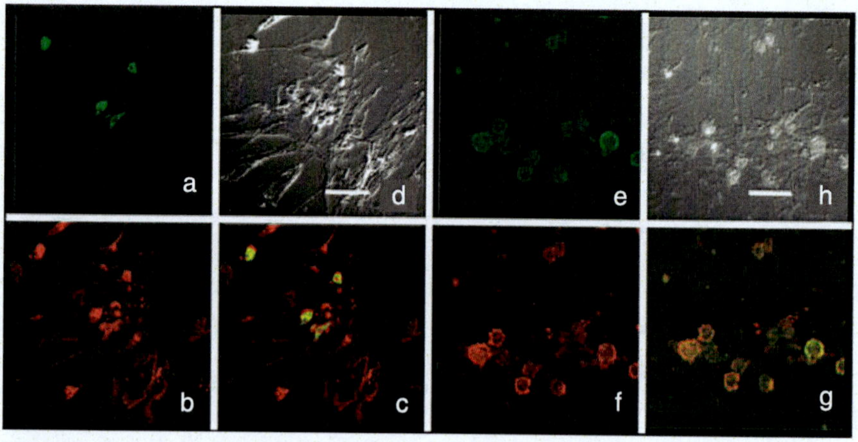

Fig. 16.4 Co-expression of H4R Protein with Macrophage-Specific Marker Proteins. (**a**) mouse anti-CD68 (*green*); (**b**) rabbit anti-H4R then Cy3 anti-rabbit (*red*); (**c**) superposition of a over b; (**d**) NPCMI; (**e**) mouse anti-CD163 (*green*); (**f**) rabbit anti-H4R then Cy3 anti-rabbit (*red*); (**g**) superposition of e on f; h: NPCMI. Bar: 50 μm. Figure reproduced with permission from the Pharmaceutical Society of Japan

sites. Consequently, we examined protein level H4R expression in RA synovial cell cultures, and used fluorescent immunoassay (Ohki et al. 2007) to determine the types of the cells in which expression occurred by identifying co-expression of cell type-specific proteins: human PH and human CD55 for fibroblast-like cells; human CD68 and human CD163 for macrophage-like cells, and human CD1a and human CD208 for dendritic cells.

First, we examined the expression patterns of PH (red) and CD68 (green). There are two morphologically distinct cell types: fibroblast-like and macrophage-like cells. In similar experiments, expression of human dendritic cell markers (either CD1a or CD208) was not detectable. Subsequent assays for fibroblast and macrophage markers showed that human H4R protein is expressed in both fibroblast-like and macrophage-like cells in RA synovial tissues (Figs. 16.3 and 16.4).

Other groups have also reported identification of H4R in synovial tissue of RA patients (Grzybowska-Kowalczyk et al. 2007). These observations indicate that H4R is a target of novel potential pharmacotherapeutic agents for RA; H4R functional analysis may be useful in developing such treatments.

16.3 Expression of H4R in Human Dermal Tissue

Following detection of H4R-expression in synovial tissue, we also analyzed H4R expression in human dermal tissue (Yamaura et al. 2009). Our immunoassays revealed that H4R is expressed in both human dermal fibroblasts and epidermal tissues.

Dermal fibroblasts are a major component of the dermis. When the skin is damaged, they perform important roles including production of extra cellular matrix (e.g. collagens). Keratinocytes are the major constituent of the epidermis. In our study, immunohistochemical staining showed strong H4R expression in K10-positive differentiated keratinocytes in the prickle cell and granular layers of the epidermis (Fig. 16.5a). In contrast, H4R expression was less in K14-positive proliferating keratinocytes in the basal layer (Fig. 16.5b).

Keratinization proceeds by keratinocytes dividing in the basal lamina and moving to the upper layer as they mature. K10 is expressed in keratinocytes in the early stages following differentiation, whilst K14 is the keratin expressed in undifferentiated keratinocytes. Correspondingly, results of this study suggest that keratinocytes increase expression of H4R following differentiation; further work is necessary to determine the expression mechanism and the receptors' physiological role.

Increased H4R expression has been reported in $CD4^+$ T cells of patients with atopic dermatitis (Gutzmer et al. 2009), and skin mast cells have been shown to express H4R (Lippert et al. 2004). These findings suggest that dermal cells may play an important role, via H4R, in dermal disorders.

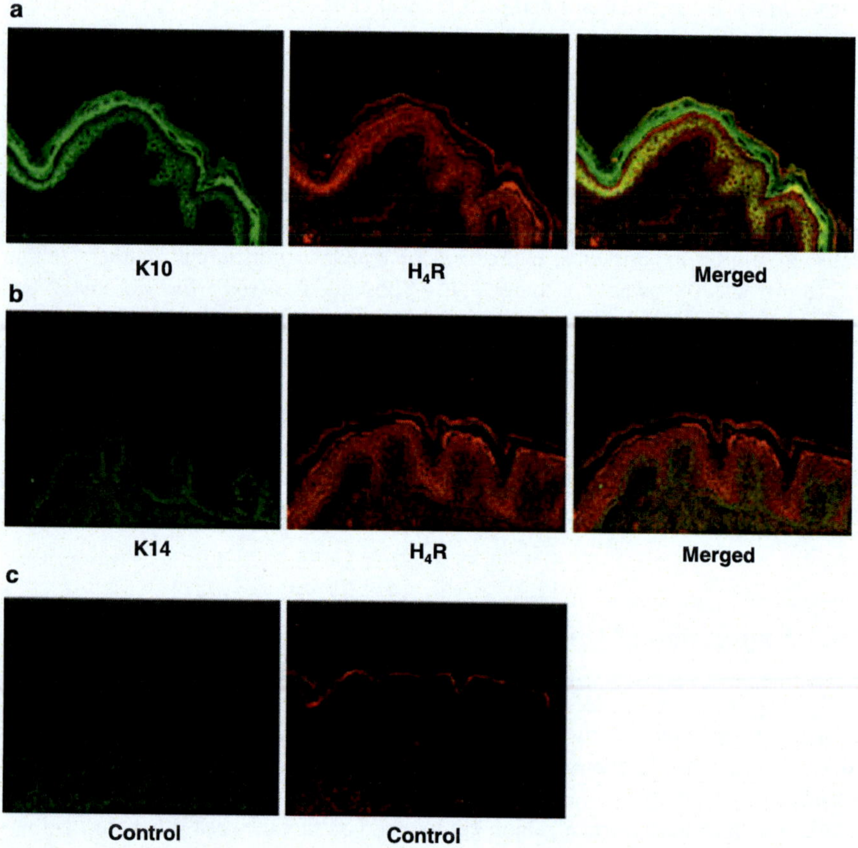

Fig. 16.5 H4R expression in human epidermal tissues. Double immunofluoresence staining of human epidermal tisses with anti- human H4R antibody followed by Cy2-conjugated anti-rabbit secondary antibody (*red*), and anti-K10 (**a**) or anti-K14 (**b**) antibody followed by Cy2-conjugated anti-mouse secondary antibody (*green*). (**c**) Negative control tissues were only exposed to the secondary antibody. Figure reprinted with permission from the Japanese Society of Toxicology

16.4 Effect of H4R Antagonists on Pruritus Model

Pruritus, associated with chronic diseases such as atopic dermatitis, is poorly controlled clinically and has a major effect on the quality of life of patients. Recent studies have raised the possibility that H4R may be an additional histamine receptor contributing to histamine-mediated pruritic responses in mice (Bell et al. 2004). Both specific H4R agonists and histamine were shown to induce pruritic responses which could be blocked by pretreatment with H4R antagonists; the response was also found to be markedly attenuated in H4R-deficient mice. We thus examined the effectiveness of selective H4R antagonists as antipruritc drugs by their effect on histamine H1R antagonist-resistant pruritus in mice, induced by substance P.

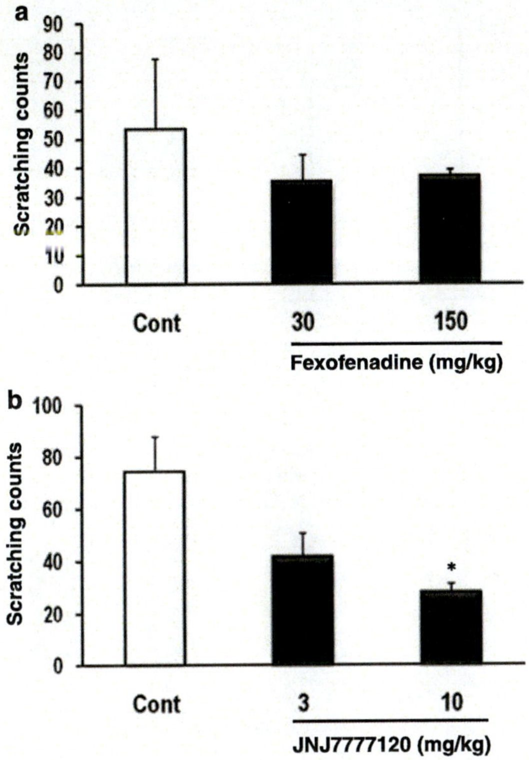

Fig. 16.6 Effect of H4R on scratching behavior induced by histamine. Histamine (300 nmol) was injected intradermally into shaved skin on the back of each mouse. Immediately after the injection of pruritogen, scratching events were counted for 30 min using MicroAct. Fexofenadine (**a**) or JNJ7777120 (**b**) was administered orally 20 min before the pruritogen injection. Values represent the mean ± SEM of four mice. *$p<0.05$ vs. control (Dunnett's multiple comparisons). Figure reprinted with permission from the Japanese Society of Toxicology

We first investigated the effect of the H1R antagonist, fexofenadine, and H4R antagonist, JNJ7777120, on histamine-induced pruritus (Yamaura et al. 2009). Oral administration of fexofenadine caused a slight reduction in scratching, whereas JNJ7777120 showed a significant reduction (Fig. 16.6). We then examined the effect of these antagonists in substance P-mediated pruritus. Fexofenadine showed no reduction in substance P-induced scratching. In contrast, JNJ7777120 at 10 and 30 mg/kg doses reduced substance P-induced scratching by an amount dependent on the dose (Fig. 16.7). Although JNJ7777120 crosses the blood-brain barrier, it does not cause sedation in rodents (Dunford et al. 2007); hence its pruritic inhibitory action is not a secondary effect of sedation. The results suggest that H1R has only limited involvement in histamine-induced pruritus; in contrast, the significant effect of the JNJ7777120 suggest that H4R has a large involvement. Substance P-induced pruritus is resistant to H1R antagonists (Togashi et al. 2002); given its occurrence

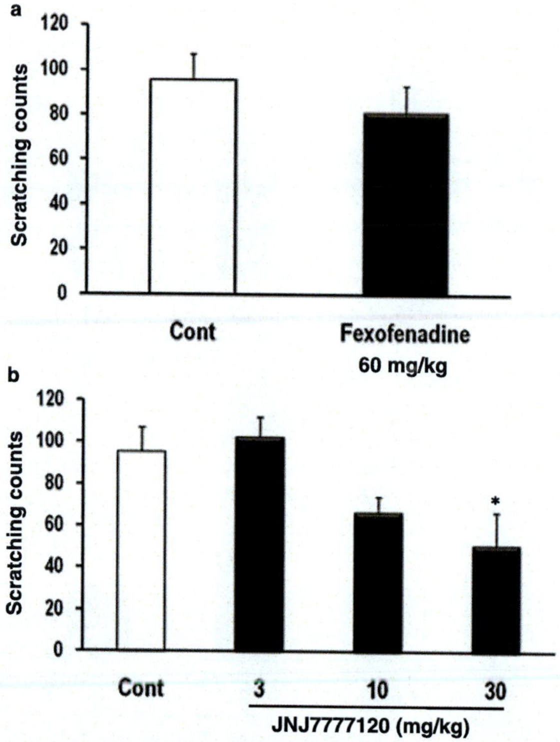

Fig. 16.7 Effect of H4R on scratching behavior induced by substance P. Substance P (100 nmol) was injected intradermally into shaved skin on the back of each mouse. Immediately after the injection of pruritogen scratching events were counted for 30 min using MicroAct. Fexofenadine (**a**) or JNJ7777120 (**b**) was administered orally 20 min before the pruritogen injection. Values represent the mean ± SEM of four mice. *$p<0.05$ vs. control (Dunnett's multiple comparisons). Figure reprinted with permission from the Japanese Society of Toxicology

in mast cell deficient mice (Andoh et al. 2001), histamine of mast cell is thought not to be involved. The role of H1R is also thought to be small, with fexofenadine having no observable effect. However, the suppression of the pruritic response by JNJ7777120 suggests that histamine may have an involvement via H4R rather than H1R.

16.5 Conclusion

We reported the expression of H4R in human synovial cells from RA patients and dermal tissues and demonstrated that H4R antagonist inhibits both histamine- and substance P-induced scratching in a mouse model. These results suggest that H4R may be a likely target for treatments for either RA or pruritus.

References

Andoh T, Katsube N, Maruyama M et al (2001) Involvement of leukotriene B(4) in substance P-induced itch-associated response in mice. J Invest Dermatol 117:1621–1626

Bell JK, McQueen DS, Rees JL (2004) Involvement of histamine H4 and H1 receptors in scratching induced by histamine receptor agonists in Balb C mice. Br J Pharmacol 142:374–380

de Esch IJ, Thurmond RL, Jongejan A et al (2005) The histamine H4 receptor as a new therapeutic target for inflammation. Trends Pharmacol Sci 26:462–469

Dunford PJ, Williams KN, Desai PJ et al (2007) Histamine H4 receptor antagonists are superior to traditional antihistamines in the attenuation of experimental pruritus. J Allergy Clin Immunol 119:176–183

Fonseca JE, Cortez-Dias N, Francisco A et al (2005) Inflammatory cell infiltrate and RANKL/OPG expression in rheumatoid synovium: comparison with other inflammatory arthropathies and correlation with outcome. Clin Exp Rheumatol 23:185–192

Frewin DB, Cleland LG, Jonsson JR et al (1986) Histamine levels in human synovial fluid. J Rheumatol 13:13–14

Grzybowska-Kowalczyk A, Wojtecka-Lukasik E, Maslinska D et al (2007) Distribution pattern of histamine H4 receptor in human synovial tissue from patients with rheumatoid arthritis. Inflamm Res 56(Suppl 1):S59–S60

Gutzmer R, Mommert S, Gschwandtner M et al (2009) The histamine H4 receptor is functionally expressed on T(H)2 cells. J Allergy Clin Immunol 123:619–625

Ikawa Y, Suzuki M, Shiono S et al (2005) Histamine H4 receptor expression in human synovial cells obtained from patients suffering from rheumatoid arthritis. Biol Pharm Bull 28:2016–2018

Lippert U, Artuc M, Grützkau A et al (2004) Human skin mast cells express H2 and H4, but not H3 receptors. J Invest Dermatol 123:116–123

Nagata Y (1991) The role of histamine in human synovial fibroblasts. Med J Kinki Univ 6:117–126 (in Japanese)

Oda T, Matsumoto S (2001) Identification and characterization of histamine H4 receptor. Nippon Yakurigaku Zasshi 118:36–42

Oda T, Morikawa N, Saito Y et al (2000) Molecular cloning and characterization of a novel type of histamine receptor preferentially expressed in leukocytes. J Biol Chem 275:36781–36786

Ohki E, Suzuki M, Aoe T et al (2007) Expression of histamine H4 receptor in synovial cells from rheumatoid arthritic patients. Biol Pharm Bull 30:2217–2220

Sweeney SE, Firestein GS (2004) Rheumatoid arthritis: regulation of synovial inflammation. Int J Biochem Cell Biol 36:372–378

Tanaka M (2005) Autoimmune abnormality. Nippon Rinsho 63(Suppl 1):80–83 (in Japanese)

Togashi Y, Umeuchi H, Okano K et al (2002) Antipruritic activity of the kappa-opioid receptor agonist, TRK-820. Eur J Pharmacol 435:259–264

Yamaura K, Oda M, Suwa E et al (2009) Expression of histamine H4 receptor in human epidermal tissues and attenuation of experimental pruritus using H4 receptor antagonist. J Toxicol Sci 34:427–431

Part XI
Role of Histamine in Reproductive Function

Chapter 17
Novel Role for Histamine Through Classical H1 and H2 Receptors: Regulation of Leydig Cell Steroidogenesis and its Implications for Male Reproductive Function

Carolina Mondillo and Omar Pedro Pignataro

Abstract Most of the physiological functions of HA described to date have been linked to the well-characterized H1 and H2 receptors. Nevertheless, extensive research is continuously going on to elucidate new roles for these receptors. In this respect, recent reports have indicated expression of H1 and H2 receptors in germinal and peritubular cells of the testis, as well as in macrophages and Leydig cells. Interestingly, HA plays a role as autocrine/paracrine modulator of Leydig cell steroidogenesis in several experimental models, both in vivo and in vitro. It was demonstrated very recently that this modulatory effect is concentration-dependent and biphasic: while H1 receptor activation would be responsible for HA-mediated negative modulation of steroidogenesis, H2 receptor activation would lead to stimulation of steroid synthesis. Because antihistamine drugs target HA receptors, the novel role of HA as modulator of testicular steroidogenesis will surely attract more attention to possible unexpected side-effects of such drugs, which might alter the local balance and in turn enhance or decrease androgen production. Considering that HA has been implicated in spermatogenesis, penile erection and sexual behavior as well as steroidogenesis, it appears that the amine plays an integral role in the regulation of male reproductive functions which certainly deserves further investigation.

C. Mondillo (✉)
Laboratory of Molecular Endocrinology and Signal Transduction, Institute of Biology and Experimental Medicine (IByME – CONICET), Vuelta de Obligado 2490, C1428ADN, Buenos Aires, Argentina
e-mail: mondillo@dna.uba.ar

Part of the data reported in this chapter is reprinted with permission from 'Histamine: Biology and Medical Aspects'. Falus A, Darvas S and Grossman N (eds), SpringMed Publishing Ltd, Budapest, 2004.

M. Shahid et al. (eds.), *Biomedical Aspects of Histamine*,
DOI 10.1007/978-90-481-9349-3_17, © Springer Science+Business Media B.V. 2010

Keywords Histamine · Histamine H1 receptor · Histamine H2 receptor · Leydig cell · Male reproductive function

Abbreviations

HA	histamine
HDC-KO	histidine decarboxylase knockout
LH/hCG	luteinizing hormone/human chorionic gonadotropin
AC	adenylate cyclase
PLC	phospholipase C
IP_3	inositol 1, 4, 5-trisphosphate
STAR	steroidogenic acute regulatory
NO	nitric oxide
NOS	NO synthase
cGMP	cyclic guanosine-3′,5′-monophosphate
GC	guanylate cyclase
NAME	N (G)-nitro-L-arginine methyl ester

Contents

17.1 Introduction

Histamine (HA) is undoubtfully one of the most important biogenic amines in medicine and biology. It is an extremely versatile molecule with a wide range of physiological functions, including smooth muscle contraction, vascular permeability regulation, stimulation of gastric acid secretion, neurotransmission, immunomodulation and cell proliferation, among others (Falus et al. 2004). The physiological versatility of HA resides in its capacity to activate at least four different receptors (H1, H2, H3 and H4). These are all G protein-coupled molecules which, upon HA binding, initiate the activation of diverse signaling cascades (Hough 2001, Igaz 2004).

Most of the physiological functions of HA described above have been linked to the well-characterized H1 and H2 receptors (H1R and H2R, respectively), for which potent agonists and antagonists have already been developed. Nevertheless, extensive research is continuously going on to elucidate new roles for these receptors. With particular regard to the male reproductive system, although evidence accumulated in the last three decades strongly suggested the existence of functional H1R and H2R (Cara et al. 1995, Kim et al. 1995, Mayerhofer et al. 1989, Nemetallah et al. 1983), it was not until recently that the expression of these receptors was demonstrated in specific cell types. In this respect, H1R and H2R have been identified in germinal and peritubular cells of the testis, as well as in macrophages and Leydig cells (Albrecht et al. 2005, Khan and Rai 2007, Mondillo et al. 2005, 2007).

17.2 Histamine and Male Reproductive Functions

To date, there are good reasons to suppose that the presence of HA is required for normal male reproductive functions: (1) HA plays a role as autocrine/paracrine modulator of Leydig cell steroidogenesis in several experimental models in vitro (Khan and Rai, 2007, Mayerhofer et al. 1989, Mondillo et al. 2005, 2009). There is also evidence for an in vivo modulation of testicular steroid synthesis by HA. Pap et al. (2002) have reported HA deficiency in histidine decarboxylase knockout (HDC-KO) mice leads to altered testicular and serum steroid levels compared to wild type mice, with no differences in hypothalamic GnRH mRNA expression; (2) HA has been demonstrated to induce penile erection in humans, mice and rabbits (Cara et al. 1995, Kim et al. 1995, Martinez et al. 2006, Nimmegeers et al. 2008); (3) Safina et al. have suggested HA synthesis by mouse male germ cells. Their observations indicate that HA can be produced in and from the acrosomes (Safina et al. 2002); (4) HA has been implicated in the regulation of sexual behavior. In this regard, Pár et al. (2003) have reported impaired reproduction in HDC-KO mice, caused predominantly by a decreased male mating behavior. Moreover, long term disruption of male reproductive behavior as well as reduced testis weight was observed in rats exposed perinatally to astemizole, a H1R antagonist (Almeida et al. 1996).

17.2.1 Unraveling the Mechanism of Histamine Action on Leydig Cell Steroidogenesis

It was demonstrated very recently that the modulatory effect of HA on steroidogenesis is concentration-dependent and biphasic, at least in mouse, rat and wall lizard Leydig cells: while 1 nM HA can stimulate basal steroid production and significantly increase the response to Luteinizing Hormone/human Chorionic Gonadotropin (LH/hCG), 10 μM HA exerts an inhibitory effect (Khan and Rai 2007, Mondillo et al. 2005, 2009). These findings appear to be at variance with the reported effects of HA in the golden hamster, where low concentrations had no effect on steroidogenesis, while high concentrations were stimulatory (Mayerhofer et al. 1989). It could be speculated that hamster Leydig cells have a lower sensitivity to HA than mouse, rat or wall lizard Leydig cells and thus respond to higher concentrations of the amine. Whether this is in fact the case is a question that requires further investigation. From a physiological perspective, having opposing effects on steroidogenesis HA could possibly contribute to the homeostatic control of steroid levels within the testis. Interestingly, HA is known to have biphasic effects on other, non-steroidogenic target cells (Martinez et al. 2000, Mikkelsen et al. 1984).

Recent studies employing selective H1R and H2R agonists/antagonists in mammalian and non-mammalian experimental models have shed light on the mechanism of HA action in Leydig cells (Khan and Rai 2007, Mondillo et al. 2005, 2009). On the basis of these studies, the response to stimulatory HA concentrations would be mainly mediated by H2R. Agonist activation of H2R leads to an augmentation of intracellular cAMP production in Leydig cells, suggesting H2R couples to the adenylate cyclase (AC) system. Considering cAMP is the main second messenger for LH/hCG action on steroidogenesis, such increase in cAMP concentration would partly explain the potent stimulatory effect of HA on basal and gonadotropin-induced steroid formation. In agreement, previous reports have documented HA-induced enhancement of ovarian steroidogenesis via H2R activation and increased cAMP production (Schmidt et al. 1987). Figure 17.1 shows a schematic

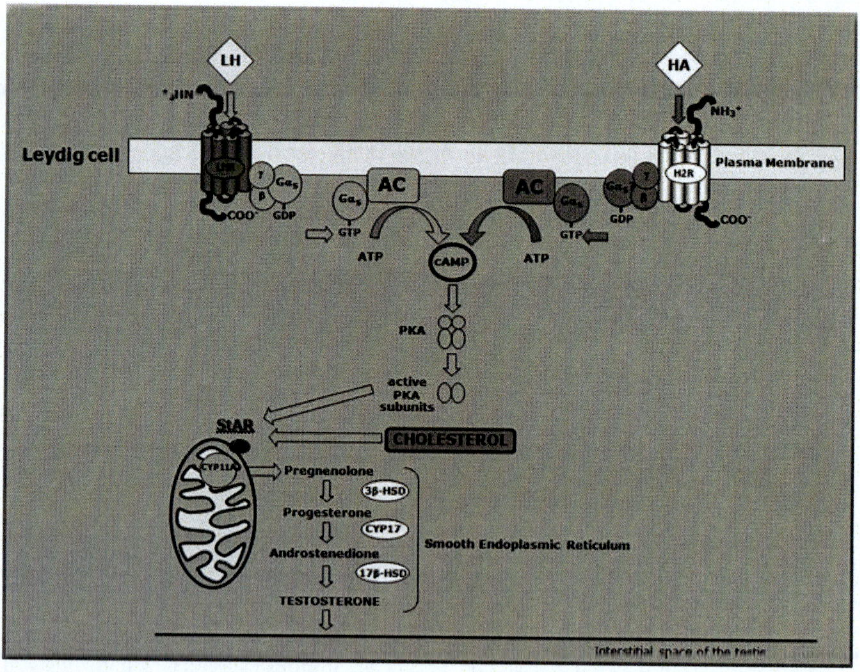

Fig. 17.1 Schematic representation of the possible signal transduction pathway involved in HA-induced stimulation of steroidogenesis via H2R. LH, luteinizing hormone; LHR, LH receptor; HA, histamine; H2R, histamine receptor subtype 2; AC, adenylate cyclase; PKA, protein kinase A; StAR, steroidogenic acute regulatory protein; CYP11A, cholesterol side chain cleavage enzyme (P450scc); 3β-HSD, 3β-hydroxisteroid dehydrogenase Δ(5)-Δ(4) isomerase; CYP17, 17 alpha-hydroxylase/17,20-lyase; 17β-HSD, 17-β-hydroxysteroid dehydrogenase

representation of the possible signal transduction pathway involved in HA-induced stimulation of steroidogenesis via H2R.

Reduction of Leydig cell steroidogenesis by inhibitory HA concentrations (10 μM) would be mediated via H1R (Khan and Rai 2007, Mondillo et al. 2005, 2009). H1R couples to phospholipase C (PLC) via the GTP-binding protein Gq in a wide variety of tissues (Leurs et al. 1995). In this regard, H1R activation induces inositol 1, 4, 5-trisphosphate (IP_3) production in MA-10 Leydig cells (Mondillo et al. 2005, 2009). Importantly, very recent evidence indicates that the PLC/IP_3 pathway plays a major role in HA-induced inhibition of Leydig cell function, as demonstrated by the ability of the specific PLC inhibitor U73122 to completely block the antisteroidogenic actions of HA in basal or gonadotropin-stimulated conditions (Mondillo et al. 2009). Activation of H1R in MA-10 cells and rat Leydig cells decreases cAMP levels stimulated by LH/hCG (Mondillo et al. 2005, 2009). These observations indicate a negative cross talk with LH/hCG activated cAMP/PKA signaling pathway, and provide a possible explanation for the inhibitory effect of HA on gonadotropin stimulated steroidogenesis. Acting via H1R, HA also antagonizes LH/hCG action at biochemical steps located beyond cAMP formation. In this regard, HA was shown to decrease db-cAMP-stimulated steroidogenic acute regulatory (STAR) protein expression in MA-10 cells, implying that HA would affect intramitochondrial cholesterol transport. Furthermore, HA was shown to inhibit steps catalyzed by P450-dependent enzymes in the steroidogenic pathway, mainly the conversion of cholesterol to pregnenolone by cholesterol side-chain cleavage enzyme (CYP11A) (Mondillo et al. 2009).

Nitric oxide (NO) is a diffusible and short-lived free radical gas known to have a diverse range of cellular targets (Bredt and Snyder 1994, Moncada et al. 1991). It is synthesized from L-arginine by the action of NO synthase (NOS), an enzyme existing in three isoforms: neuronal NOS (nNOS or NOS I, official symbol NOS1), endothelial NOS (eNOS or NOS III, official symbol NOS3) and inducible NOS (iNOS or NOS II, official symbol NOS2) (Morris and Billiar 1994, Nussler et al. 1994). Among its numerous and diverse biological actions, NO has been shown to regulate several functions within the male reproductive system under physiological and pathological conditions (Rosselli et al. 1998). With particular regard to the testis, NO has been demonstrated to reversibly inhibit LH/hCG-induced steroidogenesis in MA-10 cells and rat Leydig cells by directly affecting cytochrome P450-dependent enzymes involved in the steroidogenic pathway, mainly cholesterol side-chain cleavage enzyme (CYP11A) (Del Punta et al. 1996). Also, there is evidence to suggest an intracellular NO-mediated inhibition of STAR protein expression in Leydig cells (Diemer et al. 2003, Herman and Rivier 2006). Of particular interest, very recent reports have shown that the widely used NOS inhibitor L-NAME can markedly attenuate the inhibitory effects of HA on basal and hCG-stimulated steroid synthesis. Moreover, 10 μM HA treatment augments NOS activity in MA-10 cells (Mondillo et al. 2009). In view of these findings, it has been proposed that endogenously produced NO may at least partially account for the inhibitory effects of HA on the expression of STAR protein, as well as the activity of CYP11A. The significant decline in LH/hCG-stimulated cAMP production provoked by HA in MA-10 cells and rat Leydig cells is probably not mediated by NO, considering that the gas does not modify basal or hCG-stimulated cAMP levels in MA-10 cells (Del Punta et al. 1996). It is therefore possible that such decreased cAMP generation may exert some contribution to HA-induced reduction in steroid synthesis under hormonal stimulation independent of NOS activation. Stimulation of several receptor systems that lead to endothelial or neuronal NO synthesis has been shown to involve G protein-coupled signaling via PLC activation and production of IP_3 (Jaureguiberry et al. 2004, Joshi et al. 2007). NOS1 and NOS3 isoforms are expressed in Leydig cells (Ambrosino et al. 2003, Davidoff et al. 1995, Zini et al. 1996). Thus, it could be speculated that a similar pathway may be responsible for the augmentation of NOS activity by HA in these cells.

In diverse cellular types, NO activates a soluble guanylate cyclase (GC), increasing the levels of cyclic guanosine-3′,5′-monophosphate (cGMP). It has been reported that cGMP stimulates a specific phosphodiesterase in adrenal zone glomerulosa cells, leading to decreased levels of cAMP and aldosterone (MacFarland et al. 1991). Nevertheless, cGMP analogs are incapable of inhibiting steroid synthesis in MA-10 cells (Del Punta et al. 1996) or rat Leydig cells (Reche et al. 2003). Moreover, NO donors do not elevate cGMP levels in MA-10 cells (Del Punta et al. 1996). Based on these observations, it is unlikely that the reported inhibitory effect of HA on hCG-stimulated cAMP production would be due to the activation of a phosphodiesterase in response to the increased levels of NO induced by the amine. In addition, the NOS inhibitor N (G)-nitro-L-arginine methyl ester (L-NAME) attenuates the effect of HA on hCG-induced steroid synthesis, but it cannot completely block it (Mondillo et al. 2009). Figure 17.2 shows a schematic representation of the possible signal transduction pathways involved in HA-induced inhibition of steroidogenesis via H1R.

Interestingly, recent reports indicate that LH/hCG exerts a significant inducing effect on the expression levels of H1R and H2R genes in Leydig cells (Mondillo et al. 2007). This finding reinforces the hypothesis that HA acts as a local modulator of LH actions on Leydig cell function. Importantly, evidence from experiments using the HDC-KO mouse model strongly suggests that HA also plays a role in LH dependent development of Leydig cells. Pap et al. (2002) have reported that HDC-KO mice show significantly reduced testis weight and elevated testicular steroid levels compared with wild-type mice. Moreover, Leydig cell ultrastructure is severely altered in these mice already at the age of 7 days, when the testes have not yet descended from the abdomen. Indeed, isolated HDC KO Leydig cells in culture show lower hCG-induced testosterone production compared with wild type Leydig cells, and hCG does not increase expression levels of H1R and H2R genes (Mondillo et al. 2007). Based on these findings, it appears that prolonged HA deficiency in HDC KO mice affects various aspects of Leydig cell physiology, interfering with normal sexual development.

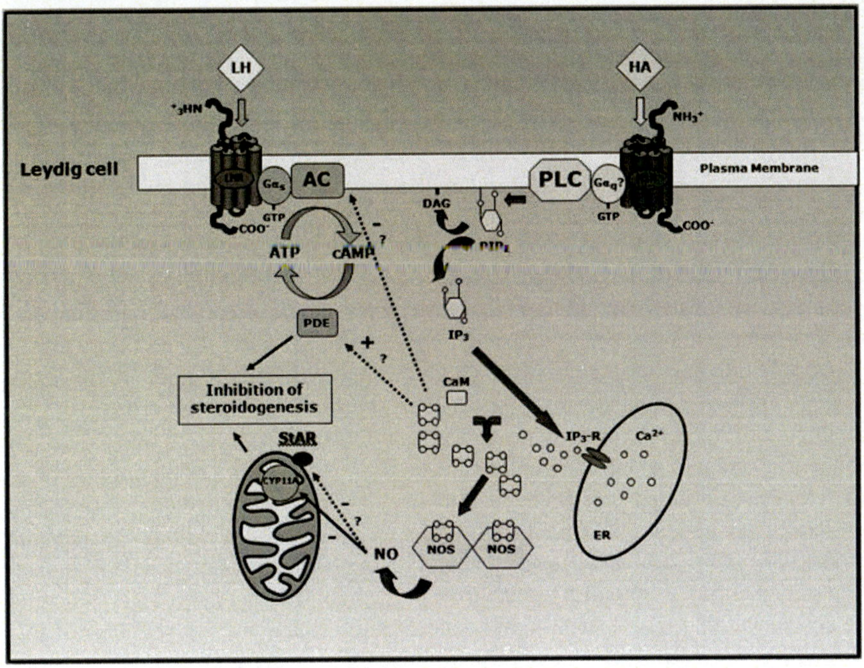

Fig. 17.2 Schematic representation of the possible signal transduction pathways involved in HA-induced inhibition of steroidogenesis via H1R. LH, luteinizing hormone; LHR, LH receptor; HA, histamine; H1R, histamine receptor subtype 1; AC, adenylate cyclase; PLC, phospholipase C, DAG, diacylglycerol, PIP_2, phosphoinositol 4,5-bisphosphate; IP_3, inositol 1,4,5-trisphosphate; IP_3-R, IP_3 receptor; CaM, calcium/calmodulin-dependent protein kinase; NOS, nitric oxide synthase; NO, nitric oxide; StAR, steroidogenic acute regulatory protein; CYP11A, cholesterol side chain cleavage enzyme (P450scc)

17.2.2 Dynamic Interplay Between Testicular Mast Cells and Leydig Cells to Regulate Gonadal Functions

Mast cells are considered to be the main source of HA in the testis (Albrecht et al. 2005). In rodents, mast cells are located near the testicular capsule, while in humans they are frequently encountered in the interstitial spaces (Gaytan et al. 1989, Nistal et al. 1984). A physiological role for these mast cells has not yet been described. However, Gaytan et al. (1992) have reported simultaneous proliferation and differentiation of mast cells and Leydig cells in the rat testis, suggesting the existence of dynamic interactions between the two cell types. This finding is in good agreement the hypothesis that HA may be involved in testicular development. Given that LH can cause ovarian mast cell degranulation in the female (Krishna and Terranova 1985), a similar situation might exist in the male gonad as well. Thus, testicular mast cell-related HA would act in a paracrine way to modulate LH actions on Leydig cells. HA production has also been reported in testicular macrophages (Albrecht et al. 2005, Khan and Rai 2007, Safina et al. 2002), as well as in germ cells (Safina et al. 2002). Because these cell types reside in the vicinity of Leydig cells, they might be sources of HA to regulate Leydig cell function. If this were the case, it would in part resemble the situation in the female mammary gland and uterus, in which two pools of HA modulate physiological functions: mast cell-related and epithelial cell-related HA (Paria et al. 1998, Wagner et al. 2003). To complicate the picture, Lima et al. (2000) have reported testosterone at low concentrations can stimulate peritoneal mast cell maturation or trigger an increase in mast cell numbers in pubertal male rats, while testosterone at high concentrations shows an inhibitory effect. Thus, although mast cells from different tissues may respond differently to the same biological factors, Lima's findings pose a tough question: does testosterone also play an important role in the control of the testicular mast cell population to regulate HA influences on Leydig cell function? Interestingly, Gaytan et al. (1989) have reported the existence of Leydig cell-related inhibitory factors for mast cells in the adult rat testicular interstitium, but not in the interstitium of 30-day-old rats (Nemetallah et al. 1983). These findings are consistent with the fact that testicular HA is considerably higher in the immature gonad than in the adult (Zieher et al. 1971). It could be speculated that HA at such higher concentrations may have a physiological role as negative modulator of testicular steroidogenesis in the immature testis, while HA at lower concentrations would positively influence testosterone synthesis in the mature gonad. Considering that testosterone regulates germ cell maturation through its paracrine effects on Sertoli cells, local regulation of LH actions on Leydig cells is essential to maintain spermatogenesis.

17.3 Concluding Remarks

Because antihistamine drugs target HA receptors, the novel role of HA as modulator of testicular steroidogenesis will surely attract more attention to possible unexpected side-effects of such drugs, which might alter the local balance and in turn enhance or decrease androgen production. In this regard, cimetidine, a potent histaminic H2R antagonist extensively prescribed for ulcers has been found to be a reproductive toxicant in male rats (Franca et al. 2000).

The more we know about HA receptors and their multiple functions, the more opportunity there will be for rational drug design. In this regard, the identification of H3 and H4 receptors (H3R and H4R, respectively) some years ago revived interest in HA research and exposed attractive perspectives for the potential therapeutic exploitation of these new drug targets. However, still very little is known regarding expression of functional H3R or H4R within the male reproductive system. So far, H4R mRNA has been documented to be expressed in an unpurified rat testis cell preparation (Nguyen et al. 2001). This constitutes the only evidence available to support the existence of H4R in the male gonad.

Considering HA has been implicated in spermatogenesis, penile erection and sexual behavior as well as steroidogenesis, it appears that the amine plays an integral role in the regulation of male reproductive function which certainly deserves further investigation. Of note, several reports have linked testicular mast cells with the pathogenesis of testicular disorders (Hussein et al. 2005, Meineke et al. 2000, Schell et al. 2008). Also, there is evidence to indicate that testicular HA concentration can increase significantly under stress conditions (Tuncel et al. 1996, 1997). Bearing this in mind, a potential role of HA in testicular pathology associated with infertility should also be evaluated.

Acknowledgements Supported by grants PICT 05-06381 and 05-38281 from ANPCYT, grant PIP 5525 from CONICET, grant X814 from UBA to OP, grant Carrillo-Oñativia to OP and CM, and a research grant from Fundación Roemmers to CM.

References

Albrecht M, Frungieri MB, Gonzalez-Calvar S et al (2005) Evidence for a histaminergic system in the human testis. Fertil Steril 83:1060–1063

Almeida RG, Massoco CO, Spinosa HS et al (1996) Perinatal astemizole exposure in the rat throughout gestation: long-term behavioral and anatomic effects associated with reproduction. Comp Biochem Physiol C Pharmacol Toxicol Endocrinol 114:123–127

Ambrosino A, Russo D, Lamanna C et al (2003) Isoforms of nitric oxide synthase in the pig testis. Acta Vet BRNO 72:493–498

Bredt DS, Snyder SH (1994) Nitric oxide: a physiologic messenger molecule. Annu Rev Biochem 63:175–195

Cara AM, Lopes-Martins RA, Antunes E et al (1995) The role of histamine in human penile erection. Br J Urol 75:220–224

Davidoff MS, Middendorff R, Mayer B et al (1995) Nitric oxide synthase (NOS-I) in Leydig cells of the human testis. Arch Histol Cytol 58:17–30

Del Punta K, Charreau EH, Pignataro OP (1996) Nitric oxide inhibits Leydig cell steroidogenesis. Endocrinology 137:5337–5343

Diemer T, Allen JA, Hales KH et al (2003) Reactive oxygen disrupts mitochondria in MA-10 tumor Leydig cells and inhibits steroidogenic acute regulatory (StAR) protein and steroidogenesis. Endocrinology 144:2882–2891

Falus A, Darvas S, Grossman N (2004) Histamine: biology and medical aspects. SpringMed, Budapest

Franca LR, Leal MC, Sasso-Cerri E et al (2000) Cimetidine (Tagamet) is a reproductive toxicant in male rats affecting peritubular cells. Biol Reprod 63:1403–1412

Gaytan F, Aceitero J, Lucena C et al (1992) Simultaneous proliferation and differentiation of mast cells and Leydig cells in the rat testis. Are common regulatory factors involved? J Androl 13:387–397

Gaytan F, Carrera G, Pinilla L et al (1989) Mast cells in the testis, epididymis and accessory glands of the rat: effects of neonatal steroid treatment. J Androl 10:351–358

Herman M, Rivier C (2006) Activation of a neural brain-testicular pathway rapidly lowers Leydig cell levels of the steroidogenic acute regulatory protein and the peripheral-type benzodiazepine receptor while increasing levels of neuronal nitric oxide synthase. Endocrinology 147:624–633

Hough LB (2001) Genomics meets histamine receptors: new subtypes, new receptors. Mol Pharmacol 59:415–419

Hussein MR, Abou-Deif ES, Bedaiwy MA et al (2005) Phenotypic characterization of the immune and mast cell infiltrates in the human testis shows normal and abnormal spermatogenesis. Fertil Steril 83:1447–1453

Igaz PHH (2004) Histamine receptors: H1, H2, H3, H4, and the putative "Hic" (intracellular) receptor. Coding genes and gene products, "in silico" and experimental data. In: Falus A, Darvas S, Grossman N (eds) Histamine: biology and medical aspects, SpringMed, Budapest

Jaureguiberry MS, di Nunzio AS, Dattilo MA et al (2004) Endothelin 1 and 3 enhance neuronal nitric oxide synthase activity through ETB receptors involving multiple signaling pathways in the rat anterior hypothalamus. Peptides 25:1133–1138

Joshi MS, Ferguson TB Jr, Johnson FK et al (2007) Receptor-mediated activation of nitric oxide synthesis by arginine in endothelial cells. Proc Natl Acad Sci USA 104:9982–9987

Khan UW, Rai U (2007) Differential effects of histamine on Leydig cell and testicular macrophage activities in wall lizards: precise role of H1/H2 receptor subtypes. J Endocrinol 194:441–448

Kim YC, Davies MG, Lee TH et al (1995) Characterization and function of histamine receptors in corpus cavernosum. J Urol 153:506–510

Krishna A, Terranova PF (1985) Alterations in mast cell degranulation and ovarian histamine in the proestrous hamster. Biol Reprod 32:1211–1217

Leurs R, Smit MJ, Timmerman H (1995) Molecular pharmacological aspects of histamine receptors. Pharmacol Ther 66:413–463

Lima AP, Lunardi LO, Rosa ESAA (2000) Effects of castration and testosterone replacement on peritoneal histamine concentration and lung histamine concentration in pubertal male rats. J Endocrinol 167:71–75

MacFarland RT, Zelus BD, Beavo JA (1991) High concentrations of a cGMP-stimulated phosphodiesterase mediate ANP-induced decreases in cAMP and steroidogenesis in adrenal glomerulosa cells. J Biol Chem 266:136–142

Martinez AC, Garcia-Sacristan A, Rivera L et al (2000) Biphasic response to histamine in rabbit penile dorsal artery. J Cardiovasc Pharmacol 36:737–743

Martinez AC, Hernandez M, Prieto D et al (2006) Enhanced histamine-mediated contraction of rabbit penile dorsal artery in diet-induced hypercholesterolemia. Vascul Pharmacol 44:34–41

Mayerhofer A, Bartke A, Amador AG et al (1989) Histamine affects testicular steroid production in the golden hamster. Endocrinology 125:2212–2214

Meineke V, Frungieri MB, Jessberger B et al (2000) Human testicular mast cells contain tryptase: increased mast cell number and altered distribution in the testes of infertile men. Fertil Steril 74:239–244

Mikkelsen E, Sakr AM, Jespersen LT (1984) Studies on the effect of histamine in isolated human pulmonary arteries and veins. Acta Pharmacol Toxicol (Copenh) 54:86–93

Moncada S, Palmer RM, Higgs EA (1991) Nitric oxide: physiology, pathophysiology, and pharmacology. Pharmacol Rev 43:109–142

Mondillo C, Falus A, Pignataro O et al (2007) Prolonged histamine deficiency in histidine decarboxylase gene knockout mice affects Leydig cell function. J Androl 28:86–91

Mondillo C, Pagotto RM, Piotrkowski B et al (2009) Involvement of nitric oxide synthase in the mechanism of histamine-induced inhibition of Leydig cell steroidogenesis via histamine receptor subtypes in Sprague-Dawley rats. Biol Reprod 80:144–152

Mondillo C, Patrignani Z, Reche C et al (2005) Dual role of histamine in modulation of Leydig cell steroidogenesis via HRH1 and HRH2 receptor subtypes. Biol Reprod 73:899–907

Morris SM Jr, Billiar TR (1994) New insights into the regulation of inducible nitric oxide synthesis. Am J Physiol 266:E829–839

Nemetallah BR, Howell RE, Ellis LC (1983) Histamine H1 receptors and prostaglandin-histamine interactions modulating contractility of rabbit and rat testicular capsules *in vitro*. Biol Reprod 28:632–635

Nguyen T, Shapiro DA, George SR et al (2001) Discovery of a novel member of the histamine receptor family. Mol Pharmacol 59:427–433

Nimmegeers S, Decaluwe K, Van de Voorde J (2008) Characterization of the effect of histamine on mouse corpus cavernosum. Inflamm Res 57(Suppl 1):S59–S60

Nistal M, Santamaria L, Paniagua R (1984) Mast cells in the human testis and epididymis from birth to adulthood. Acta Anat (Basel) 119:155–160

Nussler AK, Billiar TR, Liu ZZ et al (1994) Coinduction of nitric oxide synthase and argininosuccinate synthetase in a murine macrophage cell line. Implications for regulation of nitric oxide production. J Biol Chem 269:1257–1261

Pap E, Racz K, Kovacs JK et al (2002) Histidine decarboxylase deficiency in gene knockout mice elevates male sex steroid production. J Endocrinol 175:193–199

Pár G, Szekeres-Bartho J, Buzas E et al (2003) Impaired reproduction of histamine deficient (histidine-decarboxylase knockout) mice is caused predominantly by a decreased male mating behavior. Am J Reprod Immunol 50:152–158

Paria BC, Das N, Das SK et al (1998) Histidine decarboxylase gene in the mouse uterus is regulated by progesterone and correlates with uterine differentiation for blastocyst implantation. Endocrinology 139:3958–3966

Reche C, Mondillo C, Patrignani Z et al (2003) Effects of nitric oxide on steroidogenesis and expression of nitric oxide synthase isoforms in rat Leydig cells. In: The Endocrine Society's 85th meeting. Program and abstracts: 515 The Endocrine Society, Philadelphia, PA

Rosselli M, Keller PJ, Dubey RK (1998) Role of nitric oxide in the biology, physiology and pathophysiology of reproduction. Hum Reprod Update 4:3–24

Safina F, Tanaka S, Inagaki M et al (2002) Expression of L-histidine decarboxylase in mouse male germ cells. J Biol Chem 277:14211–14215

Schell C, Albrecht M, Mayer C et al (2008) Exploring human testicular peritubular cells: identification of secretory products and regulation by tumor necrosis factor-alpha. Endocrinology 149:1678–1686

Schmidt G, Ahren K, Brannstrom M et al (1987) Histamine stimulates progesterone synthesis and cyclic adenosine 3′,5′-monophosphate accumulation in isolated preovulatory rat follicles. Neuroendocrinology 46:69–74

Tuncel N, Aydin Y, Kosar M et al (1997) The effect of vasoactive intestinal peptide (VIP) on the testicular tissue histamine level of immobilized + cold stressed rats. Peptides 18:913–915

Tuncel N, Gurer F, Aral E et al (1996) The effect of vasoactive intestinal peptide (VIP) on mast cell invasion/degranulation in testicular interstitium of immobilized + cold stressed and beta-endorphin-treated rats. Peptides 17:817–824

Wagner W, Ichikawa A, Tanaka S et al (2003) Mouse mammary epithelial histamine system. J Physiol Pharmacol 54:211–223

Zieher LM, Debeljuk L, Iturriza F et al (1971) Biogenic amine concentration in testes of rats at different ages. Endocrinology 88:351–354

Zini A, O'Bryan MK, Magid MS et al (1996) Immunohistochemical localization of endothelial nitric oxide synthase in human testis, epididymis, and vas deferens suggests a possible role for nitric oxide in spermatogenesis, sperm maturation, and programmed cell death. Biol Reprod 55:935–941

Chapter 18
Possible Effect of Histamine in Physiology of Female Reproductive Function: An Updated Review

Nasreen Noor, Trivendra Tripathi, Shagufta Moin, and Abdul Faiz Faizy

Abstract Histamine belongs to the biogenic amines and is synthesized by the pyridoxal phosphate (vitamin B-6)- containing *L*-histidine decarboxylase (HDC) from the amino acid histidine, and is stored by mast cells, basophils, platelets, histaminergic neurons and enterochromaffine cells in intracellular vesicles. It is released on immunological and non-immunological stimuli. Histamine is an important mediator of several biologic reactions and exerts its effects by binding to its four histamine receptors (H1R, H2R, H3R, and H4R) on target cells in various tissues. Recently accumulating evidences have highlighted significant effects of histamine in normal ovulation, blastocyst implantation, placental blood flow regulation, lactation and contractile activity of uterus, and also in pathological processes such as pre-eclampsia or preterm delivery. However, there is paucity of comprehensive literature covering briefly reviewed imperative findings of histamine in female genital system. This chapter will highlight the important effects of histamine, histamine-metabolizing enzymes and histamine receptors in physiology of female reproductive biology, and it is hoped that this would definitely stimulate further discussions and research on this important aspect.

Keywords Histamine · Histamine intolerance · Pregnancy · Female reproduction

Abbreviations

HDC	histidine decarboxylase
CHO	chinese hamster ovary
hCG	human chorionic gonadotropin
hPL	human placental lactogen
PKC	protein kinase C
MMC	mucosal mast cell

N. Noor (✉)
Department of Obstetrics and Gynaecology, Jawaharlal Nehru Medical College and Hospital, Aligarh Muslim University, Aligarh 202002, UP, India
e-mail: nasreen_71@rediffmail.com

M. Shahid et al. (eds.), *Biomedical Aspects of Histamine*,
DOI 10.1007/978-90-481-9349-3_18, © Springer Science+Business Media B.V. 2010

DAO oxidative deamination
HNMT histamine-*N*-methyltransferase
HIT histamine intolerance

Contents

18.1 Introduction

L-histidine decarboxylase (HDC; EC 4.1.1.22) catalyzes the decarboxylation of *L*-histidine to form histamine (Shahid et al. 2009). Histamine (2-{4-imidazolyl} ethylamine), a monoamine, was discovered in 1910 (Dale and Laidlaw 1910) and plays an important role in both central and peripheral tissues (Hill 1990). The role of histamine in menstrual cycle and pregnancy has been studied for a long period, which is most likely based on interplay between histamine and reproductive steroids and its vasoactive, cell growth- and differentiation promoting properties (Maintz et al. 2008, Matsuyama et al. 2006). On one hand histamine is required during pregnancy in processes such as embryo development, implantation and decidualization (Matsuyama et al. 2006), on the other hand, high levels of circulating maternal blood histamine is harmful to human pregnancy and is involved in a number of complications including pre-eclampsia, spontaneous abortion, preterm labor, and hyperemesis gravidarum (Brew and Sullivan 2006). Thus, it has been suggested that histamine may have dual effects in pregnancy.

18.2 Role of Histamine in Placenta

The placenta, an organ, is essential for successful pregnancy. Placenta arbitrates the physiological exchange between mother and fetus, and exudes hormones, growth factors, cytokines and other bioactive molecules, and protects the fetus from harmful agents getting into the fetal circulation (Matsuyama et al. 2006). The placental villi, which bathe in maternal blood, consists of the outer trophoblasts layer with multinuclear syncytium on the outside and mononuclear cytotrophoblasts on the inside followed by a connective tissue layer consisting of macrophages, fibroblasts, and fetal blood vessels (Benirschke and Kaufmann 2000, Matsuyama et al. 2006). The placenta has been known to contain large amount of histamine and suggesting that histamine plays a role in placenta during pregnancy (Matsuyama et al. 2006). Pap et al. (2006) demonstrated that HDC knockout mice have problems in pregnancy; their birth rate is low, their litter size is small, and their resorption rate is high compared to wild-type mice. Thus histamine is thought to participate in the fine tuning of the process of pregnancy (Matsuyama et al. 2006). The expression of histamine receptors in placenta would be expected. However, there is only limited information on histamine receptors in human placenta. Histamine has four subtypes of its receptors such as H1-, H2-, H3- and H4-receptors (Shahid et al. 2009). However, H1-receptor has been demonstrated to exist in human placenta. On the basis of northern blot analysis, it has been showed that a high level of H1-receptor mRNA exists in human placenta tissues (Fukui et al. 1994). In situ hybridization study also demonstrated the expression of H1-receptor mRNAs in cultured human placental tissues (Brew and Sullivan 2001). In a recent study, Matsuyama et al. (2006) showed that H1-receptor was specifically expressed in syncytiotrophoblast cells in human placenta organ on the basis of following results:

(i) The ligand binding study with stereoisomers of the selective H1-receptor antagonist chlorpheniramine showed that H1-receptors are expressed in human placenta tissue.
(ii) The anti-human H1-receptor antibody has demonstrated to be specific to H1-receptor by Western blot analysis and immunohistochemical analysis of two types of Chinese hamster ovary (CHO) cells, one that expressed recombinant human H1-receptor (CHO- H1-receptor) and the other that did not (CHO[−]).
(iii) The anti-H1-receptor antibody stained the marginal regions of chorionic villus of human placenta, that is, syncytiotrophoblast regions (Boyd and Hamilton 1970).
(iv) The double staining study using the antibody to H1-receptor and that to human chorionic gonadotropin (hCG) demonstrated that H1-receptor and hCG were expressed in the same cells. Because hCG is specifically expressed in placental syncytiotrophoblast cells (Hoshina et al. 1982).

Thus, these results have indicated that H1-receptor is solely expressed in syncytiotrophoblast cells in placenta. The syncytium is a major transport, polarized, secretory epithelium that is essential for establishment and maintenance of pregnancy. However, defects in this formation can be seen in several pregnancy complications (Benirschke and Kaufmann 2000, Boyd and Hamilton 1970, Frendo et al. 2000, Matsuyama et al. 2006).

18.2.1 *Mechanism of Histamine and H1-Receptor in Syncytium Function*

An important mechanism has been explained to demonstrate "How are histamine and H1-receptor involved in syncytium function?" This mechanism explains two possibilities:

(a) First possibility demonstrates that H1-receptor regulate the production of placental peptide hormones such as hCG and human placental lactogen (hPL). These hormones are thought to be involved in the establishment and continuation of pregnancy. For example, hCG that is mainly produced in syncytiotrophoblast cells has been demonstrated to be involved in the differentiation of cytotrophoblasts to syncytium. Furthermore, activation of H1-receptor leads to induction of c-Fos that forms activator protein-1 which binds to promoter regions of various genes, and regulates their expression. Thus, it is possible that H1-receptor regulates the production of placental peptide hormones that play significant roles in pregnancy (Matsuyama et al. 2006).
(b) Second possibility demonstrated that H1-receptor in the syncytium is to regulate the transport of nutrients such as amino acids and glucose from the maternal body to the fetus. It is well known that amino acids and glucose are transported in placenta by several types of amino acid transporters (Jansson 2001, Kudo and Boyd 2002) and glucose transporters (Baumann et al. 2002), respectively. Albeit little is known about the regulation of these transporters, several studies have suggested that protein kinase C (PKC) is involved in some types of amino acid transport (Karl 1995, Roos et al. 2004). Since stimulation of H1-receptor activates PKC (Shahid et al. 2009), it is possible that H1-receptor regulates some types of amino acid transporters in syncytiotrophoblast cells. Thus H1-receptor regulates amino acids transport in the placenta (Matsuyama et al. 2006).

Several studies have shown that in the human placenta, a subpopulation of stem cytotrophoblasts differentiates along two pathways that produce either syncytiotrophoblasts or invasive extravillous trophoblasts (Cross et al. 1994, Fisher and Damsky 1993). Cultured human cytotrophoblast cells (HTR-8/SVneo cells) express H1-receptor, and stimulation of H1-receptor by histamine augments trophoblast invasion. Thus H1-receptor may be involved in the production of invasive extravillous trophoblast that is required for early pregnancy (Matsuyama et al. 2006).

18.3 Effects of Histamine in Mammary Gland

High level of histamine in mouse mammary glands has been observed by Maslinski and Kierska (1991). It has been suggested a possible role of histamine in mammary gland function and development (Wagner et al. 2003). Several in vitro studies have demonstrated the effects of HDC inhibitors and H2-receptor-antagonists on a growth of mammary cancer cells (Hegyesi et al. 2001, Rivera et al. 1994). Maslinski et al. (1993) have showed the first study on the metabolism of histamine in mammary glands, and were demonstrated that the mammary histamine system changes markedly during the estrous cycle as well as during pregnancy and lactation. Furthermore, in vivo and in vitro study was demonstrated the potent physiological effects of histamine on mammary glands (Maslinski et al. 1997a). Histamine receptors-agonists on their own or in the presence of oxytocin enhanced milk secretion. The main histamine immune reactive sites in mammae were mast cells, however some histamine positive signals were found in glandular epithelium and in the stroma (Maslinski et al. 1997b). Previous biochemical studies have shown the active HDC and histamine in mammary glands, and indicated the major changes of mammary system during various physiological states (Maslinski et al. 1997). It was well known that mast cells are rich in histamine (Maslinski 1975a, b). Both HDC and histamine positive mast cells were localized immunohistochemically in mammary glands (Wagner et al. 2003). It was evident from the subcellular analysis that HDC- positive immunoprecipitation is exhibited in granules. The latter observation was agreed well with the study of Japanese group (Tanaka et al. 1998). These authors have been studied the intracellular localization of the 74 and 53-kDa forms of HDC in RBL-2H3 cell line and demonstrated that posttranslationally processed HDC as 53 kDa form is originally localized in the endoplasmic reticulum and Golgi system and then moved and stored in the granules. It should be mentioned that the mast cells found in lactating glands seem to have a different appearance than the cell population in glands from pregnant animals (Wagner et al. 2003). The former cells were rather elongated and have an irregular shape, the latter have a regular and oval shape, were more compact giving stronger histamine signals. Epithelial cells were considered as a second source of histamine (Wagner et al. 2003). The data of several studies have suggested that the epithelial histamine stimulates mammary gland growth and differentiation as well as function during lactation by a paracrine pathway and an autocrine loop (Cricco et al. 1994, Davio et al. 1994, Rivera et al. 2000, Wagner et al. 2003).

In the complex immunochemical study, Wagner et al. (2003) have characterized the mammary epithelial cells and HDC enzyme protein expression. They have demonstrated the HDC protein expression in cultured epithelial cells, especially in dividing and non differentiated cells. Furthermore, it has been showed that the enzyme protein expression was relatively higher than in mammary gland tissue, in which the immunopositive epithelial structures were only found after the use of the more sensitive immunofluorescence method (Wagner et al. 2003). Presence of H1-receptor in resting, pregnancy and lactation stages of mammary gland has been documented. The distribution of H1-receptor in mammary gland has been suggested due to epithelial cells as the density of H1-receptors was significantly higher in isolated mucosal mast cell (MMC) population than in the whole gland (Wagner et al. 2003). Wagner et al. (2003) have been demonstrated the presence of H3-receptors in mammary gland which might be associated with blood vessels and mast cells (Rouleau et al. 1994). Moreover, it was worth noting that the H3-receptor antagonist (FUB 181) had an additive effect on oxytocin stimulated milk secretion from goat mammary glands (Eriksson et al. 1999). However, no evidence was found for the presence of H2-receptors in whole gland preparations or in epithelial cell fractions. Thus, histamine mostly of glandular origin was suggested to be involved in pregnancy mammary outgrowth as well as lactation (Wagner et al. 2003).

18.4 Histamine and Histamine-Degrading Enzyme in Pregnancy

Histamine has been known to contribute to embryo-uterine interactions due to its vasoactive, differentiation and growth-promoting properties. However, its exact functions in pregnancy are unclear (Maintz et al. 2008). Histamine can be metabolized by two alternative pathways:

(a) Oxidative deamination by DAO (former name: histaminase),
(b) Ring methylation by histamine-*N*-methyltransferase (HNMT) (Shahid et al. 2009, Schwelberger 2004).

Whether histamine is catabolized by DAO or HNMT, is supposed to depend on the localization of histamine (Maintz et al. 2008). The DAO protein is stored in plasma membrane-associated vesicular structures in epithelial cells of kidney and intestine and is secreted into the circulation upon stimulation. It has been proposed that DAO might be responsible for scavenging extracellular histamine after mediator release. On the contrary, HNMT, the second important enzyme inactivating histamine, is a cytosolic protein, which can convert histamine only in the intracellular space of cells (Maintz et al. 2008). The DAO also catabolizes other polyamines such as putrescine and spermidine. The highest expression of DAO has been observed in the intestine, kidney and placenta. DAO has been supposed to act as a metabolic barrier to prevent excessive entry of bioactive histamine from the placenta into the maternal or fetal circulation (Maintz et al. 2008).

18.5 Connection of Histamine and its Metabolism in Pregnancy

The equilibrium between histamine and the histamine-metabolizing enzyme DAO appears to be crucial for a normal pregnancy (Brew and Sullivan 2001). Reduced or precipitously falling DAO activities have been observed in high-risk pregnancies, whereas maternal plasma enzyme titers within the normal range have been mostly related with a favorable pregnancy outcome. DAO at the feto-maternal interface has been supposed to operate as a metabolic barrier to prevent excessive entry of histamine from the placenta into the maternal or fetal circulation. An important role of histamine and histamine degrading enzyme has been reported in pregnancy (Maintz et al. 2008). Briefly these important studies explain the significant effects of histamine in pregnancy such as:

(i) Maternal blood histamine levels are comparable to non-pregnant values in the first trimester and decrease during the second and third trimester of normal pregnancies (Maintz et al. 2008).
(ii) High expression of the histamine-producing enzyme HDC in the placenta, histamine receptors at the feto-maternal interface and the existence of an embryonic histamine-releasing factor (EHRF) suggest a physiological role of histamine during gestation (Maintz et al. 2008).
(iii) Histamine functions as a paracrine oxytocic directly on gestational myometrium and indirectly by an increased production of the uterotonic prostaglandin (PGF2α) (Maintz et al. 2008).
(iv) Excessive histamine levels had fatal effects on pregnancy in animal models. It stresses the impact of sufficient histamine degradation during pregnancy. Thus, low activities of the histamine-degrading enzyme DAO might indicate high-risk pregnancies, although high intra- and inter- individual variations limit its value as a screening tool (Maintz et al. 2008).

18.6 Histamine Intolerance (HIT) in Female

HIT results from a disequilibrium of accumulated histamine and the capacity for histamine degradation. Ingestion of histamine-rich food, alcohol or drugs releasing histamine or blocking DAO may provoke diarrhoea, headache, in particular premenstrual headache, dysmenorrhoea, congestion of the nose, asthmatoid wheezing, hypotension, arrhythmia, urticaria, pruritus, flushing etc. in these patients. Symptoms can be reduced by a histamine-free diet or be eliminated by antihistamines, mast cell stabilizers or substitution of DAO (Maintz et al. 2008). It has been reported that in the female genital tract, histamine is mainly produced by mast cells, endothelial cells, and epithelial cells in the uterus and ovaries. HIT women often suffer from premenstrual headache and dysmenorrhea. Besides the contractile action of histamine, these symptoms may be elucidated by the interplay of histamine and hormones (Maintz and Novak 2007). Histamine has been demonstrated to stimulate, in a dose dependent manner, the synthesis of estradiol through H1-receptor; meanwhile, only a moderate effect on progesterone synthesis was noticed (Bodis et al. 1993). The painful uterine contractions of primary dysmenorrhea are mainly caused by an augmented mucosal production of prostaglandine F2α stimulated by estradiol and attenuated by progesterone. Therefore, histamine may enhance dysmenorrhea by escalating estrogen concentrations. In reverse, estrogen can influence histamine action (Maintz and Novak 2007). A significant increase in weal and flare size in response to histamine has been shown to correspond to ovulation and peak estrogen concentrations (Kalogeromitros et al. 1995). In pregnancy, DAO is produced at very high concentrations by the placenta, and its concentration may become 500 times that when the woman is not pregnant. This increased DAO production in pregnant women may be the reason why food intolerance, frequently occur during pregnancy (Maintz and Novak 2007).

18.7 Effects of Histamine in Pregnancy Stages

18.7.1 Early Pregnancy

It has been suggested that histamine plays a part in the decidualization of the endometrium at the beginning of pregnancy (Shelesnyak 1952). This effect can be showed in the rat by the injection of histamine or histamine liberators (Marcus et al. 1963). Kraicer et al. (1963) has been reported that decidualization cannot be induced in the histamine-depleted rat. Several studies have suggested that the fall in the uterine content of histamine which occurs at the time of implantation indicates the specific release of endogenous histamine (Shelesnyak 1959, 1960). Gunther and Paton (1960) have demonstrated important supporting evidence from human pregnancy that the histamine content of the human uterus, like that of the rat, falls when pregnancy occurs. The very great differences between the rat and man in their metabolism of histamine are an indication for extreme caution in making inferences about human pregnancy from observations on the rat. The possibility nevertheless remains that histamine may transform endometrial stroma cells into decidual cells at the onset of human pregnancy and may thus play a part in the nidation of the human ovum (Mitchell 1965). In early pregnancy, histamine was present in "measurable amounts" in blood plasma from the carotid and umbilical arteries of human fetuses (Kahlson and Rosengren 1959), and they concluded from these data that the fetus forms histamine at a high rate (Kahlson et al. 1960). However, the evidence of increased histidine decarboxylase activity in the tissues of fetuses of less than 28 weeks' gestation could not observed, and was therefore unable to confirm that the human fetus produces enhanced amounts of histamine in early pregnancy (Mitchell 1964).

18.7.2 Late Pregnancy

The role of histamine in pregnancy was originated in the discovery by Kahlson et al. (1960). They have demonstrated that in the rat, there is an enormously increased output of histamine in the urine in the last third of pregnancy, and that this histamine is formed by a specific HDC in the fetal liver (Kahlson et al. 1960, Kameswaran and West 1962). However, there was no good evidence that such a phenomenon occurs in human pregnancy. Reports on the urinary excretion of histamine by women in late pregnancy are conflicting but there was no to support record consistently high rate of excretion comparable with that in the rat (Mitchell 1965). Thus, several reports have been demonstrated the normal adult levels of histamine excretion during pregnancy (Rockenschaub 1953, Wicksell 1949), while other studies have observed a modest increase in a proportion of gases (Bjuro et al. 1961). Furthermore, small amounts of a non-specific HDC in the kidney and liver of newborn infants with very little activity in the spleen have been observed (Mitchell 1963). However, Lindberg et al. (1963) have demonstrated the greatest histamine formation in the human fetus using 14C-labelled histidine at term to be in the spleen, with much less in liver and very little in kidney. These differences are probably attributable to the different in vitro methods used, and there is no evidence of the extent to which they reflect in vivo activity. Neither of these studies shows a rate of histamine production by the human fetus comparable with that by the fetal rat. There is diminutive information on the plasma histamine level of the human fetus in later pregnancy (Mitchell 1965). Mitchell and Cass (1959) and Bjuro et al. (1961) measured histamine in whole blood from the umbilical vein of newborn infants. The mean values were higher than the values usually found in adults. Moreover, Bjuro et al. (1961) have also been examined umbilical arterial blood from newborn infants and found that the mean level was higher than the mean for venous blood of normal for adults. These results are suggestive, but since most of the histamine in human blood is in the basophil leukocytes, high levels in whole blood may merely reflect a basophil leucocytosis (Mitchell 1965). Mitchell and Cass (1959) were unable to find any histamine activity, using a relatively insensitive method in a small number of observations on umbilical venous plasma. This could have been due to removal of abnormal quantities of histamine during passage through the placenta. In future studies on newborn infants it should be borne in mind that the results are likely to be complicated by the effects of intra-partum anoxia, which may cause release of histamine into the plasma, thus giving high values which may not correspond with plasma levels under intrauterine conditions (Mitchell 1965) leading to poor pregnancy outcome.

18.8 Conclusion

Histamine is a vital chemical during pregnancy in processes such as embryo development, implantation and decidualization. Thus, the knowledge of the precise mechanism of histamine actions in pregnancy is necessary for treating the complications in pregnancy. It provides significant information about persuade of various drugs related to histamine actions on pregnancy. Therefore, further investigations of histamine effects in pregnancy, the knowledge of the expression and the precise location of histamine receptors in human placenta is essential.

References

Baumann MU, Deborde S, Illsley NP (2002) Placental glucose transfer and fetal growth. Endocrine 19:13–22

Benirschke K, Kaufmann P (2000) Pathology of the human placenta, 4th edn. Springer, New York

Bjuro T, Lindberg S, Westling H (1961) Observations on histamine in pregnancy and the puerperium. Acta Obstet Gynec Scand 40: 152–173

Bodis J, Tinneberg HR, Schwarz H et al (1993) The effect of histamine on progesterone and estradiol secretion of human granulosa cells in serum-free culture. Gynecol Endocrinol 7:235–239

Boyd JD, Hamilton WJ (1970) The human placenta. MacMillan, London

Brew O, Sullivan MH (2006) The links between maternal histamine levels and complications of human pregnancy. J Reprod Immunol 72:94–107

Brew OB, Sullivan MH (2001) Localisation of mRNAs for diamine oxidase and histamine receptors H1 and H2, at the feto-maternal interface of human pregnancy. Inflamm Res 50:449–452

Cricco GP, Davio CA, Martin G et al (1994) Histamine as an autocrine growth factor in experimental mammary carcinomas. Agents Actions 43:17–20

Cross JC, Werb Z, Fisher SJ (1994) Implantation and the placenta: key pieces of the development puzzle. Science 266:1508–1518

Davio C, Martin G, Cricco G et al (1994) Effect of histamine on growth and differentiation of the rat mammary gland. Agents Actions 41:C115–C117

Eriksson L, Fogel WA, Eklund-Uusitalo S (1999) Is histamine involved in milk ejection in goats? Inflamm Res 48(Suppl 1):S90–S91

Fisher SJ, Damsky CH (1993) Human cytotrophoblast invasion. Semin Cell Biol 4:183–188

Frendo JL, Vidaud M, Guibourdenche J et al (2000) Defect of villous cytotrophoblast differentiation into syncytiotrophoblast in Down's syndrome. J Clin Endocrinol Metab 85:3700–3707

Fukui H, Fujimoto K, Mizuguchi H et al (1994) Molecular cloning of the human histamine H1 receptor gene. Biochem Biophys Res Commun 201:894–901

Gunther M, Paton WDM (1960) The histamine content of the human uterus. J Physiol (Lond) 154:417–420

Hegyesi H, Somlai B, Lia Varga V et al (2001) Suppression of melanoma cell proliferation by histidine decarboxylase specific antisense oligonucleotides. J Invest Dermatol 117: 151–153

Hill SJ (1990) Distribution, properties, and functional characteristics of three classes of histamine receptor. Pharmacol Rev 42:45–83

Hoshina M, Boothby M, Boime I (1982) Cytological localization of chorionic gonadotropin alpha and placental lactogen mRNAs during development of the human placenta. J Cell Biol 93: 190–198

Jansson T (2001) Amino acid transporters in the human placenta. Pediatr Res 49:141–147

Kahlson G, Rosengren E (1959) The prevention of foetal development by enzyme inhibition. Nature (Lond) 184:1238–1239

Kahlson G, Rosengren E, White T (1960) The formation of histamine in the rat foetus. J Physiol (Lond) 151:131–138

Kalogeromitros D, Katsarou A, Armenaka M et al (1995) Influence of the menstrual cycle on skin-prick test reactions to histamine, morphine and allergen. Clin Exp Allergy 25:461–466

Kameswaran L, West GB (1962) The formation of histamine in mammals. J Physiol (Lond) 160:564–571

Karl PI (1995) Insulin-like growth factor-1 stimulates amino acid uptake by the cultured human placental trophoblast. J Cell Physiol 165:83–88

Kraicer PF, Marcus GJ, Shelesnyak MC (1963) Studies on the mechanism of decidualization, III. Decidualization in the histamine-depleted rat. J Reprod Fertil 5:417–421

Kudo Y, Boyd CA (2002) Human placental amino acid transporter genes: expression and function. Reproduction 124:593–600

Lindberg S, Lindell SE, Westliig H (1963) Formation and inactivation of histamine by human foetal tissues *in vitro*. Acta Obsret Gynec Scand 42:49–58

Maintz L, Novak N (2007) Histamine and histamine intolerance. Am J Clin Nutr 85:1185–1196

Maintz L, Schwarzer V, Bieberl T et al (2008) Effects of histamine and diamine oxidase activities on pregnancy: a critical review. Human Repro Update 14:485–495

Marcus GJ, Kraicer PF, Shelesnyak MC (1963) Studies on the mechanism of decidualization, II. Histamine releasing action of pyrathiazine. J Reprod Fertil 5:409–415

Maslinski C (1975a) Histamine and its metabolism in mammals. Part I: chemistry and formation of histamine. Agents Actions 5:89–107

Maslinski C (1975b) Histamine and its metabolism in mammals. Part II: catabolism of histamine and histamine liberation. Agents Actions 5:182–225

Maslinski C, Kierska D (1991) Histamine in C3H/W mice carrying spontaneous tumors of the mammary gland. Agents Actions 33:192–194

Maslinski C, Kierska D, Fogel WA (1997a) Histamine stimulates milk release from mammary gland slices. J Physiol Pharm 48:22–26

Maslinski C, Kierska D, Fogel WA et al (1993) Histamine: its metabolism and localization in mammary gland. Comp Biochem Physiol 105C:269–273

Maslinski C, Kierska D, Fogel WA et al (1997b) Histamine in mammary gland: pregnancy and lactation. Comp Biochem Physiol 116A:57–64

Matsuyama K, Ichikawa T, Nitta Y et al (2006) Localized Expression of Histamine H1 Receptors in Syncytiotrophoblast Cells of Human Placenta. J Pharmacol Sci 102:331–337

Mitchell RG (1963) Histidine decarboxylase in the newborn infant. J Physiol (Lond) 166:136–144

Mitchell RG (1964) Histidine decarboxylase in hyaline membrane disease. Arch Dis Childh 39: 73–78

Mitchell RG (1965) Histamine in Human Development. Develop Med Child Neurol 7:278–284

Mitchell RG, Cass R (1959) Histamine and 5-hydroxytryptamine in the blood of infants and children. J Clin Invest 38:595–604

Pap E, Falus A, Mihalyi D et al (2006) Histamine regulates placental cytokine expression-in vivo study on HDC knockout mice. Placenta 28:239–244

Rivera ES, Cricco GP, Engel NI et al (2000) Histamine as an autocrine growth factor: an unusual role for a widespread mediator. Seminars Cancer Biol 10:15–23

Rivera ES, Davio CA, Venturino A et al (1994) Histamine receptors in an experimental mammary carcinoma. Biomed Pharmacother 48:8–9

Rockenschaub A (1953) The urinary excretion of histamine in pregnancy and pre-eclampsia. J Obster Gynec Brit Emp 60:398

Roos S, Powell TL, Jansson T (2004) Human placental taurine transporter in uncomplicated and IUGR pregnancies: cellular localization, protein expression, and regulation. Am J Physiol Regul Integr Comp Physiol 287:R886–R893

Rouleau A, Tuong MD, Newlands GF et al (1994) Fasting or dexamethasone treatment reduce protease content in rat lung mast cells and modulation of histamine synthesis by H3 receptors. Agents Actions 42:7–12

Schwelberger HG (2004) Diamine oxidase (DAO) enzyme and gene. In: Falus A (ed) Histamine: biology and medical aspects, Spring Med, Budapest, pp 43–52

Shahid M, Tripathi T, Sobia F et al. (2009) Histamine, histamine receptors, and their role in immunomodulation: an updated systematic review. Open Immunol J 2:9–41

Shelesnyak MC (1952) Inhibition of decidual cell formation in the pseudo-pregnant rat by histamine antagonists. Am J Physiol 170:522–527

Shelesnyak MC (1959) Fall in uterine histamine associated with ovum implantation in pregnant rat. Proc Soc Exp Biol Med 100:380–381

Shelesnyak MC (1960) Nidation of the fertilized ovum. Endeavour 19:81–86

Tanaka S, Nemoto K, Yamamura E (1998) Intracellular localization of the 74- and 53- kDa forms of L-histidine decarboxylase in a rat basophilic/mast cell line, RBL-2H3. J Biol Chem 273: 8177–8182

Wagner W, Ichikawa A, Tanaka S et al (2003) Mouse mammary epithelial histamine system. J Physiol Pharmacol 54:211–223

Wicksell F (1949) Observations on histamine and histaminolysis in pregnancy. Acta Physiol Scand 17:395–414

Part XII
Other Biomedical Aspects of Histamine Agonists, Antagonists, and Inverse Agonists

Chapter 19
Histamine Role in Malaria

Adil Raza, Haris M. Khan, and Fatima Shujatullah

Abstract Histamine, a biogenic amine derived from the decarboxylation of amino acid histidine by an enzyme histidine decarboxylase. It involves the local immune responses as well as regulating physiological functions. As part of an immune response to foreign pathogen (including malarial parasite infection), histamine is produced by basophils and by mast cells found in nearby connective tissue. Elevation in immune mediators such as IL-1, IL-6, IL-8, TNF-α, NO and histamine have been associated with disease severity in malarial infection. Histamine releasing factor (HRF) is a peptide described in mice and humans, causes the release of histamine from basophils. HRF belongs to a class of protein called translationally controlled tumour protein (TCTP) homologs. Recently a *Plasmodium falciparum* TCTP is identified. This protein has a high homology to human HRF. The central nervous system signs and symptoms such as drowsiness, coma, multiple seizures, destruction of blood brain barrier etc are supposed to be due to histamine secretion in CNS during *Plasmodium falciparum* infection. In this chapter we will discuss the pathophysiological effects of histamine in severe malaria infection.

Keywords Histamine · Histamine releasing factor (HRF) · Plasmodium falciparum · Translationally controlled tumour protein (TCTP)

Abbreviations

TNF-α	tumor necrosis factor-α
IFN-γ	interferon-γ
IL	interleukin
HRF	histamine releasing factor (HRF)
BBB	blood brain barrier
TCTP	translationally controlled tumour protein (TCTP)

A. Raza (✉)
Department of Microbiology, Jawaharlal Nehru Medical College and Hospital, Aligarh Muslim University, Aligarh 202002, UP, India
e-mail: dradil786_786@yahoo.co.in

M. Shahid et al. (eds.), *Biomedical Aspects of Histamine*,
DOI 10.1007/978-90-481-9349-3_19, © Springer Science+Business Media B.V. 2010

HDC	histidine decarboxylase
NMDA	*N*-methyl-D-aspartate

Contents

19.1 Introduction

Each year, 300–500 million people have a malarial illness, and as many as 2.7 million individuals, mostly African children, die (Trigg and Kondrachine 1998). *Plasmodium falciparum* is the parasite responsible for the majority of fatal malarial infections. Malaria infections can cause fever, severe anaemia, coma, and renal failure in children and adults (White 1998) and poor birth outcomes in pregnant women (McGregor 1987).

Cerebral malaria, affects more than 500,000 children in Sub-Sharan Africa per year and it kills more than 100,000 of these children (Murphy and Breman 2001). It is an established fact that cerebral malaria is a result of sequestration of RBCs in the brain parenchyma leading to ischemia, hypoxia, haemorrhage and immunological responses to *P. falciparum* including cytokine responses (Hunt et al. 2006). The role of cytokines and chemokines might be the protection from the direct and indirect effects of the *P. falciparum* (Maheshwari 1990, Schofield et al. 1987), but cytokines and chemokines may also contribute to disease via recruitment of inflammatory cells (Grau et al. 1989a), increased production and activity of other cytokines (Grau et al. 1989b), and direct toxicity to the cells and tissues (Lou et al. 1997, Wassmer et al. 2006). Animal models of cerebral malaria demonstrated involvement of brain parenchyma with activation of microglial cells (Medana et al. 1997a, Schluesener et al. 1998), damage to astrocytes (Ma et al. 1997) and increased mRNA expression of genes regulating tumor necrosis factor-α (TNF-α) (Medana et al. 1997b) and interferon-γ (IFN-γ) (de Kossodo and Grau 1993). This suggests that there would be complex mechanism in the development of cerebral malaria. Several studies have documented the role of histamine in the development of cerebral malaria. The following chemical mediators may involve directly or indirectly in the pathogenesis of cerebral malaria.

i. IL-1
ii. IL-4
iii. IL-6
iv. IL-8
v. IL-13
vi. TNF-α
vii. Nitric oxide
viii. Histamine-releasing factor (HRF)
ix. Histamine, derived from basophils, mast cells and erythrocytes
x. IgE
xi. Translationally controlled tumor protein (TCTP)

Elevations in immune mediators such as IL-1, IL-6, IL-8, TNF-α and nitric oxide have been associated with disease severity in numerous studies (Butcher et al. 1990, Clark and Rockett 1996, Friedland et al. 1993, Grau et al. 1989b, Ho et al. 1998, Kwiatkowski et al.1990, Mordmuller et al. 1997). Eosinophils, basophils, and mast cells also seem to play important roles. Increase in plasma and tissue histamine, derived from basophils and mast cells, have been associated with disease severity in human *P. falciparum* infections and in several animal malarias (Bhattacharya et al. 1988, Enonwu et al. 2000, Maegraith and Fletcher 1972, Srichaikul et al. 1976). In addition, elevated plasma levels of IgE which binds to basophils and mast cells have been associated with severity of *P. falciparum* infection (Perlmann et al. 1999). Furthermore, increased eosinophil counts have been associated with recovery from infection (Camacho et al. 1999, Davis et al. 1991, Kurtzhals et al. 1998). Despite these observations, little is known about the relationship between these cells types and pathogenesis of malaria.

19.2 Histamine: A Brief Account

19.2.1 Histamine

Histamine, a biogenic amine derived from the decarboxylation of amino acid histidine by an enzyme histidine decarboxylase (HDC). It involves the local immune responses as well as regulating physiological functions. It can cause inflammation directly as well as indirectly. Histamine is abundant in skin, lung and gastrointestinal tract. Mast cells are one of the best sources of histamine, but histamine is also secreted by a number of other immune cells (Shahid et al. 2009).

19.2.2 Histamine Receptors

There are four histamine receptors all of which are G protein-coupled. These different receptors are present on various cell types and work through diverse intracellular signalling mechanisms, which explain the diverse effects of histamine in miscellaneous cells and tissues (Shahid et al. 2009), as shown in Table 19.1.

19.3 Cerebral Malaria and Histamine

Toxic effects of histamine were first described by Dale and Richards (1918). The amine has a profound direct effect on vascular smooth muscle (Krogh 1929, Lewis 1927) and it also induces changes in vascular reactivity as an endogenous chemical mediator in bacterial infections. Schayer (1960) and Hinshaw et al. (1961) also documented the release of histamine by bacterial endotoxins.

Histamine causes acute inflammation and it is suggested that it would act in similar manner in case of malaria also. It produces vasodilatation, slowing the local circulation and increasing endothelial permeability in brain of the infected individual. This will result in loss of protein and retention of water resulting brain oedema as shown in Fig. 19.1.

Recent studies have documented that HRF is a peptide, described in mice and humans which causes the release of histamine, IL-4 and IL-13 from basophils (MacDonald et al. 1995, Schroeder et al. 1997). More recently, HRF was shown to promote IL-8 secretion and a calcium response in purified human eosinophils (Bheekha-Escura et al. 2000). Thus, HRF plays an important role in regulating basophils and eosinophils refer to Fig. 19.1.

HRF belongs to a class of proteins that is called the translationally controlled tumor protein (TCTP) homologs. Recently, a *P. falciparum* TCTP was identified (Bhisutthibhan et al. 1998). This protein has a high homology to human HRF, their amino acid sequences found to be 33% identical and 54% similar to human HRF (MacDonald et al. 2001).

Excess of histamine has been demonstrated in venous blood returning from tissues subjected to reactive hyperaemia and from ischaemic tissues (Barsoum and

Table 19.1 Table showing the location and major biologic effects

Histamine receptors	Major tissue locations	Major biologic effects
H1	Smooth muscle, endothelial cells	Acute allergic responses
H2	Gastric parietal cells	Secretion of gastric acid
H3	Central nervous system	Modulating neurotransmission
H4	Mast cells, eosinophils, T cells, dendrite cells	Regulating immune responses

Source: Shahid et al. (2009)

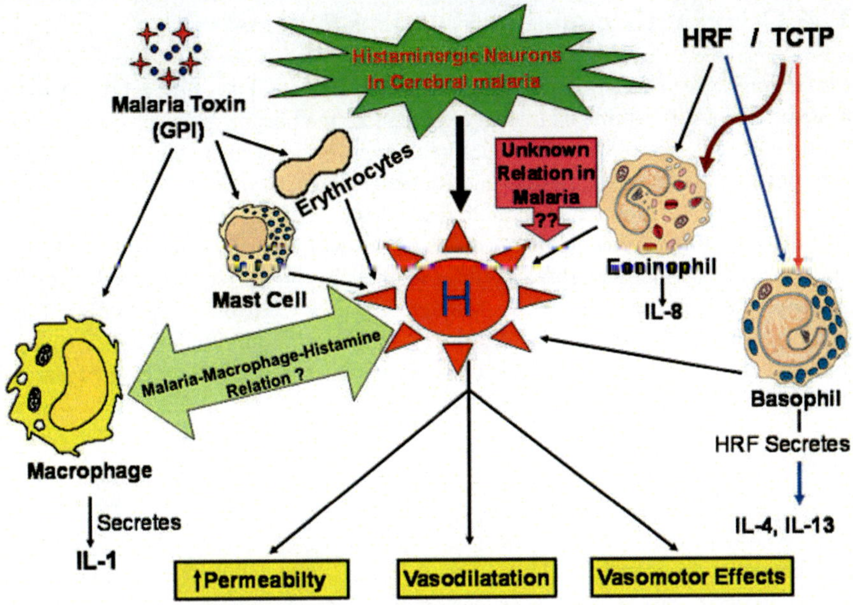

Fig. 19.1 Showing the interrelationship among TCTP, HRF, Malaria toxin (GPI) and various interleukins

Gaddum 1935, Billings and Maegraith 1938). This substance is responsible for the increased permeability observed in acute inflammation.

Breakdown in the blood brain barrier in the acute stages of *P. knowlesi* and *P. berghei* infections in animals (Maegraith and Onabanjo 1970). They suggested that this effect might be due to pharmacologically active substances released into the circulation and acting on the smooth muscles. Later on Maegraith and Onabanjo (1970) extracted histamine from the infected *Macaca mulatta* by *P. knowlesi* and suggested that histamine may be one of the agents responsible for the disturbances of the integrity of the blood vessels in the brain and elsewhere. The experimentally Maegraith and Onabanjo (1969, 1970) injected the extracts from the infected monkey into the guinea pig subdurally. After few hours blueing occurred throughout the brain. This indicated the passage of plasma proteins and water into the perivascular and cerebrospinal fluid. The extracts from the blood of control monkey produced no such effect under similar conditions.

An increase in histamine concentration in the blood of *P. knowlesi*-infected rhesus monkeys (*Macaca mulatta*) is primarily concerned, among other vaso-active substances released during the advanced stages of the disease, in the inflammatory "stasis" that often occurs in local vessels. This inflammatory stasis is particularly evident in the brain vessels, and leads to overall disturbances of the blood circulation, which in turn leads to pathophysiological effects such as coma (Maegraith 1966).

19.4 Origin of Histamine in Malarious Patients

Plasmodium species destroy the inhabited erythrocytes and it is thought that certain protein residues of peptide nature are released into the plasma of infected patients at the time of schizogony which includes kallikarein, which acts on the phospholipase A to produce histamine (Goodwin and Richards 1960).

Histamine is a product of pathological chain reactions and once produced it will produce its pharmacological effects which will contribute to the vasodilatation, increase in permeability of the endothelium of the small vessels and to vasomotor effects in *P. knowlesi*-infected monkeys (Skirrow et al. 1964). In a study, plasma concentration of histamine and neutral amino acids such as histidine and phenylalanine was increased in children of cerebral malaria (Enonwu et al. 2000).

19.4.1 Factors Responsible for Increase in Histidine Level in Malaria

As haemoglobin comprises of histidine residues, the metabolism of haemoglobin during malaria causes release of histidine, which eventually will increase in histamine concentration in the malarious patients (Kreier 1980). Waterlow and Fern (1981) stated hydrolysis of carnosine (β-alanyl histidine) to β-alanine and L-histidine during malaria infection. Pre-erythrocytic schizogony causes the destruction of liver cells resulting hepatic dysfunctions resulting increase in the blood histidine level (Sowunmi 1996). Schmid et al. (1978) reported increase in histamine level in the brains of hyperuremic rats due to renal insufficiency (90% nephrectomised rats). Enwonwu et al. (1999) reported significant rise in the levels of phenylalnine and histidine in the children suffered from falciparum malaria. Folic acid and vitamin B-12 deficiency also leads to increase in histidine level in malaria (Migsena and Areekul 1987).

19.4.2 Histamine, its Origin and Physiological Effects

Histamine in brain does not originate from histamine in plasma, it is rather synthesized in-situ by a specific histidine decarboxylase (Schwartz et al. 1991). Histaminergic neurons are concentrated in the tuberomammillary nucleus of the posterior hypothalamus, and it project efferent fibers to almost all part of brain (Wada et al. 1991). Histamine is also detected in perivascular mast cells and isolated cerebral microvessels (Edvinsson and Fredholm 1983). It acts in brain as a neuromodulator through G-protein coupled receptor subtypes (H1, H2 and H3) (Hill 1990). Various activities in brain are also regulated by histaminergic neuronal system (Beaven 1978, Schwartz et al. 1991). These activities may include arousal state, energy metabolism, locomotor activity, emesis, intence hypotension, analgesia, neuroendocrine and vestibular functions. Intracerebral histamine regulates cerebral blood flow (Edvinsson and Fredholm 1983), increases vascular endothelial permeability, enhances release of prostacyclin as well as platelet activating factor from endothelial cells, it also affects trans-endothelial transport and blood brain barrier (BBB) permeability (Joo et al. 1992, Wahl and Schilling 1993) and contributes to formation of ischaemic brain edema (Boertje et al. 1989). The above mentioned histamine related features are very relevant to the well documented features suggestive of severe or cerebral malaria in human beings (Crawley et al. 1996, Marsh et al. 1996, Molyneux et al. 1989, Newton et al. 1994, Walker et al. 1992, White and Ho 1992).

The increase in capillary permeability of brain, lungs, kidney and intestines may be due to increase in plasma histamine in severe malaria (Migsena and Areekul 1987). The increased histamine in lungs may cause severe respiratory distress in severe malaria. It is due to histamine mediated endothelial and septal capillary injuries (Duarte et al. 1985). This is well documented that histaminergic transmission through H1-receptors regulates the seizure activity in brain (Lintunen et al. 1998).

19.5 Antihistaminics and Malaria

Cerebral malaria, the commonest cause of death in severe malaria (Debron et al. 1994). Clinical signs and symptoms of cerebral malaria have a variable degree of cerebral component with headache at one end and deep unarousable coma at the other (Desowitz 1987). Tonic-clonic seizures have also been reported following intake of chloroquine and some other antimalarials prophylactically (Fish and Espir 1988). In various studies such as in Malawai (Molyneux et al. 1989), Nigeria (Walker et al. 1992) and in Zambia (Mabeza et al. 1985), it was documented that 69–70% of patients presenting with severe malaria have been unsuccessfully treated with chloroquine for the present illness, an observation showing high prevalence of chloroquine resistance in the communities (Mabeza et al. 1985). However, there was a reversal of chloroquine resistance if chloropheniramine (histamine H1-receptor blocker) was used prophylactically along with chloroquine (Peters et al. 1990, Sowunmi et al. 1998). Similarly, antihistaminic agents inhibit growth in Swiss mice of pre-erythrocytic stages of *Plasmodium yoelii nigreriensis* (N-67), a strain innately resistant to chloroquine (Singh and Puri 1998).

19.6 Role of Other Neurotransmitters in Malaria

Various neurotransmitters (monoamines, amino acids, peptides) and their receptors are implicated in initiation and termination of seizures (Gietzen et al. 1996). Depletion of the catecholamines and 5-hydroxytryptamine or blockade of their receptors elicits an increase in seizure susceptibility (Enonwu et al. 2000), while an increase in their concentration and turnover leads to a decrease. There are also reports that histaminergic transmission through H1-receptor is involved in regulation of seizure activity (Lintunen et al. 1998). Additionally, histamine modulates glutamatergic functions by interacting with *N*-methyl-*D*-aspartate (NMDA) receptors (Bekker 1993).

Therefore, it can be depicted that altered concentration of monoamines in the brain causes cerebral malaria. It is documented in several reports that cerebral malaria is more common in the well nourished and very less common in children suffering from protein energy malnutrition (Edington 1967, Hendrickse et al. 1971). It is also reported in some reports that dietary supplementation of specific essential amino acids intensified the severity of experimentally induced malaria infection in animals (Bakker et al. 1992, Fern et al. 1984).

19.7 Histamine H1-H4-Receptors in Malaria: A Critical View

Beghdadi et al. (2008) estimated the significant rise in serum histamine level in the mice. They infected the mice by *Plasmodium berghi* (ANKA strain), which is a lethal strain causes cerebral malaria. They conducted experiments on different groups of mice. In their experiments, they used $H1R^{-/-}$ (H1R deficient) mouse, $H2R^{-/-}$ (H2R deficient) mouse, $HDC^{-/-}$ (histidine decarboxylase deficient mouse) and wild mouse. They infected above mentioned group of mice by *P. berghi* and observed delayed mortality in all the groups except wild mouse. They also infected groups of wild mouse on antihistaminics (H1R-Cetrizine, H2R-Cimetidine, H3R-Imetit and H4R-JNJ7777120). They observed that mice treated with either levocetrizine or cimetidine died significantly later than similarly infected but untreated mice. In contrast imetit and JNJ7777120 had no effect on mice survival as compared with untreated mice. It is also reported that sensitivity of seizures is inversely correlated with histamine concentration in plasma (Tuomisto and Tacke 1986). Linuma et al. (1993) reported that histamine is involved in the termination of seizures (White and Ho 1992). Also, seizures sometimes may induce in childhood epilepsy through administration of an antihistaminic (Schwartz and Patterson 1978).

19.8 Concluding Remarks and Future Prospects

Malaria is one of the most important health hazards worldwide. In this chapter we discussed the role of histamine in the pathogenesis of malaria and the role of antihistaminics in the treatment protocol or preventive strategies of deadly malaria. But, when antimalarials are used along with antihistaminics, low concentration of histamine leads to seizures in childhood therefore, use of antihistamine in malaria must be judicious.

References

Bakker NPM, Eling WMC, DeGroot AMTh et al (1992) Attenuation of malaria infection, paralysis and lesions in the central nervous system by low protein diet in rats. Acta Tropica 50:285–293

Barsoum GS, Gaddum JH (1935) The pharmacological estimation of adenosine and histamine in blood. J Physiol (Lond) 85:1–14

Beaven MA (1978) Histamine: its role in physiological and pathological processes. In: Karger S (ed) Monographs in allergy, vol 13. Munchen Paris, New York, p 36
Beghdadi W, Porcherie A, Schneider BS et al (2008) Inhibition of histamine-mediated signalling confers significant protection against severe malaria in mouse models of disease. JEM 205(2):395–408
Bekker JM (1993) Enhancement by histamine of NMDA-mediated synaptic transmission in the hippocampus. Science 261:104–106
Bhattacharya U, Roy S, Kar PK et al (1988) Histamine and kinin system in experimental malaria. Ind J Med Res 88:558–563
Bheekha Escura R, MacGlashan DW Jr, Langdon JM et al (2000) Human recombinant histamine-releasing factor activates human eosinophils and the eosinophilic cell line. Blood 96:2191–2198
Bhisutthibhan J, Pan XQ, Hossler PA et al (1998) The *Plasmodium falciparum* translationally controlled tumor protein homolog and its reaction with the antimalarial drug artemisinin. J Biol Chem 273:16192–1619
Billings GFT, Maegraith B (1938) Chemical changes in tissues following obstruction of the blood supply. Quart J Exp Physiol 27:249–269
Boertje SB, LeBeau D, Williams C (1989) Blockade of histamine stimulated alterations in cerebrovascular permeability by H2-receptor antagonist cimetidine. Neuropharmacology 28: 749–752
Butcher GA, Garland T, Ajdukiewicz AB et al (1990) Serum tumor necrosis factor associated with malaria in patients in the Solomon Islands. Trans R Soc Trop Med Hyg 84:658–661
Camacho LH, Wilairatana P, Weiss G et al (1999) The eosinophilic response and haematological recovery after treatment for *Plasmodium falciparum* malaria. Trop Med Int Health 4:471–475
Clark IA, Rockett KA (1996) Nitric oxide and parasitic diseases. Adv Parasitol 37:1–56
Crawley J, Smith S, Kirkham F et al (1996) Seizures and status epilepticus in childhood cerebral malaria. Q J Med 89:591–597
Dale HH, Richards AN (1918) The vasodilator action of histamine and some other substances. J Physiol Lond 52:110–165
Davis TM, Ho M, Supanaranond W (1991) Changes in the peripheral blood eosinophils count in falciparum malaria. Acta Trop 48:243–246
Debron P, Dumont N, Nyongabo T et al (1994) Immunologic and biochemical alterations in severe falciparum malaria: relation to neurological symptoms and outcome. Clin Infect Dis 19: 450–455
de Kossodo S, Grau GE (1993) Profiles of cytokine production in relation with susceptibility to cerebral malaria. J Immunol 151:4811–4820
Desowitz RS (1987) The pathophysiology of malaria after Maegraith. Ann Trop Med Parasitol 81:599–606
Duarte MIS, Corbert CEP, Boulos M et al (1985) Ultrastructure of the lung in the falciparum malaria. Am J Trop Med Hyg 34:31–35
Edington GM (1967) Pathology of malaria in West Africa. Br Med J 1:715–718
Edvinsson L, Fredholm BB (1983) Characterization of adenosine receptors in isolated cerebral arteries of cat. Br J Pharmacol 80:631–637
Enwonwu CO, Afolabi BM, Salako LA et al (1999) Hyperphenylalaninemia in children with falciparum malaria. Q J Med 92: 495–503
Enonwu CO, Afolabi BM, Salako LO et al (2000) Increased plasma levels of histidine and histamine in falciparum malaria: relevance to severity of infection. J Neural Transm 107: 1273–1287
Fern EB, Edirisinghe JS, Targett GAT (1984) Increased severity of malaria infection in rats fed supplementary amino acids. Trans Roy Soc Trop Med 78:839–841
Fish DR, Espir MLE (1988) Convulsions associated with prophylactic antimalarial drugs: implications for people with epilepsy. Br Med J 297:526–527
Friedland JS, Ho M, Remick DG et al (1993) Interleukinin-8 and Plasmodium falciparum malaria in Thiland. Trans R Soc Trop Med Hyg 87:54–55

Gietzen DW, Dixon KD, Truong BG et al (1996) Indispensible amino acid deficiency and increased seizure susceptibility in rats. Am J Physiol 271:R18-R24

Goodwin LG, Richards WH (1960) Pharmacologically active peptides in the blood and urine of animals infected with *Babesia rodhaini* and other pathogenic organisms. Br J Pharmac Chemother 15:152–159

Grau GE, Heremans H, Piguet PF et al (1989a) Monoclonal antibody against interferon gamma can prevent experimental cerebral malaria and its associated overproduction of tumor necrosis factor. Proc Natl Acad Sci USA 86: 5572–5574

Grau GE, Taylor TE, Molyneux ME et al (1989b) Tumor necrosis factor and disease severity in children with falciparum malaria. N Engl J Med 320:1586–1591

Hendrickse RG, Hasan AH, Olumide LO et al (1971) Malaria in early childhood. An investigation of five hundred seriously ill children in whom a "clinical diagnosis of malaria was made on admission to the children's emergency room at University College Hospital, Ibadan". Ann Trop Med Parasitol 65:1–20

Hill SJ (1990) Distribution, properties and functional characteristics of three classes of histamine receptor. Pharmacol Rev 42:45–83

Hinshaw LB, Jordan MM, Vick J (1961) Mechanism of histamine release in endotoxin shock. Am J Physiol 200:987–989

Ho M, Schollaardt T, Snape S et al (1998) Endogenous interleukinin-10 modulates proinflammatory response in *Plasmodium falciparum* malaria. J Infect Dis 178:520–525

Hunt NH, Golenser J, Chan-Ling T et al (2006) Immunopathogenesis of cerebral malaria. Int J Parasitol 36: 569–582

Joo F, Leagyel I, Kovacs J et al (1992) Regulation in transendorhelial transport in cerebral microvessels: the role of second messenger generating systems. Prog Brain Res 91:177–197

Kreier JP (1980) Malaria: epidemiology, chemotherapy, morphology and metabolism, vol 1. Academic, New York, p 363

Krogh A (1929) The anatomy and physiology of capillaries, revised edn. Yale University, New Haven

Kurtzhals JAL, Reimert CM, Tette E et al. (1998) Increased eosinophil activity in acute Plasmodium falciparum infection association with cerebral malaria. Clin Exp Immunol 112:303–307

Kwiatkowski D, Hill AV, Sambou I et al (1990) TNF concentration in fatal cerebral, non-fatal cerebral, and uncomplicated Plasmodium falciparum malaria. Lancet 336:1201–1204

Lewis T (1927) The blood vessels of the human skin and their responses. Shaw and Sons, London

Lintunen M, Sallmen T, Karisredt K et al (1998) Postnatal expression of Hi-receptor mRNA in the rat brain: correlation to L-histidine decarboxylase expression and local upregulation in limbic seizures. Eur J Neurosci 10:2287–2301

Linuma K, Yokoyama H, Otsuki T et al (1993) Histamine H1 receptors in complex partial seizures. Lancet 341:238

Lou J, Donati YR, Juillard P et al (1997) Platelets play an important role in TNF-induced microvascular endothelial cell pathology. Am J Pathol 151:1397–1405

Ma N, Madigan MC, Chan-Ling T et al (1997) Compromised blood-nerve barrier, astrogliosis, and myelin disruption in optic nerves during fatal murine cerebral malaria. Glia 19: 135–151

Mabeza GF, Moyo VM, Thuma PE et al (1985) Predictors of severity of illness on presentation in children with cerebral malaria. Ann Trop Med Parasitol 89:221–228

MacDonald S, Bhisutthibhan J, Shapiro TA et al (2001) Immune mimicry in malaria: *Plasmodium falciparum* secrets a functional histamine-releasing factor homolog *in vitro* and *in vivo*. PNAS 98(19):10829–10832

MacDonald SM, Rafnar T, Langdon J et al (1995) Molecular identification of an IgE-dependent histamine-releasing factor. Science 269:688–690

Maegraith B, Fletcher A (1972) The pathogenesis of mammalian malaria. Adv Parasitol 10:49–75

Maegraith BG (1966) Pathogenic processes in malaria. In: The pathology of parasitic diseases, Fourth Symp, Br Soc Parasitology Oxford, Blackwell

Maegraith BG, Onabanjo AO (1969) The involvement of histamine in malaria. Br J Pharmacol 37:535–536

Maegraith BG, Onabanjo AO (1970) The effects of histamine in malaria. Br J Pharmacol 39: 755–764

Maheshwari RK (1990) The role of cytokines in malaria infection. Bull World Health Organ 68(Suppl):138–144

Marsh K, English M, Crawley J (1996) The pathogenesis of severe malaria in African children. Ann Trop Med Parasitol 90:221–228

McGregor IA (1987) Thoughts on malaria in pregnancy with consideration of some factors which influence remedial strategies. Parassitologia 29:153–163

Medana IM, Hunt NH, Chan-Ling T (1997a) Early activation of microglia in the pathogenesis of fatal murine cerebral malaria. Glia 19:91–103

Medana IM, Hunt NH, Chaudhri G (1997b) Tumor necrosis factor-alpha expression in the brain during fatal murine cerebral malaria: evidence for production by microglia and astrocytes. Am J Pathol 150:1473–1486

Migsena P, Areekul S (1987) Capillary permeability function in malaria. Ann Trop Med Parasito 81:549–560

Molyneux ME, Taylor TE, Wirima JJ et al (1989) Clinical features and prognostic indicators in paediatric cerebral malaria: a study of 131 comatose Malawian children. Q J Med 71: 441–459

Mordmuller BG, Metzger WG, Juillard P et al (1997) Tumor necrosis factor in Plasmodium falciparum malaria: high plasma level is associated with fever, but high production capacity is associated with rapid fever clearance. Eur Cytokine Network 8:29–35

Murphy SC, Breman JG (2001) Gaps in childhood malaria burden in Africa: cerebral malaria neurological sequelae, anemia, respiratory distress, hypoglycaemia and complications of pregnancy. Am J Trop Med Hyg 64:57–67

Newton CRJC, Peshu N, Kendal B et al (1994) Brain swelling and ischaemia in Kenyans children with cerebral malaria. Arch Dis Childh 70:281–287

Perlmann P, Perlmann H, Eighazali G et al (1999) IgE and tumor necrosis factor in malaria infection. Immunol Lett 65:29–33

Peters W, Ekong R, Robinson BL et al (1990) The chemotherapy of rodent malaria. XLV. Reversal of chloroquin resistance in rodent and human plasmodium by antihistaminic agents. Ann Trop Med Parasitol 84:541–551

Schayer RW (1960) Relationship of induced histidine decarboxylase activity and histamine synthesis to shock from stress and endotoxin. Am J Physiol 198:1187–1192

Schluesener HJ, Kremsner PG, Meyermann R (1998) Widespread expression of MRP8 and MRP14 in human cerebral malaria by microglial cells. Acta Neuropathol (Berl) 96:575–580

Schmid G, Przuntek H, Fricke L et al (1978) Increased histidine and histamine content in the brain of chronic uremic rats. Cause of enhanced cerebral cyclic adenosine monophosphate in uremia? Am J Clin Nutr 31:1665–1668

Schofield L, Ferreira A, Altszuler R et al (1987) Interferon-gamma inhibits the intrahepatocytic development of malaria parasites *in vitro*. J Immunol 139:2020–2025

Schroeder JT, Lichtenstein LM, MacDonald SM (1997) Recombinant histamine-releasing factor enhances IgE-dependent IL-4 and IL-13 secretion by human basophils J Immunol 159: 447–452

Schwartz JC, Arrang JM, Garbarg M et al (1991) Histaminergic transmission in the mammalian brain. Physiol Rev 71:1–51

Schwartz JF, Patterson JH (1978) Toxic encephalopathy related to anthistamine-barbiturate antiemetic medication. Am J Dis Child 132:37–39

Shahid M, Tripathi T, Sobia F et al (2009) Histamine, histamine receptors, and their role in immunomodulation: an updated systematic review. Open Immunol J 2:9–41

Singh N, Puri SK (1998) Casual prophylactic activity of antihistaminic agents against *Plasmodium yoelii nigriensis* infection in swiss mice. Acta Tropica 69:255–260

Skirrow MB, Chongsuphajaisiddhi T, Maegraith BG (1964) The circulation in malaria.II. Portal angiography in monkeys (*Macaca mulatta*) infected with *Plasmodium knowlesi* and in shock following manipulation of the gut. Ann Trop Med Parasit 58:502–510

Sowunmi A (1996) Hepatomegaly in acute falciparum malaria in children. Trans Roy Soc Trop Med Hyg 90:540–542

Sowunmi A, Odula AMJ, Ogundahunsi OAT et al (1998) Enhancement of the antimalarial effect of chloroquine by chloropheniramine *in vivo*. Trop Med Int Hlth 3:177–183

Srichaikul T, Archararit N, Siriasawakul T et al (1976) Histamine changes in falciparum malaria. Trans R Soc Trop Med Hyg 70:36–38

Trigg PI, Kondrachine AV (1998) The current global malaria situation. In: Sherman IW (ed) Malaria: parasite biology, pathogenesis, and protection. Am Soc Microbiol. Washington, DC, pp 11–22

Tuomisto L, Tacke U (1986) Is histamine an anticonvulsive inhibitory transmitter? Neuropharmacology 31:503–509

Wada H, Inagaki N, Yamatodani A et al (1991). Is the histaminergic neuron system a regulatory centre for whole brain activity? TINS 14:415–418

Wahl M, Schilling L (1993) Regulation of cerebral blood flow: a brief review. Acta Neurochir 59(Suppl):3–10

Walker O, Salako LA, Sowunmi A et al (1992) Prognostic risk-factors and post-mortem findings in cerebral malaria in children. Trans Roy Soc Trop Med Hyg 86:491–483

Wassmer SC, Combes V, Candal FJ (2006) Platelets potentiate brain endothelial alterations induced by *Plasmodium falciparum*. Infect Immun 74:645–653

Waterlow JC, Fern EB (1981) Free amino acid pools and their regulation. In: Waterlow JC, Stephen JML (eds) Nitrogen metabolism in man. Appl Science, London, pp 1–16

White NJ (1998) In: Malaria pathophysiology Sherman IW (ed) Malaria: parasite biology, pathogenesis, and protection, Am Soc Microbiol. Washington, DC, pp 371–385

White NJ, Ho M (1992) The pathophysiology of malaria. Adv Parasitol 31:83–173

Chapter 20
Histamine-Cytokine and Histamine-Antibody Network in Immune Regulation

Trivendra Tripathi, Richa Pandey, Adil Raza, Mohammed Shahid, Haris M. Khan, Mashhatullah Siddiqui, and Rahat Ali Khan

Abstract Histamine has tremendous influence over a variety of pathophysiological processes through the activation of four receptors: H1, H2, H3 and H4 and is known to participate in allergic, inflammation, gastric acid secretion, immunomodulation and neurotransmission. In recent years, accumulating evidences have witnessed the importance of histamine-cytokine and histamine-antibody network in immunoregulation. Moreover, histamine immunobiology pertaining to histamine-receptors is elementary in the existing literature in contrast to increasing frequency of allergic diseases. In this chapter, we tried to elaborate the newer discoveries in the current field and also discussed our recent studies on the immunobiology of histamine receptors. We hope that this article would stimulate discussions and active research on this important aspect.

Keywords Histamine · Histamine-receptors · Cytokines · Antibody · Immunobiology

Abbreviations

AD	atopic dermatitis
CU	chronic urticaria
MS	multiple sclerosis
IFN	interferon
Th	T helper
IL	interleukin
Ig	immunoglobulin
MHC	major histocompatibility complex
GM-CSF	granulocyte macrophage-colony stimulating factor

T. Tripathi (✉)
Department of Biochemistry, Jawaharlal Nehru Medical College and Hospital, Aligarh Muslim University, Aligarh 202002, UP, India
e-mail: tripathiamu@gmail.com

M. Shahid et al. (eds.), *Biomedical Aspects of Histamine*,
DOI 10.1007/978-90-481-9349-3_20, © Springer Science+Business Media B.V. 2010

TGF	transforming growth factor
HRs	histamine receptors
H1R	histamine H1-receptor
H2R	histamine H2-receptor
H3R	histamine H3-receptor
H4R	histamine H4-receptor
T-cells	T-lymphocytes
B-cells	B-lymphocytes
CD	cluster of differentiation
LPS	lipopolysaccharide
SEA	staphylococcal enterotoxin A
PMA	phorbol 12-myristate 13-acetate
TNF	tumor necrosis factor
PGE2	prostaglandin E2
CXCL12	chemokine (C-X-C motif) ligand 12
DC	dendritic cells
pDC	plasmacytoid DC
TGFβ1	transforming growth factor type β1
TLR4	toll-like receptor 4
PBMC	peripheral blood mononuclear cell
ICAM	inter-cellular adhesion molecule
GAD	glutamic acid decarboxylase
OVA	ovalbumin
SRBC	sheep red blood cells
post-I	post-immunization
pre-I	pre-immunization
b.i.d.	bis in die

Contents

20.1 Introduction

Histamine (a biogenic amine) has broadest spectrum of activities in various physiological and pathological conditions including the cell proliferation, differentiation hematopoiesis, embryonic development, regeneration, wound healing, aminergic neurotransmission and various brain functions (sleep/nociception, food intake and aggressive behavior), secretion of pituitary hormones, regulation of gastrointestinal, cardiovascular system (vasodilation and blood pressure reduction). It also regulates inflammatory reactions, modulation of the immune response, functioning of endocrine system and homeostasis (Shahid et al. 2009). Accumulating evidences have also been postulated its significant role in various other pathological conditions such as increased level in bronchoalveolar lavage fluid from patients with allergic asthma and this increase is negatively correlated with airway function. An increase in histamine levels has been noticed in skin and plasma of patients of atopic dermatitis (AD), chronic urticaria (CU), multiple sclerosis (MS) and in psoriatic skin (Thurmond et al. 2008).

The biological pleiotropic effects of histamine are mediated by four subtypes of histamine receptors (H1, H2, H3 and H4) transducing extracellular signals through different G-proteins: $G_{q/11}$ for H1, $G_{\alpha s}$ for H2, $G_{i/o}$ for H3 and H4-receptors (Shahid et al. 2009). Specific activation or inhibition of histamine receptors has led to a tremendous increase in the knowledge of the roles of histamine in physiology and pathology of disease conditions (Jutel et al. 2005, Shahid et al. 2009).

Thus, after a century of histamine discovery, the existing literature has provided intensive knowledge about its synthesis, metabolism, receptors, signal transduction, and physiological and pathological effects. However, the complex interrelationship and cross talk by histamine and its receptors in immunobiology remained to be elucidated. In the present chapter, we will discuss histamine-cytokine and histamine-antibody network in immunoregulation and immunomodulation in allergic and inflammatory conditions.

20.2 Immunobiological Aspects of Cytokine

Cytokines are low molecular weight proteins released from the cells that regulate significant biological processes including cell growth, cell activation, inflammation, immunity, tissue repair, and fibrosis. Interferons (IFN-α, IFN-β and IFN-γ) are cytokines associated with antiviral activity. However, IFN-γ possesses the least antiviral activity but this cytokine is important for the activation of T-cells and plays an important role in immunoregulation and immunomodulation. Interleukins are released from leukocytes and further act on the same (Packard and Khan 2003). Immunological stimuli arouse naïve Th cells, which exude specific cytokines, control the differentiation of naïve Th cells into Th1 and Th2 cells, and regulate several immunological events in the immune system (Fig. 20.1). Th1 cells secrete primarily IL-2, IFN-γ, IL-3, and GM-CSF, while Th2 cells mainly secrete IL-3, IL-4, IL-5, IL-10, IL-13, and GM-CSF. The pathogenesis of several allergic diseases is

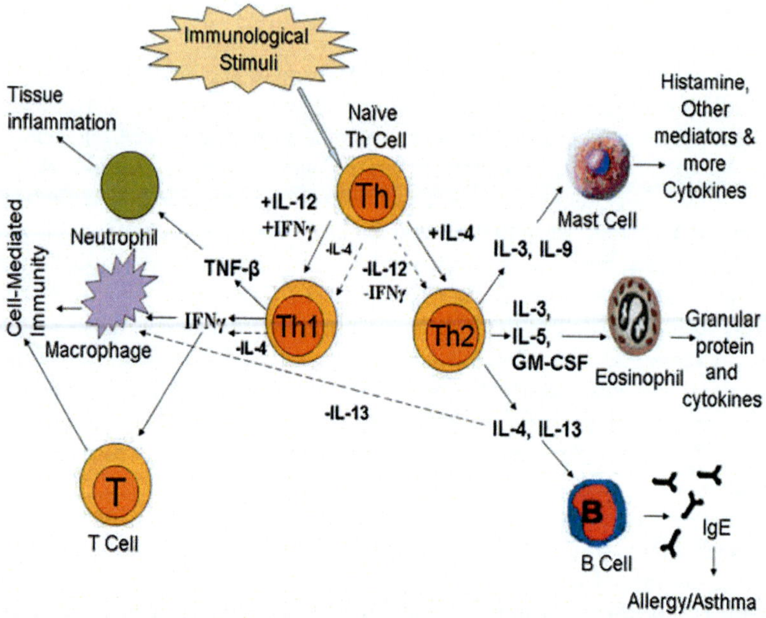

Fig. 20.1 Various immunological stimuli arouse naïve Th cells, which exude specific cytokines and control the differentiation of naïve Th cells into Th1 and Th2 cells and regulate several immunological events in the immune system. Th1 cytokine IFN-γ and monokine IL-12 are responsible for the differentiation of naïve T helper cells into Th1 cells, while Th2 cytokine IL-4 is important for the differentiation into Th2 cells. Each T helper subset has its own unique cytokine secretion profile. Th1 cells secrete predominantly IL-2, IL-3, IFN-γ, TNF-β, and GM-CSF that ultimately leads to tissue inflammation, cytotoxic response and delayed hypersensitivity, and Th2 cells secrete IL-3, IL-4, IL-5, IL-10, IL-13, and GM-CSF that ultimately perpetuate allergic diseases and asthma

perpetuated by an imbalance of cytokines released from Th cells (Packard and Khan 2003). The primary actions of the individual interleukins are variable and range from proliferation, activation, division, and differentiation of various immunological cells. IL-2, a Th1 cytokine, controls the differentiation of naïve Th cells into Th1 cells while IL-4, a Th2 cytokine, controls the differentiation of naïve Th cells into Th2 cells. IL-4, along with Th2 cytokine IL-13, also plays a vital role in the promotion of an allergic inflammatory eosinophilic reaction in allergic diseases through IgE isotype switching (Levy et al. 1997). It has been reported that IL-13 inhibits the production of inflammatory cytokines, induces B-lymphocytes proliferation and differentiation, including IgE production. It also enhances expression of CD23 and major histocompatibility complex class II molecules (MHC class II) (Defrance et al. 1994, De Vries and Zurawski 1995). Th2 cytokine IL-5 plays an imperative role in allergic disease by controlling the movement, maturation, and proliferation of eosinophils. Th2 cytokine interleukin-10 downregulates cellular immune response and affects the outcomes of viral diseases by inhibition of the production of Th1 cytokines (Packard and Khan 2003). Important cytokines such as GM-CSF regulate hemopoiesis, and inhibitory cytokines, such as transforming growth factor (TGF), stimulate connective tissue and collagen formation; however, both of them down-regulate immune function (Packard and Khan 2003). Cytokines exert their actions via binding to cytokine receptors on cells. Many cytokine receptors show sequence homology and even share identical subunits (Packard and Khan 2003).

20.3 Immunobiology of Histamine-Cytokine Network

Histamine, originally considered as a mediator of immediate hypersensitivity, might play a more complex role than expected by superseding in the cytokine network. Indeed, the cells involved in the regulation of immune responses and hematopoiesis express histamine receptors (HRs) on their surface, and most of them can also produce the mediator (Shahid et al. 2009). It has been demonstrated that histamine can modulate and/or induce cytokine synthesis in allergic inflammation. Two types of effects have been described: (a) direct effects of histamine on cytokine production and (b) modulation of cytokine synthesis induced by immunologic stimuli (Shahid et al. 2009).

Thus, the complex effects of histamine on immune cells in cytokine production are mediated by the activation of histamine receptors (H1R, H2R, H3R and H4R) (Cameron et al. 1986, Elenkov et al. 1998, Ogden and Hill 1980, Sirois et al. 2000, Thurmond et al. 2008). The immunobiology of histamine-cytokine network on different cells involved in immune regulation is as follows.

20.3.1 T Lymphocytes

T lymphocytes, especially T helper type 1 cells (Th1) and T helper type 2 cells (Th2) play distinctive roles in the development, initiation, and regulation of the immune response. Histamine have direct effects on T-cells as H1-, H2- and H4-receptors are expressed on $CD4^+$ and $CD8^+$ T cells. Th1 cells mainly express H1Rs while Th2 cells express H2Rs. Thus, this biogenic amine (histamine) enhances Th1-type responses by triggering the H1R. However, both Th1 and Th2 cells are negatively regulated through H2R. There is now contradictory data from in vivo and in vitro studies (Shahid et al. 2009, Thurmond et al. 2008). Histamine also induces chemotaxis of human T cells in vitro and there is evidence for both H1R and H4R involvement (Thurmond et al. 2008). It downregulates the proliferation of Th1 cells by inhibiting cytokines production such as IL-2, IFN-γ and monokine IL-12, which controls cytotoxic response and delayed-type hypersensitivity, while it upregulates the proliferation of Th2 cells (which control asthma and allergic disease by enhancing the cytokines secretion such as IL-4, IL-5, IL-10 and IL-13, and also by activating B-cells and regulating IgG and IgE secretion) (Elliott et al. 2001, Osna et al. 2001a, b, Packard and Khan 2003, Sirois et al. 2000, Weltman 2000, see Chapter 6 of this book). In vitro study using polarized T-cells showed that histamine inhibits IL-4 and IL-13 production by Th2 cells, but stimulates IFN-γ production in Th1 cells, although the differences are small (Jutel et al. 2001).

In vivo studies demonstrated that T-cells from H1R-deficient mice produce lower levels of IFN-γ and higher levels of IL-13 (Banu and Watanabe 1999, Jutel et al. 2001, Kobayashi et al. 2001). However, Banu and Watanabe (1999) showed that T-cells also produce lower levels of IL-2 and higher levels of IL-4, whereas Jutel et al. (2001) found no change in these cytokines (IL-2 and IL-4). Therefore, it is difficult to determine whether there is true skewing to a Th-2 phenotype in H1R-deficient animals and it would be a point of research and debate in near future. In H2R-deficient mice, T-cells increase levels of IFN-γ and IL-4 suggesting that H2R plays a general inhibitory role (Jutel et al. 2001). In a recent study, the activation of $CD4^+$ and $CD8^+$ T-cells from both H1- and H2-receptor-deficient mice was observed and it was found that $CD4^+$ cells from either H1R or H2R-deficient mice expressed increased levels of IL-4 but lower levels of IL-10 and IL-2. In $CD8^+$ cells, H1- or H2-receptor deficiency leads to increase in IFN-γ, but still lower levels of IL-10 and IL-2 were observed. Furthermore, activation of H4- or H2- receptors on human $CD8^+$ T-cells can lead to IL-16 release (Gantner et al. 2002, Thurmond et al. 2008). In addition, histamine has been shown to enhance the proliferative response of mouse T- and B-lymphocytes, in a dose dependent manner. This activity is mediated through H1R, since it does not occur in H1R-deficient mice (Dy and Schneider 2004). However, T-cell proliferation in response to cytokines was normal in these mutant mice, suggesting that H1R activation contributes primarily to antigen receptor-mediated signaling pathways that lead to cytokine production such as IL-12, IL-27 and IL-23 for Th1, and IL-4 for Th2 differentiation. The role of these $CD4^+$ T-cell subsets in the control of delayed type hypersensitivity or humoral allergic responses has been shown in existing literature. These fascinating findings have suggested that histamine, traditionally considered a chemical mediator of acute inflammation, plays a more complex role than was thought earlier in the modulation of the cytokine network (Dy and Schneider 2004).

20.3.2 Mast Cells and Basophils

Mast cells and basophils are generally thought to be the major sources of histamine, although how this varies among different mast cell types is still an important point of debate. Histamine does not appear to have any direct effect on mast cell degranulation (Fokkens et al. 1992, Godot et al. 2007, Lippert et al. 2004). There are several reports regarding the effects of H1R-antagonists on mast cells, but these results may be due to off-target effects (Thurmond et al. 2008). Several hematopoietic populations devoid of mature or morphologically recognizable mast cells or basophils can generate histamine provided the presence of HDC activity (Dy et al. 1987, Schneider et al. 1993). It has been reported that increased HDC activity in myeloid cell populations is stimulated with lipopolysaccharide (LPS) or Staphylococcal enterotoxin A (SEA). It has also been reported that the HDC activity can easily be modulated both in vitro and in vivo (Schneider et al. 1987, Yoshimoto et al. 1999). Furthermore, basophil precursors generate histamine upon exposure to IL-3, GM-CSF, calcium ionophore or phorbol 12-myristate 13-acetate (PMA) (Dy et al. 1996, Schneider et al. 1999). On the other hand, IL-1, tumor necrosis factor-α (TNF-α) or LPS alone cannot induce histamine production by basophil precursors, but act in synergy with GM-CSF to enhance its immunological effect, as explained by prostaglandin E2 (PGE2) and intracellular cyclic-AMP which accumulate in response to these factors and enhance the increase in histamine synthesis induced by GM-CSF (Piquet-Pellorce and Dy 1991). Bone marrow-derived cells of the macrophage lineage can also generate histamine upon exposure to LPS (Takamatsu et al. 1996), however, in contrast to cells from the basophil lineage, they do not respond to IL-3 and/or GM-CSF alone but in synergy with LPS, these growth factors can enhance histamine production. It has been shown that IL-3-dependent murine hematopoietic progenitor cell lines synthesize histamine in response to calcium ionophore or PMA (Dy et al. 1996). Histamine synthesis in hematopoietic cells can also be a subject to negative control, as exemplified by the effect of IFN-γ on bone marrow-derived macrophages and of pro-Th1 cytokines on the basophil lineage (Dy and Schneider 2004). It has been shown that histamine acting through H4Rs can induce chemotaxis of murine mast cells in vitro and lead to changes in tissue localization in vivo, effects that may be related to the reported redistribution of mast cells to the epithelial lining of the nasal mucosa in rhinitic responses to allergens. The activation of H4Rs in human mast cell precursors can synergize with other chemo-attractants such as CXCL12 [known as chemokine (C-X-C motif) ligand 12 (stromal cell-derived factor 1)] (Thurmond et al. 2008). There are also significant reports on H3R function on mast cells, but most of the activities may be attributed to the H4R, as the ligands used are not particularly selective and studies have reported that H3R expression is not detected in some types of mast cells (Thurmond et al. 2008).

20.3.3 Dendritic Cells

Histamine not only acts on T-cells, mast cells and basophils, it can also have various effects on dendritic cells, which express H1-, H2-, and H4-receptors (Thurmond et al. 2008). Histamine induces chemotaxis of human dendritic cells (Gutzmer et al. 2005), which is primarily mediated by H4Rs with some contribution attributed to H1Rs. Caron et al. (2001a) showed that human dendritic cells (DC) express high levels of H1- and H2-receptors (which are downregulated during maturation), and low variable levels of H3-receptors. Even though DC cannot fully differentiate in response to histamine alone, they display more CD86 and increase their chemokine production (Idzdo et al. 2002). Cytokine secretion, including inhibition of interleukin 12p70(IL12p70) and enhancement of IL-10 and IL-6 production, can be modulated by histamine (Thurmond et al. 2008). Data from recent studies suggest that histamine acting on dendritic cells can drive Th2 T-cell polarization in human and mouse cells, which is mediated by H1Rs and H4Rs (Dunford et al. 2006, Idzko et al. 2002, Mazzoni et al. 2003). In combination with differentiating stimuli like LPS, histamine exerts a potent polarizing effect towards Th2-promoting DC, characterized by reduced IL-12 and enhanced IL-10 production. This effect is mainly mediated through H2Rs, although H1R activation might be involved (Caron et al. 2001b, Idzdo et al. 2002, Mazzoni et al. 2001). It has been shown that plasmacytoid DC (pDC) constitutes another subset of professional antigen-presenting cells and a major source of IFN-α. Similarly in myeloid DC, histamine modulates the cytokine production through H2Rs. Indeed, the presence of histamine during stimulation of pDC by live flu virus or CpG oligodeoxynucleotides decreases their IFN-α and TNF-α production (Mazzoni et al. 2003). This may explain why low levels of IFN-α are associated with viral infection in atopic children (Mazzoni et al. 2003).

It has also been reported that human myeloid DC derived from monocytes in response to GM-CSF and IL-4 express HDC during their differentiation process, which is impaired in the absence of endogenous histamine in HDC-deficient mice (Szeberenyi et al. 2001). Finally, it seems that the interactions between histamine and dendritic cells are not necessarily in the same fashion as in human and murine models (Pavlinkova et al. 2003, Renkl et al. 2004). This is because of the expression of functional H1Rs and H2Rs on myeloid DC and dermal dendritic cells, as opposed to that of Langerhans cells which express neither H1- nor H2-receptors mainly because of the negative effect of transforming growth factor type β1 (TGFβ1) required for their differentiation (Ohtani et al. 2003). In addition, the effects of chemokines such as thymus activation-regulated chemokine (TARC also known as CCL17), CCL22, IL10 and macrophage inflammatory protein 1α (MIP1α; also known as CCL3) could influence T-cell polarization (Thurmond et al. 2008).

20.3.4 Epithelial and Endothelial Cells

Histamine (important autacoids) is a modulator of barrier function in epithelial and endothelial cells. In vitro it can interact with epithelial cells and endothelial cells leading to increases in paracellular permeability (Rotrosen and Gallin 1986, Zabner et al. 2003). Histamine upregulates adhesion molecules on endothelial cells through H1Rs and causes adhesion, rolling and diapedesis of leukocytes such as neutrophils (Thurmond et al. 2008). Histamine is the main mediator which is responsible for secretion of pro-inflammatory signals from epithelial and endothelial cells. Activation of H1Rs on human endothelial cells stimulates the release of inflammatory stimuli such as IL-6, IL-8 and can synergize with other mediators such as LPS and TNF-α (Thurmond et al. 2008). It has been shown on human epithelial cells that H1Rs mediated activation increases the release of mediators such as IL-6, IL-8 and GM-CSF (Thurmond et al. 2008).

20.3.5 Monocytes and Macrophages

Human monocytes have been demonstrated to express H1-, H2- and H4-receptors (Thurmond et al. 2008). Histamine promotes inhibition of p40, p70 IL-12 and IL-1 but enhances IL-10 production through its H2Rs in LPS-stimulated whole blood cells or purified monocytes (Elenkov et al. 1998, Tineke et al. 1998). Histamine can inhibit LPS-induced TNF-α production by monocytes via its H2R (Vannier et al. 1991). This activity might be due to its capacity to downregulate CD14 membrane expression on monocytes without affecting Toll-like receptor 4 (TLR4) expressions (Takahashi et al. 2002). The modulation of CD14 occurs probably through post-transcriptional events since mRNA levels remain unchanged. Histamine decreases IL-18-induced IFN-γ, TNF-α and IL-12 production by human peripheral blood mononuclear cell (PBMC). IL-18 exhibits this effect through upregulation of inter-cellular adhesion molecule (ICAM) on monocytes and histamine prevents this augmentation through its H2Rs, while it has no effect in the absence of IL-18 (Itoh et al. 2002). Furthermore, histamine blocks constitutive monocyte chemo-attractant protein-1 (also known as CCL2) production by H4Rs in human monocytes (Lichtenstein and Gillespie 1975) and H1R activation appears to increase β-glucuronidase and IL-6 release from human lung macrophages (Triggiani et al. 2001).

Thus, in nutshell, histamine drives immune and inflammatory responses in several cell types as it can act through T-cells, dendritic cells, mast cells and basophils hence, helps in organization of adaptive responses. Even though most effects of histamine on cytokine network are positively mediated through classical histamine receptors, several data obtained with H1-, H2-, H3- and H4-receptor antagonists, at more than saturating concentrations, might be explained by other mechanisms and are of potential pharmacological interest. Thus, it is important to see how histamine can be a major mediator in vivo in immune and inflammatory reactions and can be pathogenic in several diseases.

20.4 Histamine-Antibody Network in Immunomodulation

Histamine receptors have previously been shown to enhance delayed hypersensitivity and antibody mediated immune responses in many pathological processes regulating several essential events in allergies and autoimmune diseases in experimental animals especially in knock out mice (either H1 or H2 deficient) (Banu and Watanabe 1999, Bryce et al. 2006, Jutel et al. 2001). It is highly significant in the field of immunomodulation that endogenous levels of histamine influence the repertoire of autoantibodies. It has been characterized that the repertoire of natural autoantibodies in HDC-deficient mice is unable to produce histamine (Ohtsu et al. 2001). HDC-deficient and wild type mice differed in the patterns of reactivity of their immunoglobulin-M (IgM) and immunoglobulin-G (IgG) natural autoantibodies (Quintana et al. 2004). The natural autoantibodies in HDC-deficient sera manifested a larger repertoire of IgM autoantibodies than did the wild type sera (Quintana et al. 2004). The self-antigens bound by IgM from HDC-deficient mice includes structural proteins, enzymes related with cellular metabolism, double-stranded DNA, single stranded DNA and tissue-specific antigens like insulin (Quintana et al. 2004). It was noted that relatively fewer differences in the natural autoantibodies repertoire of IgG autoantibodies of the mice, notably, the HDC-deficient sera reacted with glutamic acid decarboxylase (GAD) (Quintana et al. 2004), an antigen related with autoimmune diabetes (Tisch et al. 1993). It has been documented that GAD-specific antibodies in HDC-deficient mice reflect an enhanced susceptibility to develop autoimmune diabetes. Therefore, it shows that factors not directly associated to antigenic activation such as endogenous levels of histamine can influence the natural autoantibodies repertoire. Thus, disorders of immune system characterized by altered levels of endogenous histamine, such as allergies, might be reflected as specific alterations in the repertoire of natural autoantibodies (Quintana et al. 2004).

It has also been documented that B-cell proliferation in response to anti-IgM is increased in mice. However, it is diminished in H1R-deficient mice. In H1R-deficient mice, antibody production against a T-cell-independent antigen-TNP-Ficoll is diminished (Banu and Watanabe 1999) and also in another study antibody response to T-cell-dependent antigens like ovalbumin (OVA) demonstrated a different pattern (Jutel et al. 2001). H1R-deficient mice produced high OVA-specific IgG1 and IgE as compared with wild type mice. In contrast, H2R-deficient mice showed diminished serum levels of OVA-specific IgG3 and IgE in comparison to wild type mice. H1R-deficient mice produced higher amounts of OVA-specific IgE, IgG1, IgG2b and IgG3 as compared with H2R-deficient mice (Jutel et al. 2001). Thus, H1R-deficient mice display both strong systemic T-cell and efficient B-cell responses to antigen (Bryce et al. 2006).

In our recent studies, we evaluated the role of histamine in immunomodulation. Our in vivo findings, demonstrated that anti-Sheep Red Blood Cells (SRBC)-immunoglobulins (Igs), anti-SRBC-IgM and anti-SRBC-IgG profiles in pheniramine (H1R-antagonist)-treated group was completely suppressed as compared to ranitidine (H2R-antagonist)-treated and control groups, while anti-SRBC-Igs and anti-SRBC-IgM in ranitidine (H2R antagonist)-treated group was suppressed initially and enhanced in a later phase in comparison to control group, while anti-SRBC-IgG profile remained completely suppressed in comparison to the control group. These results demonstrated B-cell proliferation, in response to anti-IgM, is increased in H2R-antagonist treated rabbits and is diminished in H1R-antagonist treated rabbits, and also H1R-antagonist treated rabbits display diminished antibody production against a T-cell dependent antigen-SRBC as compared to H2R-antagonist treated and control rabbits (Tripathi et al. 2008).

Furthermore, in another recent study we have revealed the role of histamine as an immunopotentiating agents via the enhancement of immunomodulatory profile, and demonstrated that the histamine released in control group through immunological stimuli from effector cells in vivo, could influence a detectable antibodies (Igs, IgM & IgG) response to SRBC (Tripathi et al. 2009, see Fig. 20.2a–c). Exogenous histamine treated-rabbits showed immunopotentiating properties by enhancing the anti-SRBC-antibodies (Igs, IgM and IgG) titers as compared to positive control rabbits. We have noticed that histamine stimulates antibody titer (Igs and IgG) in group II and III on day 65- post-I when treated with histamine for one week (starting from the day 58- post-I) however it showed gradual decrease on day 72- post-I. While IgM titer was unaffected and showed similar pattern to group I and group V. These findings showed potential role of histamine on antibody generation specially IgG,

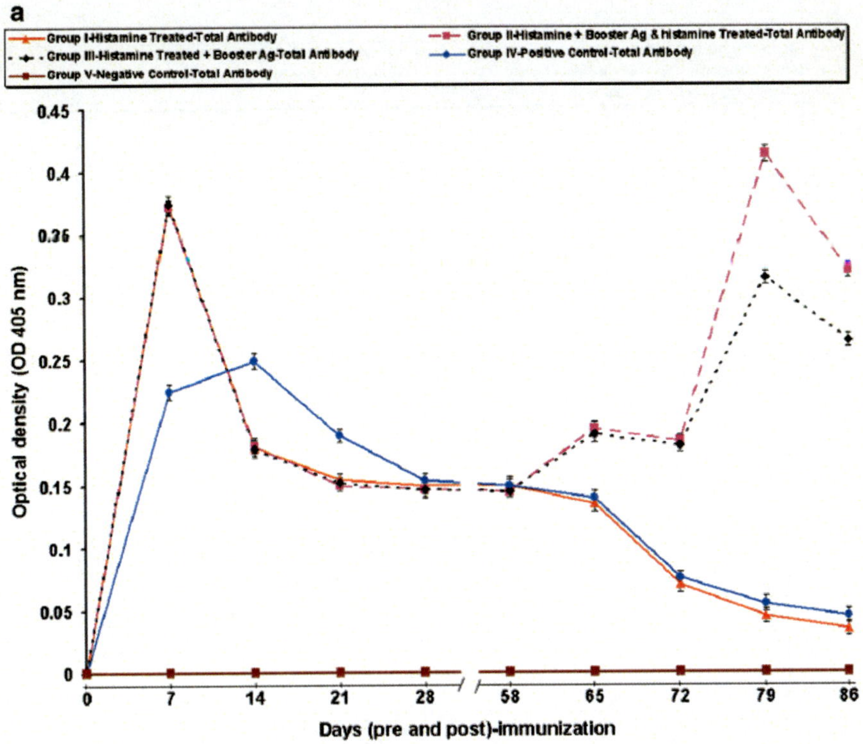

Fig. 20.2a The cohort comprised of three groups (I, II and III) containing 18 rabbits each and received subcutaneous histamine (100 $\mu gkg^{-1} \times$ b.i.d.) for 10 days (starting from day 1). Group-II and -III further received histamine (100 $\mu gkg^{-1} \times$ b.i.d.) for one week (starting from day 58) while group-II was again treated with same dose of histamine for one week (starting from day 72). They were subsequently immunized on day 3 with intravenous injection of SRBC whereas group-II and -III were further secondary immunized with SRBC at day 72. A IVth-positive control group ($n = 18$) received vehicle (sterile distilled water, 1 $mlkg^{-1} \times$ b.i.d.) and immunized on day 3 similarly, while a Vth-negative control group ($n = 18$) remained non-immunized and received only vehicle. Blood samples were collected on pre-immunization (pre-I) (day 0), as well as on days 7-, 14-, 21-, 28-, 58-, 65-, 72-, 79- and 86- post-immunization (post-I). SRBC-specific immunoglobulins (Igs), IgM and IgG production titer was measured by whole SRBC-ELISA method in duplicate 1:100 diluted sera. The results demonstrate mean ± s.d. and were found statistically significant ($p < 0.05$) (**a–c**) reprinted with permission from Applied Physiology and Allied Sciences Society, Department of Physiology, J.N.M.C., A.M.U., Aligarh, India). (**a**) SRBC-specific immunoglobulins (Igs) generation profile. (**b**) SRBC-specific immunoglobulin-M (IgM) generation profile. (**c**) SRBC-specific immunoglobulin-G (IgG) generation profile

warranting further studies on role of histamine in immunoglobulin class switching. Secondary-immunization study in group II and III, further strengthen our results of histamine role in antibody generation (see Fig. 20.2a–c). Thus, our results provide evidence that short-term effect of histamine (until it's present in the body) affects antibody class switching and potentially stimulates antibody generation titer (Tripathi et al. 2009).

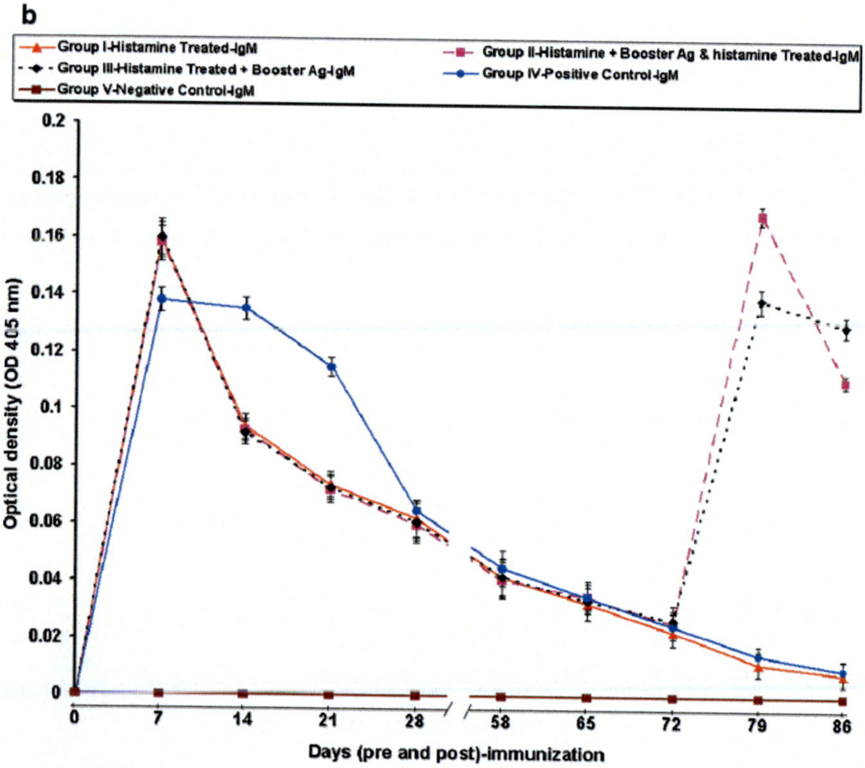

Fig. 20.2b (continued)

In addition to histamine role on antibody generation profile, recently, we have studied the effect of histamine as an immunopotentiating agent via the dose-dependent experimentations in albino rabbits (Tripathi et al. 2010). In this preliminary study, we noticed immunomodulatory effect of histamine at three different doses (50 μgkg^{-1} × b.i.d., 100 μgkg^{-1} × b.i.d. and 200 μgkg^{-1} × b.i.d.), and observed their outcome on antibody generation titer. It was interestingly noticed that 50 μg histamine-treated group affect total antibody and IgG generation titer on day 7-post-I (until histamine presence in the body). However 100 μg and 200 μg histamine-treated group on day 7-post-I (until its presence in the body) enhanced total antibody, IgM and IgG generation titer whereas; on further metabolism histamine effect disappeared on the antibody generation profile bringing it in the range of control antibody level in 50 and 100 μg histamine-treated group, while it was disappeared in 200 μg histamine-treated group. Therefore, on the basis of the present study we reached to a conclusion that the results obtained due to histamine were of short duration which disappeared in latter stage of 50 and 100 μg histamine-treated groups due to clearance of the body from these substance in rabbits (Tripathi et al. 2010).

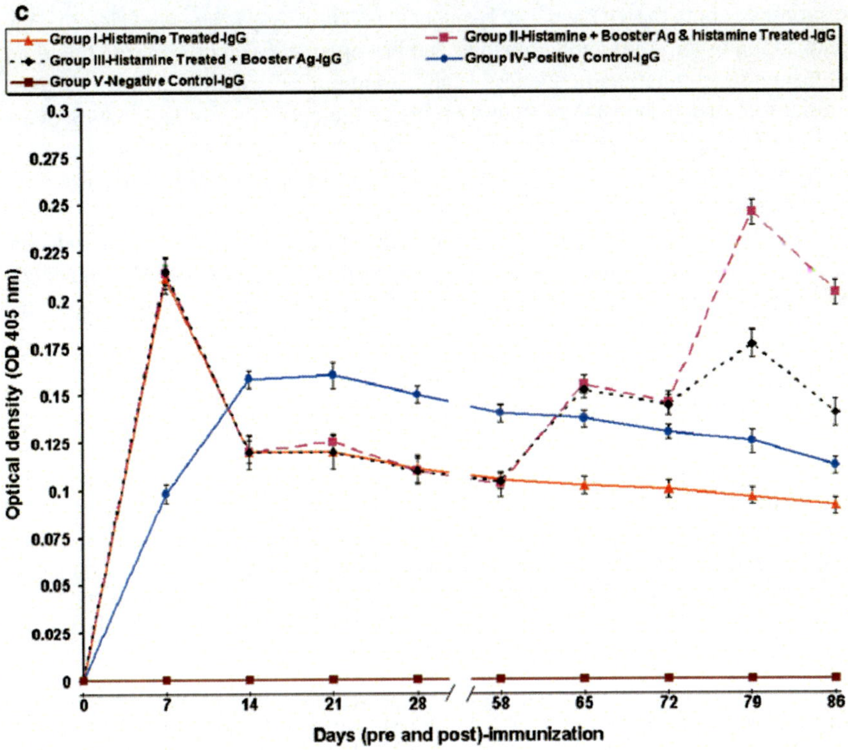

Fig. 20.2c (continued)

In summary, the recent data on the novel functions of histamine receptors have opened an interesting new chapter in immune regulation and immunomodulation in the history of histamine research and should lead to deeper relevance, and understanding treatments of pathological processes those regulating several essential events in allergies and autoimmune diseases. Thus, it is important point of research to see how histamine and its receptors-agonists/antagonists can be a major mediator for immune regulation in several diseases.

20.5 Future Prospects

Histamine receptors have been important drug targets for many years to regulate histamine-cytokine and histamine-antibody network in immune responses. Their physiological and pathological relevance and distribution in various tissues are being documented, while the exact role of histamine receptors in immunomodulation and immunoregulation is still unclear. The role of histamine in cytokine-antibody generation profile, over a span of time is still unclear or lacking in existing literatures. The scope of histamine research has been implicated in immune responses of both the Th1 and Th2 lymphocytes. The newly discovered H4-receptor, play an important role in inflammation and has opened a new way for the functions of histamine in inflammation, allergy and autoimmune diseases. Moreover, the data on the role of H3- and H4-receptors on histamine-cytokine and antibody network in immune regulation are still elementary. Thus, there is indeed an urgent need to redouble efforts performing both in vivo and in vitro studies on histamine, histamine receptors, and their role in immunoregulation and immunomodulation on cytokines and antibodies network in immune response that are potentially harmful to generate allergy/asthma and autoimmune diseases. It is also important to search for beneficial role to pursue novel strategies to cope with diagnosis and treatment of allergies and autoimmune diseases.

Acknowledgment Trivendra Tripathi acknowledges University Grants Commission, New Delhi, India for providing UGC Fellowship [UGC letter DON F. 19-33/2006 (CU)].

References

Banu Y, Watanabe T (1999) Augmentation of antigen receptor-mediated responses by histamine H1 receptor signaling. J Exp Med 189:673–682

Bryce PJ, Mathias CB, Harrison KL et al (2006) The H1 histamine receptor regulates allergic lung responses. J Clin Invest 116:1624–1632

Cameron W, Doyle K, Rocklin RE (1986) Histamine type I (H1)-receptor radioligand binding studies on normal T cell subsets, B cells, and monocytes. J Immunol 136:2116–2120

Caron G, Delneste Y, Roelandts E et al (2001a) Histamine polarizes human dendritic cells into Th2 cell-promoting effector dendritic cells. J Immunol 167:3682–3686

Caron G, Delneste Y, Roelandts E et al (2001b) Histamine induces CD86 expression and chemokine production by human immature dendritic cells. J Immunol 166:6000–6006

De Vries JE, Zurawski G (1995) Immunoregulatory properties of IL-13: its potential role in atopic disease. Int Arch Allergy Immunol 106:175–179

Defrance T, Carayon P, Billian G et al (1994) Interleukin 13 is a B cell stimulating factor. J Exp Med 179:135–143

Dunford PJ, O'Donnell N, Riley JP et al (2006) The histamine H4 receptor mediates allergic airway inflammation by regulating the activation of CD4+ T cells. J Immunol 176:7062–7070

Dy M, Arnould A, Lemoine FM et al (1996) Hematopoietic progenitors and IL-3 dependent cell lines synthetize histamine in response to calcium ionophore. Blood 87:3161–3169

Dy M, Schneider E (2004) Histamine-cytokine connection in immunity and hematopoiesis. Cytokine Growth Factor Rev 15:393–410

Dy M, Schneider E, Gastinel LN et al (1987) Histamine-producing cell-stimulating activity. A biological activity shared by interleukin 3 and granulocyte-macrophage colony stimulating factor. Eur J Immunol 17:1243–1248

Elenkov I, Webster E, Papanicolaou DA et al (1998) Histamine potently suppresses human IL-12 and stimulates IL-10 production via H2 receptors. J Immunol 161:2586–2593

Elliott K, Osna N, Scofield M et al (2001) Regulation of IL-13 production by histamine in cloned murine T helper type 2 cells. Int Immunopharmacol 1:1923–1937

Fokkens WJ, Holm AF, Blom H et al (1992) Dynamics of mast cells in the nasal mucosa of patients with allergic rhinitis and non-allergic controls: a biopsy study. Clin Exp Allergy 22: 701–710

Gantner F, Sakai K, Tusche MW et al (2002) Histamine H4 and H2 receptors control histamineinduced interleukin-16 release from human $CD8^+$ T cells. J Pharmacol Exp Ther 303:300–307

Godot V, Arock M, Garcia G et al (2007) H4 Histamine receptor mediates optimal migration of mast cell precursors to CXCL12. J Allergy Clin Immunol 120:827–843

Gutzmer R, Diestel C, Mommert S et al (2005) Histamine H4 receptor stimulation suppresses IL-12p70 production and mediates chemotaxis in human monocytes-derived dendritic cells. J Immunol 174:5224–5232

Idzdo M, La Sala A, Ferrari D et al (2002) Expression and function of histamine receptors in human monocyte-derived dendritic cells. J Allergy Clin Immunol 109: 839–846

Itoh H, Takahashi HK, Iwagaki H et al (2002) Effect of histamine on intercellular adhesion molecule-1 expression and production of interferon-gamma and interleukin-12 in mixed lymphocyte reaction stimulated with interleukin-18. Transplantation 74: 864–870

Jutel M, Blaser K, Akdis CA (2005) Histamine in chronic allergic responses. J Invest Allergol Clin Immunol 15:1–8

Jutel M, Watanabe T, Klunker S et al (2001) Histamine regulates T-cell and antibody responses by differential expression of H1 and H2 receptors. Nature 413:420–424

Kobayashi T, Koga R, Banu Y et al (2001) Immediate-type hypersensitivity and helper T cell function in histamine H1 receptor- and H2 receptor deficient mice. Int Congr Series 1224: 395–396

Levy F, Kristofic C, Heuser C et al (1997) Role of IL-13 in CD4 T cell dependent IgE production in atopy. Int Arch Allergy Immunol 112:49–58

Lichtenstein LM, Gillespie E (1975) Effects of the H1 and H2 antihistamines on allergic histamine release and its inhibition by histamine. J Pharmacol Exp Ther 192:441–450

Lippert U, Artuc M, Grützkau A et al (2004) Human skin mast cells express H2 and H4, but not H3 receptors. J Invest Dermatol 123:116–123

Marone G, Casolaro V, Patella V et al (1997) Molecular and cellular biology of mast cells and basophils. Int Arch Allergy Immunol 114:207–217

Marone G, Granata F, Spadaro G et al (2003) The histamine-cytokine network in allergic inflammation. J Allergy Clin Immunol 112:S83–S88

Mazzoni A, Leifer CA, Mullen CED et al (2003) Cutting edge: histamine inhibits IFN-a release from plasmacytoid dendritic cells. J Immunol 170:2269–2273

Mazzoni A, Young HA, Spitzer JH et al (2001) Histamine regulates cytokine production in maturing dendritic cells, resulting in altered T cell polarization. J Clin Invest 108:1865–1873

Ogden BE, Hill HR (1980) Histamine regulates lymphocyte mitogenic responses through activation of specific H1 and H2 histamine receptors. Immunology 41:107–114

Ohtani T, Aiba S, Mizuashi M et al (2003) H1 and H2 histamine receptors are absent on Langerhans cells and present on dermal dendritic cells. J Invest Dermatol 121:1073–1079

Ohtsu H, Tanaka S, Terui T et al (2001) Mice lacking histidine decarboxylase exhibit abnormal mast cells. FEBS Lett 502:53–56

Osna N, Elliott K, Khan MM (2001a) Regulation of interleukin-10 secretion by histamine in Th2 cells and splenocytes. Int Immunopharmacol 1:85–86

Osna N, Elliott K, Khan MM (2001b) The effects of histamine on interferon-gamma production are dependent on the stimulatory signals. Int Immunopharmacol 1:125–145

Packard KA, Khan MM (2003) Effects of histamine on Th1/Th2 cytokine balance. Int Immunopharmacol 3:909–920

Pavlinkova G, Yanagawa Y, Kikuchi K et al (2003) Effects of histamine on functional maturation of dendritic cells. Immunobiology 207:315–325

Piquet-Pellorce C, Dy M (1991) PGE2 potentiates GM-CSF-induced histamine synthesis in bone marrow cells: role of cAMP. Life Sci 48:2377–2378

Quintana FJ, Buzas E, Prohászka Z et al (2004) Modifying histamine production via knocking out of the histidine decarboxylase gene changes the repertoire of natural autoantibodies. J Autoimmun 22:297–305

Renkl A, Berod L, Mockenhaupt M et al (2004) Distinct effects of sphingosine-1-phosphate, lisophosphatidic acid and histamine in human and mouse dendritic cells. Int J Mol Med 13:203–209

Rotrosen D, Gallin JI (1986) Histamine type I receptor occupancy increases endothelial cytosolic calcium, reduces F-actin and promotes albumin diffusion across cultured endothelial monolayers. J Cell Biol 103:2379–2387
Schneider E, Lemoine F, Breton-Gorius J et al (1999) IL-3-induced coexpression of IL-4, IL-6 and histidine decarboxylase mRNA in basophilic myelocytes enriched in sorted-Rh-bright bone marrow cells. Exp Haematol 27:1010–1018
Schneider E, Ploemacher RE, Nabarra B et al (1993) Mast cells and their committed precursors are not required for IL-3 induced histamine synthesis in murine bone marrow: characteristics of histamine-producing cells. Blood 81:1161–1169
Schneider E, Pollard H, Lepault F et al (1987) Histamine-producing cell-stimulating activity. Interleukin 3 and granulocyte macrophage colony-stimulating factor induce de novo synthesis of histidine decarboxylase in hemopoietic progenitor cells. J Immunol 139:3710–3717
Shahid M, Tripathi T, Sobia F et al (2009) Histamine, histamine receptors and their role in immunomodulation: an updated systematic review. Open Immunol J 2:9–41.
Sirois J, Menard G, Moses AS et al (2000) Importance of histamine in the cytokine network in the lung through H2 and H3 receptors: stimulation of IL-10 production. J Immunol 164:2964–2970
Szeberenyi JB, Pallinger E, Zsinko M et al (2001) Inhibition of effects of endogenously synthesized histamine disturbs *in vitro* human dendritic cell differentiation. Immunol Lett 76:175–182
Takahashi K, Tanaka S, Furuta K et al (2002) Histamine H2 receptor-mediated modulation of local cytokine expression in a mouse experimental tumor model. Biochem Biophys Res Commun 297:1205–1210
Takamatsu SI, Nakashima I, Nakano K et al (1996) Modulation of endotoxininduced histamine synthesis by cytokines in mouse bone marrow derived macrophages. J Immunol 156:778–785
Thurmond RL, Gelfand EW, Dunford PJ (2008) The role of histamine H1 and H4 receptor in allergic inflammation: the search for new antihistamines. Nat Rev 7:41–53
Tineke CTM, van Der Pouw K, Snijders A et al (1998) Histamine inhibits the production of interleukin-12 through interaction with H2 receptors. J Clin Invest 102: 1866–1873
Tisch R, Yang XD, Singer SM et al (1993) Immune response to glutamic acid decarboxylase correlates with insulitis in non-obese diabetic mice. Nature 366:72
Triggiani M, Gentile M, Secondo A et al (2001) Histamine induces exocytosis and IL-6 production from human lung macrophages through interaction with H1 receptors. J Immunol 166: 4083–4091
Tripathi T, Shahid M, Khan HM et al (2009) Effect of histamine on antibody generation profile *in vivo*. Global J Appl Physiol Allied Sci 1:26–31
Tripathi T, Shahid M, Khan HM et al (2010) Dose-dependent effect of histamine on antibody generation *in vivo*. Asian Pacific J Trop Med 3:112–116
Tripathi T, Shahid M, Siddiqui MU et al (2008) Role and immunomodulatory profile of histamine receptors by H1 and H2 antagonists. Available from Nature Precedings. http://hdl.handle.net/10101/npre.2008.1547.1 Accessed January 24, 2010
Vannier E, Miller LC, Dinarello CA (1991) Histamine suppresses gene expression and synthesis of tumor necrosis factor alpha via histamine H2 receptors. J Exp Med 174:281–284
Weltman JK (2000) Update on histamine as a mediator of inflammation. Allergy Asthma Proc 3:125–128
Yoshimoto T, Tsutsui H, Tominaga K et al (1999) IL-18, although antiallergic when administered with IL-12, stimulates IL-4 and histamine release by basophils. Proc Natl Acad Sci USA 96:13962–13966
Zabner J, Winter M, Excoffon KJ et al (2003) Histamine alters E-cadherin cell adhesion to increase human airway epithelial permeability. J Appl Physiol 95:394–401

Subject Index

M. Shahid et al. (eds.), *Biomedical Aspects of Histamine*,
DOI 10.1007/978-90-481-9349-3, © Springer Science+Business Media B.V. 2010